# The Ocular Examination

# *Karla Zadnik, OD, PhD*

Assistant Professor
The Ohio State University
College of Optometry
Columbus, Ohio

*and*

Division of Epidemiology and Biostatistics
School of Public Health
College of Medicine
Columbus, Ohio

***Formerly***

Senior Optometrist
University of California, Berkeley
School of Optometry
Berkeley, California

*and*

Associate Clinical Professor
Director of Optometric Services
Department of Ophthalmology
School of Medicine
University of California, Davis
Davis, California

# The Ocular Examination

*Measurements and Findings*

**W.B. SAUNDERS COMPANY**
*A Division of Harcourt Brace & Company*
Philadelphia • London • Toronto • Montreal • Sydney • Tokyo

**W.B. SAUNDERS COMPANY**
*A Division of Harcourt Brace & Company*

The Curtis Center
Independence Square West
Philadelphia, Pennsylvania 19106

**Library of Congress Cataloging-in-Publication Data**

The ocular examination: measurements and findings / [edited by] Karla
Zadnik.——1st ed.

  p.    cm.

ISBN 0–7216–5209–3

1. Eye—Examination.      I. Zadnik, Karla.      [DNLM: 1. Vision Tests.
  2. Vision Disorders—diagnosis.    WW 145 021 1997]

RE75.027 1997
617.7′ 15—dc20

DNLM/DLC                                                      96–6968

THE OCULAR EXAMINATION: MEASUREMENTS AND FINDINGS          ISBN 0–7216–5209–3

Printed in the United States of America.

Last digit is the print number:     9    8    7    6    5    4    3    2    1

## *Dedication*

*This book is dedicated to my grandfather, William M. Henry, OD,*
*for inspiring me to become an optometrist*
*and to my father, Karl R. Henry,*
*for encouraging me to pursue a career in optometric research.*

Karla Zadnik

# Contributors

· · · · · · · · · · · · · · · · · · · · · · · · · · · ·

Joseph T. Barr, OD, MS

Associate Professor of Optometry and Physiological Optics,
The Ohio State University College of Optometry, Columbus, Ohio
*The Cornea*

Mark A. Bullimore, MCOptom, PhD

Assistant Professor, The Ohio State University College of Optometry, Columbus,
Ohio
*Visual Acuity; The Anterior Segment*

Robert B. DiMartino, OD, MS

Associate Clinical Professor, University of California, Berkeley, School of
Optometry, Berkeley, California
*The Posterior Segment*

David B. Elliott, BScOptom, MCOptom, PhD, FAAO

Associate Professor, Department of Optometry, University of Bradford, Bradford,
United Kingdom
*The Problem-Oriented Examination's Case History; Supplementary Clinical Tests
of Visual Function*

Karen D. Fern, OD

Associate Professor and Chief, Pediatric and Binocular Vision Service, University of
Houston College of Optometry, Houston, Texas
*Binocular Function*

Nina E. Friedman, OD, MS

Senior Optometrist, University of California, Berkeley, School of Optometry,
Berkeley, California
*The Pupil; The Anterior Segment*

Chris A. Johnson, PhD

Professor, Department of Ophthalmology and Director, Optics and Visual
Assessment Laboratory (Oval), University of California, Davis, School of Medicine,
Davis, California
*Perimetry and Visual Field Testing*

Ruth E. Manny, OD, PhD

Associate Professor and Chair, Department of Clinical Sciences, University of Houston College of Optometry, Houston, Texas
*Binocular Function*

Donald O. Mutti, OD, PhD

Senior Optometrist, University of California, Berkeley, School of Optometry, Berkeley, California
*Refractive Error*

Mark Rosenfield, MCOptom, PhD, BSc(Hons)

Associate Professor, State University of New York State College of Optometry, New York, New York
*Accommodation*

Karla Zadnik, OD, PhD

Assistant Professor, The Ohio State University College of Optometry and Division of Epidemiology and Biostatistics, School of Public Health, College of Medicine, Columbus, Ohio
*Refractive Error*

# Preface

· · · · · · · · · · · · · · · · · · · · · · · · · · · ·

*"When you can measure what you are speaking about in numbers you know something about it," declared the Victorian physicist Lord Kelvin, in 1883, "but when you cannot measure it, when you cannot express it in numbers, your knowledge is a meagre and unsatisfactory kind; it may be the beginning of knowledge. but you have scarcely, in your thoughts, advanced to the stage of science, whatever the matter may be."*

—From *Album of Science. The Nineteenth Century**
by Leslie Pearce Williams

**M**any textbooks exist for the purpose of describing primary eye care procedures and techniques. These textbooks are designed to teach eye care practitioners how to examine eyes and how to detect abnormalities in the visual system. However, no textbook has sought to combine these two—learning the techniques and sorting out what abnormal results from the techniques mean—in a manner that teaches the student or novice practitioner how to detect abnormalities and place the possible etiologies into broad diagnostic categories.

Each chapter of this textbook begins with the fundamental underlying knowledge necessary to understand that part of the eye examination. The chapter on visual acuity begins with a discussion of photoreceptor spacing as the rate-limiting step in visual resolution. The chapter on the pupil describes the relevant anatomy of the neural pupillary pathway.

A procedural guide follows the background section in each chapter and describes exactly "how to" perform the relevant measures and techniques, including alternative techniques when appropriate. The visual field chapter discusses modern automated perimetry and provides tips for performing it accurately and efficiently. The refractive error chapter presents the authors' favorite techniques as well as other well-known methods for refracting.

Each chapter concludes with a discussion of how to classify abnormal test results into broad categories of possibilities for diagnosis. The case history chapter "chats" its way through an examination, emphasizing how information gleaned from the patient can lead the doctor to a diagnosis. The chapter on binocular vision features tables depicting when binocular vision test abnormalities signify very serious underlying conditions.

The student of optometry or ophthalmology thus can learn detection and analysis of ocular anomalies initially without knowing specific diseases and their mechanisms (analogous to avoiding the need to know right off the bat how to spell a word before looking it up in the dictionary successfully). This knowledge is intended to guide diagnostic and analytical skills in a logical and retainable order.

---

*Charles Scribner's Sons, New York, 1978.

# Acknowledgments

. . . . . . . . . . . . . . . . . . . . . . . . . . . . . . . . . . . . . . . . .

This book was initiated, written, edited, and produced during what I hope proves to be the most difficult professional period I ever experience. It reflects positive interactions and relationships with people in optometry that have evolved partly as a result of negative events.

To that end, I wish to thank very specific professional colleagues, friends, confidants, and supporters who have stood by me through thick, thin, and everything in between: Don Mutti, Mark Bullimore, and Nina Friedman. Optometry is a much better profession for having them in it.

—Karla Zadnik

# Contents

• • • • • • • • • • • • • • • • • • • • • • • • • •

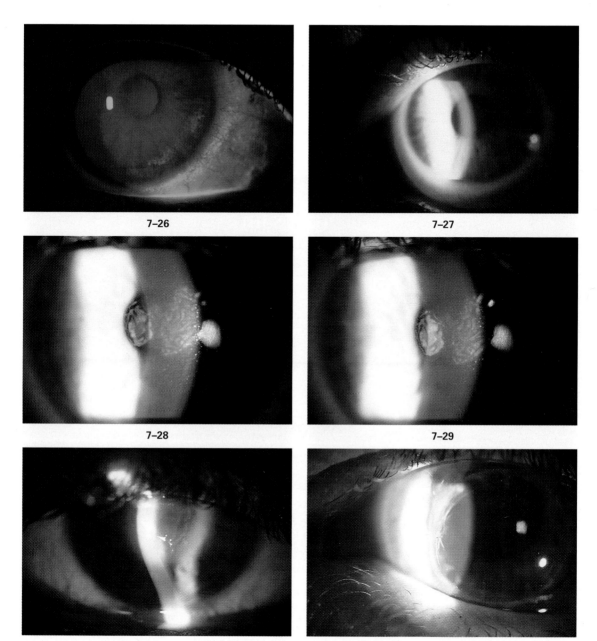

**FIGURE 7–26**   Moderate corneal and conjunctival staining.

**FIGURE 7–27**   Epithelial microcysts between slit-lamp beam and margin of iris viewed by proximal retroillumination.

**FIGURE 7–28**   Epithelial basement membrane dystrophy.

**FIGURE 7–29**   Recurrent corneal erosion in a patient with epithelial basement membrane dystrophy.

**FIGURE 7–30**   Acute corneal hydrops.

**FIGURE 7–31**   Scar from penetrating keratoplasty.

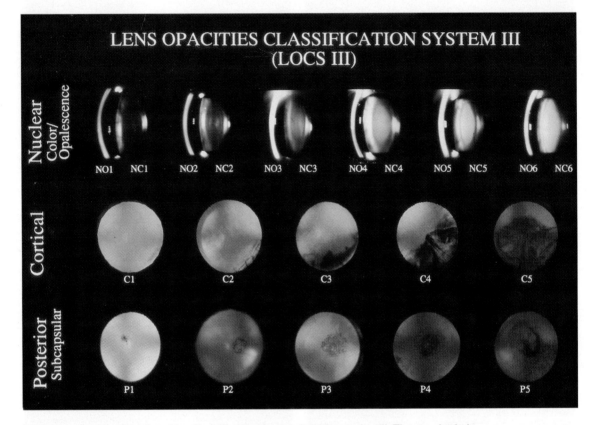

**FIGURE 8–10** The Lens Opacities Classification System (LOCS), version III. The standard photographs illustrate varying severity of nuclear, cortical, and posterior subcapsular opacities. Nuclear opacities are shown by direct focal illumination. Cortical and posterior subcapsular opacities are shown by retroillumination such that a bright red fundus reflex is observed. Any opacities appear as dark or translucent shadows against the bright background.

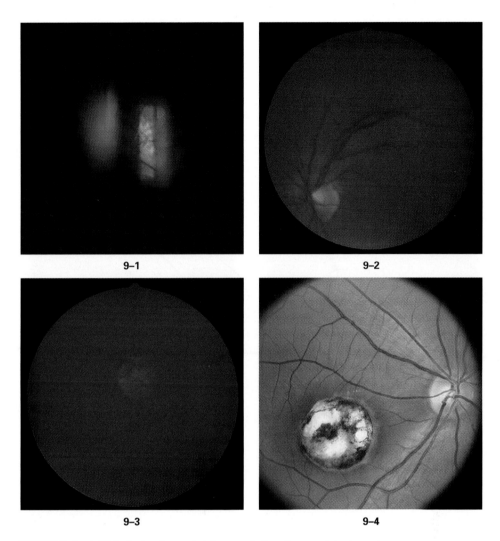

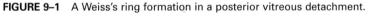

**FIGURE 9–1**  A Weiss's ring formation in a posterior vitreous detachment.

**FIGURE 9–2**  A benign choroidal nevus.

**FIGURE 9–3**  A circular absence of the retinal pigment epithelium, referred to as a window defect. Note the increased detail of the choroidal vasculature and the pale pink fundus appearance.

**FIGURE 9–4**  A macular lesion resulting from a retinal choroiditis, presumably *Toxoplasma gondii*.

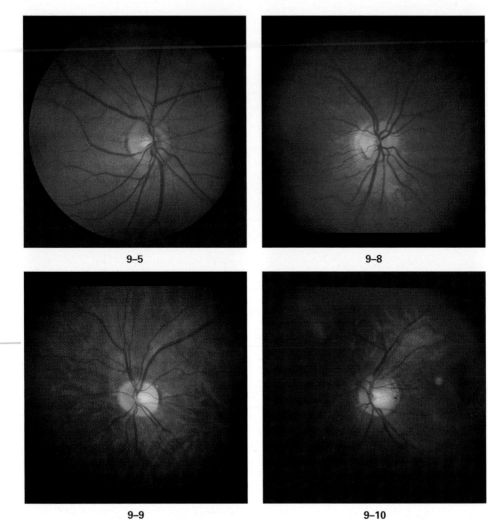

9–5

9–8

9–9

9–10

**FIGURE 9–5** Linear radial hyperplasia of the retinal pigment epithelium resulting from a connective tissue disorder referred to as angioid streaks.

**FIGURE 9–8** Physiological optic nerve head cupping 0.0 C/D.

**FIGURE 9–9** Physiological optic nerve head cupping 0.2 C/D.

**FIGURE 9–10** Physiological optic nerve head cupping 0.4 C/D.

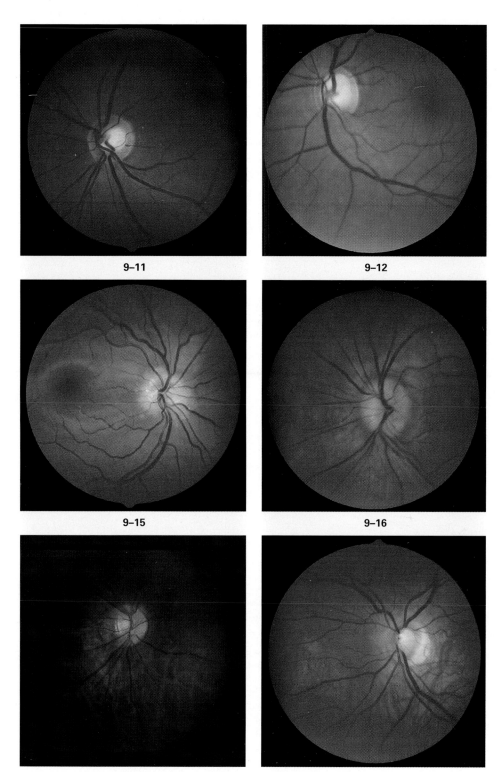

**FIGURE 9–11**  Physiological optic nerve head cupping 0.6 C/D.

**FIGURE 9–12**  Non-physiological optic nerve head cupping 0.8 C/D.

**FIGURE 9–15**  Surface optic nerve head drusen. Note the blurred margins of the disc.

**FIGURE 9–16**  Buried optic nerve head drusen. Note the blurred margins of the disc.

**FIGURE 9–17**  Choroidal crescent.

**FIGURE 9–18**  Scleral crescent.

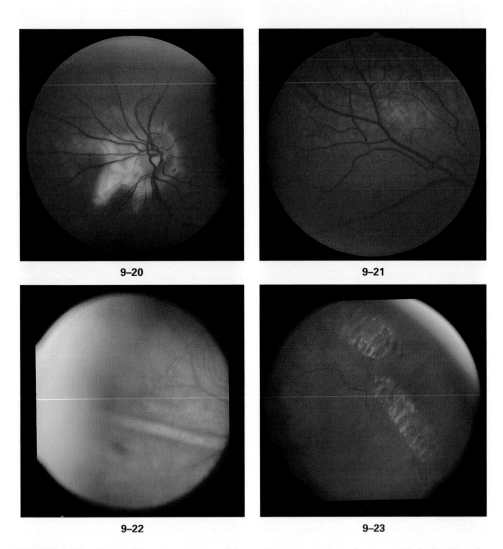

**9–20**         **9–21**

**9–22**         **9–23**

**FIGURE 9–20** Peripapillary atrophy, possibly a mild presentation of geographic helicoid peri-papillary choroiditis.

**FIGURE 9–21** Hollenhorst's plaques. Note the location and reflective nature of this calcific embolus.

**FIGURE 9–22** Long posterior ciliary nerve. Note the appearance of a linear cream-colored structure bounded by a pigment band on either side.

**FIGURE 9–23** Lattice degeneration of the retinal periphery.

*David B. Elliott, BScOptom,
MCOptom, PhD, FAAO*

1

# The Problem-
Oriented
Examination's
Case History

The case history is arguably the most important aspect of an eye examination. It is not surprising that it is one of the most difficult aspects of an examination to master, and clinicians continually add to their knowledge about case history investigation throughout their careers. Investigational skills and proper interpretation can be fully developed only by examining many patients with a variety of problems and repeatedly comparing the information given in the case history with the subsequent clinical findings. It is also necessary to keep current about all the signs and symptoms associated with the myriad of ocular abnormalities. Students may therefore find the case history investigation and analysis difficult. It is common for clinical supervisors to have to ask several additional questions of a patient after a student has completed the examination. Students can often underestimate the value of history taking simply because they are still learning what questions should be asked and how much information can be gleaned from a proper case history. They may also have a misplaced belief that the technical ocular testing itself should provide all the relevant information about the patient's problems and solutions, so why question the patient extensively? For these reasons it is essential for educators and students alike to learn case history techniques well.

# The Problem-Oriented Approach

Appreciation of the case history has grown with the increased use of the problem-oriented approach to the ocular examination.[1] The concept of the problem-oriented approach was introduced into medicine in the early 1970s.[2,3] Its introduction into optometry was in the form of the problem-oriented record, which numerically listed the patient's problems.[4-6] A plan of action was then devised to address each numbered problem. The acronym SOAP, standing for Subjective, Objective, Assessment, and Plan, was initially used for follow-up visits and progress notes but has now become closely associated with the whole problem-oriented approach. The SOAP record-keeping format is complete and provides a logical framework for the steps in an ocular examination.

Not surprisingly, the problem-oriented approach aligns the examination around the expressed problem(s) of the patient. However, this is not exclusive. For example, it is not sufficient to perform only case history, visual acuity, and refraction on a patient who complains of blurred distance vision. There are many obvious reasons why such an approach is flawed, including the fact that sight-threatening conditions that must be detected can be symptomless. Some patients may not disclose all the relevant symptoms, for example because they do not believe their headaches are associated with their eyes, or they believe that their slightly blurred vision, headaches, or diplopia is a normal consequence of aging. Optometrists also have a legal obligation to assess the entire visual system in a comprehensive examination: refractive, oculomotor, sensory, and ocular health. The assessment of ocular health must also include the assessment of ocular manifestations of systemic diseases.

What advantages does the problem-oriented examination have over a traditional data-oriented examination? The main advantage is increased efficiency. A data-oriented examination uses essentially the same set of clinical procedures in every examination. A large, "complete" database of information is collected to ensure that most patients' problems can be addressed most of the time using the information provided. By design, a data-oriented examination often collects excess data that do not address the patient's problem. The expanding scope of optometric practice continues to add extra procedures to the traditional basic optometric examination. At the same time, the advent of managed care in eye care mandates increased efficiency. Providing comprehensive contemporary optometric care that includes new procedures requires selective streamlining of the examination routine. The problem-solving approach is one way to manage this streamlining of the examination without compromising the quality of patient care. One important question is obvious: What constitutes the essential optometric "database" for a first-time patient encounter and for subsequent examinations of the same patient?

The *minimal* database must meet the medicolegal requirements for the state, province, or country in which the optometrist is practicing. These legislative statutes rarely stipulate specific tests to be performed, but they typically describe the practitioner's responsibility to evaluate each of the recognized systems involved in healthy, comfortable, efficient sight. These invariably include the refractive, sensory, motor, and ocular health systems. What constitutes an acceptable assessment of any of these systems is open to debate. A summary of the tests that would adequately assess a particular system is given in Table 1-1.[7] Note that a relevant case history is

| TABLE 1–1 The Tests/Procedures That Assess the Four Systems Involved in the Oculovisual Examination | | | |
|---|---|---|---|
| **Refractive** | **Sensory** | **Motor** | **Ocular Health** |
| Case history | Case history | Case history | Case history |
| Autorefraction | Visual acuity | Accommodation | Pupil reflexes |
| Visual acuity | Stereoacuity | Cover test | Ophthalmoscopy |
| Keratometry | Color vision | Pursuits | Biomicroscopy |
| Retinoscopy | Contrast sensitivity | Saccades | Tonometry |
| Subjective refraction | Visual fields | Motility | Gonioscopy |
| | | Pupillary responses | |

an important part of the assessment of each system. Each patient appointment slot provides a finite amount of time to conduct various tests. Many tests are available to the optometrist, who must decide which tests should provide the most useful information for each individual patient. Amos[8] offers excellent questions that an optometrist should consider when deciding which tests to include in an examination.

1. Do I really understand what the tests are measuring, and do they provide significant decision-making information?
2. Am I using the minimum number of procedures to yield the maximum amount of information?

Another relevant question, discussed by Borish,[9] among others, is:

3. Which procedures can be performed by an optometric assistant?

There has been no professional agreement and little discussion about what constitutes an adequate optometric examination.[1, 5, 6] Every practitioner should consider and evaluate the minimum number of tests or procedures required for each category of patient presentation—the new patient, the follow-up patient, and so forth. All tests should be constantly assessed in light of new technology, new research developments, and the changing modes of optometric practice. For example, can contemporary autorefractors be used instead of static retinoscopy? Given the evidence that tonometry results alone cannot diagnose glaucoma,[10, 11] should tonometry be augmented or replaced by visual field screening? Should optometric assistants be used? If so, what tests should they perform?

Although the problem-oriented examination requires a minimal database as discussed above, this is obviously not its major characteristic.

Rather, it is distinguished by its variability. For example, if a 12-year-old patient complains of frontal headaches and eyestrain when reading, the most likely tentative diagnosis is uncorrected hyperopia or a significant near heterophoria. Depending on results from other tests, additional tests used might include measuring fusional reserves, AC/A and CA/C ratio, fixation disparity, suppression, and cycloplegic refraction. If a 30-year-old patient presented complaining of sudden painless vision loss in one eye, the most likely tentative diagnoses would include a unilateral change in refractive error (i.e., suddenly noticed vision loss rather than one of sudden onset), optic neuritis, and central serous choroidopathy. None of the additional tests used in the previous example would be used. Instead, fundus biomicroscopy, photostress recovery, Amsler grid, red cap, and contrast sensitivity testing would be appropriate additional tests.

# Collection of Case History Information by an Assistant?

An assistant- or patient-completed questionnaire can be used to collect the patient's name, date of birth, address, home and work telephone numbers, and possibly his or her occupation. It is not possible for a clinical assistant to complete the full case history because history taking continues throughout the examination. However, assistants could record a baseline history which could be reviewed and augmented by the optometrist. This approach makes it less likely that a good rapport will be established between the patient and the clinician, which is vital for an optimal examination result. When patients feel at ease and confident with their optometrist, they are more likely to provide accurate and complete case history information and better subjective responses during the examination. In addition, from the patient's perspective, a "good examination" is one in which the optometrist appeared interested in his or her problem, appeared to know what he or she was doing, and provided a rational explanation of what he or she intends to do about the problem. Subsequently, of course, the end-product should "work." Unfortunately, a brief review by the optometrist of an interview conducted primarily by an assistant does not suggest an intense interest in the patient's problem. Further, if it is not a *brief* review, then little time is saved by having the assistant complete the baseline case history. It could be argued that checking the first-time patient's family and personal history of ocular and systemic disorders could be performed by an assistant in a checklist style. Alternatively, a questionnaire could be provided to the patient, and he or she could fill in this information. However, some patients are sensitive about providing this information to anyone other than the doctor, and the doctor loses some insight into the patient's *manner* as he or she answers even the simplest questions.

## Patient Introduction

The patient should always be welcomed and addressed by name. This is essential for establishing a good rapport with the patient. Some doctors take a picture of the first-time patient to insert in the patient's record. Others jot down information about the patient's family or hobbies for future reference at subsequent office visits.

## Information on Demographics

Demographic information provides vital information to the clinician—the patient's age, gender, and race. Many refractive changes and ocular diseases are age-dependent. Symptoms of distance blur in a 14-year-old patient strongly suggest myopic changes, whereas in a 75-year-old patient they are more likely to suggest cataract or age-related maculopathy.

The most common reason for a young teenager

to present for examination is myopia. The prevalence of myopia is about 2% at the age of 5 to 6 years, increases dramatically at the age of 9 or 10 years,[12] and settles to about 25% by the age of 15.[13] Myopia, with an onset in these years, tends to increase until the progression slows in the late teens.[14] Therefore, many young myopes present for examination with symptoms of blurred distance vision with eyeglasses prescribed the year before owing to the progression of the myopia. American studies have shown that myopia has an earlier onset and is slightly more common in females than in males[14] and is more prevalent in whites than blacks.[13] Another category of myopia, called adult-onset myopia, is typified by individuals doing a great deal of near work. The myopia develops for the first time or progresses significantly at the ages of 18 to 20 years. During the middle to late 20s, few patients continue to increase in myopia and there is a tendency for a slight decrease.[15] Older patients can show a sudden increase in myopia associated with nuclear sclerotic changes in the lens.[16]

Clinically significant levels of hyperopia are much less prevalent than myopia in young patients.[17] Hyperopia is more prevalent in African-Americans and in Native Americans, although no gender differences have been reported. The prevalence of clinically significant hyperopia increases after the age of about 40 years, and a hyperopic (and presbyopic) change in refractive correction is by far the most common change after this age.[17]

About 75% of patients have some astigmatism (greater than 0.25 D).[18, 19] However, this is generally low in magnitude, and only about 20% have astigmatism of 0.75 D or more. Most young patients have with-the-rule astigmatism which changes with age so that most older patients have against-the-rule astigmatism. This change is very slow, only about 0.25 D change for every 10 years. Therefore symptoms due to astigmatic changes are rare in eyeglass wearers, and large changes in astigmatism often indicate pathological changes such as keratoconus or cataract.[16]

Presbyopia, defined as insufficient accommodation for satisfactory near vision without the use of a reading addition, tends to occur between the ages of 42 and 48. Some patients present with presbyopia before others, such as patients with shorter working distances (often those with shorter arms) and/or with larger amounts of detailed close work.[20] Several studies have shown that various races and ethnic groups, including Asians and Africans, tend to become presbyopic slightly earlier, in their late 30s and early 40s. Women tend to report presbyopic symptoms earlier than men, possibly because of shorter arm lengths in women.[20]

There are many gender and age differences in non-refractive ocular conditions. Color vision deficiencies are found in 8% of North American males, yet only 0.05% of females. A sudden, painless loss of vision in a 35-year-old man is likely to suggest central serous choroidopathy (a M:F ratio of about 10:1), but in a woman, optic neuritis is more likely (F:M ratio about 3:2). The male:female ratios for common ocular disorders are shown in Table 1–2. Race is also important. Glaucoma and sarcoidosis are more prevalent among blacks, but presumed ocular histoplasmosis syndrome is more prevalent among whites,[21] as is age-related maculopathy.

A few of the considerations that come to mind with regard to a patient's demographic informa-tion are described above. It is important to know the particular characteristics of the more common ocular abnormalities, but it is essential to know the characteristics of conditions of low prevalence which have a high risk of severe consequences.[22]

# Patient Observation

When patients enter the examination room, this is a very useful opportunity to observe them carefully. Observe their stature, walking ability, and overall physical appearance. For example, a thin, "twitchy" patient may have an overactive thyroid; an overweight, ruddy-faced, and slightly sweaty older patient may be hypertensive; and

| TABLE 1–2 Estimated Prevalences of Common Eye Abnormalities Approximately Stratified by Age at First Presentation | | |
|---|---|---|
| **Age Group and Disease** | **Prevalence** | **Male:Female Ratio** |
| *<10 Years* | | |
| Strabismus | 3:100 | |
| Coloboma | 1:5,000 | |
| Congenital glaucoma | 1:10,000 | 2:1 |
| Albinism | 1:12,500 | 1.6:1 |
| Retinoblastoma | 1:20,000 | |
| Aniridia | 1:75,000 | |
| *10–20 Years* | | |
| Color defective | 8:100 | 17:1 |
| Insulin-dependent diabetes mellitus | 1:500 | |
| Keratoconus | 1:3,000 | 1.8:1 |
| Retinitis pigmentosa | 1:3,500 | 2.7:1 |
| *20–40 Years* | | |
| Pathological myopia | 2:100 | |
| Thyroid ophthalmopathy | 1:3,400 | 1:2.5 |
| Optic neuritis | 1:5,000 | 1:3 |
| *40–60 Years* | | |
| Hypertension | 10–15% | |
| | ~25% of 70+ years | |
| Primary open-angle glaucoma of 40+ years | ~1% | 1.8:1 |
|    52–64 years | 1.2% | |
|    65–74 years | 2.3% | |
|    75+ years | 3.5% | |
| Primary angle-closure glaucoma | 0.15% | 1:3 (Caucasian) |
| *60+ Years* | | |
| Age-related cataract | | |
|    52–64 years (worse than 20/30 [6/9]) | 4% | 1:1.3 |
|    65–74 years | 13% | |
|    75+ years | 41% | |
| Dry age-related maculopathy | | |
|    52–64 years (worse than 20/30 [6/9]) | 1% | 1:1.8 |
|    65–74 years | 6% | |
|    75+ years | 20% | |
| Non–insulin-dependent diabetes mellitus | 1:50 | |

Approximate male:female ratios are provided in some cases. Data from Leibowitz et al.,[33] Lyle,[34] and François.[35]

type II diabetics are often slightly obese. Early arthritic changes found in the elderly often affect the knee and hand joints and manifest as a slight limp requiring the use of a cane. Later changes include deformity of the fingers, difficulty walking, and the typical "ski posture" of ankylosing spondylitis. If you had been Abraham Lincoln's optometrist, his tall stature and long graceful fingers may have helped you to diagnose his Marfan's syndrome (Fig. 1-1).[23] Lincoln is also reported to have had strabismus and hyperopia of +5.75 D (possibly due to subluxated crystalline lenses).

Pay particular attention to any head tilt or obvious abnormalities of the face, eyelids, and eyes which require further investigation (such as facial asymmetry, acne, lid lesions, epiphora, entropion, ectropion, a red eye, or strabismus). Telling the patient about such an anomaly early in the case history may seem like a good idea. It indicates that the doctor is observant and knowledgeable. However, patients can be very sensitive to the fact that their strabismus or epiphora, for example, is so obvious; bringing it to their attention must be done tactfully.

# Communicating with Patients

A few clinical "pearls" may help novice practitioners communicate with their patients. First, remember that the patient is a person and not a "case."[8, 24, 25] Avoid being aloof and believing that technical expertise can provide all the answers. It cannot. Patients want to be listened to and want their practitioner to solve their problem(s), not necessarily to obtain a diagnosis. It is essential to be a good listener and to be interested in what the patient has to say. The patient should be given the opportunity to describe all his or her visual and ocular problems. Technical jargon should be avoided. Some words are so commonly used by practitioners that they forget that the words have little or no meaning for the average

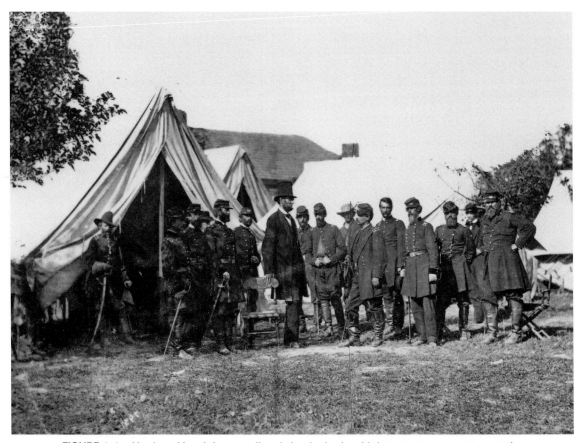

**FIGURE 1-1** Abraham Lincoln's very tall and slender body with long arms supports a putative diagnosis of Marfan's syndrome. He is seen here towering over soldiers at the camp at Antietam (also known as Sharpsburg). (Courtesy of the Library of Congress.)

**TABLE 1–3** Technical Words Commonly Used by Practitioners Which Should be Avoided When Communicating with Patients, with Suggested Lay Alternatives

| To Avoid | Suggested |
| --- | --- |
| Accommodation | Focusing |
| Acuity | How well you can see the letter chart |
| Addition | Bifocal power |
| Binocular | With both eyes |
| Foreign body | Piece of dust/glass |
| Refraction | Test to determine the power of glasses you need |
| Visual field | Peripheral vision or vision out the corner of your eye |

patient.[17] Some examples with suggested alternatives are listed in Table 1–3. Providing an explanation to the patient of his or her problem or an answer to some question in terms he or she can understand is generally appreciated by the patient.

Similarly, some words that are commonly used by optometrists can be emotive and phobic to patients and should be avoided,[25] such as those listed in Table 1–4. Some of these words, like *senile*, have already been replaced in our clinical vocabulary. (Age-related maculopathy used to be called senile macular degeneration.)

# The Chief Complaint

· · · · · · · · · · · · · · · · · · · · · · · · · · · · ·

The first step in a problem-oriented examination is to elicit the patient's problems, and most importantly the chief complaint or primary problem. This is done at the beginning of the case history by asking a very general, open-ended question, such as, "Why have you come to see me today, Mr. Jones?" or "What is the reason for your visit, Ms. Smith?" Do not ask a series of simple direct questions about blurred vision, headaches, and diplopia because this approach may not provide the relative importance that each symptom has to the patient and may fail to uncover more obscure problems such as a floater or twitching eyelids. A checklist approach also develops little rapport with the patient, because it suggests that the doctor is more interested in ticking off boxes than in the patient's problems.

## CLARIFYING THE CHIEF COMPLAINT

Having obtained information about the patient's chief complaint, the doctor must then explore

the patient's chief complaint with further questions. The number of subsequent questions depends on the complexity of the problem and the completeness of the patient's description of the chief complaint. Between initial description and subsequent questions, the following information is often obtained:

1. *The onset of the problem.* A sudden onset (hours or days) is more likely to indicate a pathological problem. An onset many months (or years) prior to the examination often indicates that the patient realizes that eyeglasses are needed and does not really want to wear them and/or that the problem is not having a severe effect on the patient's life.

2. *The frequency and occurrence of the problem.* If the symptoms are usually associated with reading, then there is obviously a high probability that they have a visual origin. Similarly, symptoms that occur most on weekdays and less often on weekends, or start in the middle of the day and gradually get worse, are more likely to be due to a visual problem.

3. *The type and severity of the problem.* For example, the type and severity of headaches are important for differential diagnosis (see "Headache," page 11). Whether diplopia is horizontal or vertical and monocular or binocular also provides important diagnostic information (see "Diplopia," page 12).

4. *The location and laterality of the problem.* If the chief complaint is blurred vision, it should be determined whether the blur is worse in one eye than the other. The specific location of a headache can also help in differential diagnosis (see "Headache," page 11). Whether diplopia is associated

**TABLE 1–4** Emotive or Phobic Words Commonly Used by Practitioners Which Should be Avoided When Communicating with Patients, with Suggested Lay Alternatives

| To Avoid | Suggested |
| --- | --- |
| Abnormal | Not quite average |
| Atrophy | Become smaller |
| Color defective | Modified form of color vision |
| Hemorrhage | Slight leak from a blood vessel |
| Hysteria | Confusion |
| Paralysis | Cannot move normally |
| Stronger prescription | Prescription modification or change |
| Tumor, growth | New tissue |

with a specific position of gaze must be determined.

5. *The effect on the patient.* This is often indicated by the patient after the initial question. If not, it is essential to determine. There are many examples of the importance of this information, including the following:

   a. Does the patient's blurred vision mean that he or she cannot see the blackboard or overhead projections at school and that his or her schoolwork is suffering? Or does it mean that he or she squints and consequently gets headaches? Or that he or she has to sit near the front of the class? This information gives some indication of severity, but it also demonstrates interest in the patient's problem. It is also reassuring to the patient to be told that the prescribed eyeglasses will solve his or her specific symptom or problem rather than just clear his or her vision. The additional information can also help suggest when the prescribed eyeglasses should be worn. There are no "magic numbers" (of acuity or dioptric power) above which eyeglasses should be worn all the time, or just for specific tasks (apart from driving). It is often useful to suggest that patients wear their eyeglasses for those situations in which they have indicated that they have problems. There may be minimal need to wear them at other times.

   b. This additional information is also essential when determining presbyopic corrections. A patient who has "blurred near vision" for reading music or looking at the computer screen requires a different near addition than one who has blurred near vision for crocheting or sewing.

   c. In patients with cataract, this information can be the basis for referral. Patients should be referred when their reduced vision is having a significant effect on their lifestyle, not when their vision is reduced to some arbitrary acuity level.[26]

   d. In low vision examinations, this information also determines the type of low vision aid prescribed. For example, there is little point in prescribing a telescope if the patient does not complain of problems seeing things in the distance. One must also determine whether referral (for mobility-orientation instruction, for example) is necessary.

   e. Is an adult patient with longstanding strabismus bothered about the cosmetic appearance? It would be pointless to make a referral for surgery if he or she is not.[24]

6. *Self-treatment and its effectivity.* This information is linked with that obtained in the patient's ocular history (described below) and refers to treatment instituted by the patient rather than another eye care specialist or health care practitioner. For example, the most common self-treatment for near vision blur and headaches is to refrain from reading. It is especially important to learn whether an older patient is changing his or her reading habits simply because he or she believes that being unable to read for long periods of time is a normal consequence of growing old. Some older patients also believe that they have only a certain amount of "reading reserve" left in their eyes, and they try to conserve it as much as possible. These are important factors if these patients are to be counseled effectively. If the doctor has developed a good rapport with the patient, the patient may say that his or her distance vision seems fine when he or she wears a brother's eyeglasses or that he or she had previously tried ready-made reading eyeglasses with little success. Prior to obtaining his first eyeglasses, a myopic patient of mine succeeded in watching soccer on television through a hole in a cracker! This may also provide a useful indication of the severity of the problem. If the patient has done nothing about his or her headaches and does not even take analgesics (e.g., aspirin), then the headaches are likely a minor problem to him or her. If he or she has seen a physician and has had a full physical examination and laboratory test battery, including referral to a neurologist, then it is most likely a much bigger problem. This also provides useful differential diagnostic information, as the optometrist can ask about the results of visits to other health care practitioners.

## Tentative Diagnoses

Knowing a patient's chief complaint allows the practitioner to mentally review the most likely tentative diagnoses. This listing should start with the most prevalent condition given the patient's symptoms, age, gender, and race. For example, a 12-year-old patient with symptoms of blurred distance vision with no other problems suggests myopia (with possible small cylindrical correction) as the most likely cause. Less likely possibilities include malingering, ocular hysteria, pseudomyopia, diabetes, and ocular pathology (e.g., Stargardt's disease).

Another example is sudden painless vision loss in one eye. In a 35-year-old patient, a possible list of tentative diagnoses could be unilateral change in prescription (i.e., suddenly noticed rather than sudden onset), idiopathic central serous choroidopathy, optic neuritis, central chorioretinopathy (presumed ocular histoplasmosis syndrome), retinochoroiditis (including toxoplasmosis), retinal detachment (high myope, trauma), branch retinal vein occlusion, and HIV-related infection. If the patient is female, optic neuritis is more likely than idiopathic central serous choroidopathy, given the higher prevalence of optic neuritis and the lower prevalence of idiopathic central serous choroidopathy in women (Table 1–2). If the patient is black, histoplasmosis is much less likely, whereas in a patient from the Ohio-Mississippi area, histoplasmosis is higher up the list. At this point, appropriate supplementary questions could be asked to begin differential diagnosis during the case history. Ask about other symptoms associated with idiopathic central serous choroidopathy (metamorphopsia, distortion, prolonged afterimages), optic neuritis (pain with large eye movements, overheating or possible vision changes in warm weather, sauna, or bath), and recent head trauma, as well as the region where the patient grew up. The mental list of tentative diagnoses becomes refined as more information is gained from further questioning in the case history.

# Secondary Complaints

Secondary complaints are often included when a patient is describing his or her chief complaint. Secondary complaints may be associated with the chief compliant. A chief complaint may be blurred distance vision, and an associated secondary complaint could be frontal headaches due to squinting to see writing on the blackboard. Sometimes secondary complaints are unrelated to the chief complaint. A patient may have a chief complaint of blurred near vision and

be worried about the little floater that he or she has just noticed recently. Give the patient the chance to talk about any secondary complaints by asking another open question: "Do you have any other problems with your eyes or vision?" All secondary complaints should be worked up in the same way as the chief complaint.

# Checklist

As stated earlier, some patients may not tell the optometrist all their symptoms. They may believe that their headaches are not associated with their vision or their eyes or that their symptoms are an inevitable and therefore unremarkable consequence of getting older. It is therefore important to ask patients about specific aspects of their vision. This investigation should obviously include only those aspects that were not described in the patient's chief and secondary complaints. For a patient stating that he or she has no complaints and has presented for a routine eye examination, you could ask about the following:

## Vision at Distance and at Near

It is often best for the doctor to first give an example so that the patient understands what the doctor is trying to ascertain. A student could be asked whether he or she can see the overhead projections or chalkboard clearly before a more general question of whether he or she can see other things in the distance clearly. A presbyope could be asked, "Can you read newspapers easily? What about telephone numbers or details on medicine bottles?" before a general question about the clarity of near vision.

Symptoms of blurred distance vision indicate myopia. The effect of myopia is evident in some of the paintings of the famous French impressionist artist Edgar Dégas (1834–1917). In his *The Ballet from 'Robert le Diable,'* the distant dancers are blurred, whereas the nearer orchestra is painted in fine detail (Fig. 1–2). Myopia is usually of gradual onset beginning at around age 10 or age 18 (adult onset). Typically the younger group presents with symptoms of not being able to see the blackboard, and adult patients may have difficulty driving, particularly at night. This can be accompanied by frontal headaches if the patient squints to improve his or her vision. Accompanying low astigmatism (0.50 to 1.00 D) can result in asthenopic symptoms, particularly with

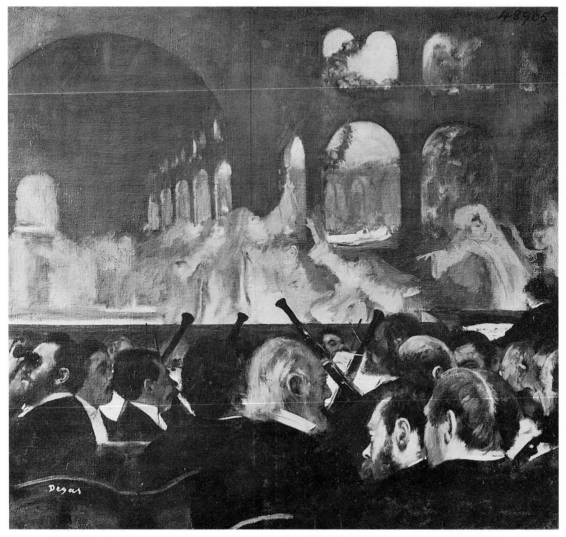

**FIGURE 1–2**   Degas' myopia is evident in his *The Ballet from 'Robert le Diable'* (1876). (Courtesy of the Board of Trustees of the Victoria and Albert Museum. London, United Kingdom.)

close work, and near vision blur can occur with greater amounts of astigmatism. Myopic eyeglass wearers often complain only of blurred distance vision, and asthenopic symptoms and near blur are much more rare, as astigmatic changes tend to be negligible. Case history can help to differentiate between myopia and pseudomyopia. In the latter case distance blur is intermittent and is commonly associated with a lot of close work. The myopia of young diabetics is also variable.[16] Patients over 60 years of age who complain of distance blur may have increased myopia due to nuclear sclerotic changes.[16] They usually indicate that they can read at some distance with or without eyeglasses. Indeed, some of these patients can now read without eyeglasses (the "second sight" of the elderly). Patients with both reduced distance and near vision are more likely to have age-related cataract or maculopathy.

Uncorrected hyperopia is usually associated with symptoms of asthenopia or headache while reading and more rarely with blurred near vision. Near vision blur associated with uncorrected hyperopia tends to be intermittent, and it is most often found in patients approaching presbyopia. Significant astigmatism with hyperopia can lead to blurred vision at both distance and near.

Presbyopic patients most commonly report near vision blur. They may indicate that they have trouble only with small print ("They're making telephone book numbers smaller these days.") and that they have to hold their reading material farther away ("My arms are too short.")

and use bright light ("I can see fine during the day.").

## Headaches

An optometric examination is a logical primary care entry point into the health system for headaches. This could be instigated by the patient or by his or her physician. Even if a headache is not the reason for the patient's visit, it must be of concern to the optometrist. Do not always give up asking about headaches if the patient suggests they "have nothing to do with my eyes" or "they are due to stress," because the patient should not always decide whether the headaches are of any interest to the doctor. Even if the headaches are not eye- or vision-related, they may have ocular manifestations (e.g., vascular and cranial lesion headaches). In any case, as the primary health care provider, the optometrist should be able to counsel patients regarding any headaches and to refer them appropriately when necessary.

If the headaches occur shortly after a demanding visual task such as reading classroom overheads or printed material, then obviously a strong chance exists that they are caused by a visual problem, such as ametropia (most often uncorrected hyperopia), accommodative dysfunction, or a binocular anomaly. Similarly, symptoms that occur more frequently on weekdays and less often on weekends, or start in the middle of the day and gradually worsen toward the end of the day, are more likely to be visually related. Vision-related headaches are usually described as mild or moderate rather than severe, dull rather than sharp, non-throbbing, and arising behind or above the eyes. Occasionally these headaches may arise occipitally or temporally, but rarely at the vertex. Anisometropes often have a headache above one eye more than the other. Surprisingly, low uncorrected myopes can also complain of headaches. Often these patients admit to continually squinting to see the chalkboard, and the headaches are likely due to muscular stress. The only certain diagnosis of a visually related headache is when the headaches disappear after successful vision training and/or wearing of eyeglasses. Even then, an initial placebo effect with eyeglasses can occur, so that the headaches return after a short period.

Other relatively common causes of headaches encountered by an optometrist are stress, muscular tension, anxiety, depression, overwork, insomnia, fatigue, constipation, undue physical activity, the various forms of migraine, hypertension, oral or sinus infection, minor trauma, and adverse effects of medications, drugs, toxins, and the like.[25] It is very helpful to ask patients what they believe to be the cause, although their opinions may not be accepted at face value. Ask how they arrived at their "diagnosis," as their explanation may make sense. Some of the headaches listed above may also occur on most weekdays and less so on weekends, or start in the middle of the day and gradually worsen, making differential diagnosis from a vision-related headache difficult. The situation is especially problematic in the presence of a small refractive error. Is the headache caused by stress, overwork, or fatigue, or could it be due to the small refractive error? The best approach may be to explain the findings to the patient and indicate that the only sure way to determine whether the refractive correction could help is to try it. The patient then becomes involved in the decision of whether to prescribe eyeglasses, which he or she may elect to defer for a short period. Monitoring the situation for a short period to determine whether the symptoms persist is a useful approach.

One classic situation in which it is usually best not to prescribe is that of the student undergoing examinations.[25] In this case, the overwork, stress, hurried meals, and late nights may cause headaches and ocular discomfort. However, the symptoms often disappear after the examination period, and prescribing eyeglasses before this time may lead to unnecessary eyeglasses dependency. Tension headaches are probably the most common type of headache. They are often at the back of the neck or feel like a ring around the head and can be associated with sleeplessness.

A throbbing headache is often associated with a vascular disorder, which suggests that blood pressure measurement is important in older patients with any form of headache. Migraine headaches are often severe, throbbing unilateral headaches, and patients report having to stay in the dark for a few hours until the pain passes. There may be associated nausea and vomiting and various visual effects such as flashes of light or scotomas, consisting of scintillating zigzag lines and patterns.[27] They often occur in patients with a meticulous, obsessional, or compulsive personality. Surprisingly, some patients with migraine have not heard of the possible links with foods containing beta-phenylethylamine or tyramine, such as chocolate, wine, cheese, and yogurt. It is useful to suggest that patients keep a diary of when these foods were eaten to determine whether there is any link with the timing of the migraines. Other causes of migraine include various drugs. Headaches caused by sinus problems occur with tenderness around the sinus area and a transillumination defect. A more thorough discussion of headaches is provided by Stelmack.[27]

## Ocular Discomfort

This covers a variety of symptoms including dull ache, pain, tired eyes, and heavy or tender eyes. The patient's exact description of the discomfort is often more personality dependent than diagnostically significant. If any ocular disease has been ruled out, these symptoms can be caused by ametropia (most often uncorrected hyperopia), accommodative dysfunction, or a binocular anomaly. Discomfort that occurs shortly after a demanding visual task such as reading, occurs on weekdays and less so on weekends, or starts in the middle of the day and gradually worsens is more likely to be due to a visual problem.

## Burning or Dry Eyes

Many older patients complain of dry, burning eyes. In such cases it is obviously essential to check for possible ocular inflammation. However, it is common for such patients to have "dry eye" symptoms due to reduced aqueous or mucin production. This can be idiopathic or a side effect of various medications, particularly oral antihypertensives. It can also be linked to various systemic diseases, particularly arthritis and other connective tissue disorders. These patients may also complain of their eyes feeling "filled to the brim," although not of frank epiphora. This is known as pseudoepiphora and is counterintuitively caused by reflex tearing induced by the dry eye.

## Diplopia

First ask whether the double vision disappears when one eye is closed. If it does, then the diplopia is caused by a binocular vision problem. If it persists with one eye covered, then it is likely due to an optical problem, such as cataract or irregular corneal astigmatism, although diplopia can occur monocularly in multiple sclerosis. Diplopia due to pathology or trauma tends to have a sudden onset, is more usually vertical than horizontal, and varies with the position of gaze but is always present.[28] The patient may also adopt an abnormal head posture. Diplopia due to heterophoria or a remote near point of convergence is usually intermittent, horizontal, and associated with prolonged visual tasks.[28]

## Other

Some texts suggest inquiring directly about more obscure symptoms such as haloes, flashes, and floaters.[7, 8] However, these visual symptoms are usually quite dramatic, particularly when associated with ocular disease, and the patient tends to be readily forthcoming with such symptoms. In addition, the diseases causing these symptoms are rare. My own experience with routinely asking about these symptoms is that positive responses often lead to lengthy discussion and examination and a diagnosis of physiological haloes, environmental haloes (steamy windows or misted windshields), afterimages of bright lights, and phosphenes.

A positive response to any of the above questions requires a full inquiry into the problem. Ask about the onset, frequency, type, severity, location, laterality, effect on the patient, and the nature and effectiveness of any treatment. Throughout the investigation of secondary complaints and other aspects of vision not mentioned by the patient, the doctor's mental list of tentative diagnoses should be updated as required, and any questions relevant to the tentative diagnoses should be asked.

# Present Refractive Correction

The doctor often asks for information about the present correction while discussing the chief complaint. If the patient is new and wears eyeglasses, you need to know the age when eyeglasses were first worn, the age of the present eyeglasses, when they are worn, who prescribed them, who supplied them, and how satisfactory they are for both function and fashion. In a young myope, the age when eyeglasses were first prescribed can give some indication about when the myopic progression will cease, a question often asked by these patients or their parents. In a patient with strabismus, anisometropia, or high astigmatism, this information can help sort out the presence and level of amblyopia. The longer the delay before eyeglasses were first worn after the critical period, the greater the amount of amblyopia. The age of the present eyeglasses can indicate whether the patient will want a change in frames. Practitioners rely heavily on the patient's reported satisfaction with his or her current eyeglasses when deciding whether to prescribe new lenses when the change in refraction is small. Asking the patient when he or she wears his or her eyeglasses is important. Does the low myope wear his or her eyeglasses all the time or just for driving? Does he or she take them off for reading? If eyeglasses are removed for driving, does the patient meet the required legal visual standards for driving? If eyeglasses are removed for reading, it is important to measure near acuity (for the presbyopic myope) and to perform screening binocular tests without the eyeglasses. Does the patient wear his or her eyeglasses for sport activities? If not, what does he or she wear?

When a new patient is a contact lens wearer, even more information is required: the lens material, type of lenses, who prescribed them, solutions and cleaning regimen, the number of years lenses have been worn, the age of the current lenses, the average wearing time, the maximum wearing time, whether the patient ever sleeps with the lenses in, and the length of time the lenses were worn on the examination day. When both eyeglasses and contact lenses are worn, it is necessary to investigate any problems the patient experiences with either correction modality.

# Ocular History

The time elapsed since the last eye examination provides some indication of the importance the patient attaches to eye care. An appointment with another practitioner within the year suggests possible unhappiness with the last examination, and this should be investigated. Patients must also be asked whether they have ever had any eye injuries, disease, treatment, or surgery. If any indications of any of these conditions exist, additional questions should be asked about the specific condition under consideration. This can save a great deal of time in unnecessary supplementary testing. Students must be aware that

some elderly patients may forget that they had cataract surgery. Patients should be asked whether they have had any previous vision training or patching. Previous problems can reappear (e.g., remote near point of convergence, accommodative infacility, various types of conjunctivitis, recurrent corneal erosions, anterior uveitis) and should be included in the list of differential diagnoses when they are suggested by the patient's symptoms. The success of previous treatment in these situations must also be determined, because this information may suggest subsequent management.

## FAMILY OCULAR HISTORY

One reason why some patients seek an examination is to check for a condition that a close family member has or that "runs in the family" (Table 1-5). In these circumstances it is important to ask questions and conduct tests that are pertinent to the condition. For example, when there is a family history of glaucoma, patients should be asked about possible symptoms of closed-angle glaucoma (particularly if the patient is hyperopic). Testing should include fundus biomicroscopy, tonometry, visual field testing, and gonioscopy. In a routine case history, an open-ended question such as, "Has anybody in your family had any eye problem or disease?" should be asked. This can be clarified by providing examples such as glaucoma or a lazy eye. A checklist style of questioning tends to make the case history stilted and does not appear to provide any increased efficiency or effectiveness.

# Medical History

A general question such as, "How is your general health?" can be misleading because some pa-

| TABLE 1–5 Approximate Prevalence of Common Hereditary Eye Abnormalities and Indications of the Increase in Prevalence with a Family History of the Disorder |||
|---|---|---|
| Disease | Prevalence | Inheritance |
| Hypertension | 10–15% | No parent (3%), one parent (25%), both parents (40%) |
| Color defective | 8% | X-linked |
| Strabismus | 3% | No parent (1%), 2 siblings (20%), 1 parent (10–20%), 2 parents (30–40%) |
| Non–insulin-dependent diabetes mellitus | 2% | 1 parent (4–10%), both parents (5–35%), sibling (3–11%) |
| Insulin-dependent diabetes mellitus | 0.2% | Sibling (5–20%), 1 parent (3%) |
| Primary open-angle glaucoma | 1% of 40+ | First-degree relative (~10–20%) |
| Primary angle-closure glaucoma | 0.1% of 40+ | First-degree relative (2–5%) |
| Retinitis pigmentosa | 1:3,500 | Type dependent (25–45%) |
| Retinoblastoma | 1:20,000 | First-degree relative (bilateral 5–40%; unilateral 5%) |

Data from Lyle[34] and François.[35]

**TABLE 1–6**  Ocular Side Effects of Systemic Drugs Most Commonly Encountered by the Optometrist in Practice, with Suggestions for Management

*Amiodarone:* For severe, life-threatening cardiac arrhythmias

Whorl-like epithelial deposits, sometimes referred to as vortex keratopathy. These probably occur in all patients on this drug within a few weeks. There is also a risk of papilledema. Perform fundus biomicroscopy and central field testing at the start of medication and every 3 months thereafter. The effects on the optic nerve can be reversible.

*Anticancer Drugs*

Irritation and severe dry eye. These symptoms can be responsive to regular use of unpreserved artificial tears. Anticancer drugs can also cause optic neuropathy, which should be monitored.

*Antihistamines (Especially Those Used for Seasonal Allergies)*

Can result in tear film deficiency. Artificial tears usually provide relief.

*Antituberculosis Drugs (e.g., Ethambutol, Isoniazid, Rifampin)*

Side effects are generally found with high dosage (>35 mg/day) for greater than 6 months and are especially found with alcoholics and diabetics. Central/paracentral scotomas are found, especially to red stimuli, so use the red Amsler or Humphrey VFA red 10-2. These drugs can also cause red-green color vision changes and optic neuropathy. Visual field and color testing before treatment starts are important, and patients at risk should be monitored frequently (every month). Reversal generally occurs within about 6 months if caught early. Rarely, an irreversible optic atrophy occurs.

*Atropine-like Drugs (e.g., Scopolamine, Hyoscine, Atropine):* For gastrointestinal upset, motion sickness

Large pupils (slightly reduced vision, glare), reduced accommodation (difficulty reading, changing focus), and dry eyes. The effects are reversible. Because of the mydriatic effect, acute closed-angle glaucoma is always a possibility.

*Blood Pressure Medication (Especially Beta Blockers)*

The tear film can be affected in 25 to 50% of patients, leading to irritation, dry eye, and the like. Artificial tears probably provide adequate relief. These patients may be poor candidates for contact lens wear.
Intraocular pressure can be reduced. This reduction is greater in ocular hypertensives than normals; normals show a 2- to 3-mm Hg reduction. Patients with high blood pressure and elevated intraocular pressure can have ~15 mm Hg reduction. When glaucomatous discs or field changes are suspected in such patients, intraocular pressure should be measured immediately before the drug is taken. Also, two to three measurements should be taken over a period of a few weeks.

*Corticosteroids:* For arthritis or inflammatory disorders of the bowels and respiratory tract

There is a variable time and dosage dependency. Side effects are most likely with high and long-term oral dosage, especially in the elderly.
*Systemic:* Posterior subcapsular cataracts and associated vision and glare problems. A much less common side effect is increased intraocular pressure and is more likely to occur in children.
*Topical:* Glaucoma: The response of intraocular pressure to steroids appears genetically determined. "Responders" might include patients with primary open-angle glaucoma, a family history of primary open-angle glaucoma, diabetes, or high myopia. Use topical steroids with caution in these patients. The effect occurs within a few weeks. Intraocular pressure returns to normal within a few weeks. Damage to the optic nerve must not be allowed to occur.

*Digitalis:* For congestive heart failure

Side effects generally occur about 2 to 3 weeks after treatment starts, generally in those on higher doses. They are usually transitory and reversible. The most common includes flashes of light, glare, brilliant snowballs, and changes in color vision (especially "yellow" vision). More rarely it can cause bilateral central scotomas. It can also cause a slight reduction in intraocular pressure.

*Hydroxychloroquine, Chloroquine:* For collagenous diseases, e.g., rheumatoid arthritis, actinic dermatitis, lupus erythematosus (daily doses used ~250–500 mg)

Side effects occur after about 2 to 3 years on above daily dosage. The first eye examination of these patients should be about 9 months after the start of treatment, and subsequently at 4- to 6-month intervals.
Side effects include bilateral corneal deposits, which can start as punctate, yellowish, intraepithelial inclusions, and progress to larger whorl-like deposits. Rarely, the corneal epithelium can become edematous, giving symptoms of glare. In rare cases a toxic maculopathy can develop. In the pre-maculopathy stage, ring scotoma to red at about 4° to 9° can be found. Tests to use include the red Amsler chart and the Humphrey VFA red 10-2. Blue-yellow color vision changes may also occur. The Ishihara is not sensitive to these effects, and the 100-Hue and D-15 are not good because patients are arthritic. Loss of foveal reflex and fine macular pigment dots may be noticed, but these changes can be difficult to differentiate from normal aging changes. Visual field and color testing before treatment starts is important. These effects may be reversible with removal of the drug at this point.
In the later stages, a "bull's-eye" maculopathy and loss of visual acuity occur. Later still, narrowing of the retinal arteries and optic atrophy occur. These changes are not reversible and can progress despite removal of drugs because these drugs remain bound to the retinal pigment epithelium.

**TABLE 1–6** Ocular Side Effects of Systemic Drugs Most Commonly Encountered by the Optometrist in Practice, with Suggestions for Management *Continued*

*Isotretinoin (Acutane):* For severe acne problems

Irritable dry eyes. The condition may be eased by the use of artificial tears. The effects are reversible.

*Nonsteroidal Anti-inflammatory Drugs (NSAIDs):* For arthritis

Perimacular pigmentary disturbances that may not be reversible. There are color vision deficits, and macular edema may develop. Optometrists must screen for color deficiencies and dilate and use fundus biomicroscopy to screen for macular edema.

*Phenothiazines (e.g., Chlorpromazine):* For epilepsy, major depression, schizophrenia

Chronic use gives ~30% ocular side effects. With long-term use (>10 years), virtually all patients have ocular side effects. Cholinergic blocking effects can lead to mydriasis and reduced accommodation, with symptoms of blurred near vision, difficulties changing focus, and glare. Closed-angle glaucoma can also occur. Pigmentary deposits can occur in the eye, especially on the anterior lens surface (where a spokelike pattern develops) and more rarely on the corneal endothelium and Bowman's layer.

*Toxic Amblyopia (Found in Pipe Smokers [1/2 oz. Tobacco Daily for 15+ Years] and/or Heavy Drinkers)*

Bilateral, progressive centrocecal scotomas. Can be of sudden onset if the scotoma invades the fixation area. Red fields are reduced earlier, so use red Amsler or Humphrey VFA red 10-2. Blue-yellow color vision defects have also been reported. It is generally reversible with vitamin $B_{12}$ (tobacco) or B-complex (alcoholic) treatment provided that the patient stops drinking or smoking.

tients think that systemic diseases are not relevant when they are borderline or are controlled by medication. It is better to give some examples of what is being specifically sought after, such as "Do you have high blood pressure or diabetes?" Another alternative is to ask whether the patient is under medical care for anything. In addition, it is important to ask patients whether they are taking any medication even if they indicate that their general health is fine. Patients may be taking medications, but they are unsure why because the medical diagnosis was not properly explained or was poorly understood. Female patients may not consider birth control pills to be medication, but because the agents in these pills can have adverse ocular effects, they should be asked about specifically. Allergies and hypersensitivities to drugs, any other ingredients of medications, or foods should also be ascertained at this point.

General health and medication information are important for several reasons. Many systemic diseases have ocular manifestations. The most common conditions include diabetes, hypertension, arthritis and other connective tissue disorders, thyroid disorders, embolic disease, and AIDS. Optometrists need to be familiar with the more common manifestations of these ocular disorders and which tests would be most appropriate to identify any problems.

The use of certain diagnostic and therapeutic drugs is contraindicated in certain systemic diseases and conditions. For example, phenylephrine, commonly used as a diagnostic pharmaceutical agent (usually in combination mydriatics), is contraindicated in patients with cardiac disorders, marked systemic hypertension, any history of aneurysm or stroke, concurrent use of certain medications for cardiac arrhythmias or high blood pressure, and sensitivity to the drug. There is also a need to stay current with recommendations in a pharmaceutical directory (e.g., *Physicians' Desk Reference*[29]). For example, when introduced in the 1970s for glaucoma management, beta blockers were widely considered to be free of major systemic side effects, yet experience has clearly shown otherwise. Current guidelines indicate that beta blockers are contraindicated in patients with bronchial asthma or a history of bronchial asthma, chronic pulmonary obstruction, sinus bradycardia, second- or third-degree atrioventricular block, overt cardiac failure, cardiogenic shock, and sensitivity to any component of the product.[29]

Obtaining specific and detailed information about medications is also essential for two reasons: First, many systemic medications can affect vision or cause adverse side effects on the eye and visual system. There are many examples of these.[30] Some of the more commonly encountered examples are shown in Table 1–6, along with their impact on the optometric examination.

The second essential reason for determining details of a patient's medication is to be able to identify and manage any interactions among drugs. The types of interactions that are especially relevant to the optometrist relate to topical diagnostic pharmaceutical agent and topical and oral therapeutic pharmaceutical agent use, but general systemic interactions between drugs (usually leading to over-reactions) should not be ignored. An appropriate pharmaceutical directory (e.g., *Physicians' Desk Reference*[29]) should be consulted for full details.

As examples, the use of phenylephrine (as a mydriatic) should be approached cautiously in patients with moderately high blood pressure who are taking any other sympathomimetics because elevated pulse blood pressure and syncope can result. The same applies to the use of "eye whiteners," which generally contain direct or indirect sympathomimetics. Although such interactions between drugs are well known, the practitioner again needs to stay current. For example, it has recently become apparent that some patients may over-react to even simple over-the-counter antihistamines (for allergies and colds) if they are also taking erythromycin (for bronchial, urinary tract, or ear infection) or ketoconazole (for vaginal infection). These antibiotics can reduce the bioelimination of the antihistamines, thereby causing an "overdose" even with standard antihistamine dosing. At high doses the antihistamines can precipitate arrhythmias. This is particularly important for optometrists given that antihistamines are part of standard therapy for rhinoconjunctivitis. Another example is that caution should be used in prescribing beta blockers if the patient is taking catecholamine-depleting drugs such as reserpine, because of possible additive effects leading to hypotension and/or marked bradycardia, which may be accompanied by vertigo, syncope, and postural hypotension.[30]

## FAMILY MEDICAL HISTORY

If a patient has a first-degree relative with certain systemic abnormalities, the eye care practitioner must look very carefully for appropriate symptoms and signs. This is particularly important because some hereditary diseases can first manifest in the eye or visual system. Common examples include refractive error fluctuations in diabetes, characteristic retinal vessel changes in hypertension, optic neuritis in multiple sclerosis, and exophthalmos in hyperthyroidism.

# Occupation and Hobbies

· · · · · · · · · · · · · · · · · · · · · · · · · · ·

Determining how patients use their vision is extremely important, especially when they are presbyopic. A patient who primarily reads music or works on a computer requires a prescription (or lens type) that is very different from that for a patient who primarily crochets or sews as a hobby. A patient who does all four of these visual tasks requires a different correction again. A presbyopic patient whose occupation involves a great deal of reading probably requires a larger reading segment in his or her bifocals than someone who simply uses his or her bifocals to read the newspaper.

It is also useful to ask all patients about any hobbies or sports activities. For presbyopes, this can again determine the lens prescription and the lens type. For all patients, it leads to a discussion of optical needs for various sports. Special eyeglass designs are available for a variety of sports including billiards, shooting, skiing, and basketball. Contact lenses can provide an enormous benefit to some young ametropic football, rugby, soccer, and baseball players. Even patients without a refractive correction require protective eyewear for some sports, such as squash and badminton.

# The Problem-Plan List

· · · · · · · · · · · · · · · · · · · · · · · · · · ·

The problem-oriented record is completed by a problem-plan list.[1, 4-7] Each separate problem is listed in a column and given a numerical value. The order of the problem-plan list communicates the relative importance of the problem to the patient. For each problem, a plan or a series of actions to be taken is outlined. Problems are defined at the highest level of understanding. For example, if a 48-year-old patient reporting difficulties reading the newspaper is found to have reduced near acuity and a 3.00 D amplitude of accommodation, the problem should be diagnosed and recorded as presbyopia. The individual symptoms and signs that led to this diagnosis need not be listed. If abnormal symptoms or test results do not lead to some diagnosis, they should be listed. In this way problems that are not immediately understood remain open for further investigation. A "plan" can usually be placed in one of three categories, requiring either treatment, further diagnostic procedures, or counseling. An example of a problem-plan list is shown in Table 1-7.

# Final Discussion with the Patient

· · · · · · · · · · · · · · · · · · · · · · · · · · ·

The baseline case history investigation occurs at the beginning of the examination, and subsequent questions are usually asked during the ex-

| Number | Problem | Plan |
|---|---|---|
| | **TABLE 1–7** Example of a Problem-Plan List | |
| 1 | Presbyopia | a. Prescribe bifocal prescription. |
| | | b. Counsel patient regarding bifocal use and difficult situations such as climbing stairs. |
| | | c. Educate patient regarding typical progression of presbyopia and future changes in prescription. |
| 2 | Suspect primary open-angle glaucoma (high intraocular pressure and vertical disc cupping OS with open angles) | a. Glaucoma work-up: Humphrey 30-2 visual fields, dilated fundus examination to assess nerve fiber layer and optic disc. Appointment booked in 1 week. |
| | | b. Explain glaucoma work-up. |

amination as prompted by test results and clinical observations. At the end of the examination, the findings must be discussed with the patient, particularly those that relate to the patient's chief complaint and other secondary complaints. What is the cause (if known) of the chief complaint? A full explanation of the diagnoses in terminology that is appropriate to the patient's perceived knowledge should be given. It is generally best to discuss the findings in order of the patient's ranking of his or her problems rather than according to the doctor's opinion of the relative importance of the diagnoses.

If the cause of the chief complaint is not known, the patient should be told what conditions have *not* been detected to reassure the patient.[31] For example, if a patient's chief complaint is headache, and no visual reason could be found on examination, negative findings should be presented in a positive manner: "I do not believe that your headaches are due to a problem with your eyes or vision, Ms. Waterloo. Your eyesight is excellent, and there is no need for eyeglasses; your eye muscles and 'focusing muscles' are all working normally and are working well together, and there is no sign of any eye disease from any of the tests I performed." If the baseline case history indicated that a particular disease is of concern to the patient (perhaps due to a positive family history), it is particularly important to indicate that this was not detected and even to indicate how this was determined. For example, in a patient with a family history of glaucoma, it is useful to tell the patient that the tests used to detect primary open-angle glaucoma—intraocular pressure, optic nerve head appearance, and visual fields (using appropriate terminology)—did not reveal any signs of the disease. This reassures the patient that his or her doctor is knowledgeable about the disease and that appropriate diagnostic tests were performed.

The patient should then become involved in a discussion about possible treatment options, the prognosis, and recommended follow-up. As always, the doctor's part of this discussion must be in terminology that the patient can easily understand. Prescribing and therapeusis are as much art as science because they depend on many factors, including the optometrist's overall assessment of the patient. A small cylindrical correction may be absolutely crucial to the visual well-being of one patient, whereas another patient may be perfectly happy for several months after breaking his or her $-2.00$ D eyeglasses. This depends heavily on a patient's occupation and hobbies but is also affected by personality.[32] More extensive discussions of reassurance therapy and prescribing low-powered lenses are given elsewhere.[31, 32]

In summary, the case history provides the framework within which to conduct an eye examination. It sets the stage for identifying the patient's problems, directs the specific testing and flow of the examination, and requires a satisfactory explanation and conclusion.

### ACKNOWLEDGMENTS
I thank the following faculty of the School of Optometry, University of Waterloo, for helpful comments on earlier versions of this chapter: Drs. Graham Strong, Michael Doughty, Patricia Hrynchak, and Lisa Prokopich.

# References

1. Amos JF: The problem-solving approach to patient care. *In* Amos JF: Diagnosis and Management in Vision Care. Boston: Butterworths, 1987.
2. Weed LL: Medical records that guide and teach. N Engl J Med 1968; 278:652–657.
3. Hurst JW, Walker HK: The Problem-Oriented System. New York: Medcom Press, 1972.
4. Sloan PG: A "problem-oriented" optometric record? Am J Optom Physiol Opt 1978; 55:352–357.
5. Maino JH: The problem-oriented optometric record. J Am Optom Assoc 1979; 50:915–918.
6. Barresi BJ, Nyman NN: Implementation of the problem-

oriented system in an optometric teaching clinic. Am J Optom Physiol Opt 1978; 55:765-770.

7. Hrynchak P: Procedures in Clinical Optometry, 5th ed. University of Waterloo: School of Optometry, 1994.

8. Amos JF: Patient history. *In* Eskridge JB, Amos JF, Bartlett JD: Clinical Procedures in Optometry. Philadelphia: JB Lippincott, 1991.

9. Borish IM: Teaching the traditional optometry with the new optometry. Optom Vis Sci 1993; 70:637-639.

10. Tuck MW, Crick RP: Relative effectiveness of different modes of glaucoma screening in optometric practice. Ophthal Physiol Opt 1993; 13:227-232.

11. Tuck MW, Crick RP: Use of visual field tests in glaucoma detection by optometrists in England and Wales. Ophthal Physiol Opt 1994; 14:227-231.

12. Blum HL, Peters HB, Bettman JW: Vision Screening for Elementary Schools: The Orinda Study. Berkeley: University of California Press, 1959.

13. Sperduto RD, Siegel D, Roberts J, Rowland M: Prevalence of myopia in the United States. Arch Ophthalmol 1983; 101:405-407.

14. Goss DA, Winkler RL: Progression of myopia in youth: Age of cessation. Am J Optom Physiol Opt 1983; 60:651-658.

15. O'Neal MR, Connon TR: Refractive error change at the United States Air Force Academy—Class of 1985. Am J Optom Physiol Opt 1987; 64:344-354.

16. Locke LC: Induced refractive and visual changes. *In* Amos JF: Diagnosis and Management in Vision Care. Boston: Butterworths, 1987.

17. Ball G: Symptoms in eye examination. London: Butterworths, 1982.

18. Bannon RE, Walsh R: On astigmatism. Am J Optom Arch Am Acad Optom 1945; 22:162-181, 263-277.

19. Saunders H: Age-dependence of human refractive errors. Ophthal Physiol Opt 1981; 1:159-174.

20. Patorgis CJ: Presbyopia. *In* Amos JF: Diagnosis and Management in Vision Care. Boston: Butterworths, 1987.

21. Alexander LJ: Primary Care of the Posterior Segment, 2nd ed. Norwalk, CT: Appleton & Lange, 1994.

22. Werner DL: Teaching clinical thinking. Optom Vis Sci 1989; 66:788-792.

23. Schwartz H: Abraham Lincoln's Marfan syndrome. *In* Sorsby A: Tenements of Clay. New York: Charles Scribner & Sons, 1974.

24. Bannon RE: Symptoms and case history—the patient as a person. Am J Optom Arch Am Acad Optom 1952; 29:275-285.

25. Ball G: Symptoms in Eye Examination. London: Butterworths, 1982.

26. AHCPR Report: Cataract Management Guideline Panel. Cataract in Adults: Management of Functional Impairment. Clinical Practice Guideline, No. 4. Rockville, MD: US Department of Health and Human Services, Public Health Service, Agency for Health Care Policy and Research. AHCPR Publication No. 93-0542, February 1993.

27. Stelmack TR: Headache. *In* Amos JF: Diagnosis and Management in Vision Care. Boston: Butterworths, 1987.

28. Pickwell D: Binocular Vision Anomalies. London: Butterworths, 1984.

29. Physicians' Desk Reference. Montvale, NJ: Medical Economics Data Production Co., 1994.

30. Onofrey BE: Clinical Optometric Pharmacology and Therapeutics. Philadelphia: JB Lippincott, 1993.

31. Blume AJ: Reassurance therapy. *In* Amos JF: Diagnosis and Management in Vision Care. Boston: Butterworths, 1987.

32. Blume AJ: Low-power lenses. *In* Amos JF: Diagnosis and Management in Vision Care. Boston: Butterworths, 1987.

33. Leibowitz HM, Krueger DE, Maunder LR, et al.: The Framingham Eye Study Monograph. An ophthalmological and epidemiological study of cataract, glaucoma, diabetic retinopathy, macular degeneration, and visual acuity in a general population of 2631 adults, 1973-1975. Survey Ophthalmol 1980; 24(Suppl):335-610.

34. Lyle WM: Genetic Risks. Waterloo, Ontario: University of Waterloo Press, 1990.

35. François J: Multifactorial or polygenic inheritance in ophthalmology. Devel Ophthalmol 1985; 10:1-39.

2

*Mark A. Bullimore, OD, PhD*

# Visual Acuity

Visual acuity is a measure of the ability of the patient's visual system to resolve fine detail. It is sometimes the only measurement of visual function made by the clinician and nearly always the first measurement in the examination sequence. The typical letter chart contains a number of lines of letters which decrease in size from the top to the bottom.

The term "20/20 vision" is familiar to most patients and, to them, signifies perfect vision (equivalent to 6/6 in most non-US countries). To the clinician, good visual acuity provides assurance of an adequate spectacle correction. Because visual acuity can be affected by disruptions in the ocular media, retina, or optic nerve, good visual acuity also implies that the key structures in the eye are intact. Visual acuity is also the criterion for a person's fitness to drive and ability to gain entrance into some professions.

# Physiological Limits of Visual Acuity

Both optical and retinal factors limit visual acuity in the normal eye. The optics of the emmetropic eye form an in-focus image on the retina. The quality of this image is limited by aberrations of the cornea and crystalline lens (see Charman[1] for an excellent overview) and the size of the pupil. The pupil serves to modulate the intensity of light incident on the retina but also influences the quality of the retinal image. Two factors work in opposition: Too large a pupil degrades the image as a result of increased spherical aberration and other aberrations; too small a pupil can degrade an in-focus image by diffraction, although this is significant only at very small pupil diameters.

Let us consider a patient viewing two point sources of light. Rayleigh's criterion states that the diffraction limit of resolution (in radians) for an optical system is given by the formula 1.22 $\lambda$/d, where $\lambda$ is the wavelength of light and d is the pupil diameter (both in meters). For a 3-mm pupil and a wavelength of 578 nm, Rayleigh's criterion predicts a resolution limit of 50 seconds of arc, or that the centers of the two spots of light are separated by just under 1 minute of arc.

In normal emmetropic subjects, visual acuity is constant across a wide range of pupil diameters. In subjects with imperfect optics due to refractive surgery[2] or keratoconus,[3] visual acuity may be poorer at the larger pupil sizes associated with dim illumination. Patients may express this in their history as "problems with night driving."

The retinal image must be interpreted by the photoreceptors. Visual acuity is thus limited by photoreceptor spacing, in the same way that the quality of a television picture is constrained by the raster or pixel density. At normal light levels, the retinal cones determine resolution. Let us again consider a patient viewing two point sources of light. If their respective images fell on two adjacent cones, they would be perceived as a single point of light. Conversely, if the images fell on two cones separated by an unilluminated cone, then the points of light would be perceived as two distinct sources and would be said to be *resolved*. At the fovea, the cones are separated by about 2 $\mu$m, corresponding to a visual angle of 25 seconds of arc. The two illuminated cones would thus be 50 seconds of arc apart. This corresponds to the optical limits of the image imposed by diffraction described above.

An increase in photoreceptor spacing leads to poorer visual acuity. Moving from the fovea into the less densely packed periphery is one manifestation of this relationship. Figure 2–1 shows the variation in both visual acuity and receptor spacing with retinal eccentricity. Conditions such as age-related maculopathy, which result in a loss of foveal function, force the patient to adopt eccentric retinal locations for crucial visual tasks. This visual strategy is associated with a concurrent drop in visual acuity.[4] Furthermore, the reduction in visual acuity that occurs late in retinitis pigmentosa is believed to be due to loss of photoreceptors and hence an increase in their spacing.

## THE EFFECTS OF LUMINANCE AND CONTRAST

Visual acuity is relatively constant at high luminances. Sheedy et al.[7] found that over a "normal"

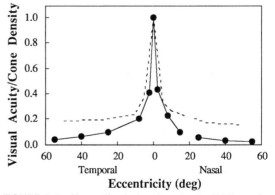

**FIGURE 2–1** Normalized visual acuity (*solid line,* after Anderson et al.[5]) and receptor spacing (*dashed line,* after Curcio et al.[6]) as a function of retinal eccentricity.

photopic range of 40 to 600 cd/m², visual acuity varied by less than one line. Within this range, a doubling of the luminance improves visual acuity by approximately one letter for a five-letter row on the acuity chart. As luminance is reduced, visual acuity decreases and is increasingly facilitated by the retinal rods. Figure 2-2 shows the change in visual acuity across a wide range of luminances. Note that both scales are logarithmic.

Reducing letter contrast has a similar effect on visual acuity. The measurement of visual acuity using low-contrast letter charts is becoming widespread in clinical research and practice, particularly in patients with corneal disease and those who have undergone refractive surgery. This is discussed in Chapter 11.

## VISUAL ACUITY AND AGE

We are not born with 20/20 vision, but rather visual acuity at birth is on the order of 20/200 and improves rapidly with age in the normal developing eye. Clearly, measurement of visual acuity in the infant requires special testing techniques, discussed later in this chapter. Electrophysiological data suggest that visual acuity may approach adult levels by the age of 6 months (Fig. 2-3). Similarly, visual acuity declines with age, even in a healthy eye. Elliott et al.[8] pooled data from a number of sources and found that visual acuity decreased by approximately one line on the letter chart across the third and sixth decades of life (Fig. 2-4).

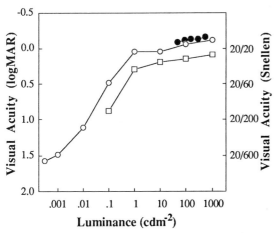

**FIGURE 2–2** Visual acuity as a function of luminance. Note that the visual acuity scale is inverted. The closed circles are replotted from Sheedy et al.[7] The open circles and squares are the author's unpublished data for a young normal subject and a retinitis pigmentosa patient, respectively.

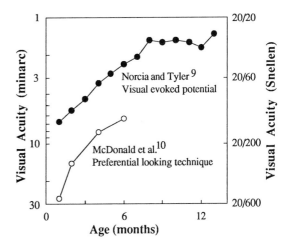

**FIGURE 2–3** The development of visual acuity in infants. Data are shown for both electrophysiological and behavioral methods.

# Units of Measurement

## SNELLEN NOTATION

In clinical practice, visual acuity is usually expressed as a fraction where the numerator represents the test distance in meters or feet and the denominator represents the letter size. Letter size is defined as the distance at which the overall letter height subtends 5 minutes of arc. Because the typical letters on a chart have a stroke width one-fifth their height, this definition could be modified to the distance at which the limb of the letter subtends 1 minute of arc (Fig. 2-5). Hence, a measured visual acuity of 20/20 (6/6) means that the test was conducted at 20 feet (6 meters) and that the limbs of the smallest letters read subtend 1 minute of arc at 20 feet (6 me-

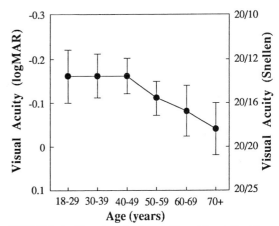

**FIGURE 2–4** Visual acuity in adulthood (replotted from Elliott et al.[8]). Note that the visual acuity scale is inverted. Vertical bars represent ±1 standard deviation.

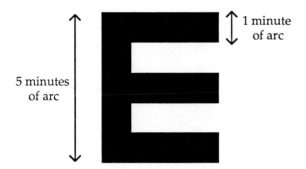

5 minutes of arc

1 minute of arc

**FIGURE 2–5**   A typical Snellen letter. The height of the letter is defined by the distance at which it subtends 5 minutes of arc (or the limbs subtend 1 minute of arc).

ters), which in this case is also the test distance. Similarly, a visual acuity of 20/50 (6/15) means that the test was conducted at 20 feet (6 meters) and the limbs of the smallest letters read subtend 1 minute of arc at 50 feet (15 meters), but at 20 feet subtend 2.5 minutes of arc.

The physical height of a given letter can be converted into a visual angle, and vice versa, by simple trigonometry. For a 6-meter letter, subtending 5 minutes of arc (or 0.083°) at 6 meters, the height of the letter is given by 6 meters × (tan 0.083), which equals 8.75 mm. Similarly, the width of each limb or the stroke width would be 1.75 mm.

A best-corrected visual acuity of 20/200 in the better eye, which happens to be the criterion for legal blindness, means that the patient can read 200-foot letters only at a test distance of 20 feet. If placed at 200 feet, the limbs of these letters would subtend 1 minute of arc. At 20 feet, however, they subtend 10 minutes of arc, and the letter height is 87.5 mm.

## PARTIAL CREDIT

Frequently a patient reads all of the letters on a given line and then a subset of the letters on the next line. There is an accepted convention for recording this scenario using superscripts such as +2, −1, +3, etc. A patient, for example, who reads all of the letters on the 25-foot line and one letter on the following line at a test distance of 20 feet would be assigned a Snellen visual acuity of 20/25[+1]. Similarly, a patient who reads all but one letter on the 40-foot line at 20 feet would be assigned an acuity of 20/40[−1].

## M UNITS

Letter size is sometimes specified in *M units*. This merely represents the denominator of the

Snellen fraction specified in meters. Hence a 6 M letter is the same as a 20-foot letter (because 20 feet approximates 6 meters) and is 8.75 mm tall (subtending 5 minutes of arc at 6 meters). The most common use of this notation is in the measurement of near visual acuity; many near vision charts specify the size of the letters in M units. Clinicians often record near visual acuity as 0.4/0.4, which implies that at 40 cm (0.4 m), the patient could read 0.4 M print. Given that this Snellen fraction is equal to one, this is equivalent to a distance visual acuity of 20/20.

## DECIMAL ACUITY

The Snellen fraction may be converted to a *decimal acuity*. Decimal acuity is calculated by simply converting the Snellen fraction into a decimal, that is, by dividing the test distance by the letter size. A Snellen acuity of 20/40 thus corresponds to a decimal acuity of 0.5 (Table 2–1). This notation has the advantage that a higher number represents better vision. It is popular in Europe.

## MINIMUM ANGLE OF RESOLUTION (MAR)

We have already discovered that the denominator in the Snellen fraction is a measure of the angular subtense of the letter size and its stroke width. We can thus specify visual acuity in terms of the *minimum angle of resolution* (MAR). This is calculated by dividing the letter size (as specified in the Snellen fraction) by the test distance. A Snellen acuity of 20/40 thus corresponds to an MAR of 2 minutes of arc (Table 2–1). The MAR is also the reciprocal of the decimal acuity. Notice that the MAR is half the limit of resolution predicted by Rayleigh's criterion, which corresponds to two stroke widths.

### logMAR

A derivative of the minimum angle of resolution is the *logarithm of the minimum angle of resolution* (logMAR). Several authors have advocated that acuity charts should contain lines of letters that follow a logarithmic (or geometric) size progression. Furthermore, Westheimer[11] demonstrated that such a logarithmic scale was most appropriate in the specification of visual acuity. The use of logMAR has been popularized by Ian Bailey, codeveloper of the Bailey-Lovie chart.[12] A Snellen acuity of 20/40 thus corresponds to a

| | | | | | Cycles per |
|---|---|---|---|---|---|
| Snellen | Decimal | MAR* | logMAR† | VAR‡ | Degree |
| 20/10 | 2 | 0.5 | −0.3 | 115 | 60 |
| 20/12 | 1.67 | 0.6 | −0.2 | 110 | 50 |
| 20/16 | 1.25 | 0.8 | −0.1 | 105 | 38 |
| 20/20 | 1 | 1 | 0 | 100 | 30 |
| 20/25 | 0.8 | 1.25 | 0.1 | 95 | 24 |
| 20/30 | 0.67 | 1.5 | 0.2 | 90 | 20 |
| 20/40 | 0.5 | 2 | 0.3 | 85 | 15 |
| 20/50 | 0.4 | 2.5 | 0.4 | 80 | 12 |
| 20/60 | 0.33 | 3 | 0.5 | 75 | 10 |
| 20/80 | 0.25 | 4 | 0.6 | 70 | 7.5 |
| 20/100 | 0.2 | 5 | 0.7 | 65 | 6 |
| 20/200 | 0.1 | 10 | 1.0 | 50 | 3 |
| 20/400 | 0.05 | 20 | 1.3 | 35 | 1.5 |

**TABLE 2–1** Relationship Between Different Visual Acuity Notations

*MAR, minimum angle of resolution.
†logMAR, logarithm of the minimum angle of resolution.
‡VAR, visual acuity rating.

logMAR of 0.3 ($=\log_{10} 2$). Equal steps on a logarithmic scale represent a constant geometric progression (Table 2-1). By default, the smaller lines of letters on most letter charts have a size progression that is close to equal logarithmic steps.

## GRATINGS AND CYCLES PER DEGREE

Some 30 years ago visual scientists recognized the benefits of using gratings, series of light and dark stripes with a sinusoidal luminance profile, in studying vision.[13, 14] Although such stimuli are widely used for testing contrast sensitivity (see Chapter 11), they are rarely employed for visual acuity measurement in adults. They have, however, found a niche for the testing of infants. The size of the grating and thus the visual acuity of the patient are specified in cycles per degree. A 30 cycle per degree grating would have 60 alternating light and dark stripes per degree of visual angle. The ability to see such a grating would, therefore, correspond to a minimum angle of resolution of 1 minute of arc (the width of one stripe) and a Snellen fraction of 20/20 (Table 2-1).

## VISUAL EFFICIENCY SCALES

Some authors have attempted to convert visual acuity values into *visual efficiency* scores to reflect, for example, an individual's visual capacity for employment. The most widely used is the *Snell-Sterling scale*,[15, 16] where 20/20 corresponds to 100% efficiency, 20/100 represents 50%, and 20/200 equates to 20%. Bailey[17] recognized that the Snell-Sterling scale was logarithmic over a wide range but had some inadequacies. He proposed an alternative which he terms *visual acuity rating* (VAR). VAR values may be calculated from logMAR by the formula:

$$VAR = 100 - (50 \times logMAR)$$

or from the denominator of a Snellen fraction of the form 20/d by the formula:

$$VAR = 165 - (50 \times \log d)$$

On this scale a VAR of 100 represents a visual acuity of 20/20, a VAR of 50 is 20/200, and a VAR of 0 represents 20/2000. This scale is particularly easy to use in conjunction with the Bailey-Lovie chart, where one line corresponds to five points and one letter is worth one point (Table 2-1).

## NOTATIONS FOR POOR VISION

Some patients are unable to read even the largest letters on the chart. In this case the clinician can hold up a number of fingers at a given distance and ask the patient "How many fingers am I holding up?" If the patient can perform this task, then visual acuity is recorded as "count fingers." The abbreviation CF@50 cm indicates that the patient could count fingers at 50 cm. A criticism of this technique is that fingers come in various sizes and colors. A preferable approach is to move the patient closer to the letter chart or the letter chart closer to the patient until he or she can read the largest letter. The visual acuity can then be recorded using the conventional Snellen notation, such as 3/400 or 8/200.

For patients unable to make any meaningful spatial discriminations, the clinician can wave his or her hand in front of the eye being tested. An ability to perform this test is signified as "hand motion" vision or HM. If the patient is unable to see a moving hand, a bright light can be shone into his or her eye. If he or she is aware of the light, the level of vision is "light perception" or LP. If the patient has no sense of the presence of the light, his or her vision is described as "no light perception" or NLP.

## Clinical Measurement Procedure

Visual acuity should be measured under controlled and constant testing conditions. The test distance should be measured and is usually constrained by the patient being seated in the examination room chair. In any case, a few inches backward and forward does not matter when the test distance is 20 feet.

Visual acuity measurements are usually made monocularly, particularly at the beginning of the eye examination, and thus the fellow eye must be occluded. Occlusion is not mandatory when measuring the better eye in a patient who has severely decreased vision in the fellow eye or an artificial fellow eye. Binocular measurement of visual acuity can be made following monocular measurement. Binocular visual acuity may be a line or so better than the monocular measures when the monocular values are equal. A specified level of binocular visual acuity (or visual acuity in the better eye) is required for driving licensure and for entry into some professions.

A specially purchased occluder is best for covering a patient's eye for monocular testing. Handing the occluder to the patient obviates the need for the examiner to keep his or her arm extended and still for the duration of the measurement and increases the patient's sense of participation. Some patients need to be told to keep both eyes open, particularly the eye being tested.

The eye care practitioner or visual acuity technician usually has a crude idea of the patient's visual acuity from his or her history or previous examination. Where possible, the patient is asked to read a line of letters slightly larger than the examiner's initial estimate. Starting at very large letters can waste valuable examination time and is not recommended. The task of reading the chart is familiar to most patients and little instruction is needed. It is important, however, to impose a consistent criterion for allowing the patient to stop reading letters. Many older patients, for example, stop after reading the 30-foot line but when encouraged read all of the 20-foot letters. Patients should be encouraged to "try the next line" and to "guess if not sure." In most cases, the patient should not be forced to keep guessing when he or she is clearly below threshold, as this can be both annoying and frustrating to the patient. A good time to stop is when the patient has missed at least half of the letters on a given line.

It can be illuminating to observe the patient while he or she is reading the chart. This becomes easier once the examiner has memorized all of the letters on the visual acuity chart. Some patients may, for example, "squint" or narrow their eyes, indicating the potential for uncorrected refractive error. Low vision patients frequently adopt unique head postures in an attempt to place the test chart's image on the best functioning part of their retina.

Finally, it is not a good tactic to show the patient too many letters that he or she cannot read. In the interest of flexibility, many projected and back-lit visual acuity charts contain some very small letters, and patients with better than 20/20 vision may still ask whether or not they ought to be able to read them.

## Letter Chart Designs

Visual acuity is usually measured with upper-case or capital letters of varying size. The typical letter chart contains 10 lines of letters or *optotypes* which decrease in size from the top to the bottom. Letters have the advantage over other symbols in that they are familiar to the patient and the response is easily verbalized. Within a given line, the thickness of the limbs, or *stroke width,* and the space between the letters is constant. Furthermore, the letters are drawn such that the aspect ratio of the letters is constant. The letters in Figure 2–6 all have an aspect ratio of 5:4. This notation indicates that the height is 5× the stroke width and the breadth is 4× the stroke width. Letters with an aspect ratio of 5:5 are also common, having both a height and breadth equal to 5 stroke widths.

The original letter charts were printed on white cardboard, since superseded by white plastic. These charts were illuminated by the con-

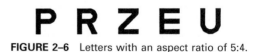

**FIGURE 2–6**  Letters with an aspect ratio of 5:4.

sulting room lights or by supplementary fixtures, and thus standardization was difficult. These have been largely replaced by rear-illuminated and projected charts. Rear-illuminated charts are popular in Europe and are constructed from opaque or translucent white plastic. Projected charts are the norm in North America.

Technological advances have resulted in the availability of computer-controlled video-based acuity charts. These have all the advantages of projected charts but also facilitate an endless supply of letter strings so that the patient has to rely on his or her vision rather than memory.

Visual acuity is typically measured at a test distance of 20 feet or 6 meters, mainly for historical reasons; it is likely that Snellen's room was this length. Although other test distances have been advocated, including 4 meters with a correction of $-0.25$ D for optical infinity, 20 feet remains one of the constants that we hold dear. Modern architecture and economies of space rarely permit the luxury of a 20-foot-long examination room. The usual solution is to use a mirror, preferably large and front-silvered, with the letter chart mounted or projected above the patient's head. Letters thus need to be reversed so that they appear vertical to the patient in the mirror.

## BAILEY-LOVIE logMAR CHARTS

The major advance in the design of letter charts has been the introduction of the Bailey-Lovie chart.[12] The chart has many elegant design features with the goal of standardizing the visual acuity measurement at each size level. Bailey and Lovie adopted ten 5:4 aspect ratio letters—DEFHNPRUVZ—which had been shown previously to have relatively equal legibility.[18] The chart has a constant number of letters, namely five, on every line and has a characteristic V shape (Fig. 2-7). This is in contrast to more widely used charts which have one 200-foot letter and up to ten 20-foot letters.

The letter size progression is constant on the Bailey-Lovie chart and geometric, such that the letters decrease in size by a factor of $\sqrt[10]{10}$, which equals 1.2589 and approximates a ratio of 5:4. This progression may also be expressed as 0.1 $\log_{10}$ units, and the charts are frequently referred to as "logMAR charts" because of this constant logarithmic size progression. This choice of progression means that a 10-line progression down the chart corresponds to a $10\times$ reduction (or 1 $\log_{10}$ unit), such as from 200 feet to 20 feet. Similarly, a three-line change corresponds to a $2\times$ reduction, a five-line change approximates a

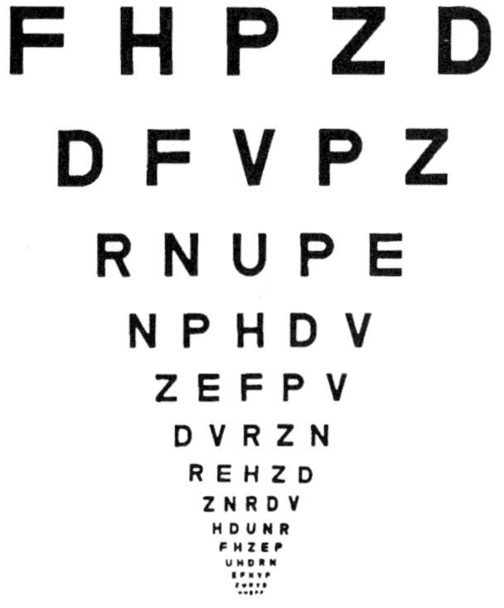

**FIGURE 2–7** Bailey-Lovie Letter Chart.

$3\times$ reduction, and a seven-line change corresponds to a $5\times$ reduction. In order to equalize any contour interaction effects,[19] the spacing between letters on a given line is also constant, being equal to the letter width. The spacing between two adjacent lines is equal to the height of the letters on the lower line and therefore equal to the width of the letters on the upper line.

The design principles inherent in the Bailey-Lovie chart have spawned several derivatives, for example, the ETDRS chart, which uses the 10 equally legible 5:5 aspect ratio Sloan letters (CDHKNORSVZ).[20] Another chart is the Waterloo chart, which has the distinction of having the letters, which are more closely spaced, decrease in size from left to right, and also has contour interaction bars to equalize crowding effects within a given line.[21] The Waterloo chart has also been translated into Chinese. Regan and Neima[22] have developed logMAR charts that have eight letters per line and are available in a range of contrasts. Taylor[23] introduced an illiterate E version of the Bailey-Lovie chart, a chart used successfully with aborigines in Australia.

## Charts for Pediatric and Special Populations

Pediatric and special populations require special charts and testing techniques.[24, 25] These rely on a child being asked either to describe the orientation of a symbol, to match a letter or shape to a reference, or merely to track or preferentially fixate a target.

## LANDOLT C's AND TUMBLING E's

*Landolt C* charts consist of a series of C's with an aspect ratio of 5:5 in four or eight orientations. The gap in the C is equal to the stroke width (one fifth of the letter size). One drawback of the Landolt C chart is that it is easy for the clinician, or indeed the patient, to lose track of where he or she is on the chart, particularly when used in conjunction with a mirror. Furthermore, uncorrected astigmatism can render some orientations less visible than others, although the astute clinician would use this information to his or her advantage.

The tumbling E test employs a series of E's with an aspect ratio of 5:5 in four orientations. This test is useful for both young children and patients unfamiliar with Arabic letters. The E's may be arranged in a letter chart format or in a hand-held flip chart.

Some tests resemble conventional letter charts but are made more friendly to the child by the inclusion of a matching card. Rather than naming the letter, the child merely matches each letter on the chart with the correct one on the card. Examples of these tests include the *Glasgow Acuity Cards*,[26] the *STYCAR test*, the *Sheridan-Gardner test*, and the *HOTV chart*. (See Fern and Manny[24] for an extensive list.)

## LETTER AND SYMBOL TESTS

An alternative to letters is symbols or objects that are familiar to children. Charts that use this approach include the *Lighthouse Chart* (Lighthouse, NY) and *LEA Symbols* (Precision Vision), formerly known as the LH test.[27] These tests are more fun for children. Examples are shown in Figure 2–8.

## POINTING TESTS

Some tests require the child to compare two shapes or pictures and point at the one that contains a particular feature. *The Broken Wheel test*[28] depicts two cars, one of which has complete wheels, the other incomplete wheels (which resemble Landolt C's). The *Bailey-Hall Cereal Test* consists of pairs of cards, one of which depicts a Cheerio and the other a square. The child may be rewarded for a correct response by being given a piece of Cheerio cereal. This is an effective way of maintaining a child's interest in any acuity test.

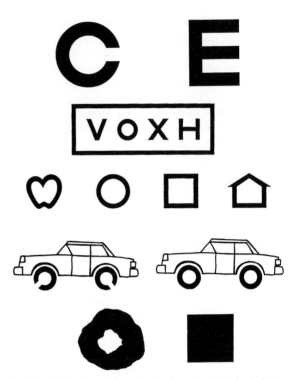

**FIGURE 2–8** Examples of visual acuity tests for infants and toddlers. From top to bottom: Landolt C and Tumbling E; Glasgow Acuity Cards; Lea Symbols; Broken Wheel Test; Bailey-Hall Cereal Test.

## PREFERENTIAL LOOKING TESTS

Infants are unable to respond even by pointing, so other strategies must be used. Emerging as the most accepted clinically are tests that use the *preferential looking* technique, which relies on infants' preference to fixate patterns over plain stimuli.[10] In the Acuity Card Procedure (ACP), an adult observer shows the infant a series of cards that contain gratings of various spatial frequencies. The grating is printed on one half of the card only, with the remainder being a uniform gray. The observer watches the eye movement patterns and behavior of the infant from behind the card and judges whether the infant fixates the grating or the blank area, or shows no preference, for each card in the series. Visual acuity is estimated from the highest spatial frequency that the infant is judged to see. The cards can be presented in an intact part of the visual field for visually impaired infants or rotated so that the stripes are horizontal for infants with nystagmus in order to obtain optimal visual acuity.

## ELECTROPHYSIOLOGICAL TESTS

In some infants and children the level of development or cooperation precludes testing using any of the aforementioned tests. Visual evoked potentials (VEP) to grating or checkerboard stimuli can be measured by attaching surface electrodes to the back of the child's head. Clinically viable techniques, notably the sweep VEP method, have been developed by Norcia and Tyler[9] and others. High-contrast gratings are presented on a screen and flickered in counterphase for a 10-second period, during which the spatial frequency of the grating increases. The amplitude of the VEP decreases with increasing spatial frequency and a visual acuity value is computed by extrapolation.

## WHEN ALL ELSE FAILS

Very crude estimates of visual abilities can be obtained by observing an infant's behavior. A child's extreme resistance to having his or her right eye occluded can indicate poorer vision in the left eye. An infant's ability to fixate can also give useful information. The clinician should observe whether the infant is fixating centrally or eccentrically. Is the fixation steady and maintained, and can the child track a moving target? These measures are purely qualitative but, in some cases, may be all the clinician can observe. In this instance, the clinician would record "fix and follow" (F&F) for each eye in the patient's chart.

# Contour Interaction and Crowding

The *crowding* phenomenon results in difficulty reading letters on a line of an acuity chart when single letters of the same size can be readily discriminated. Also termed *contour interaction*,[19] it is most commonly seen in strabismic amblyopia and macular disease. This can manifest itself when using a letter chart, wherein the patient is able to correctly identify the end letters on each line. Some tests, such as the HOTV chart, the Waterloo chart,[21] and the Glasgow Acuity Cards,[26] attempt to control this effect by having surrounding contours or bars at the end of each line.

Care must be taken in comparing visual acuity values from different charts. In particular, low vision and multihandicapped patients may show substantially better visual acuity for gratings or single letters than for letters on a closely spaced chart.[25, 29]

# Near Visual Acuity

An important component of any optometric examination is an evaluation of the patient's near vision. This serves to determine whether his or her near vision is adequate for everyday needs. This usually entails establishing that he or she is able to comfortably read the smallest print likely to be encountered at his or her habitual working distance. In patients of all ages, near visual acuity is typically measured at 40 cm. Failure to read newsprint at this distance is likely to drive the clinician to modify the patient's near eyeglass prescription.

## SPECIFICATION OF PRINT SIZE

Print size for near vision testing may be specified in a number of ways. The most logical approach is to adopt the same system as for distance charts, namely M units. A letter that subtends 5 minutes of arc at 1 meter would thus be specified as 1 M in size. This allows near visual acuity to be specified in exactly the same fashion as a distance measurement and thus facilitates easy comparison.

M units may be used for lower-case letters as well as upper-case. Print size for lower-case letters is specified by the height of a lower-case "x," often referred to as the *x-height*. A 1 M letter "x" would be 1.45 mm high (tan 0.083 × 1 meter). By measuring the height of this letter "x" in millimeters, one could calculate its size in M units by multiplying by tan 0.083 ($1.45 \times 10^{-3}$) and dividing by 1000. The page could then be moved to a point where the patient could just read the prose and the distance measured in meters. The resultant Snellen fraction should be comparable to the distance visual acuity.

Another common specification of print size is *point size,* or *N units.* These are used by printers and anyone who uses a computer with an up-to-date word processing program. A problem with using this notation is that letter height varies with the font such that Helvetica letters are taller than Times. Because a large proportion of material is printed in Times print, it is useful to remember that lower-case 8-point print (or N8) is equivalent to 1 M. This 8 times conversion factor from N to M notation holds for all print sizes.

Two other approaches are worth mentioning but are not recommended. The first is the *Jaeger* or J system. The size progression is haphazard—for example, J1 print is not half the size of J2 print—so no easy conversion factor exists. It is probably sufficient to remember that J2 is equivalent to N5. The second irrational approach is *reduced Snellen* notation. This propagates the use of such phrases as "20/20 equivalent at near" but assumes a fixed viewing distance (usually 14 inches/35 cm). The system becomes meaningless when confronted with a patient with a +5.00 reading addition or a tall patient who enjoys reading at 3 feet. In summary, it should be more intuitive, meaningful, and rational to use a Snellen fraction that contains the actual viewing distance and the actual print size.

## CHARTS FOR NEAR TESTING

As with distance visual acuity, a wide range of test types may be employed for measuring near visual acuity. Some charts are merely minified versions of distance charts, containing upper-case letters in a similar configuration. Preferable are charts made up of lower-case text such as shown in Figure 2–9. The advantage of these charts is that they contain a font, in this case Times Roman (often abbreviated to Times), that is familiar to the patient, resembling text in books and newspapers. The design considerations of these near charts are no different from those for distance charts in that they contain a broad range of sizes, a logical size progression, and appropriate specification of print size.

One near chart worthy of mention is the *Bailey-Lovie Word Reading Chart.*[30] As one might expect, the chart follows the same design principles as its distance cousin but contains unrelated words, as opposed to continuous text, in lower-case Times Roman print (Fig. 2–9). The charts, more than 20 of which are available, contain print sizes ranging from 0.25 M (2 point) to 10 M (80 point), making them useful for both normal- and low-vision patients. For the 11 smallest sizes (0.25 M to 2.5 M) there are six words per row, two four-letter words, two seven-letter words, and two ten-letter words.

Near charts are also available that are facsimiles of materials that patients may encounter at work or leisure. These include sheet music, stock market reports, and telephone books. These serve mainly to convince the patient that he or she will be able to function with the new or existing spectacle prescription. Rather than storing a wide range of materials in the examination room, the patient can be asked to bring samples. Alternatively, given the accessibility of desktop publishing, any clinician can easily produce his or her own personalized near vision test materials.

With appropriate measurement and specification of print size, there should be good agreement between measurements taken using different targets. One exception is patients with macular disease, for whom visual acuity measurements made with widely separated upper-case letters may be substantially better than those taken using words or text.[29] This is probably another manifestation of the contour interaction effects seen in amblyopia.[19] Care should be taken,

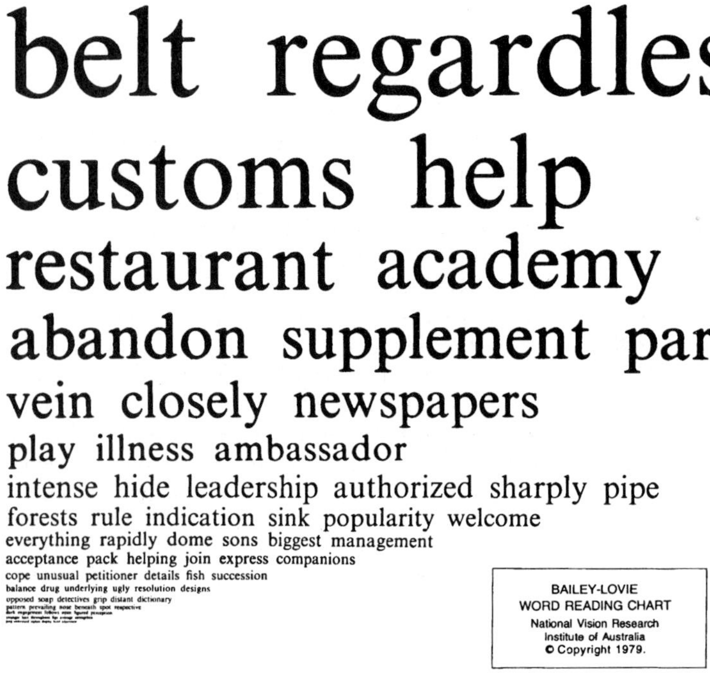
belt regardless
customs help
restaurant academy
abandon supplement park
vein closely newspapers
play illness ambassador
intense hide leadership authorized sharply pipe
forests rule indication sink popularity welcome
everything rapidly dome sons biggest management
acceptance pack helping join express companions
cope unusual petitioner details fish succession
balance drug underlying ugly resolution designs
opposed soap detectives grip distant dictionary
pattern prevailing nose beneath spot respective
BAILEY-LOVIE
WORD READING CHART
National Vision Research
Institute of Australia
© Copyright 1979.

**FIGURE 2–9** Bailey-Lovie Word Reading Chart.

therefore, to ensure that the test type reflects the task that the patient is most interested in performing at near distance; in most cases, this means reading newspaper print.

# Reduced Visual Acuity: What Could It Mean?

. . . . . . . . . . . . . . . . . . . . . . . .

So, the patient's visual acuity is somewhat below par. What could be causing this reduction? The first obvious candidate is refractive error. In the case of a teenager with reduced distance visual acuity, the first thought should be myopia! A good rule of thumb is that one line of visual acuity loss corresponds to $-0.25$ diopter of myopia (Table 2-2). In younger patients, visual acuities of 20/15 are common, and patient's presenting with 20/20 may still have low levels of uncorrected myopia. Hyperopia or presbyopia rarely manifests as a reduction in visual acuity. The patient, regardless of age, is more likely to complain of discomfort, eyestrain, asthenopia, or headaches associated with near work.

Astigmatism tends to have a much less predictable effect on visual acuity. A patient with 2.00 diopters of simple with-the-rule astigmatism (Plano $= -2.00$ DC $\times$ 180) may still present with an uncorrected visual acuity of 20/20, particularly if the patient reduces the retinal blur by narrowing the eyes or squinting. Conversely, oblique astigmatism may have a more pronounced effect on visual acuity. Another rule of thumb is that one line of visual acuity loss corresponds to 0.50 diopter of astigmatism (Table 2-2).

## PINHOLE ACUITY TESTING

A test that is elegant in its simplicity is the pinhole test. In uncorrected refractive error, reducing the effective pupil size by placing a pinhole in front of the eye reduces the size of the blur circle on the retina and hence improves visual acuity. The pinhole test enables the clinician to determine whether the reduced visual acuity is due to refractive error or to more serious ocular pathology. If the pinhole improves visual acuity, then the cause is refractive error. Theoretically, that eye can be refracted to the same acuity level as that achieved through the pinhole. No improvement suggests a problem with the ocular media, retina, or optic nerve.

## DIAGNOSTIC CONTACT LENS ACUITY TESTING

The pinhole test does not apply when visual acuity is reduced by irregularities in the refracting surfaces of the eye, principally the cornea. Common examples include keratoconus, in which the cornea assumes a conelike shape, and corneal lacerations, which induce surface irregularities. The clinician can identify that corneal irregular astigmatism is the cause of the reduced vision by placing a rigid contact lens on the eye. For an irregular cornea, the tears cancel out the irregularities, giving a spherical refracting surface, and visual acuity should improve to near-normal levels with appropriate over-refraction. A topical anesthetic is a good idea for this procedure.

## OCULAR DISEASE

When visual acuity appears to be reduced from ocular disease, it is wise to first consider the obvious and to eliminate possibilities in a logical fashion. The clarity of the media can be assessed quickly by observing the light reflex with a retinoscope or ophthalmoscope. A bright orange reflex is a sign that the media are clear. Likewise, the view into the eye with a direct ophthalmoscope through an undilated pupil should approximate the patient's view out through the same optical system.

If the ocular media are clear, attention can be directed to retinal and neural problems. Again, common diagnoses should be considered first. In an elderly population, *age-related maculopathy* accounts for over half of all cases of vision loss.[31, 32] The vast remainder of incident cases in the elderly are attributable to *vascular problems* such as venous occlusion associated with hypertension or diabetes. For patients in the 20 to 50 years age range, *optic neuritis* should be considered.

| TABLE 2–2  Visual Acuity as a Function of Spherical and Cylindrical Blur | | |
|---|---|---|
| **Visual Acuity** | **Spherical Blur** | **Cylindrical Blur** |
| 20/15 | — | — |
| 20/20 | 0.25 | 0.50 |
| 20/25 | 0.50 | 1.00 |
| 20/30 | 0.75 | 1.50 |
| 20/40 | 1.00 | 2.00 |
| 20/50 | 1.25 | 2.50 |
| 20/60 | 1.50 | 3.00 |
| 20/80 | 1.75 | 3.50 |
| 20/100 | 2.00 | 4.00 |

In children, a primary concern is *amblyopia,* or "lazy eye." This is classically defined as reduced vision in the presence of a full optical correction and the absence of ocular pathology. Amblyopia is usually monocular and associated with *strabismus,* an eye turn, or *anisometropia,* unequal refractive error in the two eyes.

Occasionally a child or adult presents with reduced visual acuity that has no apparent cause. It is possible that the patient may be *malingering.* This presentation is also referred to as *hysterical amblyopia* and may be the manifestation of emotional problems. In the case of a child, the parents should be questioned about the home and school situations. The malingerer can be exposed by a variety of methods. An easy method is to halve the viewing distance and measure visual acuity. The non-malingerer reads letters that are half as big, but the malingerer may insist that he or she can still read no further down the chart. Other techniques that can expose a malingerer claiming poor acuity in one eye include the use of polaroid glasses and test targets, fogging the better eye in the phoropter, and stereopsis testing (good stereopsis implies two good eyes).[33]

## Visual Acuity Standards

. . . . . . . . . . . . . . . . . . . . . . . . . . . . . .

The measurement of visual acuity has many implications. The most common is obtaining and retaining a driver's license. The visual acuity standard in most states is 20/40 in at least one eye, although patients with poorer vision may in special circumstances drive, for example with the aid of an eyeglass-mounted telescope.[34]

Many professions, such as police and firefighters, require a certain level of vision in order to gain entry.[35] These standards typically require a binocular uncorrected visual acuity of 20/40 or better. Applicants may undergo refractive surgery in order to meet these standards.[36]

Finally, in the United States the criterion for legal blindness is "20/200 in the better eye with best correction." In the United States and other western countries, around 0.2% of the population fall into this classification. The majority of the legally blind population are over the age of 65 but have some useful vision. These patients can frequently read when given the appropriate low vision aids such as magnifiers.

## Summary

. . . . . . . . . . . . . . . . . . . . . . . . . . . . . .

Visual acuity measurement is usually a quick and familiar test that can provide valuable information to the clinician. Good visual acuity does not, of course, guarantee an intact and healthy visual system, as the tests and techniques described in subsequent chapters demonstrate. Nonetheless, as a clinician I place a great deal of emphasis on the patient's presenting visual acuities when finalizing my management plan. This is, after all, information taken before the patient has been tired and worn out by our barrage of tests and observations.

### ACKNOWLEDGMENTS
Much of the material presented here was absorbed during the years in which I have worked with Ian Bailey at UC Berkeley. I wish to thank Ruth Manny and Deborah Orel-Bixler for their comments on testing pediatric and special populations.

## References

. . . . . . . . . . . . . . . . . . . . . . . . . . . . . .

1. Charman WN: The retinal image in the human eye. *In* Osborne N, Chader G (eds): Progress in Retinal Research, Vol 2. Oxford: Pergamon, 1983, pp 671–713.
2. Applegate RA: Acuities through annular and central pupils after radial keratotomy. Optom Vis Sci 1991; 68:584–590.
3. Zadnik K: Keratoconus. *In* Bennett ES, Weissman B (eds): Clinical Contact Lens Practice. Philadelphia: JB Lippincott, 1991.
4. Whittaker SG, Budd J, Cummings RW: Eccentric fixation with macular scotoma. Invest Ophthalmol Vis Sci 1988; 29:268–277.
5. Anderson SJ, Mullen KT, Hess RF: Human peripheral spatial resolution for achromatic and chromatic stimuli: Limits imposed by optical and retinal factors. J Physiol 1991; 442:47–64.
6. Curcio CA, Sloan KR, Kalina RE, Hendrickson AE: Human photoreceptor topography. J Comp Neurol 1990; 292:497–523.
7. Sheedy JE, Bailey IL, Raasch TW: Visual acuity and chart luminance. Am J Optom Physiol Opt 1984; 61:595–600.
8. Elliott DB, Yang KCH, Whitaker D: Physiological changes in logMAR visual acuity throughout adulthood: Seeing beyond 6/6. Optom Vis Sci 1991; 72:186–191.
9. Norcia AM, Tyler CW: Spatial frequency sweep VEP: Visual acuity during the first year of life. Vision Res 1985; 25:1399–1408.
10. McDonald MA, Dobson V, Sebris SL, et al.: The acuity card procedure: A rapid test of infant acuity. Invest Ophthalmol Vis Sci 1985; 26:1158–1162.
11. Westheimer G: Scaling of visual acuity measurements. Arch Ophthalmol 1979; 97:327–330.
12. Bailey IL, Lovie JE: New design principles for visual acuity letter charts. Am J Optom Physiol Opt 1976; 53:740–745.
13. Campbell FW, Green DG: Optical and retinal factors affecting visual resolution. J Physiol 1965; 181:576–593.
14. Campbell FW, Robson JG: Application of Fourier analysis to the visibility of gratings. J Physiol 1968; 197:551–566.
15. Snell AC, Sterling S: The percentage evaluation of macular vision. Arch Ophthalmol 1925; 54:443–461.
16. American Medical Association: Council on Industrial Health: Special report: Estimation of loss of visual efficiency. Arch Ophthalmol 1955; 54:462–468.

17. Bailey IL: Measurement of visual acuity—towards standardization. *In* Vision Science Symposium: A tribute to Gordon G. Heath. Bloomington: Indiana University, 1988.

18. Bennett AG: Ophthalmic test types. A review of previous work and discussions on some controversial questions. Br J Physiol Opt 1965; 22:238-271.

19. Flom MC, Heath G, Takahashi E: Contour interaction and visual resolution: Contralateral effects. Science 1963; 142:979-980.

20. Ferris FL III, Kassoff A, Bresnick GH, Bailey I: New visual acuity charts for clinical research. Am J Ophthalmol 1982; 94:91-96.

21. Strong G, Woo GC: A distance visual acuity chart incorporating some new design principles. Arch Ophthalmol 1985; 103:44-46.

22. Regan D, Neima D: Low-contrast letter charts as a test of visual function. Ophthalmology 1983; 90:1192-1200.

23. Taylor HR: Applying new design principles to the construction of an illiterate E chart. Am J Optom Physiol Opt 1978; 55:348-351.

24. Fern K, Manny RE: Visual acuity of the preschool child: A review. Am J Optom Physiol Opt 1986; 63:319-345.

25. Haegerstrom-Portnoy G: New procedures for evaluating vision functions of special populations. Optom Vis Sci 1993; 70:306-314.

26. McGraw PV, Winn B: Glasgow Acuity Cards: a new test for the measurement of letter acuity in children. Ophthal Physiol Opt 1993; 13:400-404.

27. Hyvarinen L, Nasanen R, Laurinen P: New visual acuity test for pre-school children. Acta Ophthalmol 1980; 58:507-511.

28. Richman JE, Petito GT, Cron MT: Broken wheel acuity test: A new and valid test for preschool and exceptional children. J Am Optom Assoc 1984; 55:561-565.

29. Bullimore MA, Bailey IL, Wacker RT: Face recognition in age-related maculopathy. Invest Ophthalmol Vis Sci 1991; 32:2020-2029.

30. Bailey IL, Lovie JE: The design and use of a new near-vision chart. Am J Optom Physiol Opt 1980; 57:378-387.

31. Grey RHB, Burns-Cox CJ, Hughes A: Blind and partial sight registration in Avon. Br J Ophthalmol 1989; 73:88-94.

32. Sommer A, Tielsch JM, Katz J, et al.: Racial differences in the cause-specific prevalence of blindness in east Baltimore. N Engl J Med 1991; 325:1412-1417.

33. Keltner JL, May WN, Johnson CA, Post RB: The California syndrome. Functional visual complaints with potential economic impact. Ophthalmology 1985; 92:427-435.

34. Bailey IL: Bioptic telescopes. Arch Ophthalmol 1985; 103:13-14.

35. Sheedy JE, Keller JT, Pitts D, et al.: Recommended vision standards for police officers. J Am Optom Assoc 1983; 54:925-930.

36. Bullimore MA, Sheedy JE, Owen D, and the Refractive Surgery Study Group: Diurnal visual changes in radial keratotomy: Implications for visual standards. Optom Vis Sci 1994; 71:516-521.

*Nina E. Friedman, OD, MS*

3

# The Pupil

Although pupil testing is considered a necessary part of every eye examination, it is probably the least understood and most underutilized part of the optometric test battery. Performed with care, the pupil examination can be of immense value in providing a gross assessment of visual function, aiding in the differential diagnosis of acuity loss, testing the patency of the visual system behind a cataract, and detecting neoplasm, inflammation, and systemic disease. It takes minutes to perform and requires only a transilluminator and an attentive clinician.

The key to effective pupil testing lies in its physical *and* intellectual integration into the examiner's test battery. Too often the pupil examination goes by like a familiar car trip: You can't remember it when it is over, but you assume that if something important had happened you would have noticed. Unfortunately, anisocoria and afferent pupillary defects can be subtle, and detection requires the examiner's conscious attention. The information gathered in the preceding parts of the examination sequence—history, acuity, cover test, and perhaps confrontation visual fields—provides a context and a focus for the evaluation of pupil function. It tells the clinician what to look for and how to think about what he or she finds. In this way the process becomes active, rather than merely reactive, and missing something important is much less likely. The results help guide the remainder of the examination and should be consistent with refraction, visual fields, anterior segment findings, intraocular pressure, and fundus appearance.

For example, consider a young, myopic, apparently healthy female contact lens patient complaining of blurred vision in one eye. Her acuity is reduced and cannot be improved with over-refraction or a pinhole. Even before refraction, a careful pupil test showing a relative afferent defect in the eye with reduced acuity alerts the clinician to the possibility of optic neuritis, or perhaps a retinal problem. At this point the emphasis of the examination, which at first seemed to rest on the anterior segment, shifts to visual field and posterior segment assessment.

## Overview of the Pupil Examination

. . . . . . . . . . . . . . . . . . . . . . . . . . .

The pupil examination can be divided into two parts: static and dynamic. The static phase tests the motor component of the pupillary pathways and consists of simple observation of pupil size in both normal and dim room illumination. Is the overall size of the pupils normal for the patient's age? Are the pupils equal in size? If not, is one pupil constricted, or is the opposite pupil dilated? Is either of the pupils anatomically disrupted as a result of, for example, previous surgery, trauma, or an anterior chamber intraocular lens? In the absence of mechanical disruption, pupil size provides information about the balance of autonomic motor influences on the iris; deviations from the status quo may indicate central nervous system or systemic pathology.

The dynamic phase of the examination tests the sensory pathways via the pupillary light reflex. Because fibers carrying sensory information destined for the pupillary centers share the same neural pathway as visual fibers in the retina, optic nerve, chiasm, and most of the optic tract, many lesions affecting vision cause an abnormal pupillary reaction to light; the pupillary response serves as a surrogate indicator of the visual pathway's health. Although certain motor problems also affect the pupil's ability to constrict in response to light (influencing pupil behavior during dynamic testing), they affect both the direct and consensual response equally and are not confused with an afferent defect (which affects the direct, but not the consensual, response).

Detecting a pupil abnormality is the first challenge; deciding what it means is the next. In order to understand the clinical behavior of the pupil, some familiarity with the the anatomy of pupillary pathways is essential.

## Anatomy of the Pupillary Pathways

. . . . . . . . . . . . . . . . . . . . . . . . . . .

The pupillary system can be roughly organized into three components: (1) the iris musculature, (2) the autonomic motor pathways that innervate the muscles, and (3) the sources of input—sensory stimulation and higher level processes—that modulate the autonomic output to the iris muscles.

### MUSCLES OF THE IRIS

Like smooth muscle elsewhere in the body, the iris musculature is controlled by the autonomic nervous system. Iris muscle fibers are arranged into two groups: the sphincter muscle, the stimulation of which tends to *reduce* pupil size, and the dilator muscle, which when stimulated acts to *increase* pupil size. As antagonists, reduction in the level of stimulation to one muscle favors the action of the other.

The iris sphincter muscle—primarily innervated by the parasympathetic nervous system—is composed of a layer of circumferentially oriented muscle fibers running around the pupillary margin. When stimulated, these fibers act together like a drawstring to constrict the pupil. Disruption of these fibers (either locally or anywhere along the parasympathetic pathway) results in a reduced or absent response to light exposure to either eye and relative dilation of the pupil—except when the pupil is mechanically fixed.

The iris dilator muscle, oriented radially inward in a sheet-like layer from the iris root to the sphincter, is innervated primarily by the sympathetic nervous system. Lesions along the sympathetic pathway result in relative miosis.

## THE EFFERENT PATHWAYS

### Pupillary Constriction: The Parasympathetic Pathway

Excitation of the iris sphincter muscle is transmitted via a two-neuron parasympathetic chain from the midbrain to the iris. Although numerous influences modulate the output from the midbrain nuclei, no matter what the stimulus to constriction (e.g., light and near), the neural impulse to the muscle travels the same route.[1] Damage along any part of this two-neuron pathway results in an ipsilateral pupil deficit: mydriasis and a poor or absent response to light or near. That is, disruption to the parasympathetic outflow pathway gives rise to both a static pupil sign (anisocoria

or unequal pupil size) and a dynamic pupil sign (inability to constrict upon light stimulation of *either* eye). This effect on the dynamic behavior of the pupil is a direct result of the fact that the parasympathetic outflow path constitutes the second half of the reflex arc for the pupillary light response. An *efferent* defect is easily distinguished from an *afferent* defect by noting the robust constriction of the contralateral eye when the eye with the motor problem is stimulated with light.

The first order, or preganglionic, fiber originates in the third nerve motor nucleus of the midbrain* and terminates just behind the globe in the ciliary ganglion. Preganglionic fibers travel from the midbrain as part of the oculomotor nerve (cranial nerve III), which passes from the middle cranial fossa (at the cavernous sinus) into the orbit through the superior orbital fissure. Within the orbit the nerve divides; the pupillomotor fibers (along with fibers carrying accommodative signals to the ciliary body) follow the branch of the inferior division of the nerve which supplies the inferior oblique muscle but ultimately split off to form the motor root to the ciliary ganglion (Fig. 3–1).

The ciliary ganglion, which sits just behind the globe, consists primarily (but not exclusively†) of the cell bodies of the second order, or postganglionic, parasympathetic neurons serving ac-

*Specifically, the Edinger-Westphal and anteromedian subnuclei.

†Sensory fibers from various ocular tissues, on their way to join the nasociliary branch of the trigeminal nerve, and sympathetic vasomotor fibers also pass through the ciliary ganglion, although they have no synapses there.[2] These same fibers, along with the postganglionic parasympathetic axons, make up the short ciliary nerves.[1]

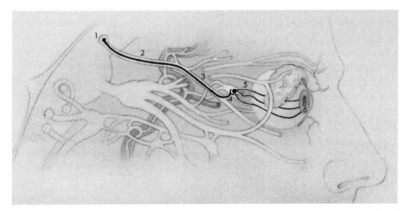

**FIGURE 3–1** Parasympathetic pathway to the iris and ciliary body. *1,* Edinger-Westphal and anterior median nuclei of the dorsal mesencephalon. *2,* Oculomotor nerve. *3,* Branch to the inferior oblique muscle. *4,* Motor root of the ciliary ganglion. *5,* Short ciliary nerves. *6,* Iris sphincter and ciliary muscle. (Chart prepared by Dr. HS Thompson and drawn by J Esperson. From Walsh FB: Walsh and Hoyt's Clinical Neuro-Ophthalmology. Baltimore: Williams & Wilkins, 1982–1985, p 414.)

commodation and pupillary constriction. The axons of these fibers enter the eye as numerous short ciliary nerves—which pierce the sclera in a circle surrounding the optic nerve—and travel anteriorly to their target muscles in the ciliary body and the iris.

The parasympathetic pupillary pathway carries only excitatory action potentials.[2] Inhibitory influences from any source—sudden dark, increased arousal—act by reducing the firing rate of the midbrain motor nuclei. That is, inhibition from elsewhere in the system acts by "turning off the tap" of excitatory impulses to the sphincter muscle.

The course of the parasympathetic outflow path remains within the cranium, leaving only to pass directly into the orbit. This is in marked distinction to the sympathetic pathway, which follows a relatively long extracranial course before re-entering the skull and reaching its target organ within the eye.

## Pupillary Dilation: The Sympathetic Pathway

The iris dilator muscle and its sympathetic innervation are secondary in determining pupil size and reactivity. However, the proximity of its long, vulnerable pathway to important structures in the neck and to the apex of the lung means that anisocoria—due to a unilateral disruption in the normal balance of autonomic stimulation to the sphincter and dilator muscles—may be the first or most obvious warning sign of serious disease.

Innervation of the dilator muscle (Fig. 3-2) is accomplished via a three-neuron chain whose components are the central (first) neuron, the preganglionic (second) neuron, and the postganglionic (third) neuron.[2] The central neurons have their cell bodies in the hypothalamus; their axons travel down the brain stem, exit the skull, and synapse with preganglionic neurons in the grey matter of the spinal cord at the level of spinal nerves C8 through T2 (the ciliospinal center of Budge and Waller).*

A general feature of the sympathetic autonomic system is that preganglionic neurons exit the spinal cord with the spinal nerves, then split off in small bundles to join the ipsilateral paravertebral sympathetic chain, which is a chain of ganglia running alongside the spinal column. The

_____

*Although the hypothalamus appears to be the source of pupillomotor sympathetic outflow, the preganglionic neurons of the ciliospinal center of Budge and Waller have their own spontaneous firing rate and are thought to be the site of reciprocal inhibition to parasympathetic excitation.[2]

sympathetic pupillomotor fibers leave the spinal cord via roots C8, T1, and T2[1] and join the paravertebral sympathetic chain in close proximity to the apex of the lung, turning and heading up toward their synapse with postganglionic fibers in the superior cervical ganglion, just below the angle of the jaw.[2] It is thought that most of the preganglionic axons loop around the subclavian artery, in the ansa subclavia of Vieussens, on their way to the superior cervical ganglion.[1] Postganglionic pupillomotor fibers leave the superior cervical ganglion, form part of the nerve plexus around the internal carotid artery, and in this form enter the skull. Traveling with the internal carotid artery up into the middle cranial fossa, they ultimately join the ophthalmic branch of the fifth cranial (trigeminal) nerve and enter the orbit. Once in the orbit, the pupillomotor fibers follow the nasociliary branch of the trigeminal nerve, splitting off to form the long ciliary nerves, which enter the globe and make their way to the iris dilator muscle (Fig. 3-3).

Other postganglionic sympathetic nerve fibers from the superior cervical ganglion innervate the sweat glands and blood vessels of the face and Müller's muscle, the smooth muscle responsible for involuntary lid tonus. Whereas the fibers serving Müller's muscle accompany the pupillomotor fibers within the internal carotid plexus, the vast majority of the sudomotor and vasomotor fibers travel in the external carotid nerve plexus.[2] This is important in the differential diagnosis of lesions in the sympathetic pathway (Horner's syndrome).

## AFFERENT CONNECTIONS TO THE PUPILLOMOTOR SYSTEM

The pathways described above are the effectors of pupil constriction and dilation. The actual size of the pupil is determined by the relative amount of neural stimulation reaching the two muscle groups, which depends on the relative output of the third nerve motor nuclei (for constriction) and the ciliospinal center of Budge and Waller (for dilation). Although each is characterized by some tonic level of output,[2] the actual output from these centers is modulated by several types of input, both excitatory and inhibitory.

## Pupillary Constriction: Parasympathetic Excitation

The two main excitatory inputs to pupil constriction are the light reflex and the near reflex. The

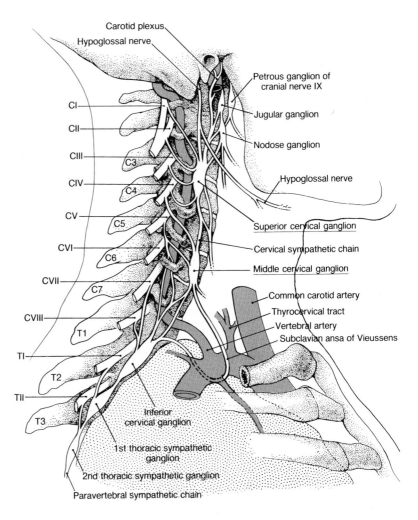

Carotid plexus
Hypoglossal nerve
Petrous ganglion of cranial nerve IX
Jugular ganglion
Nodose ganglion
Hypoglossal nerve
Superior cervical ganglion
Cervical sympathetic chain
Middle cervical ganglion
Common carotid artery
Thyrocervical tract
Vertebral artery
Subclavian ansa of Vieussens
Inferior cervical ganglion
1st thoracic sympathetic ganglion
2nd thoracic sympathetic ganglion
Paravertebral sympathetic chain

CI, CII, CIII, CIV, CV, CVI, CVII, CVIII, TI, TII

C3, C4, C5, C6, C7, T1, T2, T3

**FIGURE 3–2** Sympathetic pathways in the neck. Note the close association of the thoracic sympathetic chain and the ansa subclavia to the pleura of the pulmonary apex. (Redrawn from a chart prepared by Dr. HS Thompson. From Walsh FB: Walsh and Hoyt's Clinical Neuro-Ophthalmology. Baltimore: Williams & Wilkins, 1982–1985, p 426.)

light reflex, by far the more important of the two, is discussed in detail next.

### The Light Reflex

In describing the efferent path of pupillary constriction, we have already accomplished half the job because it is the "back end" of the pupillary light reflex pathway. The "front end," or afferent leg, of the arc coincides with the visual pathway all the way from the retina to just before the lateral geniculate nucleus. That is, light hitting the retina stimulates the photoreceptors; a signal is transmitted through the various layers of the retina to the retinal ganglion cells, the axons of which make up the optic nerve. The axons from the temporal retina continue without crossing through the chiasm to become part of the ipsilateral optic tract, whereas those from the nasal retina cross at the chiasm and join temporal fibers from the fellow eye to make up the contralateral optic tract. In the latter third of the optic tract—just before reaching the lateral geniculate

nucleus, where the fibers carrying information destined for the visual cortex have their first synapse—fibers concerned with pupil constriction split off and head for the pretectal nucleus of the midbrain. There they synapse with neurons that carry the impulse to both the ipsilateral and contralateral oculomotor nuclei, primarily the Edinger-Westphal nuclei. The entire light reflex pathway is shown schematically in Figure 3–4.

Light hitting the retina, then, stimulates both the visual cortex and the centers for pupillary constriction, and the characteristics of the stimuli that influence the pupil response have been explored in much the same ways as have those that determine visual thresholds. For example, the wavelength, intensity, size, retinal location, and duration of the light stimulus all affect the pupil response. It has been found that as detectors for the pupillary response, rods and cones behave very much as they do for the visual response: Rods are more sensitive to dim light, saturate in bright light, and show the same spec-

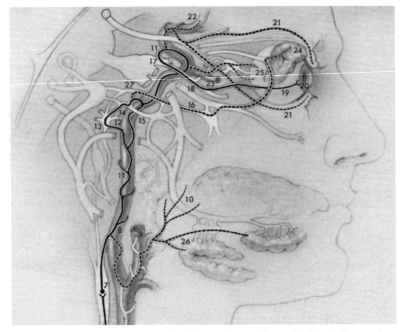

**FIGURE 3–3** Sympathetic pathways to the face and eye. The solid line indicates the pathway of the pupillary dilator fibers, and the dashed lines show some of the other sympathetic pathways to the orbit and face. *7,* Superior cervical ganglion. *8,* Internal carotid artery. *9,* External carotid artery. *10,* Sudomotor fibers to face. *11,* Carotid plexus. *12,* Caroticotympanic nerve. *13,* Tympanic plexus. *14,* Deep petrosal nerve. *15,* Lesser superficial petrosal nerve. *16,* Sympathetic contribution to Vidian nerve. *17,* Ophthalmic division of the trigeminal nerve. *18,* Nasociliary nerve. *19,* Long ciliary nerve. *20,* Ciliary muscle and iris dilator muscle. *21,* Probable pathway of sympathetic contribution to retractor muscles of the eyelids. *22,* Vasomotor and some sudomotor fibers. *23,* Ophthalmic artery. *24,* Lacrimal gland. *25,* Short ciliary nerves. *26,* Sympathetic contribution to salivary glands. *27,* Greater superficial petrosal nerve. (Chart prepared by Dr. HS Thompson and drawn by J Esperson. From Walsh FB: Walsh and Hoyt's Clinical Neuro-Ophthalmology. Baltimore: Williams & Wilkins, 1982–1985, p 427.)

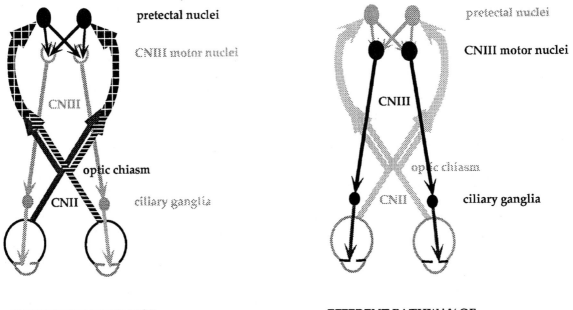

AFFERENT PATHWAY OF
PUPILLARY LIGHT REFLEX

EFFERENT PATHWAY OF
PUPILLARY LIGHT REFLEX

**FIGURE 3–4** Pupillary light reflex pathway.

tral sensitivity for the pupil response as they do for vision. Cones have a higher brightness threshold but can adapt to higher light levels and so do not saturate out as quickly; they also show the same spectral sensitivity for pupil response as they do for vision.* In fact, the behavior of the pupil is so similar to that of the visual system when these stimulus parameters are varied that the two systems must share the same set of receptors. It is in the higher level processing that the information is used differently. According to Loewenfeld:

> . . . *pupillary impulses derived from all areas of the retina are simply added in the primitive midbrain while the forebrain is capable of discriminating between different kinds of visual input, that is, of disregarding some and using other afferent information. . . . Spatial summation is generally more marked for the pupil than it is for vision.*[2]

These similarities and differences between the visual and pupillary response to light explain why certain types of acuity loss are accompanied by a diminished pupil response, why other types are not, and how it is that certain conditions that leave acuity intact can profoundly affect the pupil response. The relationship between vision loss and afferent pupillary defects is discussed in detail below.

The multiple decussations in the afferent path of the light reflex from the retina to the pupillo-motor nuclei† guarantee that anisocoria—an asymmetry in pupil size—is never caused by a lesion affecting only the afferent pathway. A reduced or absent signal from one eye (for example, from blindness in that eye) results in a reduced signal to the pretectal nuclei on both sides because of the decussation at the chiasm and therefore causes bilateral mydriasis.[1] Similarly, although a lesion in the afferent pathway beyond the chiasm reduces only the signal to the ipsilateral pretectal nucleus, because intercalated neurons connect the pretectal nuclei to oculomotor nuclei on both sides, the effect is symmetrical between the eyes. True anisocoria can come only from a disruption in the efferent pathways.

### The Near Reflex

The neural impulse that gives rise to all components of the near triad—convergence, accommo-

dation, and miosis—originates in the occipital cortex.[1] These three simultaneous actions are nevertheless independent in terms of innervation; that is, any one of them can be elicited in the absence of the others.[2] The excitatory signal from the cortex stimulates different sites of the oculomotor nuclei to cause contraction of the medial rectus muscle (convergence), contraction of the ciliary muscle (accommodation), and contraction of the pupillary sphincter muscle (miosis). Although the preganglionic fibers share the road between the oculomotor nuclei and the ciliary ganglion, those serving pupillary constriction and accommodation are distinct, originating and terminating at different sites.

The simultaneous stimulation of the components of the near triad and the anatomical proximity of their motor pathways can give rise to two interesting forms of "light-near dissociation," discussed below.

Although some textbooks speak of a "lid-closure" miosis—pupil constriction upon attempted lid closure with the eye held open—Loewenfeld makes a convincing argument against its existence, believing it to be caused by an unconsciously recruited near response.[2]

## Pupillary Constriction: Sympathetic Inhibition

Excitation of pupillary constriction in response to light is accompanied by reciprocal inhibition of the sympathetic outflow to the dilator muscle at the ciliospinal center of Budge-Waller, that is, at the level of the preganglionic sympathetic neuron.[2]

## Pupillary Dilation: Sympathetic Excitation

### Psychosensory Stimuli

Unlike the iris sphincter, which responds to light and near via specific afferent pathways, the iris dilator can respond reflexively to any form of sensory input—except for light—and to any stimulating thoughts or emotions. To quote Irene Loewenfeld, ". . . any somatic or visceral afferent nerve as well as all central connections involved in sensation or in general arousal responses can serve as an afferent path for pupillary reflex dilation."[2] In fact, psychosensory stimulation from fear or excitement can actually reduce the light reflex and should always be considered when testing the pupils of extremely apprehensive patients (especially children).

---

*Although the pupillary threshold to colored lights for both light- and dark-adapted eyes is slightly higher than the visual threshold.[2]

†Both at the chiasm and between the pretectal nuclei and the oculomotor nuclei.

### *"Light-off" Reflex, Part One*

When a light-adapted eye is suddenly exposed to dark—that is, when the light is suddenly shut off—the retina sends a "light-off" signal, which, like the other afferent stimuli, most likely works through the hypothalamus to increase the sympathetic firing rate to the dilator muscle.

## Pupillary Dilation: Parasympathetic Inhibition

### *Alertness*

The parasympathetic pathway from the midbrain to the pupil sphincter carries only excitatory impulses; it is the level of neural output from the oculomotor nuclei which governs pupil size in the awake individual. This output level is determined by the amount of stimulation coming from the pretectum as a result of light hitting the retina, from the cortex in response to a near object, and by higher level inhibition of this mesencephalic discharge. The more alert or aroused the individual, the greater the inhibition to pupillary constriction; this inhibition of the sphincter muscle works in parallel with direct sympathetic stimulation to the dilator muscle to increase pupil size. A release from this inhibitory output during drowsiness, fatigue, or sleep results in miosis.

### *"Light-off" Reflex, Part Two*

We have seen that sudden dark causes a reflex excitation of pupillary dilation through the sympathetic motor pathways to the dilator muscle. In addition to this active mechanism, passive relaxation of the sphincter muscle results from cessation of input from the light reflex pathway and probably also a reflex inhibition at the Edinger-Westphal nuclei initiated by the "light-off" signal at the retina.[2] The component of dark reflex dilation attributable to parasympathetic inhibition is slower, weaker, and longer-lasting than that due to sympathetic stimulation.[2]

## SUMMARY OF INFLUENCES ON PUPIL SIZE

Pupil size at any given moment reflects a balance between the parasympathetic and sympathetic outputs to the iris muscles, which are in turn governed by the basal firing rates of the centers for the two systems, modulated by inputs from nearly all sensory systems and the higher centers of the brain. Under ordinary conditions, the light level is the primary determinant of pupil size. However, the presence of pain, the proximity of the object of regard, and the alertness and emotional state of the individual are all capable of significantly affecting pupil size.

In addition, average pupil size changes with age. The pupils are small from birth to about 1 year of age. According to a cross-sectional study performed on 5000 subjects from birth to age 100 years, pupil size increased during childhood to a peak at about the time of puberty. After that point it decreased gradually into old age.[3]

Despite these general trends, it is not possible to know whether someone's pupil size is abnormal for his or her age unless it is grossly so, given the wide variation between individuals due to anatomical differences, alertness, and emotional factors. A difference in size between the pupils, or a diminished response to light, is a much more reliable indicator of pathology.

# The Minimum Pupil Examination

. . . . . . . . . . . . . . . . . . . . . . . .

Pupil testing should be done early in the eye examination, before exposing the patient to bright light or pharmacological agents. It is usually done just after visual acuity and cover test and before refraction. If confrontation fields are part of the test battery, pupil testing should be done afterward, to avoid creating afterimage scotomas.

## PUPIL SIZE

Observe the size of each pupil in moderate and then dim illumination.

**Technique**  Have the patient look across the room and slightly upward, to get the upper lid out of the way. Measure pupil size with a "pd ruler" or pupil gauge. After measuring pupil size in a reasonable number of patients, estimating pupil size becomes easier, but you should "calibrate" yourself frequently by measuring a series of pupils. Always measure quantitatively where anisocoria is suspected.*

Document the size of both pupils. Inspect the lid position (both upper and lower), comparing between the eyes, looking for a ptosis. Also look at the eyebrow position (a raised eyebrow may be an attempt to compensate for a lid droop).

---

*According to Zinn, a difference of 20% of pupil diameter is considered significant.[4]

Turn down the room lights and, illuminating the eyes tangentially, observe (1) the relative pupil size and (2) whether or not each pupil dilates. If there was anisocoria in moderate illumination, observe whether the difference between the pupils increases, decreases, or stays the same.

**Observation**   Record the size of each pupil in moderate illumination.

Does overall pupil size seem consistent with the age of the patient? Are the pupil diameters within 1 mm of each other? Is there a ptosis in either eye? If so, does the ptotic eye have a larger or smaller pupil than the other eye?

Did both pupils get larger in response to lowering the light level? Is there an anisocoria in dim light which was not apparent in moderate light? If there was an anisocoria, how did it change, if at all?

**Interpretation**   Bilateral small pupils in a child may indicate hyperopia. In an adult, pupils that are small and fail to dilate in dim light may signal a midbrain lesion.

A detailed discussion of anisocoria can be found below. Briefly, anisocoria that is greater in light than in dark points to a problem in innervation or function of the sphincter muscle (larger pupil abnormal), whereas a greater difference in the dark throws suspicion on the innervation of the dilator muscle (smaller pupil abnormal). In either case, the next step is to check the light reaction, because this is an important part of the differential diagnosis.

## LIGHT REFLEX

Observe how each pupil reacts to direct light stimulation.

**Technique**   Smith[5] recommends testing the direct response three times in one eye, then three times in the other. Repeating the stimulus three times in quick succession may cause fatigue—a marked diminution in response—in an abnormal eye which is nevertheless capable of an initial brisk response; normal pupils can recover quickly and reconstrict at least three times. Lowering the ambient illumination opens up the pupils and makes the constriction (or lack thereof) more obvious. Instruct the patient to fixate a distant object and bring the transilluminator up from below, to avoid contamination by the near response. (Also, avoid stimulating the contralateral eye.) With children you may need another person (e.g., a parent or technician wielding a toy) to provide a compelling distance target. Smith recommends the use of a binocular indi-

rect ophthalmoscope aimed from below, a bit farther away, for an apprehensive child.[5]

In the case of an absent or obviously diminished response in either eye, check the quality of the consensual response while stimulating the fellow eye. If the consensual response is also abnormal, check the near response as follows:

**Near Response**   With the lights just high enough to allow a good view of the pupils, have the patient look from the distant target to a near target—for example, his or her thumbnail—while you encourage him or her to focus. The success of this test depends on the effort of the patient, and it may take several tries with encouragement to teach him or her the task, particularly in older patients who have not tried to accommodate in years. (It is the accommodative *effort*, not the accommodative *amplitude*, that triggers the response.) After the pupil constricts (if it does), have the patient look back at the distant target and watch to see if redilation is brisk or slow.

**Observation**   Record the briskness of the direct response for each eye, and look for differences over time in each eye and between eyes. The response should be graded from 4+ (brisk) to 0 (no response). If fatigue is observed, grade and record all three responses for each eye.

If the direct response is abnormal (sluggish or absent), grade the consensual response as well. If near testing was done, note whether or not the constriction to near was greater than that to light and whether redilation after near effort was fast or slow. Normal results can be abbreviated: "PERRLA" (pupils equal, round, and reactive to light and accommodation).

**Interpretation**   An absent or reduced direct light response in an eye capable of a robust consensual response indicates an afferent (visual) defect. The swinging flashlight test (below) provides a more sensitive test in unilateral or asymmetrical cases.

If anisocoria is present and the eye with the larger pupil has diminished direct *and* consensual light responses, the anisocoria is due to a problem in the motor leg of the light reflex arc, that is, the third nerve,* the ciliary ganglion, or the iris, or to pharmacological block with an anticholinergic agent. A constriction to near that is greater than that to light ("light-near dissociation") points to a tonic pupil, particularly if the redilation is slow.† Light-near dissociation

---

*In general, a third nerve palsy is accompanied by strabismus, which will already have shown up on cover test.

†Although midbrain lesions may also cause non-reactive pupils with light-near dissociation, these are usually bilateral with miotic pupils and prompt redilation after near effort.

is not always present in tonic pupil syndromes, however.

In anisocoria in which both eyes react briskly to light, the differential diagnosis is between simple (idiopathic) anisocoria and a sympathetic lesion (Horner's syndrome); in the latter case the eye with the smaller pupil is the abnormal one. How to proceed with the differential diagnosis of the anisocoria is discussed below.

## SWINGING FLASHLIGHT TEST

**Technique**   With the room darkened, move the transilluminator quickly from one eye to the other across the bridge of the nose, closely watching the eye to which the light is moved. The light should be angled from below to avoid contamination by the near response and should come from roughly the same part of each eye's visual field. The light should be swung briskly from one eye to the other, left on each eye for several seconds, and then swung back. Care must be taken not to expose one eye to significantly more light than the other.

**Observation**   *Immediate* constriction or dilation of either eye upon direct stimulation is a positive result.

Record the presence of an afferent defect as a positive swinging flashlight test, grading the defect on a scale of 4+ (dramatic pupillary escape of the worse eye or full-scale direct constriction of the better eye) to 1+ (just noticeable movement), specifying the abnormal eye (e.g., "3+ APD OD").* Record the absence of an afferent defect as a negative swinging flashlight test ("—APD").

**Interpretation**   This technique compares the patency of the visual pathways of the two eyes by comparing the eye's direct response (reflecting the sensitivity of its own visual pathway) with its consensual response (reflecting the sensitivity of the other eye's visual pathway). When the light is swung quickly from one eye to the other, any significant movement in the pupil of the illuminated eye reflects a difference between its consensual response (initial state) and its di-

---

*A relative afferent defect can be quantified by performing the swinging flashlight test with progressively darker neutral density filters over the better eye until no defect is detected.

rect response (new state). Slight constriction upon illumination of *each* eye is caused by not moving quickly enough between the eyes. Slight dilation that occurs shortly *after* the initial illumination of each eye is normal pupillary escape. Marked pupillary escape indicates pathology. Small oscillatory movements are due to normal pupillary "play."

The diagnosis can be summarized as follows (see box below):

## Comments

The swinging flashlight test has several major advantages over simply looking at each eye's direct and consensual responses individually. First, the eye being observed is always the one being illuminated (as opposed to looking at the consensual response in the non-illuminated eye). Second, it is nearly impossible to see a subtle difference between pupil responses separated in time, whereas with the swinging flashlight test, the examiner is looking for an instantaneous change in a single pupil. Note, however, that because this test compares the afferent pathways of the two eyes, a completely symmetrical visual defect—a relatively rare event—does not produce a positive result.

Because more fibers contribute to the light reaction from the temporal than the nasal retina,[6] it is important that the eyes be stimulated symmetrically, that is, with the light coming from roughly the same part of each eye's visual field. If the light source were swung back and forth while held at a constant angle, such as always from the patient's left hemifield (as might occur with a right-handed clinician), then a left relative afferent pupillary defect (RAPD) could be "created" by the fact that the response from the nasal retina in the left eye was being compared to the response from the temporal retina in the right. Another way in which a clinician might "create" a relative afferent pupillary defect is if the light is held longer on one eye than the other, causing an asymmetrical retinal light adaptation. Because the important features of the swinging flashlight test are observed almost immediately upon light exposure, there is no reason to linger on one eye or the other; it is far better to "keep on swinging" when looking for a defect.

---

**Swinging Flashlight Test: Possible Outcomes and What They Mean**

No movement upon illumination ⇒ direct = consensual ⇒ no relative afferent pupillary defect (RAPD)
Dilation upon illumination ⇒ direct < consensual ⇒ ipsilateral RAPD
Constriction upon illumination ⇒ direct > consensual ⇒ contralateral RAPD

The swinging flashlight test works even in the presence of one non-functioning pupil, because a problem anywhere in the motor leg of the light reflex pathway (e.g., a third nerve problem, Adie's pupil, pharmacological block, or an iris problem) affects both direct and consensual constriction equally. Remember that a positive swinging flashlight test reveals an *unequal* response of the pupil to direct and consensual stimulation. In a patient with two functioning pupils (i.e., no motor problem), a relative afferent pupillary defect in the right eye manifests itself as a dilation of the right pupil and a constriction of the left pupil as the light is alternated between them. If, however, the right pupil is not working, the examiner still sees a constriction in the left; with a non-functional left pupil the dilation of the right upon illumination clinches the diagnosis.

Although an outflow problem itself does not cause a relative afferent pupillary defect, the anisocoria, if large enough, can give rise to a positive swinging flashlight test. Thompson and Pilley[7] explain that the greater amount of light getting to the retina of the eye with the larger pupil can result in an apparent afferent defect on the other side. Keep in mind, however, that the patient with both anisocoria and a true positive swinging flashlight test has two different problems, one visual and one motor; both must be explained.

Because a positive swinging flashlight test indicates a problem in the visual pathway, the differential diagnosis fits naturally into the optometric examination. Refraction, tonometry, biomicroscopy, funduscopy, and visual fields usually uncover the true cause of vision loss.

Anisocoria, on the other hand, points to a problem in the motor pathways, and the usual battery of tests probably does not give a conclusive diagnosis. In this case additional tests are needed to find the source of the problem, and these tests use topical drugs. The effective concentration of these drugs is absolutely crucial in differentiating one type of problem from another, so anything that affects the amount of the drug reaching the iris—that is, anything that disrupts the corneal epithelium—contaminates the results. Obviously, other mydriatic or miotic agents also interfere with the process. Pupil testing therefore must be done before applanation tonometry and the dilated fundus examination or at a return visit. Differential diagnosis of anisocoria should not be delayed, however, in suspected third nerve disease; a cranial nerve palsy of recent onset, particularly if accompanied by headache, is an ominous sign and demands an immediate neurological workup.[2]

## CLINICAL IMPLICATIONS OF THE AFFERENT PUPILLARY DEFECT

The principal value of the swinging flashlight test in uncovering an afferent pupillary defect is in the differential diagnosis of vision loss, which may be manifested as a drop in acuity, a visual field defect, or both. As a general rule, because the strength of the light reaction is directly tied to the integrity of the neural components of the afferent leg of the light reflex pathway and because the loss of these cells corresponds to a loss of part of the visual field, but not always to a loss in acuity, an afferent defect usually correlates more closely with the visual field defect.[8] However, acuity loss is more often noticed and reported by patients, so it is usually the main clue to a visual problem at the beginning of the eye examination. How the presence or absence of an afferent defect contributes to the differential diagnosis of a vision problem can be seen by considering how various ocular conditions affect the ability of the retina and optic nerve to process visual and pupillary input.

The pupillary light reflex is a mass response; any light hitting the retina gets added to the signal, as long as it falls on a functioning photoreceptor feeding into a functioning ganglion cell. The visual system is far more complex, with receptive field organization such that light can be either excitatory or inhibitory and can either contribute to the image or obscure it. Thus, a condition that affects only a small portion of the retina, or one that defocuses, disorganizes, or scatters the incoming light, does not substantially reduce the pupil response but may wreak havoc with the visual image.

The most common cause of reduced visual acuity is uncorrected refractive error. Because refractive error simply defocuses the visual image, it does not cause an afferent defect.

Although there has been some controversy about whether or not an afferent pupillary defect is associated with amblyopia, Loewenfeld concludes that any effect that may exist is quite small and does not correlate with the acuity deficit.[2] In any case, it is usually clear from the history, visual acuity, cover test, and refraction whether amblyopia is a reasonable diagnosis. A clinically observable relative afferent defect in an amblyope points to the existence of accompanying organic disease.

Lens and corneal opacities, even when fairly dense, do not cause a positive swinging flashlight test, because incoming light, although diffused, lands on some part of the retina and thus contributes to the pupil response. This is one of the simplest (and least expensive) methods of testing the integrity of the retina and optic nerve behind a cataract: a poor pupil response in an eye with cataract almost invariably indicates additional pathology.[2]

Whether or not retinal disease causes an afferent defect depends on the size of the lesion. Because the density of photoreceptors is much higher at the fovea than in the periphery, a macular lesion affects the pupil response more than a lesion of the same size elsewhere. Also, there is a fairly close correspondence between the size of a central lesion and the acuity loss associated with it. According to Thompson and Pilley,[7] no clinically observable afferent defect is caused by a macular lesion as long as the visual acuity is better than 20/100. If macular disease is severe enough to cause a pupil defect, the macular abnormality is almost certainly ophthalmoscopically visible, and the differential diagnosis is obvious. The same principle can be applied to almost all retinal disease (including detachments, inflammation, dystrophies, and degenerations), whether or not central vision is affected: If it is bad enough to cause a pupil defect, you'll see it.* On the other hand, some ophthalmoscopically obvious retinal lesions do not cause a clinically apparent afferent defect. In Walsh's judgment, "An afferent defect virtually *never* occurs in a patient with macular drusen or central serous chorioretinopathy. When an afferent defect is noted in such a patient, that patient should be evaluated for an underlying retrobulbar optic neuropathy."[1]

To summarize, in a patient with central retinal disease, an afferent pupillary defect should correlate roughly with the acuity loss; by the time the pupil defect is apparent, the differential diagnosis can be made ophthalmoscopically or, if necessary, with fluorescein angiography.

Because the same is *not* true of optic nerve disease, the swinging flashlight test is very useful. An afferent defect due to compromise of the optic nerve, chiasm, or radiations by inflammatory, neoplastic, ischemic, or demyelinating disease provides a more positive diagnostic sign than disc pallor and manifests itself long before optic atrophy becomes apparent ophthalmoscopically.[1]

Furthermore, the pupil defect can occur even in the absence of significantly reduced acuity if the central fibers are not affected and may persist after acuity has recovered in cases of optic neuri-

tis. Thompson et al.[8] found that afferent pupillary defects are so uniformly present in optic neuritis, even after acuity has recovered, that if no relative defect is found on the swinging flashlight test, the apparently "normal" fellow eye should be carefully tested, as bilateral disease almost certainly exists. They also found that the severity of an afferent defect associated with optic neuropathy is more closely correlated with the visual field loss than with acuity loss. Glaucoma provides a second example: A relative afferent defect can be seen in patients suffering from unilateral or asymmetrical disease,[1] yet visual acuity is often preserved until the final stages. One cautionary note, however: When dealing with symmetrical (bitemporal or binasal) field loss such as might occur with chiasmal lesions, the swinging flashlight test does not reveal the afferent defect because roughly the same number of fibers from each eye may be affected.

With the above information we can look at how the outcome of the swinging flashlight test adds to our differential diagnosis when a patient complains of vision loss or when reduced acuity is discovered in the examination. Depending on the age, health, and refractive status of the patient, the most likely cause of the vision loss is one of the following: uncorrected refractive error, amblyopia, hysteria/malingering, media opacity, inflammation, retinal disease, or optic neuropathy. Of these, only the optic neuropathy is capable of producing a clinically significant afferent pupillary defect without the diagnosis being obvious from the history or funduscopy.

Thus, the finding of a relative afferent pupillary defect in an eye with no *severe* retinal disease (e.g., large detachment, large macular lesion, widespread dystrophy, or significant vascular occlusive event) defines optic nerve disease and makes visual field testing a high priority.

## DIFFERENTIAL DIAGNOSIS OF ANISOCORIA†

As we have already seen, anisocoria is always caused by a motor problem. This means either a disruption in the parasympathetic pathway to the iris sphincter (including local damage to the sphincter muscle itself) or a disruption in the sympathetic pathway to the iris dilator. Both the parasympathetic and sympathetic efferent pathways to the iris musculature are overwhelmingly

---

*An important exception to this rule may be found in case of retinal vascular occlusion, in which past damage may or may not be obvious ophthalmoscopically. Smith also discusses several interesting cases of transient afferent defect associated with amaurosis fugax.[5]

†The technique for differential diagnosis set out in this section is based on the paper *Unequal Pupils. A Flow Chart for Sorting out the Anisocorias* by H. Stanley Thompson and FJ Pilley. (Surv Ophthalmol 1976; 21:45–48).

uncrossed[2]; consequently, a lesion affecting the pathway on one side causes a pupil defect on the same side.

By the end of the basic pupil examination, the clinician already has the following information essential to the differential diagnosis of anisocoria: (1) The quality of direct and consensual light response in each eye, (2) How anisocoria changes with light level, (3) The quality of reflex dilation in each eye, and (4) The presence or absence of light-near dissociation.

The first two pieces of information indicate whether the problem is in the pathway to constriction (poor light response in larger eye, anisocoria greater in light) or not (good light response in both eyes, anisocoria greater in dark), thus narrowing the differential diagnosis (Fig. 3–5).

## Anisocoria with Mydriasis and Reduced Light Response

**Differential Diagnosis** In a patient with anisocoria due to a constriction problem, the abnormal eye has a larger pupil in light; the difference in pupil size is greatest in bright light (because the other eye is constricting normally)

and diminishes as the lights are turned down (as the stimulus to constriction to the other eye is reduced). More importantly, the abnormal eye has a reduced or absent reaction to direct *and* consensual light stimuli.

The following are the four most common causes of unilateral, unresponsive, mydriatic pupil in an ambulatory patient:

**Local disruption:** Mechanical limitation of iris sphincter movement due to trauma (natural or iatrogenic) or disease.

**CN III palsy:** Third nerve lesion of any etiology from the oculomotor nuclei up to the ciliary ganglion, that is, affecting the *preganglionic* fibers; characterized by reduced or absent light response, ciliary (accommodative) paresis, and in most (but not all) cases by exotropia and ptosis.* The near response is affected to the same degree as the light response. *Recent-onset cranial nerve III palsy can be a sign of serious intracranial disease and requires a prompt neurologi-*

---

*It is also possible to have cranial nerve III lesions that spare the pupil and accommodation ("external ophthalmoplegia"), manifesting only as strabismus and ptosis. This is commonly the case with diabetic third nerve palsy.

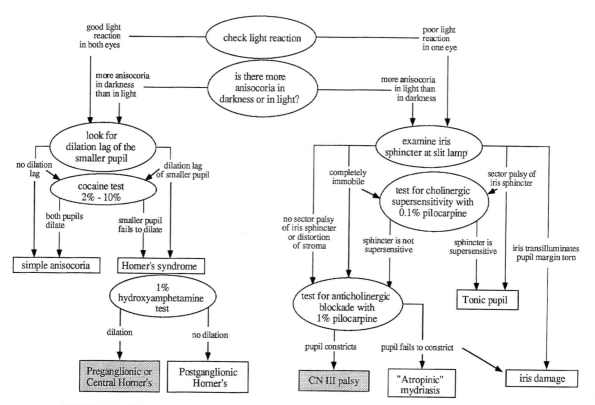

**FIGURE 3–5** Algorithm for diagnosis of anisocorias. (From Thompson HS: Unequal pupils: A flow chart for sorting out the anisocorias. Surv Ophthalmol 1976; 21:45–48.)

*cal workup, particularly if accompanied by pain.*[2]

**Tonic pupil:** A syndrome caused by damage to the *postganglionic* fibers at the ciliary ganglion or short ciliary nerves. Presents as a diminished constriction to light, which, by slit lamp, may be seen as a sector palsy of the pupillary sphincter; often accompanied by accommodative paresis, light-near dissociation (with a slow, delayed redilation after near constriction), and supersensitivity to cholinergic agents.[1]

**Pharmacological block:** Blockade of cholinergic receptors on the sphincter muscle by an atropinic agent.

The differential diagnosis among these conditions is fairly simple and proceeds as follows: First, the history of the patient can be helpful. Has there been trauma? Does the patient work in a hospital setting or come into contact with topical atropinic drugs? Does the patient complain of photophobia, trouble with reading, or blur? If so, when did these start? (Third nerve palsy, tonic pupil, and pharmacological block may all present as internal ophthalmoplegia.) Next, consider the results of the cover test and inspection of the lid position. Because cranial nerve III innervates the levator palpebrae and all the extraocular muscles except for the superior oblique and the lateral rectus, a third nerve palsy is in most—but not all—cases manifested as an exotropia with a ptosis on the side with the larger pupil. On rare occasions only the innervation to the intraocular muscles (pupil sphincter and ciliary muscle) is affected, and differentiation from a tonic pupil and pharmacological block requires further testing.

Inspect the iris using the slit lamp. If the iris is damaged secondary to trauma or surgery or adherent to the crystalline lens by posterior synechiae, the diagnosis is obvious. Check the anterior chamber angle. An acute angle-closure glaucoma also causes a fixed, dilated pupil, but the accompanying pain and redness leave little room for doubt in the diagnosis.

Use the slit lamp to check the light reaction under magnification: With the light intensity set high and the beam positioned on the edge of the pupil, under low-medium (10 to 15×) magnification, close off the slit, then open it up and watch the pupil margin closely. A tonic pupil, if it reacts at all, reacts segmentally, because only certain sections of the pupil margin are still innervated and able to constrict to light. It is possible that no movement will be seen, even under magnification. Unilateral segmental light reaction in the absence of iris trauma or inflammation

is strongly suggestive of a tonic pupil.[7] Further evidence of a tonic pupil would be the presence of a light-near dissociation with slow redilation after near constriction.

To clinch the diagnosis of tonic pupil, test for cholinergic denervation supersensitivity. In a tonic pupil the sphincter muscle has been deprived of its acetylcholine supply by destruction of the postganglionic fibers. In an effort to compensate, the muscle develops a higher than normal number of muscarinic receptors and so becomes supersensitive to any cholinergic substance in its vicinity. This is different from a third nerve palsy, in which, despite the damage to the preganglionic fibers, the postganglionic fibers and their synaptic connections remain intact. It is also not the case in pharmacological block, in which not only are there no extra receptor sites, but many of the ones that are there are already bound up by anticholinergic molecules. One-eighth per cent pilocarpine (a direct-acting cholinergic drug), although too dilute to have any effect in an eye with normal acetylcholine levels (and therefore far too weak to counteract an anticholinergic drug), causes a dramatic reaction in a pupil with postganglionic denervation. To test for supersensitivity, begin by making sure that the pupils are not constricted by near effort, as this contaminates the test results. Bourgon and Thompson[9] suggest fogging the patient with plus lenses (or removing correction in myopes) for 5 minutes prior to instilling drops. Measure each pupil. Instill one drop of 0.1% (or 0.125%) pilocarpine in each eye, wait 30 seconds, and instill a second drop in each eye.* Have the patient wait 30 minutes, emphasizing that he or she not read or focus on anything close up. After this time, measure the pupils again, making sure that the lighting conditions are the same as they were in the "before" measurement because the normal pupil's light reaction could disguise the result. Comparing before and after tells whether or not the abnormal pupil has constricted significantly more than the pupil of the other eye. If this is the case, the diagnosis is tonic pupil.

If there is no iris damage or strabismus and no segmental constriction to light or light-near dissociation and if 0.1% pilocarpine does not cause pupil constriction, then the differential diagnosis comes down to internal ophthalmoplegia due to third nerve damage versus pharmacological block. These are distinguished by instilling two drops (30 seconds apart) of 1% pilocarpine in each eye, waiting 30 minutes, and comparing

---

*Because individual sensitivities to pharmacological agents vary, always instill drops in both eyes and use the normal eye as a control.

the pupil size between eyes. Again, make sure illumination is the same before and after instilling drops. Pilocarpine 1% is strong enough to cause constriction in an eye with intact postganglionic fibers but is blocked by atropinic agents at the receptor. Therefore, in a third nerve palsy there is constriction in both eyes, and anisocoria is reduced; in a pharmacological block only the normal eye constricts, increasing the anisocoria.

To summarize, then:

1. If the larger pupil constricts to 0.1% pilocarpine, postganglionic denervation is present and the diagnosis is tonic pupil.
2. If the larger pupil constricts to 1% pilocarpine, but not to 0.1% pilocarpine, a preganglionic (cranial nerve III) problem is present.
3. If the larger pupil does not constrict to 1% pilocarpine and there is no mechanical interference, the diagnosis is pharmacological block.

It is important to keep in mind that the differential diagnosis is usually made on the basis of an entire constellation of signs and symptoms and is not based solely on pharmacological testing.

**Clinical Significance** Of the four major causes of anisocoria with a dilated, nonresponsive pupil, *third nerve palsy* is of the greatest concern. Many conditions can damage the preganglionic parasympathetic pupillomotor pathways, either at the midbrain nuclei or along the nerve as it runs in the middle cranial fossa, through the cavernous sinus, and into the orbit. Although it is beyond the scope of this chapter to discuss all the possible causes of unilateral cranial nerve III palsy, the most frequently implicated are vascular disease (stroke from atherosclerosis and/or hypertension), compressive lesion (tumor or aneurysm), demyelinating disease (multiple sclerosis), diabetes, inflammation, infection, and trauma. Different etiologies tend to affect different parts of the pathway, but localizing the lesion is obviously beyond the scope of the routine eye examination. A patient with a previously undiagnosed third nerve palsy should be referred immediately for a neurological examination.

*Tonic pupil syndrome* can be caused by any insult to the ciliary ganglion or short ciliary nerves, including local inflammation or infection, systemic neuropathies, trauma, surgery, and space-occupying lesions. The term *Adie's syndrome* is used to indicate the presence of tonic pupil in apparently healthy individuals who have no evidence of ocular or peripheral disease, with

the possible exception of abnormal deep tendon reflexes. This particular form of tonic pupil is found about twice as often in women as in men, with its age of onset between about 20 and 50 years of age; it is usually (80%) unilateral.[1]

The acute phase of tonic pupil is characterized by mydriasis, diminished or absent light *and near* response, and accommodative paresis. Patients present because they notice the difference in the size of their pupils or because their vision is blurred. With time (weeks to months), the pupil gets smaller and less reactive; accommodation tends to recover somewhat, although it usually remains somewhat slow, both in focusing and in relaxing. Along with the recovery of accommodation comes light-near dissociation, as some of the regenerating accommodative fibers find their way to the pupillary sphincter[2]; pupillary redilation after near effort is slow, however.

A sudden internal ophthalmoplegia without pain or other neurological signs that responds to dilute (0.1%) pilocarpine can be presumed to be a tonic pupil. The patient should be followed until the acute phase has given way to the tonic phase, proving the diagnosis. If there is any doubt or if pupil signs are accompanied by pain, the patient should be referred for a neurological workup.

## Anisocoria with Normal Light Response

If pupil response in both eyes is normal and if the anisocoria is greater in dim light than in bright light, the differential diagnosis is between simple anisocoria and a lesion in the sympathetic pathway to the iris dilator (Horner's syndrome). Because the first is completely benign and the second may signal life-threatening disease, the differential diagnosis is very important.

### Differential Diagnosis

*Simple Anisocoria* Benign ("simple, central," "see-saw") anisocoria is most likely an exaggerated form of the asymmetry in supranuclear inhibition to the Edinger-Westphal nuclei, thought to be present in all individuals.[2] This anisocoria is highly variable, changing from day to day or even hour to hour, sometimes going away and sometimes even reversing direction. It tends to run in families and is not associated with any type of pathology.[2] Old photographs in which anisocoria is evident show that the condition is longstanding—which is reassuring—but does not differentiate between a simple anisocoria and a congenital or an early acquired injury to the sympathetic pathway.*

***Horner's Syndrome***   Any lesion in the sympathetic pathway to the dilator muscle causes a loss of tone in the dilator muscle and thus a relative miosis on the affected side. Even with complete interruption of the sympathetic supply, the miosis is moderate† because supranuclear inhibition of constriction is still intact. Lesions affecting the sympathetic pathway proximal to the superior cervical ganglion are also likely to interfere with sympathetic innervation to the blood vessels and sweat glands of the face and to the smooth muscle of the eyelid. Thus, miosis is commonly accompanied by relative warmth and dryness of the skin, a narrowing of the palpebral aperture due to both elevation of the lower lid ("upside-down ptosis") and drooping of the upper lid. Like all sympathetic functions, these signs are highly dependent on the emotional state and alertness of the patient at the time of examination, and they may be very subtle in the morning, when the patient is fresh, but grow more obvious with fatigue. (The upper lid ptosis associated with Horner's syndrome is rarely as obvious as that due to third nerve palsy.) The anisocoria varies inversely with ambient illumination because only in dim conditions does the dilator muscle play a major role in pupil size. Because Horner's syndrome can easily be missed in normal room lighting, careful observation of relative pupil size in reduced illumination may be the only way of detecting it, unlike a parasympathetic anisocoria, which is most obvious under favorable viewing conditions and in which a reduced light reflex is an obvious adjunct sign.

Here again, history can be extremely important in differential diagnosis. Any trauma (including surgery) involving the brain stem, upper spine, neck, or head may cause disruption of the sympathetic supply to the eye. Because the sympathetic fibers to Müller's muscles accompany the pupillomotor fibers along the internal carotid artery, "upside-down" ptosis is a more dependable indicator of Horner's syndrome than are facial anhidrosis, facial flushing, or conjunctival hyperemia. Grimson and Thompson[10] describe a simple test for confirming the presence of this ptosis. Have the patient follow a target into upgaze until the lower lid on the side of the miosis is just touching the corneal limbus. Observe the lower lid of the other eye: If sclera is visible, it represents an "upside-down" ptosis.

If no clear accompanying signs of sympathetic denervation are present with which to differentiate Horner's syndrome from simple anisocoria, the first thing to look for is dilation lag, which is an increase in anisocoria in the first few seconds after turning the lights down. Although in both conditions the anisocoria is greater in dim illumination, the dynamics of redilation are quite different; in simple anisocoria, the sympathetic innervation to the dilator muscle is completely normal and reflex dilation in response to dark (or psychosensory stimuli) is brisk. In patients with simple anisocoria, both the smaller and the larger pupil should redilate at roughly the same rate. This is not the case with Horner's syndrome, however, where the innervation to the iris dilator is compromised. Although some redilation eventually occurs on the affected side as a result of reflex inhibition of the iris sphincter, this "passive" redilation is slower than on the normal side. Therefore the anisocoria is greatest just after the lights go down (for the first 4 to 5 seconds) and then decreases to some stable intermediate level after 10 to 15 seconds. Thompson and Pilley[7] suggest using flash photography for the documentation of dilation lag. Photographs are taken in normal illumination, then 5 seconds and 10 to 15 seconds after turning off the lights.

If the search for dilation lag is difficult or inconclusive, establish the differential diagnosis by administering one drop of 2 to 10% topical cocaine hydrochloride (generally available in 4% and 10% solutions) in each eye and observing both eyes after 45 minutes. Cocaine prevents the re-uptake of norepinephrine (the adrenergic neurotransmitter) at the neuromuscular junction, thus acting as a passive agent of pupil dilation *after norepinephrine has been released* by sympathetic nerve impulses. In eyes affected by denervation anywhere along the sympathetic pathway, no norepinephrine is being released; the cocaine has no effect and the miotic eye fails to dilate. In eyes with intact sympathetic innervation (e.g., simple anisocoria), cocaine enhances the effectiveness of the norepinephrine at the synapse and thus causes dilation. That is, dilation of the miotic eye indicates that the sympathetic pathways are intact and Horner's syndrome is not present. If the normal pupil dilates but the miotic eye fails to dilate, the diagnosis is Horner's syndrome.

Horner's syndrome can be caused by damage in any one of the three segments of the sympathetic pathway from the hypothalamus to the iris. Although a failure to dilate to cocaine indicates sympathetic denervation, it does not identify which of the three segments of the sympa-

---

*However, a loss of iris pigment on the affected side is an indicator of longstanding sympathetic denervation.

†Compared, for example, to miosis from Argyll Robertson syndrome.

thetic pathway is damaged. Because some causes of Horner's syndrome are life-threatening, some are relatively benign, and different etiologies cause damage in different parts of the pathway, once the presence of Horner's syndrome has been established it is important to distinguish between central or preganglionic lesions and postganglionic lesions. To do this, instill hydroxy-amphetamine (Paredine) 1% in each eye* and observe the pupils after 45 minutes. Hydroxy-amphetamine is an indirect sympathomimetic that acts by releasing stored norepinephrine from the nerve terminals of intact postganglionic sympathetic fibers. Postganglionic lesions destroy some or all of the fibers to the iris dilator muscle, along with their norepinephrine supplies, leaving the hydroxyamphetamine little or nothing to release; no significant dilation occurs. On the other hand, a central or preganglionic lesion leaves the postganglionic (third-order) neurons intact. Stored norepinephrine is thus available for release by the hydroxyamphetamine, and dilation occurs.

In summary, if the smaller pupil dilates to cocaine hydrochloride, the diagnosis is simple, central anisocoria. If the smaller pupil fails to dilate to cocaine hydrochloride but does dilate to hydroxyamphetamine, the diagnosis is central or preganglionic Horner's syndrome. If the smaller pupil fails to dilate to both cocaine hydrochloride and hydroxyamphetamine, the diagnosis is postganglionic Horner's syndrome.

**Clinical Significance**   Although pharmacological tests do not differentiate between central and preganglionic Horner's syndrome, both may reflect serious pathology and need to be referred for investigation of the cause.

Central Horner's syndromes are relatively rare[10, 11] and result from damage to the parasympathetic pathways in the brain stem or upper spinal cord. Lesions in these areas usually cause multiple neurological signs rather than an isolated pupil defect. Although vascular disorders are the most common cause of central Horner's syndrome, trauma, surgery, tumors, demyelinating disease, and infectious neuropathies can also impair the first-order sympathetic neurons on their way to their synapse with the preganglionic fibers at the ciliospinal center of Budge-Waller.[1]

Preganglionic Horner's syndrome results from damage to the second-order fibers making up the sympathetic pathway from the spinal cord to the superior cervical ganglion. Invasive tumors of the lung and breast are common causes of pre-

ganglionic Horner's syndrome. Pain in the shoulder and arm on the same side as the miotic pupil in a previously undiagnosed preganglionic Horner's syndrome patient is highly suggestive of neoplasm; such patients should be referred for appropriate diagnostic workup.[12] Other possible causes of preganglionic Horner's syndrome include brachial plexus injury (e.g., from birth trauma†) and neck trauma or surgery.

A postganglionic Horner's syndrome is least likely to reflect serious, previously undetected pathology, being most often caused by vascular headache or head trauma.[10] Loewenfeld suggests that disruption of the blood supply to the superior cervical ganglion resulting from carotid disease or neck surgery (such as lymph gland or tumor removal or thyroidectomy) can cause postganglionic Horner's syndrome.[3] This might be a source of confusion in cases in which the anatomical site of the insult seems to predict preganglionic damage but pharmacological testing reveals a postganglionic lesion.

Unlike damage to preganglionic fibers, which regenerate quickly after trauma, postganglionic damage tends to be permanent.[3]

## LIGHT-NEAR DISSOCIATION

As we have already seen, light-near dissociation—the state defined by greater pupil constriction to near stimulus than to light stimulus—is a common and diagnostically helpful sign in patients with tonic pupil syndromes. In such patients the conventional efferent pathway to the pupil sphincter has been disrupted, thus reducing or abolishing the direct light reaction on the affected side, but aberrant regeneration of damaged accommodative fibers results in some of these fibers finding their way into the pupillary pathway. As a result, accommodative impulses reach the pupil, causing constriction. A similar effect can be seen in some other cases, in which regenerated fibers from a damaged branch of the third nerve serving the medial rectus make their way into the pupil sphincter pathway, such that miosis occurs with convergence.[13]

An entirely different form of light-near dissociation occurs as a result of a lesion in the rostral midbrain. This syndrome is characterized by bi-

---

*Unless the normal eye has been previously dilated with cocaine, in which case test only the miotic pupil.

†Congenital preganglionic Horner's syndrome can interfere with development of postganglionic fibers; these patients may not dilate to hydroxyamphetamine and may thus be mistakenly diagnosed with postganglionic Horner's syndrome.[3] Heterochromia and a history of longstanding anisocoria (as evidenced by baby pictures) may help dispel confusion.

lateral miosis (more apparent in dim lighting), bilateral loss of the light reflex, irregular pupils, and an intact near response. This syndrome goes by the name of *Argyll Robertson pupil.* Although it has historically been associated with syphilis, it has many other possible causes, including neoplasm, vascular occlusion, and inflammatory disease.[14]

The presumed mechanism for the Argyll Robertson syndrome is as follows: A lesion of the rostral midbrain disrupts the connections from the pretectal nuclei to the oculomotor nuclei but does not affect the connections from the cortex to the oculomotor nuclei serving the near response. Thus, the light reflex suffers, but the near reflex does not. Walsh suggests that the miosis may be due to several factors, including compromise to the sympathetic pathways (reducing dilator tone) and abnormally increased iris sphincter tone secondary to disruption of the supranuclear inhibitory pathways of the Edinger-Westphal nuclei.[1]

Because longstanding tonic pupil syndrome can result in miotic pupils and because it can also be bilateral, it is possible to confuse these two conditions. In this case, observe the constriction and redilation of the pupils with and after near effort. Argyll Robertson pupils constrict and redilate crisply, whereas tonic pupils do both slowly.

Finally, remember that any visual problem that severely reduces the pupillary light response causes light-near dissociation. However, severe visual problems tend to increase, rather than decrease, the pupil size, so there should be no confusion.

In conclusion, the technically simple pupillary examination surveys the visual system and its innervation in all its complexity. Learning how to perform a proper pupillary examination helps the astute clinician diagnose many subtle problems and, in certain cases, may save patients' lives.

# References

1. Walsh FB: Walsh and Hoyt's Clinical Neuro-Ophthalmology. Baltimore: Williams & Wilkins, 1982-1995.
2. Loewenfeld IE: The Pupil: Anatomy, Physiology, and Clinical Applications. Detroit: Wayne State University Press, 1993.
3. Loewenfeld IE: Pupillary changes related to age. *In* Thompson HS, et al.: Topics in Neuro-Ophthalmology. Baltimore: Williams & Wilkins, 1979.
4. Zinn KM: The Pupil. Springfield, IL: Charles C Thomas, 1972.
5. Smith JL: The Pupil. Miami: JL Smith, 1976.
6. Cox TA, Drewes CP: Contraction anisocoria resulting from half-field illumination. Am J Ophthalmol 1984; 97:577-582.
7. Thompson HS, Pilley FJ: Unequal pupils. A flow chart for sorting out the anisocorias. Surv Ophthalmol 1976; 21:45-48.
8. Thompson HS, Montague P, Cox TA, et al.: The relationship between visual acuity, pupillary defect, and visual field loss. Am J Ophthalmol 1982; 93:681-688.
9. Bourgon P, Thompson HS: How to test for cholinergic supersensitivity of the iris sphincter. *In* Thompson HS, et al.: Topics in Neuro-Ophthalmology. Baltimore: Williams & Wilkins, 1979.
10. Grimson BS, Thompson HS: Horner's syndrome: Overall view of 120 cases. *In* Thompson HS, et al.: Topics in Neuro-Ophthalmology. Baltimore: Williams & Wilkins, 1979.
11. Maloney WF, Young BR, Moyer NJ: Evaluation of the causes and accuracy of pharmacologic localization in Horner's syndrome. Am J Ophthalmol 1980; 90:394-402.
12. Slamovits TL, Glaser JS: The pupils and accommodation. *In* Glaser JS: Neuro-Ophthalmology. Philadelphia: JB Lippincott, 1990.
13. Thompson HS: Light-near dissociation of the pupil. Ophthalmologica 1984; 189:21-23.
14. Thompson HS: Pupillary light-near dissociation. A classification. Surv Ophthalmol 1975; 19:290-292.

*Donald O. Mutti, OD, PhD*
*Karla Zadnik, OD, PhD*

4

# Refractive Error

The eye as a living camera is an analogy that eye care practitioners have used as an educational tool with patients for generations. The analogy works particularly well when discussing refractive error, as the concept of blur in photographs is one that all patients can understand and extend to their own vision. Clear vision at distance and near occurs in **emmetropia,** when there is a match between the length of the eye and the focal length of the dioptrics of the eye (Fig. 4-1*A*).

Defects in focus can take several forms. If the optics of the eye are too strong for the length of the eye, the images of distant objects focus anterior to the retina and result in **myopia,** or nearsightedness (Fig. 4-1*B*). Myopia can occur in an eye of normal size with high corneal or lenticular power, or in an eye with average corneal and crystalline lens power but too great a length. **Hyperopia** occurs when the optics of the eye are too weak for the length of the eye, with images of distant objects coming into focus behind the retina (Fig. 4-1*C*). Again, this occurs either when the cornea and lens are too weak in an eye of normal size or when the size is inadequate in an eye with normal cornea and crystalline lens powers.

**Astigmatism** is more difficult to explain to patients because cameras ordinarily use spherical optics. Astigmatism ("a-stigma" = not pointlike) is a refractive condition in which there is no single focal point but rather an interval between two line foci called the interval of Stürm. (Point foci occur when there is equal power in all meridians of an optical system.) Astigmatism occurs when there is a difference in focal power between meridians. The astigmatism is **regular** when the meridians containing the maximum and minimum power are 90° apart and **irregular** when some other angle or angles separate them or when the refracting surface itself is irregular. If refractive error were plotted as a function of polar angle around the line of sight, regular astigmatism may be thought of as a sine wave whose amplitude represents the amount of astigmatism and whose phase represents the axis, whereas irregular astigmatism is a more complex wave form. The majority of refractive astigma-

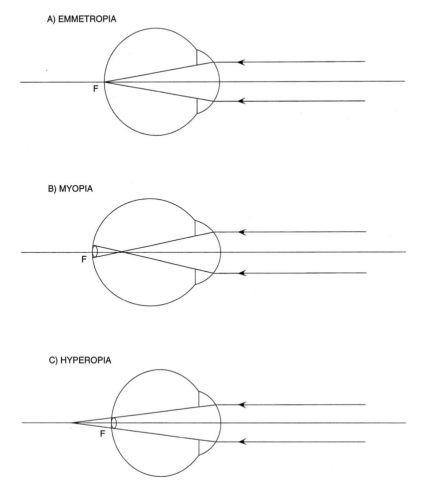

A) EMMETROPIA

B) MYOPIA

C) HYPEROPIA

**FIGURE 4–1** Diagrammatic representation of three common spherical refractive states. *A,* If the dioptric power of the eye is such that its focal length matches its axial length, the retina is in the correct position to receive focused light from a distant source. This is termed *emmetropia,* or having no refractive error. *B,* When the dioptrics of the eye are too strong for the eye's axial length or the eye is too long and the retina is beyond the eye's focal length, *myopia* results. Images of a distant point source appear as a blur circle on the retina. *C,* When the dioptrics of the eye are too weak for the eye's axial length or the eye is too short and the retina is beyond the eye's focal length, *hyperopia* results. If the patient does not accommodate to increase the eye's dioptric power, images of a distant point source also appear as a blur circle on the retina.

tism comes from corneal toricity, with other sources being tilt and decentration of the crystalline lens. Often the words "toricity" and "astigmatism" are used interchangeably; however, astigmatism more precisely refers to the differences in net refractive error or focal power between meridians, whereas toricity refers to the difference in the physical radius of curvature between meridians and produces astigmatism.

Fortunately, given the vertical and horizontal nature of the English alphabet, most astigmatism is oriented in these meridians. Many uncorrected astigmats can still read letters with fair accuracy (Fig. 4–2). Most astigmats have the vertical meridian as the more myopic; this astigmatism is called **with-the-rule.** When the horizontal meridian is more myopic, the astigmatism is **against-the-rule.** Figure 4–2 depicts with-the-rule astigmatism. The vertical meridian has the greater power, bringing light from optical infinity to a horizontal line focus. The less myopic horizontal meridian brings light to a vertical line focus closer to the retina. Because both of these line foci are in front of the retina, this is termed

**compound myopic astigmatism** (Fig. 4–2*A*). If the interval of Stürm straddles the retina, this is **mixed astigmatism** (Fig. 4–2*B*). Both line foci are located behind the retina in **compound hyperopic astigmatism** (Fig. 4–2*C*). If one meridian is focused on the retina, **simple myopic astigmatism** is produced if the other meridian is focused in front of the retina, and **simple hyperopic astigmatism** exists if the other meridian is focused behind the retina.

# Ocular Component Development

· · · · · · · · · · · · · · · · · · · · · · · · ·

Refractive error is not a physical quantity in itself but is the optical sum of the ocular components' individual mismatches. It is therefore important to understand normal ocular component development in order to understand refractive development. Data on the growth of the components from birth through the early teens are taken from several sources (Fig. 4–3). Most of the compo-

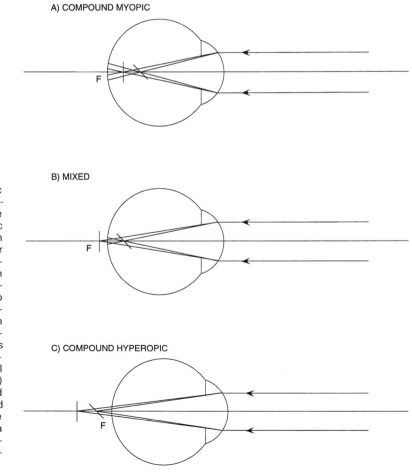

A) COMPOUND MYOPIC

F

B) MIXED

F

C) COMPOUND HYPEROPIC

F

**FIGURE 4–2** Diagrammatic representation of three common astigmatic refractive states. *A,* Compound myopic astigmatism occurs when both meridians are focused anterior to the retina. *B,* Mixed astigmatism occurs when one meridian is focused anterior and one meridian is focused posterior to the retina. *C,* Compound hyperopic astigmatism occurs when both meridians are focused behind the retina. These diagrams depict with-the-rule astigmatism because the vertical meridian (horizontal line focus) is more myopic. Compound myopic, mixed, and compound hyperopic against-the-rule astigmatisms are defined in a similar fashion, with the horizontal and vertical line foci reversed.

TOP

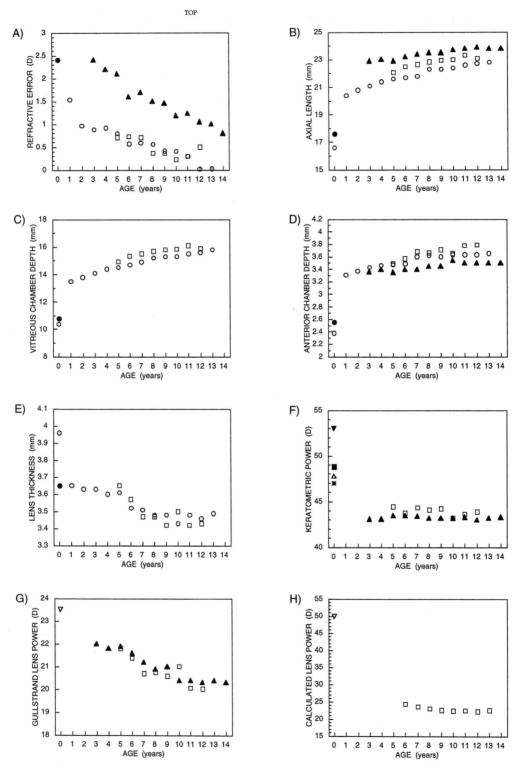

**FIGURE 4–3**  Growth curves for the various ocular components from birth through the age of 14 years. *A,* Refractive error: ● Luyckx (1966); ◯ Larsen (1971); ▲ Sorsby et al. (1961); ☐ Zadnik et al. (1993). *B,* Axial length: same with ◯ Larsen (1971). *C,* Vitreous chamber depth: same with ◯ Larsen (1971). *D,* Anterior chamber depth: same as *A. E,* Lens thickness: same with ◯ Larsen (1971). *F,* Keratometer power: same with ▼ Grignolo and Rivara (1968); △ York and Mandell (1969); ■ Mandell (1967) × Inagaki (1986); + Insler et al. (1987). *G,* Gullstrand lens power. *H,* Calculated lens power: same with ▽ Wood et al. (in preparation).

**TABLE 4–1** Newborn Refractive Errors as Measured by Retinoscopy

| Author | Number | Age | Method | Mean Refraction | Percentage Myopic |
|---|---|---|---|---|---|
| Goldschmidt (1969) | 356 infants | 2–10 days | Atropine 0.5% | +0.62 ± 2.24 D | 24.2 |
| Santonastaso (1930) | 34 infants | 0–3 months | Atropine | +1.67 ± 2.54 D | 8 |
| Luyckx (1966) | 104 eyes | 0–1 week | Cyclopentolate 1% | +2.40 ± 1.20 D | 0 |
| Cook and Glasscock (1951) | 1000 eyes | After post-delivery care | Atropine 1% ointment | +1.54 D | 25.1 |
| Zonis and Miller (1974) | 600 eyes | 48–72 hours | Mydriaticum | +1.10 ± 1.60 D | 14.5 |
| Mohindra et al. (1981) | 48 infants | 0–4 weeks | Non-cycloplegic near retinoscopy | −0.70 ± 3.20 D | Not given |
| | 27 infants | 5–8 weeks | | −0.35 ± 2.30 D | |
| | 78 infants | 9–16 weeks | | −0.52 ± 2.25 D | |
| | 70 infants | 17–32 weeks | | +0.13 ± 1.39 D | |
| | 50 infants | 33–64 weeks | | +0.78 ± 0.97 D | |

nents undergo rapid development between birth and 5 years. At birth, the typical eye is hyperopic and about 17 mm long. Over the next 5 years, vitreous chamber depth increases by 3 to 4 mm, anterior chamber depth by 1 mm, and axial length by 4 to 5 mm. Surprisingly, the crystalline lens appears to either maintain its thickness or undergo thinning despite the continual growth of new fibers and increase in weight throughout life. As the eye grows, changes in equivalent lens power are quite rapid, decreasing nearly 25.00 D by the age of 5 years. Lens power decreases several more diopters during the school years, and the equivalent refractive index of the lens decreases with age, indicating a change in the distribution of the actual gradient index structure of the crystalline lens during the growth of the eye.[1] The cornea also develops rapidly, losing 5.00 to 10.00 D of power in the first year of life, with little change after that time. Refractive error on average decreases in hyperopia by 1.00 to 2.00 D, and myopia decreases in prevalence to only about 2%.

## Refractive Error in Infancy

As seen in Table 4-1, most studies of infant cycloplegic refractive error conclude that newborns are moderately hyperopic with a fairly broad distribution of refractive errors. Myopia is also commonly, albeit sporadically, reported in newborns, with frequencies ranging from 0 to 25%. The data from Cook and Glasscock[2] (Fig. 4-4) show the normal distribution skewed toward hyperopia, typical of neonatal refractive error. Several factors may be responsible for the myopia seen in infants. One is poor response to cycloplegia. Goldschmidt[3] noted that the infant pupil responds poorly to mydriatics, a common clinical observation. If there is some immaturity

to the cholinergic receptors in the infant ciliary body, it is unknown how deeply infants may experience cycloplegia. It is clear, however, that cycloplegia may reveal latent hyperopia in many infants. Many infants who were myopic by non-cycloplegic retinoscopy were quite hyperopic following instillation of atropine.[4] Mean refractive error is less hyperopic when near (non-cycloplegic) retinoscopy is used than when cycloplegic retinoscopy is used.[5]

A second source of myopia in infancy is prematurity. Dobson et al.[6] found that the average refraction of 146 premature infants was −0.55 D, much more myopic than expected for full-term newborns. Grignolo and Rivara[7] studied both refractive error and ocular components in 58 full-

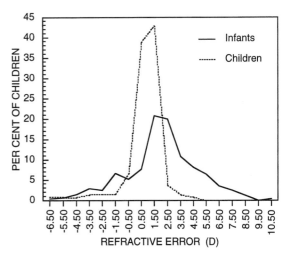

**FIGURE 4–4** Comparison of refractive error distribution from newborns (Cook and Glasscock, 1951) with that from children (unpublished data from the Orinda Longitudinal Study of Myopia: Vertical meridian cycloplegic autorefraction, 1993). Note the reduced standard deviation and higher peak near emmetropia in the data for children, indicating the process of emmetropization.

**TABLE 4–2** Prevalence of Myopia in 8- to 13-Year-Old Children as a Function of Birth Weight

| Premature Children Weight Group | Number | Prevalence of Myopia | Mean Refraction (D) |
|---|---|---|---|
| ≤1500 grams | 89 | 17% | +0.52 |
| 1501–1750 grams | 93 | 14% | +0.76 |
| >1750 grams | 118 | 10% | +0.92 |

From Fledelius H: Prematurity and the eye. Acta Ophthalmol (Suppl) 1976; 128:1-245.

term and 57 premature infants. Premature newborns had a mean refractive error of +0.50 D and were about −1.00 D less hyperopic than full-term infants. The source of this relative myopia was the premature infants' greater refractive power of the cornea and crystalline lens. The axial length of the eye in premature infants was actually 0.75 mm shorter (equivalent to about +4.50 D in an infant eye) than in full-term babies. In addition to less hyperopia and shorter axial lengths, Fledelius[8] found that premature infants had thicker lenses (3.99 versus 3.76 mm) and shallower anterior chamber depths (2.38 versus 2.65 mm) than full-term infants. These differ-

ences diminish by the age of 6 months,[7] unless retinopathy of prematurity is present, in which case myopia of prematurity tends to persist.[9] Fledelius[10] found that myopia over −6.00 D was more common (1.1%) at ages 8 to 13 years in 300 Danish children who had low birth weights (<2000 grams) than in 237 children born at full term (0.2% highly myopic). Although the distributions of refractive errors were similar between the two groups as a whole, there was an association between myopia at 8 to 13 years and birth weight (Table 4–2).

A curious feature of infant refractive error is a high prevalence of refractive astigmatism oriented against-the-rule. Anywhere from 17%[11] to 63%[12] of infants may have astigmatism greater than 1.00 DC (Table 4–3). Most reports place the orientation against-the-rule (minus cylinder axis 90°) in 40% to 100% of cases. Proposed explanations for this astigmatism have been a large angle lambda,[13] decentration or tilt of the crystalline lens, and a change in accommodative posture between measurement of the two meridians during non-cycloplegic retinoscopy. Howland and Sayles[14] showed, from photokeratometric measures, that this astigmatism is primarily corneal, especially in infants less than 1 year of age. This

**TABLE 4–3** Estimates of the Prevalence and Orientation of Astigmatism ≥1.00 DC in Infancy (Under 1 Year)

| Author | Number | Method | Age | Prevalence of Astigmatism (≥1.00 DC) | Orientation |
|---|---|---|---|---|---|
| Ingram and Barr (1979) | 296 eyes | Atropine retinoscopy | 1 year | 29.7% | Not given |
| Fulton et al. (1980) | 133 infants | Cyclopentolate 1% retinoscopy | 40–50 weeks | 20% | 71% ATR<br>21% WTR<br>8% oblique (for children 0–3 months) |
| Dobson et al. (1984) | 46 infants<br>187 infants | Cyclopentolate 1% retinsocopy | 0–6 months<br>6–18 months | 17%<br>19% | 100% ATR<br>70% ATR<br>18% WTR<br>2% oblique |
| Santonastaso (1930) | 63 infants | Atropine retinoscopy | 0–12 months | 52.4% | 15% ATR<br>85% WTR |
| Howland et al. (1978) | 93 infants | Non-cycloplegic photorefraction | 0–12 months | 47% | 70% "horizontal and vertical" |
| Gwiazda et al. (1974) | 521 infants | Non-cycloplegic near retinoscopy | 0–11 months | 53% | 44% ATR<br>39% WTR<br>16% oblique |
| Howland and Sayles (1984) | 117 infants | Non-cycloplegic photorefraction | 0–12 months | 63% | 55% ATR<br>3% WTR<br>42% oblique |
| Mohindra et al. (1978) | 276 right eyes | Non-cycloplegic near retinoscopy | <1–50 weeks | 45% | 40% ATR<br>40% WTR<br>20% oblique |

astigmatism is also transient. The prevalence of cylinders ≥1.00 DC decreases rapidly during the first year of life, reaching levels found in childhood by the age of 18 months[15] to 2 years.[16]

# Refractive Error in Childhood

. . . . . . . . . . . . . . . . . . . . . . . . . .

A fascinating process occurs in ocular development. Recall that the distribution of refractive errors at birth closely resembles a normal distribution, with some skew toward hyperopia. Figure 4-4 shows that between infancy and childhood, the eye grows in such a way that the distribution of refractive errors shifts toward emmetropia; narrows considerably, with most children emmetropic to slightly hyperopic; and shows a shift in skew toward myopia. The growth curve in Figure 4-3A depicts the slow decline in average hyperopia from infancy through childhood. This process, whereby mean refractive error shifts toward emmetropia and the entire distribution of refractive errors decreases in standard deviation, is termed **emmetropization.**

When does emmetropization stop? Between the ages of 5 and 15 years, ocular component development is much slower. The cornea is remarkably stable throughout childhood, on average. Anterior chamber depth increases only 0.1

to 0.2 mm and vitreous chamber depth and axial length by about 1 mm. Crystalline lens thinning continues its earlier trend by thinning another 0.15 to 0.20 mm. Many textbooks describe the lens as a unique part of the body in that it grows throughout life, continually laying new fibers onto the lens cortex. Studies reviewed by Larsen[17] show that the lens weighs about 65 mg at birth and doubles its weight during the first year of life, growing very slowly after age 1 year. A redoubling of weight to 258 mg does not occur until age 80 years. While the lens may grow by laying down new fibers, it does not continually grow by thickening axially. Lens power decreases by about 2.00 D, whether in the Gullstrand or the calculated form. The average hyperopia decreases by about 1.00 D. It is fascinating that during this time of relatively slow average growth compared with earlier in life, the prevalence of myopia increases more than seven times, to 15%.

As shown in Table 4-4, the prevalence of myopia remains low, under 2%, until about the age of 7 or 8 years, when there is a sudden rise in prevalence which begins to level off only in the early teens (Fig. 4-5).[18] Myopia with onset during these years is termed **juvenile onset.** This myopia typically progresses after its onset, with an average rate of increase of about −0.50 ± 0.30 D per year.[19-21] As is apparent from Figure 4-3B, the eye continues to grow throughout the teen years, suggesting that myopia progresses in these children because the crystalline lens's ability to

**TABLE 4–4**    Prevalence of Refractive Error in Children (Predominantly Caucasian Samples)

| Author | Number | Method | Age (Years) | Prevalence of Hyperopia | Prevalence of Myopia |
|---|---|---|---|---|---|
| Laatikainen and Erkkilä (1980) | 162 218 222 220 | Cyclopentolate 1% retinoscopy | 7–8 9–10 11–12 14–15 | (≥ +2.00 D) 19.1% 6.9% 11.7% 3.6% | (≤ −0.50 D) 1.9% 6.4% 7.2% 21.8% |
| Blum et al. (1959) | Not specified (>1000 children total in the study) | Non-cycloplegic retinoscopy | 5 6 7 8 9 10 11 12 13 14 15 | ≥ +1.50 D 6% for all ages | 2% 2.25% 2.5% 4% 5.5% 8% 10.5% 12.25% 13.25% 14.5% 15% |
| Kempf et al. (1928) | 1860 children | Homatropine retinoscopy | 6–8 9–11 12 or more | > +1.00 D 35.4% 25.2% 15.2% | ≤ −0.75 D 1.2% 3.4% 4.8% |
| Sperduto et al. (1983) | Not specified | Screening-based | 12–17 | Not measured | 23.9% |

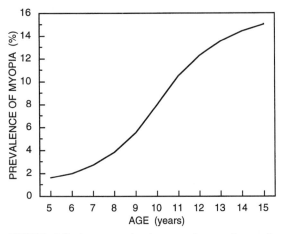

**FIGURE 4–5** Increases in the prevalence of myopia (at least −0.50 D by non-cycloplegic retinoscopy) as a function of age. (Data from Blum et al., 1959.)

compensate for axial length increases is reduced. All the millimeters of axial length increase translate directly into diopters of myopia. Sorsby et al.[22] found that the average values of components of children at 14 to 15 years of age were not different from those of young adult military recruits 19 to 21 years old. He concluded that the eye does not grow appreciably after age 13 to 14 years. The age of cessation of the progression of myopia is 14 to 15 years for girls and 15 to 17 years for boys[23] and is consistent with the cessation of ocular growth. There is clearly considerable variation around this average age of cessation, as many patients' myopia progresses well into adulthood. Additionally, many patients, perhaps another 10% of the population, become myopic for the first time after the teen years. This type of myopia, termed **adult onset,** may be the result of axial growth continuing into adulthood for a small portion of the population. These two forms of myopia bring the total prevalence of myopia in the adult population to about 25%.[24] A third classification for myopia, typically greater than −6.00 D accompanied by degenerative fundus changes, is termed **pathological myopia.**

Most infants begin life with a moderate degree of hyperopia (see Table 4–1). The process of emmetropization then results in a reduction in the amount and the frequency of hyperopia (see Table 4–4), as well as a narrowing of the distribution of refractive error. When one examines a young hyperope, one may wonder whether the hyperopia represents a failure of emmetropization or whether the initial hyperopia was so extreme that emmetropization could not overcome it. Recent longitudinal evidence on infants suggests that the former is the case. In a study

of 93 infants with more than +4.00 D of hyperopia in one meridian at age 9 months, the average change by age 3.5 years was a decrease in hyperopia, but only by −0.50 to −0.75 D.[25]

Slow ocular growth may be both the reason for the appearance of hyperopia and the reason why it does not disappear with time. Correlations listed in Table 4–6 (p. 62) indicate that hyperopic refractions are associated with shorter axial lengths, shallower anterior chamber depths, and flatter corneas. Previous literature suggests that lens power is not correlated with hyperopia, but recent work shows correlations on the order of 0.19, with hyperopes having steeper and more powerful lenses than other refractive groups (Orinda Longitudinal Study of Myopia—unpublished data).

Reports of the prevalence of refractive astigmatism in childhood vary (Table 4–5), with some estimates as high as 45% of children having ≥1.00 DC. These high prevalence estimates come from clinically based samples. When the data are population based,[26-28] the expected prevalence is under 10%. Although against-the-rule astigmatism may still be found in pre-schoolers, with-the-rule astigmatism appears to predominate during the school years. For the most part, this astigmatism appears to be stable throughout childhood in amount and orientation. A small proportion of children may develop astigmatism over the school years. In a longitudinal study, Hirsch[27] found that 81% of children have <0.25 DC at age 6 years, and only 72% have that amount by age 12.5 years. Cylinder orientation appeared to shift slowly toward against-the-rule in a small group of children, with about 8% changing in category from ±0.25 DC to −0.74 DC against-the-rule.

# Refractive Error in Adulthood

Refractive error is generally stable in adulthood. Data from Slataper[29] show a decrease in average hyperopia up to age 20 years in a large clinical sample consisting of refractions in 34,570 eyes under atropine 1% cycloplegia in children and homatropine 2% cycloplegia in adults (Fig. 4–6). Despite a greater level of hyperopia in this sample, perhaps due to the choice of cycloplegic, this trend is expected, given the notion that eye growth and the progression of myopia are largely complete. Little change is seen up to the age of 50 years. At that point, an increase in hyperopia is seen which continues up to the age of about

**TABLE 4–5** Prevalence of Astigmatism in Childhood

| Author | Number | Method | Age (Years) | Prevalence of Astigmatism ($\geq$1.00 DC) | Orientation |
|---|---|---|---|---|---|
| Fabian (1966) | 1200 children | Cyclopentolate retinoscopy | 2 | 2.3% | 70% WTR |
| Dobson et al. (1984) | 98 | Cyclopentolate 1% retinoscopy | 1.5–2.5 | 11% | 35% ATR |
| | 97 | | 2.5–3.5 | 32% | 55% ATR |
| | 105 | | 3.5–4.5 | 37% | 30% ATR |
| | 108 | | 4.5–5.5 | 50% | After age 4: |
| | 87 | | 5.5–6.5 | 41% | 50–60% WTR |
| | 93 | | 6.5–7.5 | 45% | 20–30% oblique |
| | 90 | | 7.5–8.5 | 18% | |
| | 68 | | 8.5–9.5 | 13% | |
| Ingram and Barr (1979) | 296 eyes | Atropine retinoscopy | 3.5 | 7.8% | Not given |
| Fulton et al. (1980) | 149 | Cyclopentolate 1% retinoscopy | 1–2 | 16% | 71% ATR |
| | 94 | | 2–3 | 14% | 21% WTR |
| | | | | | 8% oblique |
| Zadnik et al. (1992) | 231 children | Tropicamide 1% autorefraction | 6–12 | 8.6% | 30% ATR |
| | | | | | 50% WTR |
| | | | | | 20% oblique |
| Hirsch (1963) | 333 eyes | Non-cycloplegic retinoscopy | 6.5 | $\geq$1.25 DC = 1.8% | 100% WTR |
| | | | 8.5 | $\geq$1.25 DC = 2.7% | 100% WTR |
| | | | 10.5 | $\geq$1.25 DC = 2.7% | 100% WTR |
| | | | 12.5 | $\geq$1.25 DC = 3.0% | 100% WTR |
| Howland and Sayles (1984) | 61 | Non-cycloplegic photorefraction | 1–2 | 42% | 50–78% ATR across ages |
| | 29 | | 2–3 | 20% | |
| | 60 | | 3–4 | 10% | <10% WTR |
| | 70 | | 4–5 | 12% | 10–50% oblique |
| Gwiazda et al. (1984) | 63 | Non-cycloplegic near retinoscopy | 1–2 | 43% | 55–65% ATR up to age 4.5, then |
| | 86 | | 2–3 | 30% | |
| | 137 | | 3–4 | 22% | 20–40% ATR, |
| | 140 | | 4–5 | 18% | 60–80% WTR |
| | 53 | | 5–6 | 24% | |

65 years. The underlying cause of this refractive change has confused clinicians and researchers alike. It is well known that the crystalline lens both thickens and steepens during this time,[30] which means that eyes should become more my-

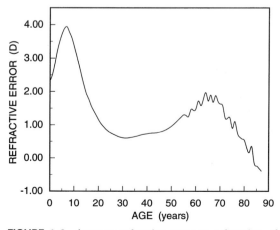

**FIGURE 4–6** Average refractive error as a function of age. (Data from Slataper, 1950.)

opic with age. This has been termed "the lens paradox." It has been suggested that the length of the eye actually shrinks with age in order to prevent this myopia.[31] Recent evidence has shown that although the length of the eye is stable over these years, the gradient refractive index structure of the lens changes so that the net equivalent index of the lens decreases, and so does its equivalent power.[32, 33] The lens radii of curvature may steepen, but this refractive index change causes a net shift toward hyperopia. Population-based estimates of the prevalence of refractive error in Beaver Dam, Wisconsin, show that myopia is much less common at age 65 to 74 years (15%) than it was at age 43 to 54 years (43%).[34] The trend late in life is toward myopia once more, presumably due to cataractous changes, which increase the refractive power of the crystalline lens.

Astigmatism in childhood tends to be with-the-rule (minus cylinder, axis 180), and this finding appears stable through much of early adulthood. Hirsch[35] studied 1606 records of patients between ages 40 and 80 years to determine the changes in refractive astigmatism during that period. Figure 4–7 shows that as in childhood, the most common finding at age 40 years is virtually no astigmatism (45.5%), with a distribution skewed toward with-the-rule orientations. With increasing age, the mean and skew of this distribution shift toward against-the-rule, reaching a prevalence of 35% ≥1.00 DC against-the-rule cylinder by age 80 years.

# Causes of Refractive Error

. . . . . . . . . . . . . . . . . . . . . . . . . .

What is responsible for emmetropization, and what causes refractive error? These two questions are tightly linked, as we can view the development of refractive error as a failure of the emmetropization process that serves most children so well through infancy. The two basic theories for both emmetropization and the development of refractive error may be broadly categorized as nature versus nurture.

## ACTIVE EMMETROPIZATION AND NURTURE

Active emmetropization proposes that the eye is a "smart organ," one that can alter the rate of its growth in response to its own optics. In other words, the axial length grows in order to compensate for errors in the eye's focal length. A hyperopic infant with a weak corneal or lens power would undergo more rapid increases in axial length, thereby reducing the hyperopia, and for a myopic infant the eye would grow more slowly. The primary evidence for such a model comes from animal experimentation. When positive and negative spectacle lenses are placed over the eye of a chick, the chick eye grows to compensate for the error of the inducing lens. When the inducing lens is positive, the myopic blur is compensated by the chick's eye becoming shorter and more hyperopic; when the inducing lens is negative, the hyperopic blur is reduced by the eye growing more quickly and becoming myopic (Fig. 4–8).[36] The degree of compensation is more pronounced for myopic blur from positive lenses than for hyperopic blur from negative lenses. The chick eye is able to reduce hyperopic blur by growing more rapidly, but surprisingly, it reduces myopic blur by increasing choroidal thickness.[37] This effectively pushes the retina forward, making the eye shorter. This type of experiment is an attractive model for active emmetropization because it demonstrates that the eye can monitor and respond to both the sign and magnitude of defocus. Major stumbling blocks to the universal acceptance of this model, however, are that changes in choroidal thickness are not seen in human refractive error,[38] and it is unclear

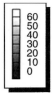

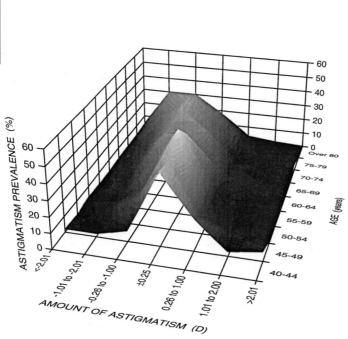

FIGURE 4–7 Three-dimensional surface representing the prevalence of astigmatism as a function of age (Hirsch, 1959). Positive values are with-the-rule, negative against-the-rule. Note how the peak of the surface changes from predominantly with-the-rule to against-the-rule with increasing age while remaining skewed toward with-the-rule at all ages.

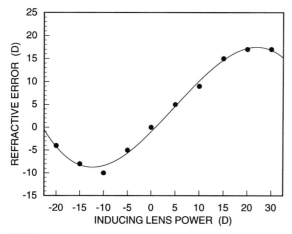

**FIGURE 4–8** The response of the chicken eye to negative and positive inducing lenses. After the chicken wears positive lenses, the eye becomes hyperopic, whereas it becomes myopic in response to negative lenses (Irving et al., 1992).

whether or not the animal is accommodating to the negative lens.[39]

Accommodation during excessive amounts of time spent in near work is the oldest and most often cited suspected environmental cause of myopia. Ware[40] is credited with making the first report in modern times of an association between level of education, near work, and myopia. He noted that only 12 of 10,000 recruits for military service over the previous 20 years had to be discharged for myopia. At a military school in Chelsea, only three schoolchildren of 1300 had myopia. Precise ages were not given. These two groups were meant to represent the prevalence of myopia among the lower, less educated classes. At Oxford, however, 32 of 127 students were myopic. In the late 1800s, Cohn[41] observed that myopia was quite common in the town schools and more rigorous gymnasia but rare in the village schools. Of 240 village schoolchildren between 6 and 13 years examined under atropine cycloplegia, only 1% were myopic. In a more intensive Breslau gymnasium of 361 students, the prevalence of myopia increased from 13% in the youngest to 60% in the oldest class.

Reports from this century echo those from the last. Young et al.[42] measured cycloplegic refractive error and ocular components in an Eskimo population in Barrow, Alaska. Mean refractive error for the younger segment of the population aged 6 to 25 years (n = 283) was − 0.12 D, whereas it was + 1.45 D for those 26 years and above (n = 225). The proportion of the population with − 0.25 D or more myopia in the younger group was 43.4% but only 13.8% in the older group. Only two subjects of the 131 over

45 years had − 0.25 D or more myopia. Young et al.[42] cited the increase in the population of Barrow around 1940 and the concurrent increase in the number of children attending school as the reasons for the higher prevalence of myopia in children than in adults. The prevalence of myopia in Asian students is reported to be as high as 40 to 60%,[43, 44] reportedly due to the near work demands of a rigorous educational system.

## PASSIVE EMMETROPIZATION AND NATURE

Passive emmetropization proposes that the eye is an elegant, if not a smart, organ: one that can alter the rate of change in its optics according to the needs of its growth and size. In other words, the focal length of the eye changes in response to the size and shape of the eye. A hyperopic infant with a weak corneal or lens power would undergo slower decreases in the power of those components as the eye grows in axial length, thereby reducing the hyperopia, and vice versa for a myopic infant. That there is some inborn relationship between size and optics is clear from the fact that eyes as different in size as those of a mouse and an elephant can both be emmetropic. Hofstetter[45] noted this, proposing that absolute size could be irrelevant if the growing eye could maintain certain relationships between its optics and its size.

Proportional growth, as in Hofstetter's model eye, takes place to some degree in the human eye, as shown by the correlations between ocular components* (Table 4-6). The strongest relationship is between refractive error and axial length, indicating that longer eyes are associated with more negative refractive errors. Because anterior chamber depth is included in axial length, they are naturally highly correlated, and anterior chamber depth is related to refraction. The negative correlation between axial length and corneal power indicates that the larger the eye, the flatter the cornea. Corneal power is also significantly related to refraction. Lens power shows little relation to refraction.

Sorsby et al.[46] examined the range of axial lengths seen in emmetropes, finding that eyes anywhere from 21 to 26 mm in length could be emmetropic. Emmetropia was not the product of having the correct axial length, but rather of having the right match between axial length and

---

*Correlation shows how strongly two factors are related, with ± 1.0 indicating perfect correlation and 0.0 indicating no correlation. Positive correlation means that as $x$ increases, so does $y$. Negative correlation means that as $x$ increases, $y$ decreases.

**TABLE 4–6**  Correlations Among Ocular Components

| | Axial Length | Anterior Chamber Depth | Corneal Power | Lens Power |
|---|---|---|---|---|
| Refraction | −0.76 | −0.34 | −0.18 | −0.00 |
| Axial length | | +0.44 | −0.31* | −0.36* |
| | | +0.48 | −0.29† | −0.49† |
| Anterior chamber depth | | | +0.10* | −0.27* |
| Corneal power | | | +0.14† | −0.47† |
| | | | | −0.12* |
| | | | | −0.07† |

From van Alphen GWHM: On emmetropia and ametropia. Ophthalmologica (Suppl) 1961; 142:1–92.
*Data from Stenström.[68]
†Data from Sorsby et al.[46]

primarily (according to Sorsby) corneal power. For ametropias up to ±4.00 D, the cause was not an incorrect axial length, but rather a mismatch with corneal power which he called **correlation ametropia.** Errors greater than ±4.00 D were called **component ametropia** because they were due primarily to excessive axial lengths; the corneas of these patients fell within a range similar to that of emmetropes.

At present, no definitive evidence is available to guide the clinician's decision between these two explanations for emmetropization and the development of refractive error. A substantial amount of evidence also supports a hereditary cause for myopia. Myopic parents tend to have myopic children. The prevalence of myopia in children with two myopic parents is 30 to 40%, whereas it is 20 to 25% in children with one myopic parent and less than 10% in children with no myopic parents.[47, 48]

In our Orinda Longitudinal Study of Myopia, we examined a group of schoolchildren without myopia (refractive error less myopic than −0.75 D in both meridians). Children who are not myopic but have a positive family history of myopia are—on average—less hyperopic, have deeper anterior chambers, and have longer vitreous chambers. In other words, children with a positive family history of myopia have eyes of a different size and shape, namely longer eyes.[47]

Monozygotic (MZ) twins also resemble each other more closely than dizygotic (DZ) twins. Sorsby et al.[49] measured refraction, corneal curvature, anterior chamber depth, lens power and thickness, and axial length in 78 MZ pairs, 40 DZ twins of the same gender, and 48 unrelated pairs. These unrelated pairs were included for comparison because they share neither genes nor the effects of a common familial environment present for both types of twins. Zygosity was determined on the similarity of physical appearance, fingerprints, tasting of phenylthiourea (if one twin could taste it and the other could

not, the twins were considered DZ), and blood type.

MZ twins were within ±1.25 D of each other 90% of the time. Only 55% of DZ twins and 52% of unrelated pairs were within ±1.25 D. MZ twins were within ±1.65 D of each other 95% of the time. Only 62% of DZ twins and 60% of unrelated pairs were within ±1.65 D. This analysis for refraction and the other ocular components is summarized in Table 4–7.

Teikari et al.[50] reported on similarities between refractions of 6314 pairs of twins from the Finnish Twin Cohort Study. Correlations in liability for refractive error between MZ twins were 0.81, compared with 0.30 to 0.40 for DZ twins. From these data, Teikari et al. obtained an estimate of heritability, or the proportion of variability in refractive error that can be accounted for by variability in genetics. Heritabilities were 0.82 for males and 1.02 for females.

If myopia is primarily inherited, then predicting which children are likely to become my-

**TABLE 4–7**  Range of Values for Refraction and the Ocular Components Over Which 95% of MZ Twin Pairs Agree and the Percentage of DZ and Unrelated Pairs That Fall Within That Interval

| | MZ 95% Interval | Percentage Within MZ 95% Interval | |
|---|---|---|---|
| | | DZ | Unrelated |
| Refraction (D) | ±1.65 | 62 | 60 |
| Corneal power (D) | ±1.25 | 72 | 56 |
| Anterior chamber (mm) | ±0.45 | 92 | 92 |
| Lens power (D) | ±1.80 | 75 | 73 |
| Axial length (mm) | ±0.85 | 58 | 65 |

From Sorsby A, Sheridan M, Leary GA: Refraction and Its Components in Twins. London, Her Majesty's Stationery Office, 1962. Crown copyright is reproduced with the permission of the Controller of HMSO.
MZ, monozygotic; DZ, dizygotic.

**TABLE 4–8**  Sensitivity and Specificity
of Various Predictive Tests

| Predictive Test | Test Sensitivity | Test Specificity |
|---|---|---|
| Refraction at school entry | 0.59 | 0.91 |
| Infant refraction (10%) | 0.81 | 0.63 |
| Infant refraction (42%) | 0.62 | 0.59 |
| Both parents myopic | 0.39 | 0.80 |
| Either parent myopic | 0.90 | 0.36 |

Sensitivity is the proportion of future myopes (assuming an eventual prevalence of myopia of 15%) whose myopia is correctly predicted from the test results. Specificity is the proportion of future non-myopes (85% of the population) who are identified correctly based on the results of the predictive test. Predictive tests are (1) refraction at school entry; (2) refraction in infancy assuming 10% of emmetropic infants become myopic; (3) refraction in infancy assuming 42% of emmetropic infants become myopic; (4) history of myopia in both parents; and (5) history of myopia in any parent.[52]

opic should be simple if one knows the refractive error of the parents. Unfortunately, this is not the case. Considering the number of known risk factors for myopia, clinicians are remarkably poor at identifying the child at risk for myopia. Three significant risk factors—parental history of myopia, retinoscopy at school entry,[51] and retinoscopy in infancy[48]—have been reported in sufficient detail to allow for calculation of sensitivity and specificity of the tests.*

Although some tests have high sensitivities, their specificities are low and vice versa. No present test has both high sensitivity and high specificity (Table 4–8). Consider parental history of myopia. If any parent was myopic (one or both), the probability is that 90% of the future myopes would be correctly identified but that 64% of the future nonmyopes would be incorrectly identified as myopic. If both parents were myopic, only 20% of the future non-myopes would be incorrectly categorized as myopic, but the correct identification of future myopes drops to 39%.[52]

What can the clinician tell a parent about whether or not a child will become myopic? If both parents are myopic, the chances are 30 to 40% that the child will develop myopia. If only one parent is myopic, the chances are reduced to 20 to 25%. If no parent is myopic, the chances are less than 10% that the child will ever become myopic. A more complete history and examination can make for a better prediction if several risk factors can be identified and combined. If a child has two myopic parents and a refraction at

school entry less hyperopic than +0.50 D, then the chances are 70% that he or she will develop myopia. Even though the chances that a child with a refraction at school entry of less hyperopia than +0.50 D will develop myopia are about 53%, it is reduced to 22% if neither parent is myopic.

Numerous other risk factors for myopia are known. High levels of near work, high IQ, against-the-rule refractive astigmatism, steep keratometric values, an introverted personality, and near point esophoria are all associated with myopia. It is hoped that data from these risk factors may be available some day in a form by which the clinician can provide each patient with an individual risk profile of the chances of developing myopia.

What can the clinician tell the parent of a child obtaining the first pair of glasses about how myopic the child may become? Predicting a child's ultimate refractive error may be as difficult as predicting its onset, but despite variation in progression of myopia, the clinician can at least provide information on the behavior of the average myopic eye. Mäntyjärvi[53] studied 214 children at ages 15 to 16 years, noting their degree of myopia at that age and the age of onset of their refractive error. As expected, the earlier the onset of myopia, the greater the myopia at ages 15 to 16 years (Table 4-9). The large standard deviations indicate that children may eventually have 2.00 to 4.00 D more or less myopia than these average values. As stated above, an average annual rate of progression of myopia in childhood tends to be $-0.50 \pm 0.30$ D per year.

The young myope and his or her parents are also concerned about when the progression of myopia might stop. Goss and Winkler[54] examined the records of 299 patients from three optometric practices, looking for the age at which juvenile-onset myopia stopped progressing. Al-

**TABLE 4–9**  Expected Amount of Myopia
at Ages 15 to 16 Years Given the
Age of Onset of Myopia

| Age of Onset (Years) | Mean Refractive Error at 15 to 16 Years of Age (D) | Number |
|---|---|---|
| 7–8 | $-5.00 \pm 1.94$ | 9 |
| 9 | $-4.43 \pm 1.87$ | 17 |
| 10 | $-4.16 \pm 1.04$ | 14 |
| 11 | $-3.16 \pm 1.30$ | 47 |
| 12 | $-2.75 \pm 1.08$ | 49 |
| 13 | $-2.54 \pm 0.90$ | 26 |
| 14 | $-2.11 \pm 1.07$ | 28 |
| 15 | $-1.15 \pm 0.62$ | 24 |

From Mäntyjärvi MI: Predicting of myopia progression in school. J Pediatr Ophthalmol Strab 1985; 22:71–75.

---

*Sensitivity is the proportion of future myopes who would have been correctly identified by the test. Specificity is the proportion of future non-myopes also correctly identified.

though four different criteria for progression were used, all methods were consistent in that over 90% of patients no longer progressed in myopia by the age of 20 years. Females tended to stop progressing earlier, with mean ages of cessation ranging from 14.44 ± 2.34 to 15.28 ± 2.04 years for girls and 15.01 ± 2.01 to 16.66 ± 2.10 years for boys, depending on the method used to judge progression.

# Assessing Refractive Error

## RETINOSCOPY

Retinoscopy is a simple, yet powerful clinical technique to assess refractive error. Not all patients can respond to a subjective refraction. If the patient is an infant or toddler, unresponsive, mentally impaired and unable to understand instructions, or speaks a different language than the examiner, obtaining answers to the standard "which is better, one or two?" may be difficult. With relatively inexpensive equipment, refractive status can be measured in these patients without the need for any verbal responses. Even if a subjective refraction is to be performed, retinoscopy is a routine part of the general examination of the eye, serving as a starting point for the subjective refraction, along with the patient's current spectacle correction. Retinoscopy also provides the clinician's first look at the clarity of the optical media. Many cataracts and cases of keratoconus can be detected during retinoscopy prior to any further specialized testing.

The principle of retinoscopy is simple: The clinician shines the retinoscope beam into the patient's eye; this beam forms an image on the patient's retina which is observed by the examiner as a red "reflex" in the patient's pupil. If this reflex moves in the same direction as the retinoscope when the retinoscope is tilted by the examiner, this is termed "with motion" and indicates that the patient is focused farther back than the peephole of the retinoscope. The patient is therefore either hyperopic, emmetropic, or less myopic than the dioptric distance at which the retinoscope is being held. For example, if the retinoscope is held at 67 cm and "with" motion is observed, the patient must be less myopic than −1.50 D. If the reflex moves in the opposite direction from the retinoscope's tilt, this is termed "against" motion and indicates that the patient is focused closer than the peephole of the retinoscope. If "against motion" is observed at a working distance of 67 cm, then

the patient must be more myopic than −1.50 D. If neither "with" nor "against" motion is observed, but the reflex in the pupil just flashes uniformly at the examiner, this is termed "neutrality" and indicates that the patient is focused at the peephole of the retinoscope. In this example, neutrality at a working distance of 67 cm indicates that the patient is a −1.50 D myope.

To refract a patient by retinoscopy, the clinician observes the movement of the reflex in the pupil and adds spectacle lenses according to the motion observed until neutrality is reached. If "with" motion is seen, either more plus-powered or less minus-powered lenses are added. If "against" motion occurs, more minus-powered or less plus-powered lenses are added. In practice, neutrality is difficult to observe. What is more typically done is to bracket the end point of neutrality within a reasonably small interval, observing "against" and "with" motion when either ±0.25 D or ±0.50 D is added. This bracketing interval may increase if the quality of the dioptrics of the patient's eye is poor. The spectacle lens that is either the midpoint of the bracketing interval and/or achieves neutrality is the power that makes the patient's retina conjugate with the peephole of the retinoscope. In order to obtain a spectacle correction, therefore, the working distance in diopters at which retinoscopy is performed must be subtracted from this lens power. For example, if neutrality is achieved with a +3.00 DS lens and retinoscopy is performed at 67 cm, then the patient's refraction is +1.50 DS. If no motion is seen at −3.00 DS and retinoscopy is performed at a working distance of 50 cm, then the patient is a −5.00 D myope.

Most patients possess some astigmatism. This is measured during retinoscopy by obtaining neutrality in both principal meridians. First, the clinician must locate these meridians by aligning the streak of the retinoscope with the streak image of the fundus reflex in the patient's pupil. If the retinoscopic streak is not aligned with a principal meridian, some disparity is seen between the orientation of the streak and the reflex (Fig. 4-9). The retinoscope is in line with the principal meridian when the streak is rotated toward this displaced reflex, toward the vertical. If using a minus cylinder phoropter, it is preferable to refract the least myopic or most hyperopic meridian first with spheres, leaving the second meridian to be neutralized with cylinders. This therefore does not affect the neutrality first obtained by spheres in the opposite meridian. The least myopic or most hyperopic meridian is the one that shows "with" motion if the other meridian is "against," or either the slower "with" or the

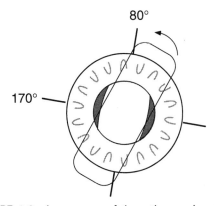

80°

170°

**FIGURE 4–9** Appearance of the retinoscopic reflex in a patient with astigmatism when the retinoscopic beam is not aligned with one of the major meridians of the eye. The reflex appears displaced toward the major meridian, indicating the direction toward which the clinician should move the axis of the beam *(arrow)*.

faster "against" motion if both meridians move in the same direction. If the incorrect meridian is neutralized first and the clinician finds that the second meridian consists of "with" motion (which, of course, cannot be neutralized with minus cylinders), he or she need only count the number of clicks until neutrality is reached with plus spheres in this second meridian. This is the number of clicks of minus cylinder that are needed when returning to the first meridian. When both meridians are neutralized, once again the working distance in diopters must be subtracted from the sphere in the phoropter. Of course, the exact reverse argument applies when using plus cylinders for retinoscopy.

In the example in Figure 4-9, if the retinoscope streak is aligned with the reflex at 80° and neutrality is obtained with a +0.50 DS, neutrality is obtained at 170° with a −2.00 DC, and retinoscopy is performed at 67 cm, the patient's spectacle correction is −1.00 = −2.00 × 170. It is important to understand that the meridian being measured is the one **perpendicular** to the long axis of the streak and **parallel** to the direction in which the streak is being moved. When the streak is aligned with 80°, the meridian at 170° is being refracted. Likewise, when the streak is oriented at 170°, the 80° meridian is being refracted. Hence, it is appropriate to place the cylinder power at 80° and its axis at 170°.

For retinoscopy, the patient should be seated comfortably and be able to fixate a distance target. If a projected visual acuity chart is used, the 20/400 chart is an adequate fixation target. The patient should relax his or her eyes and look at the distance target. The examiner uses his or her right hand and right eye to sight through the

retinoscope to examine the patient's right eye and his or her left hand and left eye to sight through the retinoscope to examine the patient's left eye. The patient can provide feedback as to when he or she cannot see the "E" when the examiner drifts too far toward the midline.

It is important for each individual to establish and maintain a consistent working distance when performing retinoscopy. Taller examiners favor a working distance of 67 cm, whereas examiners with shorter limbs are more comfortable at a working distance of 50 cm. Although a more remote working distance may slightly enhance retinoscopic repeatability, physical comfort and consistency of the selected working distance are more important factors.

Retinoscopy can be, and often is in the case of infants, performed under cycloplegia. Although such an examination stabilizes accommodation, repeatability of retinoscopy under cycloplegia is poorer than under non-cycloplegic conditions, presumably because of the irregularity of the retinoscopic reflex through the mydriatic pupil.[55]

Although it is relatively easy to grasp the principles and practice of retinoscopy, its optics have been somewhat confused through the years. The movement of the retinoscopic reflex can be simulated by taking a pencil to represent the image of the streak on the retina and holding it behind a strong plus trial lens representing the convergent dioptrics of the eye. If the pencil is held close to the lens and moved back and forth, the movement of its image is in a direction "with" the real pencil. Moving the pencil farther away from the lens, one can observe that the image becomes larger (or the field of view of the pencil becomes smaller), and the image moves more rapidly until a point is reached at which it fills the lens. No net movement of the image of the pencil is seen as the real pencil is moved; it is either present or absent in the aperture of the lens. Moving the pencil out farther past this "neutral" point, one sees an inverted image of the pencil moving "against" the direction of the real pencil. The image becomes smaller (or the field of view of the pencil enlarges), and the movement becomes slower, as the pencil is pushed farther from the lens. Describing this situation in terms of the observer, neutrality occurs when the image of the pencil is conjugate with the observer's entrance pupil. "With" motion is seen when the pencil forms an upright, virtual image to the observer, and "against" motion is seen when an inverted, real image is formed relative to the observer.

In order to apply this analogy to the optics of retinoscopy, let us first identify the aperture and field stops in a system that includes patient, ex-

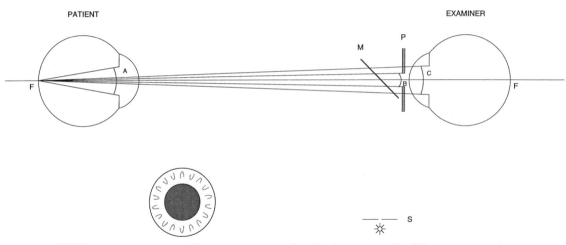

**FIGURE 4–10** Various possible aperture stops for viewing the patch of light on the retina. Angle A is formed by the patient's own pupil and is the largest. Angle B, formed by the retinoscope peephole, is usually smaller than the examiner's pupil (angle C), and therefore angle B is the system's aperture stop. M is the half-silvered mirror at 45° in the retinoscope. P is the retinoscope peephole. Inside the head of the retinoscope, S represents the light source behind an aperture for producing the retinoscope streak. In each of the subsequent diagrams, the appearance of the patient's pupil is shown in the inset.

aminer, and retinoscope. From the vantage point of the object in this system, the image of the retinoscope streak on the patient's retina, the aperture subtending the smallest angle forms the aperture stop. As seen in Figure 4-10, this is angle B formed by the peephole of the retinoscope. The field stop is formed by the aperture that subtends the smallest angle from the peephole. In Figure 4-11, this is angle D formed by the patient's pupil. Therefore, in retinoscopy, the examiner's view of the reflex, the movement of the image of the streak on the retina, is limited by the patient's pupil and not by the peephole

of the retinoscope. Although this point may seem obvious given that the examiner has a full view of the patient's pupil and head during retinoscopy, it becomes important when previous explanations of retinoscopy are presented.

Three features are of interest when analyzing the movement of the retinoscopic reflex: (1) Where is the streak on the patient's retina? (2) What is the examiner's field of view of the patient's retina? and (3) Is the streak being viewed as a virtual or a real image (i.e., where is the image of the streak on the examiner's retina)? In Figure 4-12, the streak is formed by illumina-

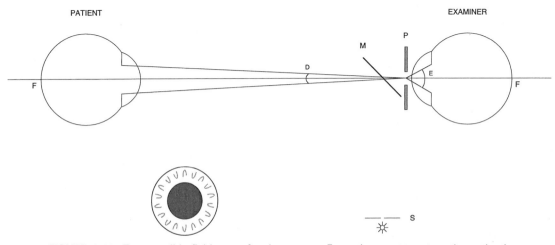

**FIGURE 4–11** Two possible field stops for the system. From the aperture stop, the patient's pupil subtends the smaller angle (D) compared with the examiner's pupil (E); therefore, the patient's pupil is the limiting aperture for the examiner's field of view of the patch of light on the retina.

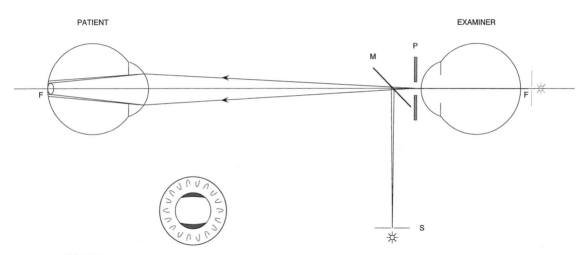

**FIGURE 4–12** Image formation and observation during retinoscopy on a patient who is hyperopic relative to the retinoscope, that is, whose refractive error is less myopic than the dioptric distance of the retinoscope from the patient (the working distance). The patch of light is upright on the retina, the field of view is slightly larger than the patch, and the patient's pupil appears to contain the horizontally oriented streak of light.

ting slit S (actually imaged near optical infinity by a condensing lens) by a light source in the head of the retinoscope. The streak, oriented horizontally, is aligned with the patient's pupil and forms an upright, blurred image on the fovea of this hyperopic patient. (Confirm this by holding a high minus lens in front of your eye while looking at a retinoscope held at arm's length. Moving a finger from above into the incoming beam produces an entoptic shadow appearing to come from below.) The field of view is somewhat larger in this example, appearing to the examiner as a horizontal streak bounded by darkness in

the patient's pupil. If the retinoscope is then tilted upward (Fig. 4–13) so that the streak beam moves up on the patient's face, the image of the streak also moves up on the patient's retina. The patient reports that the slit has appeared to move down as well. At some point, the center of the image of the streak approaches the limit of the field of view of the examiner. In this example, where the patient is hyperopic relative to the retinoscope—that is, the patient's retina is conjugate with a point behind the eye (Fig. 4–14), the image of the streak is erect and virtual. This means that a chief ray from the edge of the

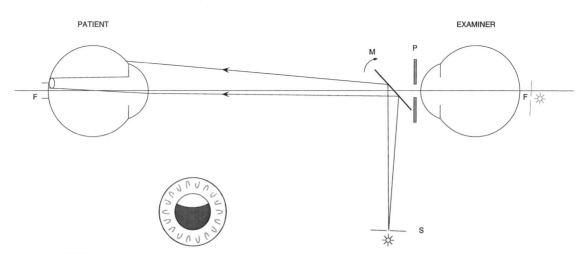

**FIGURE 4–13** For the same patient as in Figure 4–12, when the streak is tilted up, the patch of light also moves up on the patient's retina. The examiner's field of view, however, remains the same (marked by the two horizontal lines straddling the patient's fovea). The streak of light on the retina appears to move up in the patient's pupil as the retinoscope beam is moved up, out of the field of view of the examiner ("with" motion).

PATIENT

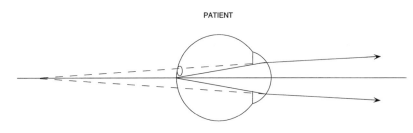

**FIGURE 4–14** In this hyperopic patient, the retina is conjugate with a point behind the patient's eye. A patch of light from the retina diverges upon leaving the patient's eye.

field of view containing the image of the streak falls on the inferior retina of the examiner and appears to be in the superior part of the patient's pupil (Fig. 4-15). The movement appears as "with" movement.

In the myopic patient, the streak forms an inverted, real, and blurred image on the patient's fovea (Fig. 4-16). (This can be confirmed by holding a high plus lens in front of the eye while looking at a retinoscope held at arm's length. Moving a finger from above into the incoming beam produces an entoptic shadow appearing to come from above.) The field of view is somewhat smaller than the image of the streak in this example, appearing to the examiner as a pupil filled with light. If the retinoscope is then tilted upward (Fig. 4-17) so that the streak beam moves up on the patient's face, the image of the streak again moves up on the patient's retina. The patient still reports that the slit has appeared to move down. At some point, the center of the image of the streak approaches the limit of the field of view of the examiner. In this case, where the patient is myopic relative to the retinoscope (Fig. 4-18), the image of the streak is inverted

and real. This means that a chief ray from the edge of the field of view containing the image of the streak falls on the superior retina of the examiner and appears to be in the inferior part of the patient's pupil (Fig. 4-19). The movement appears as "against" movement.

When the patient's myopia equals the dioptric distance of the location of the retinoscope, the image of the streak is an inverted, real blurred image on the fovea—that is, the slit is more distant than the peephole of the retinoscope. The field of view, however, is infinitely small. The view for the examiner is therefore a pupil filled with light (Fig. 4-20). The pupil continues to be filled with light as the blurred patch of light from the streak crosses this infinitely small area of retina corresponding to the field of view. Once the edge of this image crosses the border of the field of view of the examiner, the pupil appears to be completely dark (Fig. 4-21). When the image of the streak once again enters the pinpoint field of view, the pupil appears filled with light during the entire time the patch of light crosses it (Fig. 4-22). Once the other edge of the patch of light crosses the field of view, the

PATIENT                                                    EXAMINER

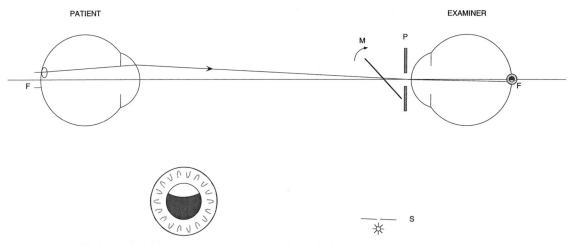

**FIGURE 4–15** A chief ray for the retinoscope (through the center of the peephole, or aperture stop) from the edge of the field of view of the patient's retina to the examiner's retina. This ray marks the location of the superior edge of the patient's pupil as well as the middle of the streak of light on the retina. As the streak moves up on the patient's retina, it moves down on the examiner's, depicted by the image of the patient's pupil on the examiner's retina. This results in the appearance of "with" motion to the examiner (inset).

PATIENT                                                                EXAMINER

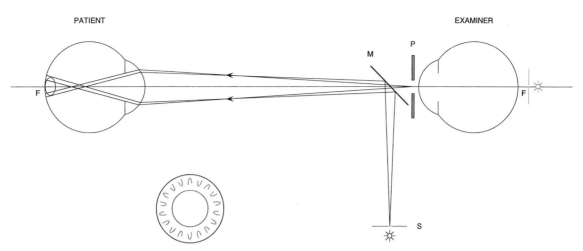

**FIGURE 4–16**   Image formation and observation during retinoscopy on a patient who is myopic relative to the retinoscope, that is, whose refractive error is more myopic than the dioptric distance of the retinoscope from the patient (the working distance). The patch of light is inverted on the retina, the field of view is slightly smaller than the patch, and the patient's pupil appears to be filled with light.

PATIENT                                                                EXAMINER

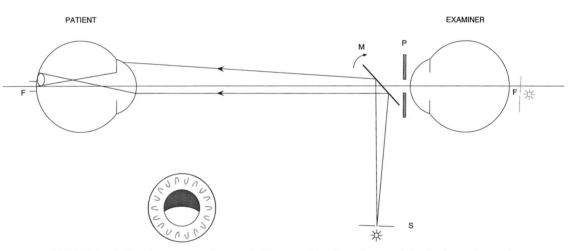

**FIGURE 4–17**   For the same patient as in Figure 4–16, when the streak is tilted up, the patch of light also moves up on the patient's retina. The examiner's field of view, however, remains the same (marked by the two horizontal lines straddling the patient's fovea). In this case, the streak of light on the retina appears to move down in the patient's pupil as the retinoscope beam is moved up, out of the field of view of the examiner ("against" motion).

**FIGURE 4–18** In this myopic patient, the retina is conjugate with a point in front of the patient's eye, between the patient and the retinoscope peephole. A patch of light from the retina converges upon leaving the patient's eye.

PATIENT

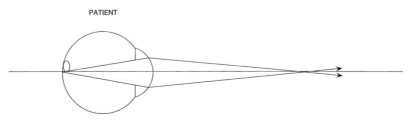

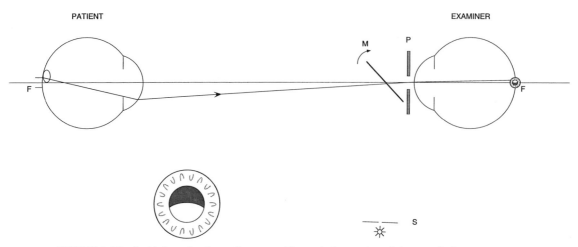

**FIGURE 4–19** A chief ray for the retinoscope (through the center of the peephole, or aperture stop) from the edge of the field of view of the patient's retina to the examiner's retina. In this case, rays conjugate with the peephole cross within the patient's eye because the myopia exceeds the working distance. This ray now marks the location of the inferior edge of the patient's pupil as well as the middle of the streak of light on the retina. As the streak moves up on the patient's retina, it also moves up on the examiner's, depicted by the image of the patient's pupil on the examiner's retina. This results in the appearance of "against" motion to the examiner (inset).

pupil again appears totally dark (Fig. 4–23). This instantaneous on-and-off flashing of light in the pupil without any visible movement is characteristic of "neutrality."

The more traditional textbook explanation of retinoscopy gives the primary responsibility for producing "with" and "against" movement to the retinoscope peephole. The appearance of the pupil in Figure 4–24 is explained as the result of vignetting of the light coming from the patient by the peephole of the retinoscope. This vignet-

ting creates the appearance of darkness at the edges of the patient's pupil with light filling the center. Given the previous explanation of the role of apertures and stops, this represents a confusion of the ability of the peephole as the aperture stop in this system to limit the field of view, a function fulfilled by the patient's pupil. This incorrect diagram implies that if the peephole were smaller, more of the patient's pupil would be dark, or if it were larger, or if there were no peephole, the patient's pupil would be

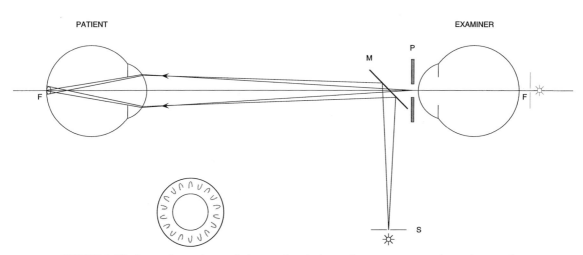

**FIGURE 4–20** Image formation and observation during retinoscopy on a patient whose retina is conjugate with the peephole of the retinoscope, that is, whose myopic refractive error equals the dioptric distance of the retinoscope from the patient (the working distance). The patch of light is inverted on the retina, the field of view is infinitely small, and the patient's pupil appears to be filled with light.

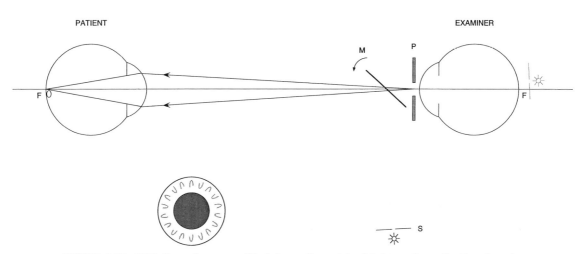

**FIGURE 4–21** With the retinoscope tilted down, the patch of light on the patient's retina also moves down, outside the infinitely small field of view of the examiner. The patient's pupil appears completely dark.

filled with light. This is clearly not the case. Perfectly adequate retinoscopy can be performed with a light source and half-silvered mirror with *no* peephole. The peephole merely serves as a device to keep the retinoscope and the observer aligned. "With" motion is produced by uncrossed rays from the hyperopic patient striking the lower portion of the peephole as the image of the streak moves up on the patient's retina. The vignetted, lower, dark portion of this beam is supposed to be referred back to the patient to make the bottom portion of the patient's pupil appear dark to the examiner (Fig. 4-25). In "against" motion, the crossed rays from the myopic patient still strike the lower portion of the peephole as the image of the streak moves up on the patient's retina. The vignetted, lower, dark

portion of these rays is now referred from the lower part of the peephole back to the upper part of the patient's pupil, giving the "against" appearance (Fig. 4-26). Again this is an inappropriate function for the peephole in this system and is not intended to be an explanation for reflex movement. Rather, it is included for the student to understand and compare the traditional diagrams with more appropriate ones.

Although retinoscopy is a useful technique in many clinical situations, several potential biases may affect the validity of retinoscopic refractions, that is, how well they may compare to subjective refractions. One is chromatic aberration. The retinoscopic reflex is typically orange-red in color, yet most of our visual life occurs either outdoors, or indoors under illumination that mimics day-

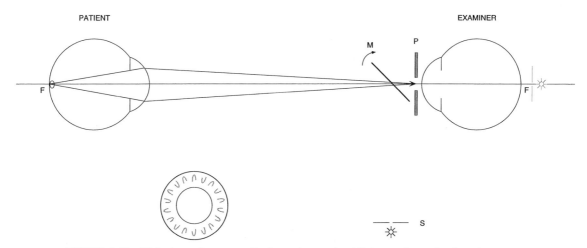

**FIGURE 4–22** With the retinoscope tilted up, the patch of light on the patient's retina moves up inside the infinitely small field of view of the examiner. The patient's pupil appears completely filled with light as long as the patch is over this point field of view.

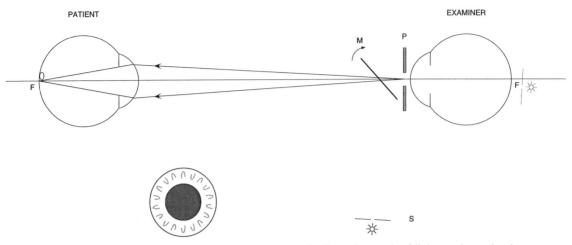

**FIGURE 4–23** As the retinoscope continues to be tilted up, the patch of light on the patient's retina crosses out of the point field of view and the patient's pupil again appears completely dark.

light. Refractions are conducted where acuity charts and examination rooms are traditionally illuminated by tungsten sources. One might expect that the discrepancy between the dominant reddish wavelength of the retinoscopic reflex and that used during subjective refraction may create hyperopic bias in retinoscopy. Although such a bias may exist, Charman and Jennings[56] have shown that it is negligible in size. If most retinoscopes operate at a color temperature between 2000 and 3000°K, then they produce a reflex with a dominant wavelength of 580 to 590 nm (wave number = 16,949 to 17,241). Subjective testing using a daylight source with a dominant wavelength of 557 nm (wave number = 17,953) produces a discrepancy of only 23 to 33 nm, or less than +0.25 D more hyperopia with retinoscopy due to chromatic aberration.

The validity of retinoscopy would be enhanced if the source of retinoscopic reflections were from a location close to the photoreceptors, the plane of reference in subjective refraction. Unfortunately, we are not certain where the origin of the retinoscopic reflex is. Glickstein and Millodot[57] proposed that the origin is at the inner limiting membrane of the retina, between the retina and the vitreous. This model was based on the observation of an increase in the hyperopia of animals with small eyes, which is inversely proportional to eye size. If reflections came from a location anterior to the photoreceptors (about 135 μ), they would be falsely hyperopic ac-

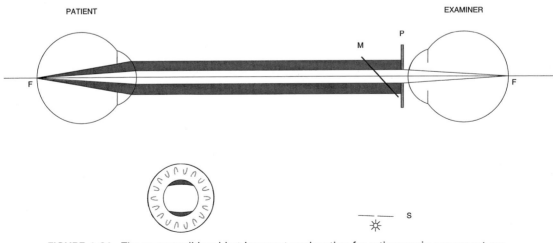

**FIGURE 4–24** The more traditional but incorrect explanation for retinoscopic movement proposes that the retinoscope peephole vignettes the entrance of light into the observation system of the retinoscope. In this emmetropic patient with the retinoscope pointed straight ahead, shadows on either side of the reflex result from restriction of light by the peephole.

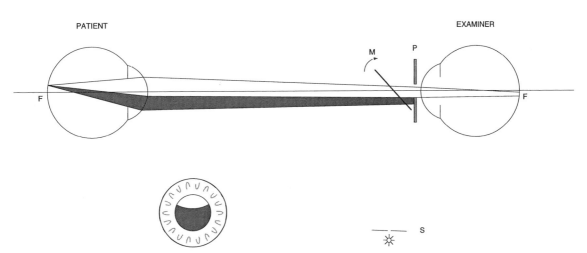

**FIGURE 4–25** Incorrect explanation of "with" motion. As the retinoscope is tilted up, the streak also moves up on the patient's retina. The inferior portion of the cone of rays leaving the eye is vignetted, creating a shadow in the inferior portion of the patient's pupil and the appearance of "with" motion.

cording to the dioptric distance from the photoreceptors to the inner limiting membrane. Although a 135-μ offset between the inner limiting membrane and the photoreceptors might be worth only +0.34 D of artifactual hyperopia in an adult human eye (2.50 D/mm), it is a substantial +9.60 D error in a small eye such as that of the rat (71.40 D/mm). Such an error might be more important clinically in the smaller eye of the human infant, where 135 μ translates into +0.64 D (4.75 D/mm).

Mutti et al.[58] compared retinoscopy with visual evoked potential (VEP) refraction in the rat, an animal with a small eye expected to have a large hyperopic artifact based on the model of Glickstein and Millodot.[57] They found that retinoscopy is only +1.81 D more hyperopic than VEP refractions, rather than the expected +9.60 D. They concluded that a probable source of the retinoscopic reflex is the external limiting membrane, at the end of the photoreceptor inner segment, about 25 μ from the pigments in the

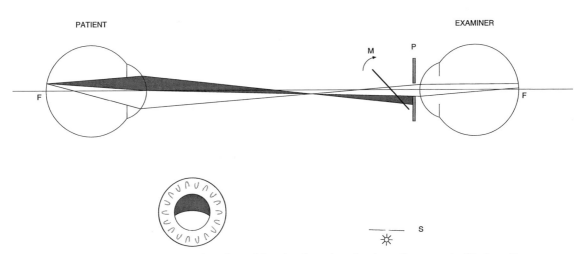

**FIGURE 4–26** Incorrect explanation of "against" motion. As the retinoscope is tilted up, the streak also moves up on the patient's retina. Because the patient is more myopic than the working distance of the retinoscope, the vignetting of the inferior portion of the cone of rays leaving the eye creates a shadow in the superior portion of the patient's pupil and thus the appearance of "against" motion. This explanation and the one for Figure 4–25 are incorrect because the retinoscope peephole produces no shadow. It serves as the aperture stop, limiting the amount of light, but not as the field stop. The examiner's view is limited by the patient's pupil, the true field stop.

outer segment. This offset translates into negligible errors in adult (+0.06 D) and infant (+0.12 D) human eyes.

Tilting of an optical system induces changes in power. Not only does the spherical power increase, but astigmatism is also induced with an axis parallel to the axis of rotation. It is therefore important for the retinoscopist to attempt to stay as close as possible to the line of sight of the patient without obscuring the patient's view of the fixation target with the eye not under regard. Substantial errors can be induced as retinoscopy is done further off-axis. As seen in Figure 4–27, 0.50 to 0.75 D of unwanted cylinder can be induced at 20° off-axis. The amount of change in the off-axis spherical equivalent depends on the shape of the eye, and, interestingly, this shape differs with refractive status. Most people have a nearly spherical globe, whereas hyperopes have a larger equator than axis (oblate) and myopes a longer axis than equator (prolate). This means that the hyperopic eye displays a relative myopia in the periphery and the myopic eye a relative hyperopia. The degree of increase in astigmatism is also less in myopia. Such patterns have been characterized diagrammatically in **skiagrams** by Rempt et al.[59] (Fig. 4–28). As seen in Table 4–10, the type I and II skiagrams with their increasing hyperopia in the periphery are more often seen in myopic eyes, whereas the type IV and V skiagrams are seen more often in hyperopic eyes. The asymmetrical type III is rarely seen. Off-axis

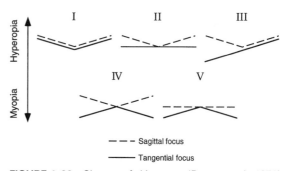

**FIGURE 4–28** Classes of skiagrams (Rempt et al., 1971) representing common patterns in peripheral refraction. As in Figure 4–27, the tangential focus is the more myopic.

errors can increase if there are distortions in the shape of the globe from conditions such as nasal fundus ectasia or retinal detachment repair procedures such as scleral buckling. Understanding the magnitude and direction of these off-axis errors may assist the clinician in interpreting off-axis retinoscopic findings obtained either accidentally or by design.

## SUBJECTIVE REFRACTION

Refractive error is one of the most common anomalies managed in optometric practice, whether for correction by spectacles or contact lenses, as part of the preoperative evaluation for refractive surgery, or as a precursor to other tests in the examination of the eye. Measurements of phoria, accommodative function, and visual fields all assume that the patient has maximum visual acuity through the best subjective correction. The subjective refraction is like an extended conversation with the patient. Rather than a rigid script of instructions and questions that might be the stereotype, the skilled examiner, like the skilled conversationalist, tailors the speed and

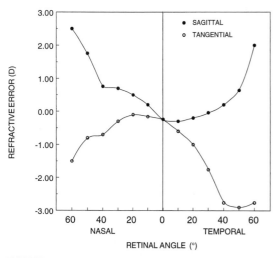

**FIGURE 4–27** Retinoscopic refractive error as a function of the angle between the retinoscopist and the line of sight. The angles are given for the nasal and temporal retina, that is, when the retinoscopist is in the patient's temporal and nasal visual fields, respectively. The amount of astigmatism increases with the angle, with the tangential focus the more myopic of the two. Data are for a near-emmetrope (from Millodot, 1981).

| Refractive Group | Peripheral Refraction Type | | | |
|---|---|---|---|---|
| | I | II | IV | V |
| Myopia (< −0.50 D) | 67 | 5 | 14 | 1 |
| Emmetropia | 38 | 53 | 150 | 16 |
| Hyperopia (> +0.50 D) | 2 | 4 | 61 | 17 |

**TABLE 4–10** Regrouping of Data From Rempt et al.[59] by Refractive Error Group and Peripheral Refraction Class

Each cell contains the number of subjects in that refractive error and peripheral astigmatism class. Note the association between type I skiagrams and myopia, types I, II, and especially IV in emmetropia, and types IV and V in hyperopia.

difficulty of his or her refraction to the individual patient. The pace and difficulty of the choices during refraction are very different depending on the age, experience, and acuity of the patient.

## Monocular Subjective Refraction

Basic steps in monocular refraction are the following:

1. Find the best sphere.
2. Find the cylinder power.
3. Find the axis.
4. Refine the cylinder power if a large change in axis occurs; further refine the axis if another large change in power occurs.
5. Refine the sphere.

The two most common starting points for a subjective refraction are (1) the latest spectacle prescription and (2) the retinoscopic findings. One eye is occluded and the monocular visual acuity is measured through the starting point lenses. While the patient looks at a suprathreshold line of Snellen letters, the best spherical equivalent is found for the amount of cylinder in the starting point refraction. As a general rule in refraction procedures, two choices are offered for the patient to make a judgment as to which is better—that is, sharper and easier to read—with the most minus or least plus choice given first, followed by the least minus or most plus, in order to control accommodation. The amount of change in each choice depends on the patient. Usually, +0.50 D is standard for a patient with normal acuity, but larger steps are required if acuity is reduced. The concept is for the clinician to offer a choice large enough that the patient can actually detect a difference. Much time can be saved and fatigue and frustration reduced with the appropriate selection of step size. Plus power is added until the patient detects the first blur to the suprathreshold Snellen letters. This indicates that the amount of plus power is excessive and must be reduced. How to reduce the amount of plus power depends on whether or not the patient is a presbyope. The ideal non-presbyopic patient responds that excess minus is no different than the best spherical equivalent. Many non-presbyopic patients, however, accept an excessive amount of minus power if given the choice, as minification of the chart appears to add contrast. This excess minus is to be avoided because it creates an unnecessary accommodative demand and alters the phoria. The clinician asks the patient, "Does the more minus choice make the letters clearer and easier to read, rather than just smaller and darker?" in order to avoid "over-minusing" the patient. More minus power is given only when it improves the ability to read letters. If the patient continues to prefer minus, the clinician may isolate a row of letters on the acuity chart, add plus to blur the patient, then begin providing choices and accepting minus power only if it allows the patient to read smaller rows of letters. The clinician should stop providing choices once the patient has received enough minus power to read a threshold row of letters. Starting from retinoscopic findings is an advantage in this procedure because the power for the working distance may either be removed all at once or in stages as acuity improves. Presbyopes are easier to examine in this respect because they report blur with excess minus as well as excess plus power. This procedure is then repeated with a smaller step size, as long as it produces changes that the patient can detect; ±0.25 D is standard for patients with normal acuity.

Table 4-11 shows how, in four choices, the sphere has been refined to ±0.25 D. The first two choices say that any less minus than −1.50 D is not adequate for best acuity. The next possible choice is to offer −2.50 D, but it is unlikely that a patient with 20/25 acuity is undercorrected by a diopter. The usual rule of thumb is one row of acuity lost per 0.25 D of blur, described in Chapter 2 as the relationship between visual acuity and optical blur. Switching to −2.25 D and finding no difference narrows the range of possible best spheres to either −1.75 or −1.50 D, with −1.75 D picked as the final choice.

## ASTIGMATISM

The starting point for determining the astigmatic correction is usually the previous spectacle correction or the retinoscopic results. Two aids may be employed to provide additional confidence in these findings. The more important is keratometry. Because the cornea is the most powerful dioptric component of the eye, the primary factor determining refractive astigmatism is corneal toricity. A simple formula relates the two and is known as Javal's rule:

$$\text{Refractive astigmatism} = (1.25 \times \text{Corneal toricity}) + (-0.50 \text{ DC} \times 90)$$

The 0.50-DC against-the-rule astigmatism represents the lenticular component of the refractive astigmatism. Grosvenor et al.[60] found that changing the corneal toricity coefficient to 1.00 provides a better fit to clinical data relating refractive astigmatism and corneal toricity. This has been

**TABLE 4–11** Flow of Lenses Shown and Responses Given by the Patient During an Uneventful Subjective Refraction

| Starting Point | Acuity | |
|---|---|---|
| −1.50 = −2.50 × 175 | 20/25 | |
| **Row of Letters Showing** | **Sphere Choices 1 and 2** | **Response** |
| 20/40 | −1.50 and −1.00 | "−1.50 better" |
| 20/40 | −2.00 and −1.50 | "−2.00 better" |
| 20/40 | −2.25 and −1.75 | "No difference" |
| 20/40 | −1.75 and −1.50 | "−1.75 better" |
| **End Point** | | |
| −1.75 = −2.50 × 175 | | |

further confirmed by Elliott et al.,[61] who found that 66% of predicted refractive astigmatism agreed within ±0.50 D to the actual measured refractive astigmatism with Grosvenor's rule, whereas only 60% agreed at that level after using Javal's rule. This simpler rule seems a sensible modification because changes in corneal power as measured by the keratometer usually translate 1:1 to changes in refractive error, ignoring vertex distance. In patients in whom retinoscopy is difficult, such as after penetrating keratoplasty, or when the patient cannot respond to a subjective refraction, keratometry can be a useful adjunct to determining the astigmatic correction.

The axis of astigmatism can also be determined during subjective refraction by having the patient view a "fan dial" chart. The fan dial chart makes use of the meridional blur created by the astigmatic interval (Fig. 4–29). The patient should be fogged with plus lenses until all the lines corresponding to the clock hours on the dial are blurred. This ensures that both foci on the interval of Stürm are in front of the retina. The amount of plus power is then reduced until the patient reports that one of the clock hours is clearer than the others. That clock hour multiplied by 30 is the approximate axis for minus cylinder correction. In Figure 4–30, the patient views a simplified fan dial target with only horizontal and vertical detail. The with-the-rule cornea refracts light to a more myopic focus in the vertical meridian than the horizontal meridian. This results in greater vertically oriented blur, which spreads out and defocuses horizontal lines (not-to-scale) at the retina. Vertical lines are therefore in better focus because the image has less horizontal defocus and spread. The patient reports that the 6 o'clock hour is the clearer, and the clinician infers that the axis of astigmatism is 180 (i.e., 6 × 30), as expected for a with-the-rule cornea. Conversely, for the against-the-rule

cornea in Figure 4–31, the horizontal meridian is the more myopic focus, which creates blur for the vertical lines due to the lateral defocus and spread of the image. The patient perceives that the 3 o'clock hour is clearer and the predicted axis of astigmatism is 90 (i.e., 3 × 30). The same sort of reasoning applies to any oblique orientation as well.

The axis and amount of astigmatism may be most precisely refined using the Jackson flip crossed cylinder after finding the best equivalent sphere. This device is a sphero-cylindrical lens that has equal and opposite power in perpendicular meridians. A ±0.25 D "flip-cross" would

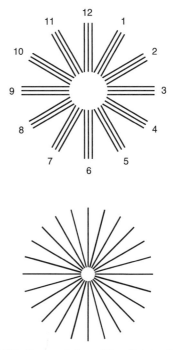

**FIGURE 4–29** Two varieties of fan dial charts, one with clock hours and one including half-hours.

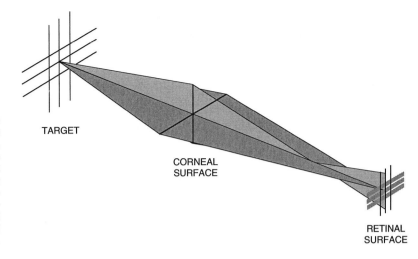

**FIGURE 4–30** Simplified view of a fan dial target for a simple myopic with-the-rule astigmat. Light is focused in front of the retina for the vertical meridian (horizontal line focus) and on the retina for the horizontal meridian (vertical line focus). Vertical lines appear in focus and the minus cylinder axis should be 180° (6 o'clock × 30 = 180).

have a "prescription" of +0.25 = −0.50 DC, and a ±0.50 D "flip-cross" would be +0.50 = −1.00 DC. The minus cylinder axis is indicated by the two red lines on the lens for Greens phoropters or two red dots for AO Ultramatic phoropters (Fig. 4–32). This lens creates an interval of Stürm that the clinician can use to present the patient with choices between more or less power, analogous to refining the sphere as described above, but now in one meridian at a time. Higher-powered crossed cylinders are available for use either in the phoropter or as a hand-held device over a trial frame for patients with reduced acuity who have difficulty making these subjective judgments.

The Jackson crossed cylinder lens is held in a ring that can be either rotated or "flipped" between one side and the other. The procedure begins with rotating the "flip-cross" so that the red lines or dots are parallel to the axis of the cylinder in the phoropter. This is done manually by aligning a scribe mark to the degrees on the cylinder ring on Greens phoropters but is indicated by a click-stop on AO Ultramatic phoropters. Because the following choices involve meridional rather than spherical defocus, they are much more confusing for the patient, and making the decision on which is preferable is more difficult. The choices are further complicated for the patient because the end point for the cylindrical refraction is not when he or she sees well. It is when the patient's astigmatism is neutralized and the interval of Stürm from the "flip-cross" straddles the retina, creating equal degrees of defocus in each meridian. Questions during this part of the examination are usually phrased, "I'm going to give you two choices. Neither may be perfect, but tell me which makes the letters look darker, rounder, and easier to read." At some point, patients almost universally complain that

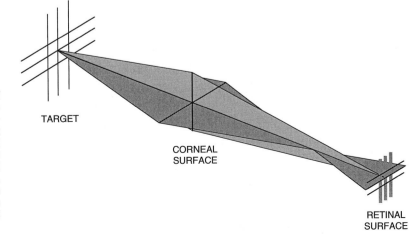

**FIGURE 4–31** The opposite of Figure 4–30 occurs for the simple myopic against-the-rule astigmat. Light is focused in front of the retina for the horizontal meridian (vertical line focus) and on the retina for the vertical meridian (horizontal line focus). Horizontal lines appear in focus and the minus cylinder axis should be 90° (3 o'clock × 30 = 90).

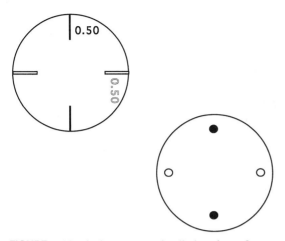

**FIGURE 4–32**  Jackson crossed cylinders for a Greens and an AO phoropter.

neither choice looks very good, but this merely means that the end point is near.

While displaying a row of letters one or two lines above the patient's acuity threshold and directing the patient's attention to one letter, such as the "B" of the 20/40 line, flip the Jackson cylinder that has been aligned with the phoropter cylinder. Note that in one position, the red lines or dots are aligned with the patient's cylinder, and the white lines or dots are aligned in the other meridian. The clinician is asking the patient to choose between more or less cylinder at this axis. In minus cylinder refraction, the rule is "follow the red." (In many ophthalmological care settings that use plus cylinder conventions and phoropters, the rule would be "follow the white.") If the patient responds that the choice when the red is aligned is better, add another $-0.25$ DC and repeat. If the patient again responds that the choice when the red is aligned is better and another $-0.25$ DC is added, then the sphere must be adjusted by adding $+0.25$ DS. For every 0.50 DC change, a compensatory change of 0.25 D of the opposite sign must be made. This is to keep the net spherical equivalent in the phoropter constant and the patient's interval of Stürm centered on the retina. If the cylindrical power were reduced, adjustments would be made by adding minus spherical power.

At some point the patient responds that the choice when the white is aligned is better. Reduce the cylinder power by 0.25 DC and make any adjustments to the sphere in order to maintain a constant spherical equivalent. The patient may also respond that the two choices are equally blurred, meaning that the patient's interval of Stürm is neutralized and the crossed cylin-

der is making an equal interval of astigmatic blur during the two choices. Either of these two responses marks the end of the first determination of cylinder power.

Suppose that no cylinder was found on retinoscopy or in the patient's previous spectacles. The clinician must determine if any astigmatism is present subjectively. This is done by searching the principal meridians with the Jackson cylinder. Place an amount of cylinder in the phoropter equal to the amount of cylinder in the "flip-cross" and orient it either horizontally or vertically. Align the Jackson crossed cylinder with the cylinder in the phoropter. This gives the patient the choice of either preferring cylinder at that orientation or not. If cylinder is rejected, that is, if the "white is better," rotate the cylinder 90° and offer the same choice to the patient. (The Jackson crossed cylinder holder remains aligned in Greens phoropters.) If cylinder is rejected again, orient the cylinder in the phoropter and the flip-cross obliquely and determine whether astigmatism is present at 45°, then 135°. If the white is preferred at all four orientations, the patient has no astigmatism. If the red is preferred at any orientation, further refine the cylinder power as described above.

In order to refine the axis of the cylindrical correction, rotate the crossed cylinder so that the white and red lines or dots straddle the cylinder axis in the phoropter. This is again done manually by aligning a second scribe mark to the degrees on the cylinder ring on Greens phoropters but is found as a second clickstop on AO Ultramatic phoropters. Now when the Jackson cylinder is flipped, the red and white lines or dots change sides across the cylinder axis in the phoropter. This asks the patient whether he or she prefers the cylinder axis more to one side or the other. Again, the rule in minus cylinder is "follow the red." Move the axis of cylinder in the phoropter toward the side where the red was preferred. Make the choice larger for small cylinders and smaller for large cylinders. For Greens phoropters, make sure that the crossed cylinder continues to straddle the cylinder axis in the phoropter. American Optical and other "Synchro-Cyl" phoropters maintain this position automatically.

What the clinician is looking for is a reversal; at some point the patient indicates that he or she prefers the choice where the axis is located in the opposite direction. Many inexperienced clinicians spend large and unproductive amounts of time at this step as patients run them "around the dial." Most patients never respond with consistent reversals in a $\pm 1°$ range. As in retinoscopy, bracketing rather than moving in 1° steps is a useful strategy. The width of the bracketing interval again depends on the amount of cylinder and the sensitivity of the patient. Zeroing in on the midpoint of reversals using large intervals at first, $\pm 10°$ to $15°$, which are sequentially reduced until the patient fails to note consistent differences, is an efficient means of refining the cylinder axis.

If refinement of the cylinder axis has changed its position substantially, the power of the cylinder must be rechecked with the Jackson "flip-cross" cylinder. With the correct cylinder power and axis in the phoropter, the "flip-cross" can be removed and the sphere refined. By maintaining the spherical equivalent, the sphere should be close to that of the final refraction. A threshold row of letters should be shown as choices of most minus/least plus first are given to the patient. The same cautions given in the previous section regarding excessive amounts of minus power also apply at this stage. The end point is the most plus power that results in maximum clarity and visual acuity.

An alternate method for determining the end point of the monocular subjective refraction utilizes the longitudinal chromatic aberration of the eye. The duochrome or bichrome test is performed by placing the red-green background behind the letters on the projected acuity chart. Chromatic aberration creates a chromatic interval, with letters on the green side focused at a more myopic location than letters on the red side. Similar to the fan dial test, the patient is asked which side has the clearer letters, the red or the green. A response of "red" indicates a need for more minus or less plus and vice versa for a response of "green." In order to control accommodation, the patient should be given increasing plus power until the letters on the red side are clearer, then this plus power is decreased until the letters are either equally clear on each side or until the first $-0.25$ change that produces greater clarity for letters on the green side.

The clinician usually encounters small discrepancies in cylinder and axis between the monocular subjective refraction and retinoscopy or the previous spectacle prescription. It is often useful to present these choices subjectively outside the phoropter to the patient at this point in the refraction, offering the more minus cylinder power choice first, to determine the patient's sensitivity to change and his or her preference for old versus new prescriptions. Which lens to prescribe depends on the amount and orientation of the astigmatism and numerous individual patient factors, making prescribing spectacle correction as much an art—involving the skill, intuition, and experience of the clinician—as a science.

## BINOCULAR BALANCE

In order to maintain clear and comfortable binocular vision, the prescription must be balanced after completing monocular refractions of the two eyes. One procedure for achieving balance is the prism dissociation or von Graefe technique. Vertical prism is placed before the patient in order to disrupt fusion, by splitting $6\Delta$—$3\Delta$ base up in front of one eye and $3\Delta$ base down in front of the other eye—with Risley prisms. While viewing a suprathreshold line of letters, the patient is fogged by the addition of $+0.75$ DS in front of each eye. The patient is then asked which of the two lines is clearer, the top or the bottom. Plus is increased for the clearer line until the point where each line is equally blurred. Many times the patient does not find a point of exact equality but rather responds that the bottom, for example, is clearer for one choice and that the top is clearer with the addition of the next $+0.25$ DS. The clinician should ask for which choice the two lines are more nearly equal and select that as the end point.

Many patients find the initial choice difficult in prism dissociation because the monocular subjective may be close to the balanced prescription and the level of blur very comparable for the two lines. A more efficient procedure is to add $+0.75$ DS for one eye and $+0.50$ DS for the other. If the monocular balance is correct, then the patient finds the $+0.50$ DS line clearer. If the lens power is then increased to $+1.00$ DS over the monocular subjective, this line appears to be more blurred. The clinician then knows that the balance end point is within $\pm 0.25$ DS and the patient has had some practice at the task. The remaining choices can be presented to the patient as described above, with the same end point criterion of finding the point of most equal blur between the two lines.

The prism is removed at this point, and fusion is restored. A threshold line of letters is given, which should appear to be blurred and unreadable. If the patient can read this threshold row, the amount of plus over the monocular subjective was inadequate; it should be increased and the balance procedure repeated. The clinician should reduce the amount of plus or increase the amount of minus in the phoropter in 0.25 DS steps simultaneously before the two eyes as the patient views the acuity chart. Once the patient can read the threshold row of letters, the clinician must take care not to provide excess minus power to the non-presbyope. More minus power may be given if it either improves acuity or makes the letters actually easier to read, rather than just smaller and darker. A response of "no difference" between two choices also denotes the same end point of maximum plus with maximum visual acuity.

The end point of the binocular subjective refraction may also be found by the duochrome test. When the vertical prism is removed and fusion is restored, the red-green bichrome filter is put in place. Because the patient is fogged after the von Graefe technique, the letters in the red should be clearer. The plus power is decreased binocularly until the letters are either equally clear on each side or until the first $-0.25$ D change that produces greater clarity for letters on the green side, as in the monocular procedure described above.

## BINOCULAR REFRACTION

What if the patient making the comparisons between the two lines during prism dissociation binocular balance has different visual acuities in the two eyes? One line will always look worse, but not because of an incorrect prescription. When the blur is equalized, too much plus power is given to the eye with the better acuity. This problem can be managed by performing a binocular refraction. Other advantages to a binocular refraction include greater efficiency because binocularly balancing the patient is automatically a part of the technique. Binocular refraction techniques also provide a more natural condition for finding cylinder power and axis because any possible cyclotorsional effects occurring under monocular conditions are removed. Binocular refraction is possible when there is fusion, but when each eye sees different letters. This can be accomplished by using a septum, as in the Turville infinity balance (TIB) technique. The patient in Figure 4–33 views a 20/40 row of letters binocularly with a septum placed at the mirror until the "B" in the middle is obscured. The clinician quickly rechecks the correct placement of the septum by asking what letters are visible with the left eye occluded by hand (D and 4), and which are visible when the right eye is occluded (F and Z). Fusion is maintained by the outline of the isolated line as well as the mirror and frame. Patients with vertical phorias may report vertical separation between the two halves, in which case TIB can become an alternate measurement of vertical phoria once that separation is neutralized with the Risley prism.

The entire refraction can then proceed with-

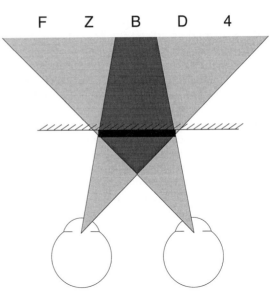

F   Z   B   D   4

**FIGURE 4–33** Patient's view of a chart with a TIB septum in place. The right eye views the right side of the chart only and the left eye views the left side of the chart only. The patient's attention is directed to the letters on the appropriate side when that eye is being refracted.

out occlusion, with the clinician directing the patient's attention to the appropriate side of the chart. The best equivalent sphere, cylinder power and axis, and refined sphere are obtained for each eye as described above for the monocular subjective refraction. After each eye is refracted, the patient has received a balanced refraction. The septum can then be removed and the sphere power rechecked binocularly using a threshold line of letters to achieve the usual criterion end point of maximum plus with maximum visual acuity. As can be guessed from the word "balance" in TIB, this technique can also be used as a balance technique after monocular subjective refraction with occlusion. Following determination of cylinder power and axis for each eye, both eyes are opened and the septum is placed so as to cover the middle of the line of letters. The sphere is then refined as in monocular subjective refraction, the septum removed, and the final sphere refined binocularly.

Another method for achieving fused conditions but different input to the two eyes is with the Polaroid feature found in AO-type phoropters. An acuity chart presents letters that are polarized in perpendicular meridians on each side of the chart. The phoropter contains auxiliary lenses that are also polarized in orthogonal planes. Fusion is maintained by an unpolarized surround and a central vertical bar between the columns of letters. The patient sees a single chart, but each eye sees only half of each row of letters on each side of the vertical bar. The clinician then conducts the refraction in the same manner as the monocular subjective refraction, directing the patient's attention to the letters on one side of the chart, then the other. Once each eye is refracted, the Polaroid filter can be removed and the final sphere refined binocularly.

Although it is an indispensable tool, the phoropter is also somewhat unnatural. The size of its apertures is small, its vertex distance is large and unstable, and it can be perceived by patients as a large, dark, and confining wall between them and the rest of the world. It is also unsuitable for examinations of young children. Recent research has shown that merely the perception of being enclosed may raise the level of open-loop or tonic accommodation.[62] It is therefore advisable to confirm the binocular subjective refraction and demonstrate it to the patient with a trial frame. This may also be done with trial lenses either held or clipped over the patient's existing spectacles. The final sphere may be checked in free space with a threshold row of letters or a real target. The patient may be shown the degree of improvement (or lack of improvement) in the clarity of real objects provided by the change in prescription, motivating him or her to change (or to maintain as need be) the current spectacles. The impact of large changes in cylindrical correction can be demonstrated to patients as they move about the examination room, attuning them to what they might expect with their new correction as they go through the adaptation process. The use of trial lenses as a last step can be a valuable tool for patient management as well as for refraction.

Trial frame refinement of the subjective refraction is required for high degrees of refractive error. In cases greater than $\pm 6.00$ D, differences between the vertex distance at which a refraction is performed and that at which prescribed spectacles sit can result in inadequate vision. For patients with moderate to high refractive error, refinement of the spherical prescription, followed by careful measurement of the vertex distance with a distometer, is mandatory. The vertex distance is then communicated as part of the prescription, so that appropriate compensation in spectacle lens power can be made.

## HYPEROPIA

The child or young adult with low degrees of hyperopia typically presents with few complaints. Distance vision remains clear as the patient uses his or her own accommodation to correct the refractive error. If the AC/A ratio is not too high or the patient is too esophoric, the use of accommodation presents no great difficulty. Asthenopia or avoidance of reading may result if the hyperopia increases accommodative demand beyond the patient's tolerance. In adulthood, hyperopic refractive error presents greater difficulty for the patient as presbyopia sets in and accommodative reserve lessens. At this point, the myope has the advantage of having a built-in reading addition as well as lens effectivity working to delay the onset of presbyopic symptoms. The hyperope has neither and complains of presbyopia sooner.

Because the hyperope habitually uses accommodation to maintain clear vision, refraction of these patients as children and pre-presbyopic adults presents special challenges. The object is to entice the hyperope to relax his or her accommodation during manifest refraction. A common technique is to blur the 20/40 line until it can no longer be read, followed by reducing plus power slowly until an end point of maximum visual acuity is reached. Often, maintaining this blur, or "fog," before the eyes may result in improvements in the hyperope's acuity as accommodation relaxes. One difficulty is that when the eye is presented with a degraded target, such as extreme blur, an empty field, or darkness, it assumes a position of rest or a tonic posture, which is myopic relative to the far point. If you hold your arm at your side without looking at it, your hand is not extended out straight (analogous to the eye being focused for infinity) but is curled somewhat by tonic muscular activity (analogous to accommodative activity or myopic focus). This level of **tonic accommodation** varies as function of refractive error, both in adults and children, with hyperopes having the highest (most myopic) levels, followed by emmetropes, and myopes with the lowest levels.[63] The hyperope may react to blur by slipping into this myopic, tonic posture, leaving the clinician back at the beginning after one click too many of the phoropter.

A cycloplegic refraction can be very useful in uncooperative patients, in patients with accommodative spasm, in patients for whom there is a need to correct all the hyperopia possible, such as in strabismus, or merely to confirm that little latent hyperopia is present compared with the manifest refraction. Caution should be used if prescribing from cycloplegic results, as many times patients do not accept the full amount of plus power determined under a cycloplegic.

Whenever a child is being examined, the clinician should inquire about difficulties in school as part of the case history. Hyperopic children are more likely to have such problems. Not only do they have the burden of using part of their accommodative reserve to correct their refractive error, but hyperopia in children is also associated with developmental delay and poorer perceptual skills. At the age of 3.5 years, 14 of 36 hyperopic children could not perform a letter matching task, compared with 2 of 33 children with normal refractive errors, because of difficulty with the concept of finding the "middle letter."[64] In a clinical sample of children between 6 and 12 years of age, 21 of 29 (72%) hyperopic children were rated as having inadequate visual perceptual skills, compared with 44 of 81 (54%) emmetropes and 20 of 52 (38%) myopes.[65]

Correcting hyperopia certainly improves visual comfort and may reduce distraction, encourage study, and improve academic performance. Spectacles may not be a panacea for reading difficulties, however, and referral for further remediation with other educational specialists may also be needed. Correcting hyperopia may have some benefit in the young patient in reducing the risk of strabismus. Of 48 children with over +4.00 D of hyperopia at age 9 months who wore a refractive correction, 3 (6%) became strabismic by the age of 4 years, compared with 16 of 76 (21%) of such children who wore no correction.[25]

## CYCLOPLEGIC REFRACTION

Cycloplegia is an extremely valuable tool in refraction when the amount of hyperopia present in a pre-presbyopic patient may be greater than what is revealed using non-cycloplegic techniques. The amount of **latent hyperopia,** the difference between the refractive error measured with and without cycloplegia, is an important piece of clinical data in the examination of infants and children, in whom the expected refractive error is a low degree of hyperopia. It is not uncommon, for example, to find that a child who is doing poorly in school has a refractive error near plano without cycloplegia, but to find +4.00 D or more hyperopia after cycloplegia. Likewise, patients with accommodative esotropia may benefit from receiving the maximum correction of their hyperopia because this provides the maximum relaxation of accommodative vergence.

The amount of cycloplegia required for an adequate cycloplegic refraction has been debated in the literature for many years. Various agents deliver differing levels of cycloplegic intensity. Topical application of 1% atropine ointment for several days prior to an ocular examination provides the greatest degree of cycloplegia for the longest duration. Cyclopentolate is probably the most commonly used cycloplegic agent for the examination of children, providing cycloplegia in 1 hour comparable to that from 3 days of atropine with a much shorter duration of action.[69] Tropicamide, a reputedly weak cycloplegic agent, has been recommended in the past only for repeat cycloplegic refractions; more often its use for cycloplegic refraction is actively discouraged.[70, 71]

Although it may be the acknowledged "gold standard" for cycloplegic effectiveness, atropine's effects are neither rapid in onset nor brief in duration. The onset of cycloplegia under atropine requires several hours and, along with mydriasis, may last for 2 weeks or longer.[72, 73] Atropine is also highly toxic; a fatal dose for a child is estimated at only 10 mg. Lesser doses may result in side effects such as redness of the skin, dryness of the mucous membranes, fever, tachycardia, and delirium.[69]

Cyclopentolate has more desirable pharmacokinetic properties than atropine, reaching maximum cycloplegia in 20 to 60 minutes and recovery in 6 to 24 hours,[74-80] but this may still be too long a period of time for many patients. In addition, noticeable mydriasis from cyclopentolate may persist for several days.[69, 77, 81] The clinician should also be aware of the possibility of psychogenic side effects in children and adults through the central nervous system action of cyclopentolate in both 1 and 2% concentrations. Visual and tactile hallucinations, ataxia, disorientation, incoherent speech, and failure to recognize familiar faces have all been reported.[82-89] Reactions consisting of two or more of these symptoms have been shown to occur in as many as 24% of children following instillation of 2% cyclopentolate[86] and in 4% of children receiving only 0.5% or 1% concentrations.[87] Dizziness, nausea, or mood changes have been reported in 15% of adults receiving 2% cyclopentolate.[84]

Tropicamide 1% is more commonly used as a mydriatic, but it has several desirable cycloplegic properties. It has a rapid onset of cycloplegia, short duration of action, minimal number of side effects, and no psychogenic adverse reactions.[9, 22, 23] Maximum cycloplegia reportedly occurs within 25 to 40 minutes and dissipates within 2 to 6 hours.[71, 80, 92, 93] Recovery from mydriasis occurs within 6 to 7 hours.[79, 80, 94] Tropicamide is virtually free of systemic side effects,[91] its minor ocular side effects are rare,[91] and the risk of more serious ocular effects such as anterior chamber angle closure is remote in children.[95] Tropicamide's value as a cycloplegic has been questioned, however. Comparison studies gener-

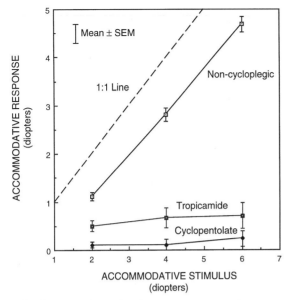

**FIGURE 4–34** Autorefraction measurement of accommodative response (average of all subjects). This graph shows the mean (± SEM) of the objectively measured responses to each stimulus before and during cycloplegia. Non-cycloplegic results show normal accommodative responses to the changes in stimulus values. For each stimulus level after cycloplegia, cyclopentolate more strongly suppresses the accommodative response to a statistically significant degree. (From Mutti DO et al: The effect of cycloplegia on measurement of the occular components. Invest Ophthalmol Vis Sci 1994; 35:515–527.)

ally report about twice the amount of residual accommodation following use of tropicamide than cyclopentolate, hence its primary use as a mydriatic agent.[71, 80, 93, 96-99] Only one study has found similar levels of residual accommodation for both agents.[79]

The amount of residual accommodation is commonly used as the benchmark for the efficacy of a cycloplegic agent. Although this may be a valid benchmark, it is also the most conservative. Does a cycloplegic agent need to eliminate accommodation to effectively reveal the full amount of latent hyperopia? The answer may be no. Residual accommodation following cyclopentolate measured by "push-up" amplitude is between 1.00 and 2.50 D.[74, 78, 79, 97, 100, 101] When measured objectively with an autorefractor, residual accommodation is greater after instillation of tropicamide 1% than after cyclopentolate 1% (Fig. 4–34), although both clearly suppress the accommodative response. This is consistent with previous results using the "push-up" technique. Milder reported average residual accommodation levels of 6.25 D in children up to 9 years old and 3.65 D in children 10 to 14 years old after instillation of two drops of tropicamide 1%.[97] Gettes found that 60% of patients between 14 and 35 years old had residual accommodation ≥3.50 D 30 minutes after instillation of one drop of tropicamide 1%.[92] Those residual levels decreased when two drops were instilled. More recently, Lovasik has reported residual accommodation of 2.00 to 4.00 D 20 minutes after instillation of one drop of tropicamide 1% and 1.00 to 2.00 D 20 minutes after instillation of one drop of cyclopentolate 1%.[76]

A more functional indicator of cycloplegic efficacy is the amount of latent hyperopia revealed. Obtaining valid measures of true hyperopia is, after all, the reason cycloplegia is used. When tropicamide and cyclopentolate 1% were compared in 20 emmetropic to moderately hyperopic, non-strabismic children aged 6 to 12 years by this criterion, tropicamide performed quite well.[102] Refractive error measured in the vertical meridian as well as the cylinder was the same for either drop, regardless of whether it was measured at 30 or 60 minutes (Table 4–12). This gives the clinician some flexibility in the time between drop instillation and patient examination. Both cycloplegic agents uncovered latent hyperopia. The difference between autorefraction in the vertical meridian with and without cycloplegia was +0.98 ± 0.58 D for cyclopentolate and +0.74 ± 0.44 D for tropicamide. The mean difference in latent hyperopia between the

**TABLE 4–12** Mean of the Differences (± 1 SD) Between Measurement Times (30 Minutes Minus 60 Minutes) for Autorefraction in the Vertical Meridian and Autorefraction Cylinder

| Mean Difference Between Measures (30–60 min) | Drug Type | |
| --- | --- | --- |
| | *Tropicamide* | *Cyclopentolate* |
| Vertical meridian refraction (D) | +0.02 ± 0.28 | −0.06 ± 0.28 |
| Cylindrical component of refraction (sphero-cylinder and axis) | +0.09 − 0.12 × 12 | −0.04 − 0.03 × 37 |

The mean of the differences between cylinders is a sphero-cylinder. Neither the vertical meridian refraction nor the cylindrical difference is significant as a function of time for either drug ($P < .74$, paired t-tests).

**TABLE 4–13** Effect of Cycloplegic Agent*

| Component | Cyclopentolate | Tropicamide | Difference (bias) Cyclopentolate-Tropicamide | P Value |
|---|---|---|---|---|
| Vertical meridian refraction (D) | 1.46 ± 0.91 | 1.26 ± 0.93 | +0.20 ± 0.30 | .008 |
| Cylindrical component of refraction | −0.16 − 0.37 × 93 | −0.21 − 0.34 × 95 | +0.06 − 0.04 × 77 | NS |

*1% cyclopentolate after 60 minutes and 1% tropicamide after 30 minutes. All values represent mean ± 1 SD.

two cycloplegic agents (+0.24 ± 0.52 D) was not statistically significant. Refractive error itself was statistically, but not clinically, significantly different. Cyclopentolate 1% revealed more hyperopia than tropicamide 1%, but the difference was only 0.20 ± 0.30 D (Table 4-13).[102]

Although cyclopentolate may be superior in minimizing accommodation, this does not translate to important differences in distance refraction. Cyclopentolate may be the clinical standard for revealing latent hyperopia, but tropicamide appears to be as effective when examining normal, non-strabismic, non-amblyopic, low to moderately hyperopic children. Cyclopentolate should remain the cycloplegic of choice for infants and strabismics, however, because full correction of hyperopia may be critical to the efficacy of any refractive correction in these groups. No comparative studies between tropicamide and cyclopentolate have been performed in infants. The efficacy of tropicamide compared with cyclopentolate in the refraction of hyperopes is further supported by the comparability of average refractive results after cyclopentolate to those using the "gold standard" of atropine. Refractive findings after either atropine or cyclopentolate are comparable in children who are categorized as normal,[103] highly hyperopic,[104, 105] or strabismic,[106] or who have darkly pigmented irides.[107]

# References

1. Mutti DO, Zadnik K, Adams AJ: The equivalent refractive index of the crystalline lens in childhood. Vision Res 1995; 35:1565-1573.
2. Cook RC, Glasscock RE: Refractive and ocular findings in the newborn. Am J Ophthalmol 1951; 34:1407-1413.
3. Goldschmidt E: Refraction in the newborn. Acta Ophthalmol 1969; 47:570-578.
4. Santonastaso A: La rifrazione oculare nei primi anni di vita. Ann Ottalmol Clin Oculistica 1930; 58:852-884.
5. Mohindra I, Held R: Refraction in humans from birth to five years. Docum Ophthalmol Proc Series 1981; 28:19-27.
6. Dobson V, Fulton AB, Manning K, et al.: Cycloplegic refractions of premature infants. Am J Ophthalmol 1981; 91:490-495.
7. Grignolo A, Rivara A: Observations biométriques sur l'oeil de la enfants nés a terme et des prématurés au cours de la première année. Ann Oculistique 1968; 201:817-826.
8. Fledelius HC: Pre-term delivery and the growth of the eye. An oculometric study of eye size around term-time. Acta Ophthalmol (Suppl) 1992; 204:10-15.
9. Quinn GE, Dobson V, Repka MX, et al.: Development of myopia in infants with birth weights less than 1251 grams. Ophthalmology 1992; 99:329-340.
10. Fledelius H: Prematurity and the eye. Acta Ophthalmol (Suppl) 1976; 128:1-245.
11. Dobson V, Fulton AB, Sebris SL: Cycloplegic refractions of infants and young children: The axis of astigmatism. Invest Ophthalmol Vis Sci 1984; 25:83-87.
12. Howland HC, Sayles N: Photorefractive measurements of astigmatism in infants and young children. Invest Ophthalmol Vis Sci 1984; 25:93-102.
13. London R, Wick BC: Changes in angle lambda during growth: Theory and clinical applications. Am J Optom Physiol Opt 1982; 59:568-572.
14. Howland HC, Sayles N: Photokeratometric and photorefractive measurements of astigmatism in infants and young children. Vision Res 1985; 25:73-81.
15. Atkinson J, Braddick O, French J: Infant astigmatism: Its disappearance with age. Vision Res 1980; 20:891-893.
16. Mohindra I, Held R, Gwiazda J, Brill S: Astigmatism in infants. Science 1978; 202:329-330.
17. Larsen JS: The sagittal growth of the eye. II. Ultrasonic measurement of the axial diameter of the lens and the anterior segment from birth to puberty. Acta Ophthalmol 1971; 49:427-440.
18. Blum HL, Peters HB, Bettman JW: Vision Screening for Elementary Schools: The Orinda Study. Berkeley: University of California Press, 1959.
19. Goss DA, Cox VD: Trends in the change of clinical refractive error in myopes. J Am Optom Assoc 1985; 56:608-613.
20. Goss DA: Effect of bifocal lenses on the rate of childhood myopia progression. Am J Optom Physiol Opt 1986; 63:135-141.
21. Grosvenor T, Perrigin DM, Perrigin J, Maslovitz B: Houston Myopia Control Study: A randomized clinical trial. Part II. Final report by the patient care team. Am J Optom Physiol Opt 1987; 64:482-498.
22. Sorsby A, Benjamin B, Sheridan M: Refraction and Its Components During the Growth of the Eye from the Age of Three. London: Her Majesty's Stationery Office, 1961.
23. Goss DA, Winkler RL: Progression of myopia in youth: Age of cessation. Am J Optom Physiol Opt 1983; 60:651-658.
24. Sperduto RD, Siegel D, Roberts J, Rowland M: Prevalence of myopia in the United States. Arch Ophthalmol 1983; 101:405-407.

25. Atkinson J: Infant vision screening: Prediction and prevention of strabismus and amblyopia from refractive screening in the Cambridge Photorefraction Program. *In* Simons K: Early Visual Development: Normal and Abnormal. New York: Oxford University Press, 1993.
26. Fabian G: Augenärztliche Reihenuntersuchung von 1200 kindern im 2. Lebensjahr. Acta Ophthalmol 1966; 44:473-479.
27. Hirsch M: Changes in astigmatism during the first eight years in school—an interim report from the Ojai Longitudinal Study. Am J Optom Arch Am Acad Optom 1963; 40:127-132.
28. Zadnik K, Mutti DO, Adams AJ: Astigmatism in children: What's the rule? *In* Ophthalmic and Visual Optics Technical Digest. Washington, DC: Optical Society of America, 1992.
29. Slataper FJ: Age norms of refraction and vision. Arch Ophthalmol 1950; 43:466-481.
30. Brown N: The change in lens curvature with age. Exp Eye Res 1974; 19:175-183.
31. Grosvenor T: Reduction in axial length with age: An emmetropizing mechanism for the adult eye? Am J Optom Physiol Opt 1987; 64:657-663.
32. Ooi CS, Grosvenor T: Mechanisms of emmetropization in the aging eye. Optom Vis Sci 1995; 72:60-66.
33. Hemenger RP, Garner LF, Ooi CS: Change with age of the refractive index gradient of the human ocular lens. Invest Ophthalmol Vis Sci 1995; 36:703-707.
34. Wang Q, Klein BEK, Klein R, Moss SE: Refractive status in the Beaver Dam Eye Study. Invest Ophthalmol Vis Sci 1994; 35:4344-4347.
35. Hirsch M: Changes in astigmatism after the age of forty. Am J Optom Arch Am Acad Optom 1959; 36:395-405.
36. Irving EL, Sivak JG, Callender MG: Refractive plasticity of the developing chick eye. Ophthalmic Physiol Opt 1992; 12:448-456.
37. Wallman J, Wildsoet C, Xu A, et al.: Moving the retina: Choroidal modulation of the refractive state. Vision Res 1995; 35:37-50.
38. Cheng H, Singh OS, Kwong KK, et al.: Shape of the myopic eye as seen with high-resolution magnetic resonance imaging. Optom Vis Sci 1992; 698-701.
39. Zadnik K, Mutti DO: How applicable are animal myopia models to human juvenile onset myopia? Vision Res 1995; 35:1283-1288.
40. Ware J: Observations relative to the near and distant sight of different persons. Philosoph Trans Soc London 1813; 103:31-50.
41. Cohn H: The Hygiene of the Eye in Schools. London: Simpkin, Marshall and Co, 1886.
42. Young FA, Leary GA, Baldwin WR, et al.: The transmission of refractive errors within Eskimo families. Am J Optom Arch Am Acad Optom 1969; 46:676-685.
43. Lam CSY, Goh WSH: The incidence of refractive errors among school children in Hong Kong and its relationship with the optical components. Clin Exp Optom 1991; 74:97-103.
44. Au Eong KG, Tay TH, Lim MK: Race, culture and myopia in 110,236 young Singaporean males. Singapore Med J 1993; 34:29-32.
45. Hofstetter HW: Emmetropization—biological process or mathematical artifact? Am J Optom Arch Am Acad Optom 1969; 46:447-450.
46. Sorsby A, Benjamin B, Davey JB, et al.: Emmetropia and Its Aberrations. London: Her Majesty's Stationery Office, 1957.
47. Zadnik K, Satariano WA, Mutti DO, et al.: The effect of parental history of myopia on children's eye size. JAMA 1994; 271:1323-1327.
48. Gwiazda J, Thorn F, Bauer J, Held R: Emmetropization and the progression of manifest refraction in children followed from infancy to puberty. Clin Vis Sci 1993; 8:337-344.
49. Sorsby A, Sheridan M, Leary GA: Refraction and Its Components in Twins. London: Her Majesty's Stationery Office, 1962.
50. Teikari JM, Kaprio J, Koskenvuo MK, Vannas A: Heritability estimate for refractive errors—a population-based sample of adult twins. Genet Epidemiol 1988; 5:171-181.
51. Hirsch MJ: Predictability of refraction at age 14 on the basis of testing at age 6—interim report from the Ojai Longitudinal Study of Refraction. Am J Optom Arch Am Acad Optom 1964; 41:567-573.
52. Mutti DO, Zadnik K: The utility of three predictors of childhood myopia: A Bayesian analysis. Vision Res 1995; 35:1345-1352.
53. Mäntyjärvi MI: Predicting of myopia progression in school. J Pediatr Ophthalmol Strab 1985; 22:71-75.
54. Goss DA, Winkler RL: Progression of myopia in youth: Age of cessation. Am J Optom Physiol Opt 1983; 60:651-658.
55. Zadnik K, Mutti DO, Adams AJ: The repeatability of measurement of the ocular components. Invest Ophthalmol Vis Sci 1992; 33:2325-2333.
56. Charman WN, Jennings JAM: Objective measurements of the longitudinal chromatic aberration of the human eye. Vision Res 1976; 16:999-1005.
57. Glickstein M, Millodot M: Retinoscopy and eye size. Science 1970; 168:605-606.
58. Mutti DO, Ver Hoeve JN, Zadnik K, Murphy CJ: Is there an artifact of retinoscopy? Comparison of retinoscopic to visual evoked potential refraction in the rat. Invest Ophthalmol Vis Sci (Suppl) 1994; 35:1804.
59. Rempt F, Hoogerheide J, Hoogenboom W: Peripheral retinoscopy and the skiagram. Ophthalmologica 1971; 162:1-10.
60. Grosvenor T, Quintero S, Perrigin DM: Predicting refractive astigmatism: A suggested simplification of Javal's rule. Am J Optom Physiol Opt 1988; 65:292-297.
61. Elliott M, Callendar MG, Elliott DB: Accuracy of Javal's rule in the determination of spectacle astigmatism. Optom Vis Sci 1994; 71:23-26.
62. Rosenfield M, Ciuffreda KJ: Effect of surround propinquity on the open-loop accommodative response. Invest Ophthalmol Vis Sci 1991; 32:142-147.
63. McBrien NA, Millodot M: The relationship between tonic accommodation and refractive error. Invest Ophthalmol Vis Sci 1987; 29:460-469.
64. Atkinson J, Braddick O: Infant precursors of later visual disorders: Correlation or causality? *In* Yonas A: 20th Minnesota Symposium on Child Psychology. Hillsdale, NJ: Erlbaum, 1988.
65. Rosner J, Rosner J: Relation between tonic accommodation and visual perceptual skills development in 6- to 12-year-old children. Optom Vis Sci 1989; 66:526-529.
66. Zonis S, Miller B: Refractions in the Israeli newborn. J Pediatr Ophthalmol 1974; 11:77-81.
67. van Alphen GWHM: On emmetropia and ametropia. Ophthalmologica (Suppl) 1961; 142:1-92.
68. Stenström S: Investigation of the variation and the correlation of the optical elements of human eyes. Am J Optom Arch Amer Acad Optom 1948; 25:218-286, 340-388, 438-496.
69. Havener WH: Ocular Pharmacology. St. Louis: CV Mosby Company, 1983.
70. Helveston E, Ellis FD: Pediatric Ophthalmology Practice. St. Louis: CV Mosby Company, 1980.
71. Gettes BC: Choice of mydriatics and cycloplegics for diagnostic examinations in children. *In* Apt L: Diagnostic Procedures in Pediatric Ophthalmology. Boston: Little, Brown and Company, 1963.

72. Marron J: Cycloplegia and mydriasis by use of atropine, scopolamine, and homatropine-paredrine. Arch Ophthalmol 1940; 23:340-350.

73. Wolf AV, Hodge AC: Effects of atropine sulfate, methylatropine nitrate (metropine) and homatropine hydrobromide on adult human eyes. Arch Ophthalmol 1946; 36:293-301.

74. Milder B, Riffenburgh RS: An evaluation of cyclogyl (compound 75 GT). Am J Ophthalmol 1953; 36:1724-1726.

75. Priestly BS, Medine MM: A new mydriatic and cycloplegic drug: Compound 75 GT. Am J Ophthalmol 1951; 34:572-575.

76. Lovasik JV: Pharmacokinetics of topically applied cyclopentolate HCl and tropicamide. Am J Optom Physiol Opt 1986; 63:787-803.

77. Jose JG, Polse KA, Holden EK: Optometric Pharmacology. Orlando: Grune and Stratton, 1984.

78. Gettes BC, Leopold IH: Evaluation of five new cycloplegic drugs. Arch Ophthalmol 1953; 49:24-27.

79. Gettes BC, Belmont O: Tropicamide: Comparative cycloplegic effects. Arch Ophthalmol 1961; 66:336-340.

80. Merrill DL, Goldberg B, Zavell S: bis-Tropamide, a new parasympatholytic. Curr Therap Res 1960; 2:43-50.

81. Barbee RF, Smith WO: A comparative study of mydriatic and cycloplegic agents in human subjects without eye disease. Am J Ophthalmol 1957; 44:617-622.

82. Simcoe CW: Cyclopentolate (cyclogyl) toxicity. Arch Ophthalmol 1962; 67:406-408.

83. Adcock EW: Cyclopentolate (cyclogyl) toxicity in pediatric patients. J Pediatr 1971; 79:127-129.

84. Awan KJ: Adverse systemic reactions of topical cyclopentolate hydrochloride. Ann Ophthalmol 1976; 8:695-698.

85. Beswick JA: Psychosis from cyclopentolate. Am J Ophthalmol 1962; 53:879-880.

86. Binkhorst RD, Weinstein GW, Baretz RM, Clahane AC: Psychotic reaction induced by cyclopentolate (cyclogel). Am J Ophthalmol 1963; 55:1243-1245.

87. Khurana AK, Ahluwalia BK, Rajan C, Vohra AK: Acute psychosis associated with topical cyclopentolate hydrochloride. Am J Ophthalmol 1988; 105:91.

88. Mark HH: Psychotogenic properties of cyclopentolate. JAMA 1963; 186:430-431.

89. Praeger DL, Miller SN: Toxic effects of cyclopentolate (cyclogel): Report of a case. Am J Ophthalmol 1964; 58:1060-1061.

90. Garston MJ: A closer look at diagnostic drugs for optometric use. J Am Optom Assoc 1975; 46:39-43.

91. Yolton DP, Kandel JS, Yolton RL: Diagnostic pharmaceutical agents: Side effects encountered in a study of 15,000 applications. J Am Optom Assoc 1980; 51:113-117.

92. Gettes BC: Tropicamide, a new cycloplegic mydriatic. Arch Ophthalmol 1961; 65:632-635.

93. Pollack SL, Hunt JS, Polse KA: Dose-response effects of tropicamide HCl. Am J Optom Physiol Opt 1981; 58:361-366.

94. Gambill HD, Ogle KN, Kearns TP: Mydriatic effect of four drugs determined with pupillograph. Arch Ophthalmol 1967; 77:740-746.

95. Keller JT: The risk of angle closure from the use of mydriatics. J Am Optom Assoc 1975; 46:19-21.

96. Mordi JA, Lyle WM, Mousa GY: Does prior instillation of a topical anesthetic enhance the effect of tropicamide? Am J Optom Physiol Opt 1986; 63:290-293.

97. Milder B: Tropicamide as a cycloplegic agent. Arch Ophthalmol 1961; 66:70-72.

98. Cable MK, Hendrickson RO, Hanna C: Evaluation of drugs in ointment for mydriasis and cycloplegia. Arch Ophthalmol 1978; 96:84-86.

99. Rosenfield M, Linfield PB: A comparison of the effects of cycloplegics on accommodation ability for distance vision and on the apparent near point. Ophthalmic Physiol Opt 1986; 6:317-320.

100. Gettes BC: Three new cycloplegic drugs: Clinical report. Arch Ophthalmol 1954; 51:467-472.

101. Stolzar IH: A new group of cycloplegic drugs. Am J Ophthalmol 1953; 36:110-112.

102. Egashira SM, Kish LL, Twelker JD, et al.: Comparison of cyclopentolate versus tropicamide cycloplegia in children. Optom Vis Sci 1993; 70:1019-1026.

103. Ingram RM, Barr A: Refraction of 1-year-old children after cycloplegia with 1% cyclopentolate: Comparison with findings after atropinisation. Br J Ophthalmol 1979; 63:348-352.

104. Zetterström C: A cross-over study of the cycloplegic effects of a single topical application of cyclopentolate-phenylephrine and routine atropinisation for 3.5 days. Acta Ophthalmol 1985; 63:525-529.

105. Robb RM, Petersen RA: Cycloplegic refractions in children. J Pediatr Ophthalmol 1968; 5:110-114.

106. Rosenbaum AL, Bateman JB, Bremer DL, Liu PY: Cycloplegic refraction in esotropic children. Cyclopentolate versus atropine. Ophthalmology 1981; 88:1031-1034.

107. Khurana AK, Ahluwalia BK, Rajan C: Status of cyclopentolate as a cycloplegic in children: A comparison with atropine and homatropine. Acta Ophthalmol 1988; 66:721-724.

*Mark Rosenfield, PhD, BSc(Hons), MCOptom*

5

# Accommodation

Accommodation refers to a temporary change in the refractive power of the crystalline lens resulting from contraction of the ciliary muscle, thereby altering the location of that point in space which is optically conjugate with the retina. This process allows diverging light from a near object to focus on the retina.[1]

# The Physiology and Anatomy of Accommodation

Early investigators proposed that temporary changes in the refractive power of the eye could be brought about either by elongation of the globe, changes in corneal curvature, or variations in pupil size.[2] However, in 1677, Descartes was the first to propose that accommodation is accomplished by a change in the shape of the crystalline lens. This hypothesis was confirmed by Porterfield, who observed that accommodation was absent in aphakic patients,[3] and later in a series of experiments by Young.[4]

In studies of Purkinje images III and IV, formed by reflection at the anterior and posterior crystalline lens surfaces, respectively, Helmholtz demonstrated that the anterior pole of the lens moves forward during accommodation, while the posterior pole remains relatively stationary.[5] In the unaccommodated state, the anterior lens surface is roughly spherical, with a radius of curvature of approximately 11 to 12 mm.[6, 7] When the eye accommodates, this anterior surface becomes approximately hyperboloid (although the central 3-mm region does remain approximately spherical, with a radius of curvature of up to 5 mm).[7] In addition, the peripheral zones of the anterior lens surface exhibit only minor changes in curvature and may even become slightly flatter during active accommodation.[7] The change in the radius of curvature of the anterior lens surface with

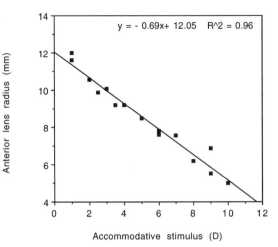

$$y = -0.69x + 12.05 \quad R^2 = 0.96$$

**FIGURE 5–1** The radius of curvature of the anterior crystalline lens surface plotted against the dioptric stimulus to accommodation in two 19-year-old male subjects. A linear relationship may be observed between these two parameters within the range of stimuli tested. (Data from Fincham, 1937.[6])

increasing accommodation is illustrated in Figure 5-1. For a summary of those physical changes occurring during accommodation, see Table 5-1.

Contraction of the ciliary muscle pulls the choroid forward and the ciliary attachment of the zonule inward, thereby producing relaxation in the tension of the zonular fibers and allowing the lens to become more convex as a result of both the elastic forces in the lens capsule[6] and the viscoelastic properties of the lens substance.[8, 9]

## INNERVATION OF THE ACCOMMODATIVE RESPONSE

The ciliary muscle is innervated by the autonomic nervous system and receives supply from both the parasympathetic and sympathetic divisions.

**TABLE 5–1** Change in Ocular Dimensions when Increasing the Accommodative Stimulus from 1.00 D to 9.00 D in Two 19-Year-Old Individuals

|  | Subject 1 | | Subject 2 | |
|---|---|---|---|---|
|  | **1.00 D** | **9.00 D** | **1.00 D** | **9.00 D** |
| Anterior lens radius of curvature (mm) | 11.62 | 6.90 | 12.00 | 5.00 |
| Anterior chamber depth (mm) | 3.68 | 3.34 | 3.33 | 3.06 |
| Relative movement of anterior pole (mm) | — | +0.34 | — | +0.27 |
| Lens thickness (mm) | 3.68 | 4.24 | 3.84 | 4.20 |
| Posterior lens radius of curvature (mm) | 5.18 | 5.05 | 5.74 | 4.87 |

Data reproduced with permission from Fincham.[6]

## Parasympathetic Innervation

The efferent pathway starts from the peristriate region of the visual cortex and travels down the internal corticotectal tract to the hypothalamus and the Edinger-Westphal nucleus. Parasympathetic fibers originate within the Edinger-Westphal nucleus. These fibers pass out of the midbrain in the main trunk of the third cranial nerve and enter the orbit via the inferior oblique branch of the oculomotor nerve. They subsequently leave this branch to form the motor root of the ciliary ganglion. Within the ganglion the parasympathetic fibers are thought to synapse,[10, 11] although Westheimer and Blair proposed that the fibers pass through the ganglion without synapsing.[12] The myelinated post-ganglionic fibers enter the globe via the short ciliary nerves around the optic nerve and pass forward in the perichoroidal space to supply the ciliary muscle.[13]

## Sympathetic Innervation

The role of sympathetic innervation to the ciliary muscle during accommodation was comprehensively reviewed by Gilmartin, who cited anatomical, physiological, pharmacological, clinical, and psychological evidence for the sympathetic supply playing a role in the control of accommodation.[14] The sympathetic fibers travel from the cervical sympathetic trunk and synapse at the superior cervical ganglion. From there they pass along the trunk of the internal carotid to the cavernous plexus. They subsequently pass forward to the eye as two long ciliary nerves[15] and the short ciliary nerves via the sympathetic root of the ciliary ganglion.[16]

The nature of sympathetic innervation to the ciliary muscle may be summarized as follows.[14]

1. The sympathetic input is inhibitory in nature and mediated via beta-adrenergic receptors, predominantly of the beta-2 subgroup.[17, 18]
2. The input is relatively small with respect to the predominant parasympathetic output[19] and has a maximum dioptric value of around $-1.50$ D.
3. The time course of sympathetic activity is significantly slower than that of parasympathetic activity, taking 10 to 40 seconds to reach its maximum effect.[19-21] In contrast, parasympathetically mediated responses are completed in approximately 1 to 2 seconds for normal visual environments.[22]
4. Sympathetic activity appears to be augmented by concurrent parasympathetic activity.[19, 20, 23-26]

## QUANTIFYING ACCOMMODATION

Both the accommodative stimulus and accommodative response are conventionally measured in diopters (D), that is, the reciprocal of the linear distance in meters from the eye to the target (for the accommodative stimulus) or the point conjugate with the retina (for the accommodative response). For example, in the case of a fully corrected subject fixating an object of regard at a viewing distance of 2 meters, the stimulus to accommodation equals 1/2 or 0.50 D.

### Effect of Uncorrected Refractive Error

In Figure 5-2, an emmetropic patient whose eye has a total refractive power of $+60.00$ D when viewing a distant object of regard wishes to view a near object at 0.5 meter. Thus, the power of the eye must be increased from $+60.00$ to $+62.00$ D, a change in refractive power (i.e., accommodative stimulus) of 2.00 D. However, if a 2.00 D uncorrected hyperope, having a total, unaccommodated refractive power of only $+58.00$ D, wishes to view this same near target,

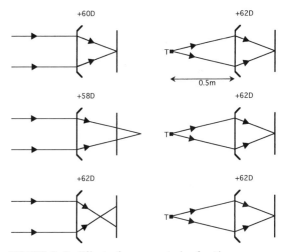

**FIGURE 5-2** Effect of uncorrected refractive error on the stimulus to accommodation. The left top, middle, and bottom diagrams indicate an emmetrope, 2.00 D hyperope, and 2.00 D myope viewing a distant target, respectively. The right top, middle, and bottom diagrams illustrate the dioptric requirement for these same subjects to observe a target at a viewing distance of 0.5 meter. The dioptric stimulus to accommodation is the required change in the refractive power of the eye when shifting fixation from the distant to the near object, which equals 2.00 D, 4.00 D, and 0.00 D for the emmetrope, hyperope, and myope, respectively. Note, for simplicity in this and subsequent figures, a simple reduced eye is used, that is, one with a single refracting surface.

then the required change in refractive power to bring the image of the near object onto the retina (i.e., the accommodative stimulus) is 4.00 D. Conversely, for a 2.00 D myope, the accommodative stimulus is zero because the target is already located at the individual's far point.

## SPECTACLE VERSUS OCULAR ACCOMMODATION

In clinical practice, most measurements of accommodation are referred to the spectacle plane. This is termed **spectacle accommodation.** However, because most of the refraction takes place at the eye, strictly speaking, the accommodative stimulus should be calculated at the principal point of the eye, that is, **ocular accommodation.**

EXAMPLE

A myopic patient is fully corrected by a thin, $-4.00$ D spectacle lens at a vertex distance of 14 mm. An object of regard is located 350 mm in front of the cornea. What is the stimulus for ocular and spectacle accommodation?

The stimulus for *spectacle accommodation* is simply the reciprocal of the distance (in meters) from the object to the spectacle plane plane, i.e., $1/0.336 = 2.98$ D.

When quantifying *ocular accommodation,* one must consider the difference between the vergence of light at the eye when viewing the near object and the vergence when viewing an object located at optical infinity.

### *Viewing a Near Object*

Because the object is being viewed through a $-4.00$ D lens, the actual stimulus to accommodation is the image formed by the spectacle lens. Accordingly, one must determine the location of this image.

$$F = 1/u' - 1/u$$
$$\text{Therefore, } -4.00 = 1/u' - (1/0.336)$$
$$1/u' = -4.00 - 2.98 = -6.98 \text{ D}$$
$$u' = -143 \text{ mm}$$

Thus the image of the near object is located $-143 - 14 = -157$ mm (in front of the eye).

Therefore, vergence of the near object at the eye $= 1/-0.157 = -6.37$ D.

### *Viewing a Distant Object*

$$F = 1/u' - 1/u$$
$$\text{Therefore, } -4.00 = 1/u' - (1/-\infty)$$

$$1/u' = -4.00 - 0 = -4.00 \text{ D}$$
$$1/u' = -250 \text{ mm}$$

Thus the image of the distant object is located $-250 - 14 = -264$ mm (in front of the eye).

Therefore, vergence of the distant object at the eye $= 1/-0.264 = -3.79$ D.

Ocular accom- = Vergence of distant object
modation        $-$ Vergence of near object
$$= (-3.79) - (-6.37)$$
$$= +2.58 \text{ D}$$

Thus for this myopic patient, ocular accommodation is less than spectacle accommodation.

If the same calculation is carried out for a 4.00 D hyperope and an emmetrope, the results would be as shown in Table 5-2. Examination of these findings indicates that the ocular stimulus to accommodation is greatest in the hyperopic patient and least in the myope when both are corrected with spectacle lenses. However, if these patients were corrected with contact lenses, then the stimulus to ocular accommodation would be equal in all cases (2.86 D). Thus, when compared with a spectacle prescription, contact lenses produce an increased accommodative demand in myopes and decreased accommodative demand in hyperopes. This can be especially relevant when prescribing contact lenses for a myopic pre-presbyope.

# Clinical Measurement of Accommodation

. . . . . . . . . . . . . . . . . . . . . . . . . . . . . .

## AMPLITUDE OF ACCOMMODATION

☐ The **far point of accommodation** is the point conjugate with the retina when accommodation is fully relaxed.

| TABLE 5–2 Comparison of Spectacle and Ocular Accommodative Stimulus When Viewing an Object of Regard at a Distance of 350 mm in Front of the Cornea (Vertex Distance = 14 mm) for a 4.00 D Myope, Emmetrope, and 4.00 D Hyperopic Patient | | |
|---|---|---|
| | Spectacle Accommodation (D) | Ocular Accommodation (D) |
| 4.00 D Myope | 2.98 | 2.58 |
| Emmetrope | NA | 2.86 |
| 4.00 D Hyperope | 2.98 | 3.20 |

□ The **near point of accommodation** is the point conjugate with the retina when accommodation is fully exerted.

□ The **amplitude of accommodation** is the dioptric distance between the far point and the near point of accommodation.

If the far point of accommodation is located at optical infinity, that is, zero diopters, then the amplitude of accommodation simply equals the near point of accommodation, or the reciprocal of the nearest distance (measured in meters) at which distinct vision can be obtained. Accordingly, when this parameter is measured clinically, it is simplest to measure the near point after the subject's refractive error has been fully corrected.

A number of techniques are available to the clinician for determining the amplitude of accommodation:

1. The push-up (and push-down) technique
2. Minus lens technique
3. Dynamic retinoscopy and other optometers

## Push-up Technique

The procedure here aims to identify the near point of accommodation, that is, the target location for which the patient is exerting his or her maximum accommodative response. Therefore, the clinician wishes to determine the closest distance at which the target remains absolutely sharp. In practice, such an end point is difficult to identify consistently. Accordingly, rather than attempting to determine this last point of clear vision, it is conventional to locate the position where the target exhibits the **first, slight, sustained blur.** Although the target location corres-

ponding to this first blur is marginally closer to the patient than the true near point, this difference is likely to be extremely small, and perhaps more importantly, this end point can be demonstrated consistently in most patients.

A diagrammatic representation of this procedure is shown in Figure 5-3. The accommodative stimulus is increased steadily in a ramplike fashion, and in a normal, pre-presbyopic individual, the subject produces an appropriate increase in the accommodative response. It should be noted from Figure 5-3 that with the exception of a single stimulus level, the accommodative response is never equal to the stimulus; for low dioptric (i.e., distant) targets, the response generally *exceeds* the stimulus (usually referred to as the lead of accommodation), whereas for higher dioptric (i.e., near) objects of regard, the response is typically *less* than the stimulus (lag of accommodation). The depth of focus of the eye allows the subject to maintain a clear image of the object despite these slight errors in accommodation. Examination of Figure 5-3 reveals that the patient reports the first slight blur when the dioptric separation of the stimulus and response exceeds one-half of the depth of focus of the eye, typically of the order of 0.40 D. It is also apparent from this figure that different measurements of the amplitude of accommodation are recorded, depending on whether the accommodative stimulus location or the actual accommodative response is measured.

An alternative end point for this procedure is that the target should be advanced toward the patient until the letters become so blurred that the patient cannot read them (also termed the blur-out end point[1]). However, the use of this blur-out end point results in a significant overestimate of the near point (probably of the order of

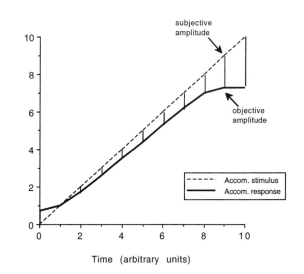

**FIGURE 5-3** Diagrammatic illustration of the push-up amplitude of accommodation procedure. The solid line indicates the accommodative response to the steadily increasing accommodative stimulus (*broken line*) plotted with respect to time. The end point (i.e., the report of the first, slight, sustained blur) of this test occurs when the separation between the accommodative stimulus and response (shown by the vertical lines) exceeds one half of the depth of focus of the eye. The objective amplitude represents the maximum, objectively measured accommodative response (not usually determined during this procedure) whereas the subjective amplitude is the accommodative stimulus that produces this maximum response.

1.00 to 2.00 D in young subjects, although this varies with age), because the target is advanced well beyond the point of maximum accommodation, which is represented by the closest distance at which the target is last seen clearly.

### Clinical Procedure

The patient observes a finely detailed test object, which is advanced toward the eye until the detail "just begins to blur and remains blurred," that is, the **first, slight, sustained blur.** The patient should always be encouraged to try and clear the target when he or she first reports blur because the goal is to achieve the maximum accommodative response. The reciprocal of the distance from the target at this position of first, slight, sustained blur to the spectacle plane (in meters) represents the near point of accommodation (in diopters).

## Push-down Amplitude of Accommodation

In the push-down procedure, the target is advanced a little beyond this point of the first sustained blur (i.e., closer than the near point) and then moved away from the patient until the target "just becomes absolutely clear." This procedure attempts to obtain a more accurate determination of the near point, that is, the closest point at which the target remains clear, rather than the first slight blur. However, care must be taken to ensure that the target is advanced only slightly beyond the first blur position. If the stimulus is moved several diopters closer than the near point, the patient may start to relax his or her accommodative response. Such relaxation would subsequently necessitate a large increase in accommodation when the decreasing stimulus does fall within the individual's amplitude of accommodation. Such a large change might be produced relatively slowly, especially in early presbyopes.

In a comparison of amplitudes determined using both the push-up and push-down techniques, Fitch reported higher amplitudes of accommodation using the push-up procedure, which were statistically significant in those subjects over 40 years of age.[27] Similarly, an additional study (Telor Ophthalmic Pharmaceuticals Inc., unpublished data, 1994) also observed a significantly greater amplitude of accommodation using the push-up procedure in a population of early presbyopes. When examining 25 subjects between 35 and 46 years of age (mean age = 42.6 years), the mean amplitudes obtained using the push-up and push-down procedures were 2.44 D (SEM = ±0.10) and 2.33 D (SEM = ±0.08), respectively. This difference was significant ($P = 0.03$).

A valuable compromise might be to take the average of the push-up and push-down findings.[28] This may provide a more accurate assessment of the near point of accommodation because it incorporates both the slight overestimate of the near point during the push-up procedure and the possible small underestimate occurring with the push-down technique.

An additional factor to consider is whether the patient or examiner moves the target. Fitch demonstrated that allowing the patient to grasp the target resulted in a significant increase in the amplitude of accommodation in all subjects under 50 years of age.[27] It seems likely that this resulted from the effect of the enhanced stimulus to proximally induced accommodation.[29]

## Minus Lens Technique

In this procedure, the target remains at a fixed position (typically 40 cm [2.50 D]), and minus lenses are introduced to move the location of the optical image of the target. This is illustrated in Figure 5-4. A near target is placed at 40 cm (2.50 D), and minus lenses are introduced in 0.25 D steps until the patient reports the first noticeable, sustained blur that cannot be cleared by further conscious effort (Fig. 5-5). The total amplitude is equal to the amount of minus lens power introduced, plus the 2.50 D required to focus initially on the target. This technique is used for each eye individually. However, it is not performed binocularly, as this would be assessing positive relative accommodation.

### Differences Between Minus Lens and Push-up Techniques

During testing with the minus lens technique, the target remains fixed; accordingly, the psycho-

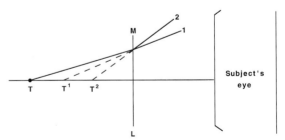

**FIGURE 5–4** Measurement of the amplitude of accommodation using the minus lens procedure. As minus lenses (ML) of increasing power are introduced before the eye, light rays from the near target (T) are increasingly diverged to produce images of T at T[1] and T[2], respectively. The increasing proximity of these images enhances the blur-stimulus to accommodation.

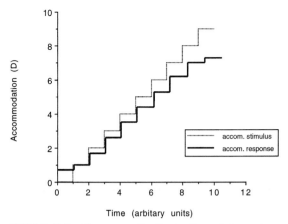

**FIGURE 5–5** Diagrammatic illustration of the minus lens amplitude of accommodation procedure. The solid line indicates the accommodative response to the step changes in accommodative stimulus (*broken line*) plotted with respect to time. Again, the end point (i.e., the report of the first, slight, sustained blur) of this test occurs when the separation between the accommodative stimulus and response exceeds one half of the depth of focus of the eye.

logical proximal stimulus to accommodation remains relatively constant. However, the target minification resulting from the minus lenses may make the target appear smaller and consequently further away as the dioptric stimulus demand is increased.[30, 31] This is in contrast to the push-up technique, in which the angular subtense of the target increases for higher dioptric stimuli. The latter situation (i.e., target size and accommodative demand changing concurrently in the same direction) is more natural than the minus lens method. Studies have recorded higher amplitudes with the push-up technique than with the minus lens procedure, probably due to the additional proximally induced accommodation stimulated by the advancing target.[32, 33] However, the increased angular subtense of the target when performing the push-up procedure at high dioptric demands should also be considered (see later section on Target Size).

## Objective Techniques

The amplitude of accommodation may also be measured using any type of optometer, an instrument that measures the actual accommodative response. Because the conventional clinical procedure determines the stimulus level that corresponds with this maximum response, one would predict that these objective measurements would obtain lower amplitudes than the subjective findings due to the lag of accommodation (Fig. 5–3).

Objective measurements may be particularly useful in those patients who are unable to cooperate in the subjective procedures for any reason, such as an inability to report the required end point. In addition, it provides a veridical measurement of the maximum accommodative response.

The most common technique used to assess the objective amplitude is dynamic retinoscopy. The accommodative response is measured for a series of increasing stimulus levels until the maximum response is achieved. This maximum response corresponds to the objective amplitude. An example of a typical series of measurements is provided in Table 5–3. However, any optometer, such as an autorefractor, may be used to determine the objective amplitude, provided that an adequate range of stimuli can be introduced.

## ADDITIONAL FACTORS AFFECTING MEASUREMENTS OF THE ACCOMMODATIVE AMPLITUDE

### Monocular Versus Binocular Measurements

Push-up and push-down measurements of the amplitude of accommodation may be obtained under both monocular and binocular viewing conditions. When testing monocularly, the limiting factor is the magnitude of blur-driven accommodation (although proximally induced ac-

| **TABLE 5–3**  Assessment of the Amplitude of Accommodation Using Dynamic Retinoscopy* | |
|---|---|
| Target at 40 cm   (AS = 2.50 D) | Neutral at 50 cm (AR = 2.00 D) |
| Target at 25 cm   (AS = 4.00 D) | Neutral at 33 cm (AR = 3.00 D) |
| Target at 20 cm   (AS = 5.00 D) | Neutral at 25 cm (AR = 4.00 D) |
| Target at 17 cm   (AS = 6.00 D) | Neutral at 20 cm (AR = 5.00 D) |
| Target at 14 cm   (AS = 7.00 D) | Neutral at 20 cm (AR = 5.00 D) |
| Target at 13.5 cm (AS = 8.00 D) | Neutral at 20 cm (AR = 5.00 D) |
| Therefore, objective amplitude of accommodation = 5.00 D. | |

*For each target distance *(i.e., accommodative stimulus [AS]), the accommodative response (AR) is determined by finding the location of the point conjugate with the retina. This may be achieved by altering the retinoscopic working distance while keeping the near object of regard fixed. Eventually a point is reached where further increases in the accommodative stimulus are not accompanied by an increase in the accommodative response. Thus the maximum response may be determined.

commodation also adds a small contribution[29, 34]). In contrast, when testing binocularly, the addition of convergent accommodation must also be considered. When measuring the binocular amplitude, subjects are required to maintain both a clear *and* single binocular image of the object of regard. Thus, both the accommodative and vergence responses must be appropriate for the target stimulus.

Duane reported that the binocular amplitude was regularly higher than the monocular finding, although this difference declined with age.[35] He reported "usual differences" of 1.00 to 2.00 D in 8- to 15-year-olds, which declined to almost zero in subjects over 40 years of age. Both Fitch and Schapero and Nadell also observed slightly higher amplitudes when assessed binocularly.[27, 36] Their findings are illustrated in Figure 5–6. Although Fitch noted that the difference between the monocular and binocular result was statistically significant in subjects above 32 years of age, inspection of this figure clearly indicates that these differences would not be clinically significant.[27] However, Otake et al., using an objective infrared optometer, recorded larger binocular amplitudes, with the difference ranging from 0.10 to 2.20 D (mean difference = 0.70 D).[37] Both Otake et al. and Fitch observed that the difference between the monocular and binocular amplitudes increased with age,[27, 37] which is not consistent with the findings of Duane.[35]

When measuring the binocular accommodative amplitude, care must be taken to measure the actual distance from the target to the spectacle plane along the visual axis. If this is measured along the midline, then it results in a shorter physical measurement and an apparently ele-

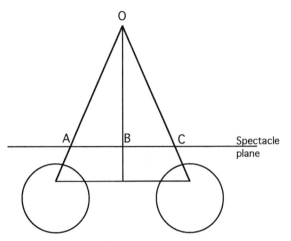

**FIGURE 5–7**  When determining the binocular amplitude of accommodation, the target distance must be measured along the visual axis, that is, distance OA (when determined with respect to the spectacle plane). If the target distance is measured along the midline (OB), then OA can be calculated using the Pythagorean theorem. This difference is particularly significant in young patients. For example, if OB equals 10 cm (10.00 D), then OA equals 10.44 cm (9.58 D) in a patient with a near centration distance of 60 mm. Thus, the midline measurement overestimates the binocular amplitude by 0.42 D.

vated accommodative amplitude (in diopters). This is particularly important in young patients (Fig. 5–7).

In contrast, the minus lens technique can be used only under monocular conditions. During the binocular push-up and push-down procedures, the disparity-vergence stimulus changes concurrently with the accommodative stimulus. However, when adopting the minus lens technique, the disparity-vergence stimulus remains fixed at approximately 2.5 meter-angles. Thus, if the procedure were performed binocularly, this would require increased accommodation while maintaining the vergence response at a relatively constant level. This is a test of positive relative accommodation.

## Angle of Gaze

Ripple examined the monocular subjective amplitude of accommodation using the push-up procedure in varying directions of gaze. He observed that when varying horizontal gaze 20° on either side of the midline, the accommodative amplitude was greatest when looking nasally (mean = 11.40 D) and least when looking temporally (mean = 9.84 D).[38] Additionally, when examining the effects of variations in vertical gaze in 56 subjects, Ripple noted that the mean

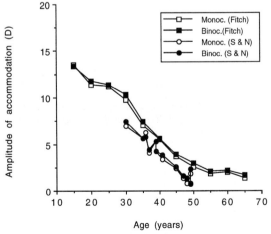

**FIGURE 5–6**  Mean monocular and binocular push-up amplitudes of accommodation versus age. (Data from Fitch[27] and Schapero and Nadell [S & N].[36])

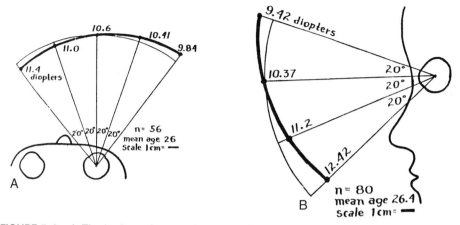

FIGURE 5–8  *A,* The horizontal near-point curve of accommodation. The broad dark line joins the mean monocular near-point of accommodation of 56 normal, pre-presbyopic individuals in the designated directions of horizontal gaze at eye level. The fine line is of equal distance from the eye. *B,* The vertical near-point curve of accommodation. (From Ripple PH: Variation of accommodation in vertical directions of gaze. Am J Ophthalmol 1952; 35:1630–1634.)

amplitude ranged from 9.42 D when looking 20° upward to 12.42 D when viewing 40° downward (Fig. 5–8). Ripple suggested that this observation of increased accommodative ability when looking down and in may be related to the output of convergent accommodation, which would be consistent with the finding of an esophoric shift in near heterophoria with downward gaze.[39]

In contrast, Takeda at al. measured the objective amplitude of accommodation in three subjects and found no significant change in the near point of accommodation with varying gaze angle; however, they did observe a myopic shift in the far point with downward gaze.[40] Nevertheless, these two studies[39, 40] indicate that the amplitude of accommodation may vary with gaze angle. Thus, the practitioner should measure the accommodation amplitude in the patient's habitual angle of gaze. Clearly this is impossible if amplitude measurements are performed only through a phoropter, and the clinician should consider the use of a trial frame and lenses to allow measurement of amplitude under naturalistic viewing angles.

## Target Size

Somers and Ford noted that when observing larger targets, the borders of the image are farther apart and there is less overlap of their blur distributions.[41] Thus, the use of larger optotypes when measuring the amplitude of accommodation may produce a delay in the patient's first appreciating the presence of blur, resulting in an erroneously elevated amplitude of accommodation. This was confirmed by Rosenfield and

Cohen, who measured the subjective push-up amplitude of accommodation using Snellen optotypes ranging in size from 20/20 (6/6) to 20/100 (6/30).[42] The mean values of amplitude of accommodation for the five target sizes are illustrated in Figure 5–9, and it is apparent that variations in target size do indeed produce significant changes in the subjective amplitude of accommodation.

Although a small target clearly represents the most suitable stimulus for the push-up procedure, caution must be exercised when choosing an appropriate stimulus size due to the age-

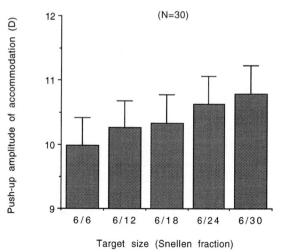

FIGURE 5–9  Mean push-up amplitude of accommodation recorded when viewing Snellen optotypes of varying sizes. All Snellen fractions are referenced to 40 cm. Error bars indicate 1 SEM. (From Rosenfield M, Cohen AS: Push-up amplitude of accommodation and letter size. Ophthalmic Physiol Opt 1995; 15:231–232.)

related recession of the near point. Because a 20/20 letter on a chart calibrated for a viewing distance of 40 cm subtends 5 minutes of arc at 40 cm and 20 minutes of arc at 10 cm, it is apparent that the same target should not be used on patients with accommodative amplitudes of 2.50 D and 10.00 D, respectively. Berens and Fonda proposed that the amplitude of accommodation should be measured using a target that subtends an angle of no more than 5 minutes of arc at the individual's near point. For patients under 30 years of age, they recommended a letter that subtends 5 minutes of arc at a distance of 20 cm (physical height of this letter = 0.29 mm).[43] However, it is evident that this target subtends 10 minutes of arc when located at the near point of a patient having a 10.00 D amplitude of accommodation. An alternative and perhaps more practical target would be the use of a series of fine lines, perhaps in the shape of a cross, which could be photographically reduced.[43] However, such a target might still be difficult to mass produce consistently.

## Age

The decline in the amplitude of accommodation with age has been well documented, with the studies of Donders and Duane being most commonly cited.[44-46] Both workers reported a decline in amplitude at a rate of approximately 0.30 D per year. In a review of these classic studies, Hofstetter noted a number of methodological differences that might account for the slight variation in findings between these two investigations.[47] These differences are summarized in Table 5-4. However, with the exception of those subjects under 20 years of age in Donders' investigations, the differences were relatively small, as may be seen in Figure 5-10.

Figure 5-11 shows that a plot of the subjective amplitude of accommodation against age may be best fitted by a second-order polynomial function. Hofstetter[47] proposed three equations to represent the minimum, mean, and maximum expected amplitudes:

$$\text{Minimum amplitude} = 15 - (0.25 \times \text{age})$$
$$\text{Mean amplitude} = 18.5 - (0.3 \times \text{age})$$
$$\text{Maximum amplitude} = 25 - (0.4 \times \text{age})$$

## Lead of Accommodation to Distant Targets

When considering the veridical objective amplitude of accommodation, one should determine not only the lag of accommodation typically found when viewing near targets but also the lead of accommodation observed when fixating far targets. This is illustrated in Figure 5-12. This may be particularly relevant when an autorefractor is used to measure the objective amplitude because autorefractors are typically calibrated to provide a zero reading for an emmetropic eye viewing a distant target.[26] However, Hamasaki et al. noted that the true amplitude of accommodation is given by the difference between the maximum and minimum accommodative responses, as indicated in Figure 5-12.[48]

## Refractive Error

A number of studies have reported variations in accommodative amplitude with refractive error,

| **TABLE 5–4** Comparison of the Methodology Used by Donders[44] and Duane[46] in Determining the Age-Related Change in the Amplitude of Accommodation | |
| --- | --- |
| **Donders** | **Duane** |
| Non-cycloplegic distance refraction. Subjects were emmetropic or near emmetropic during their early adult life. | Refractive error determined under homatropine. |
| Thin vertical wires used as test target. | Single vertical, narrow black line on white card. |
| Target distance measured to the nodal point of the eye (assumed to be 7 mm behind the cornea). | Target distance measured to the spectacle plane (13 to 14 mm in front of the cornea). |
| Plotted curves only approximate to the data points. Table of expected amplitudes is based upon these curves. | Plotted curves showing average and range of normal limits based upon general inspection. |
| Near point values measured with "maximum" amount of convergence (i.e., converging to within 8 Parisian inches or approx. 22 cm). | Measured monocularly (although used repeated testing to ensure that maximum effort was achieved). |
| Used spectacle lenses when the near point fell beyond 20 cm. | Used spectacle lenses when the near point fell beyond 50 cm. |
| N = 130 | N = 4200 |

After Hofstetter HW: A comparison of Duane's and Donders' table of the amplitude of accommodation. Am J Optom Arch Am Acad Optom 1944; 21:345–363.

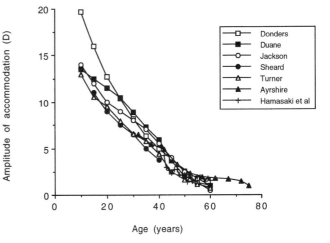

FIGURE 5–10 Mean amplitude of accommodation as a function of age. Values are taken from the investigations of Donders,[44] Duane,[45, 46] Jackson,[185] Sheard,[186] Turner,[181] the Ayrshire Study Circle,[179] and Hamasaki et al.[48] All data were collected under monocular viewing conditions with the exception of the study by Jackson, who obtained binocular measurements. It should be noted that with the exception of the results of Donders for the 20- to 30-year-old subjects, all data show relatively limited variation.

particularly in myopes. Fledelius observed mean amplitudes in groups of juvenile myopes, emmetropes, and hyperopes of 13.80 D, 11.60 D, and 10.70 D, respectively.[49] In addition, both Maddock et al. and McBrien and Millodot subdivided their myopic population into either low (< 3.00 D) and high (> 3.00 D) myopes, or early- (myopia onset at 13 years of age or earlier) and late- (myopia onset at 15 years of age or later) onset myopes. Because the late-onset myopes are also typically low myopes, both studies reported similar findings, with low myopes having higher amplitudes than high myopes.[50, 51] However, both myopic subgroups had higher amplitudes than either emmetropes or hyperopes. In contrast, Fisher et al. did not observe any significant variation in the near point of accommodation with refractive error.[52]

When considering the amplitude of accommodation in different refractive error groups, care must be taken to consider the stimulus to ocular accommodation. For example, if the near point is located 10 cm in front of the spectacle plane of a fully corrected 5.00 D hyperope and a 5.00 D myope (vertex distance = 14 mm), the ocular stimulus to accommodation is 10.05 D and 7.72 D, respectively. Conversely, if both of these patients have ocular accommodative amplitudes of 10.00 D, the near point of the hyperope and myope would be located 100.6 mm and 74.3 mm in front of their respective spectacle planes. Thus, the myopic patient could appear to have a higher accommodative amplitude when, in fact, they are identical. It should be noted that the findings of McBrien and Millodot are indeed ocular accommodative amplitudes.[51] Although the study by Maddock et al. did not specify whether the measurements were spectacle or ocular accommodation, the observation of higher amplitudes in low myopes compared with high myopes cannot be explained with respect to ocular accommodation.[50]

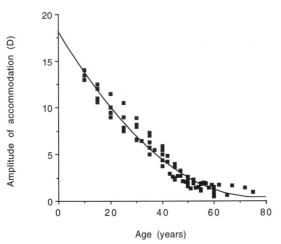

FIGURE 5–11 Composite plot of the data illustrated in Figure 5–10 with the exception of those data from the investigation of Donders[44] for subjects under 30 years of age. The data may be best fitted (r = 0.98) by a polynomial function having the equation $y = 18.17 - 0.46x + 0.003x^2$. However, it is also well fitted (r = 0.95) by the linear equation $y = 14.2 - 0.22x$.

## Effects of Race and Climate

There is some suggestion that both the amplitude of accommodation and the clinical onset of presbyopia vary with geographic location.[53-58] For example, it has been proposed that presbyopia occurs earlier in people living closer to the equator.[54] Factors such as ambient temperature,[59] solar radiation,[54, 55] increased pigmentation within the ciliary body,[60] and nutritional differences[28] have all been suggested to account for these

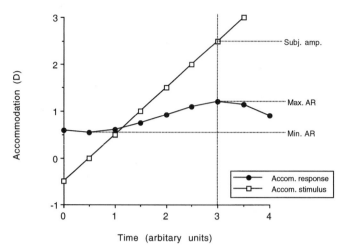

**FIGURE 5–12** Diagrammatic illustration of the objective amplitude of accommodation procedure. The closed circles indicate the objectively determined accommodative response (measured with an optometer) to the steadily increasing accommodative stimulus (*open squares*) plotted with respect to time. The subject typically exhibits a lead of accommodation (i.e., accommodative response exceeds the accommodative stimulus) to distant targets and a lag of accommodation (i.e., stimulus exceeds response) to nearer targets. The true amplitude of accommodation is given by the difference between the maximum and minimum accommodative responses (AR). For comparison, the subjective amplitude of accommodation (subj. amp) would be taken as the magnitude of the accommodative stimulus that elicits the maximum accommodative response. Thus, in this example, the maximum AR ≈ 1.15 D, minimum AR ≈ 0.60 D, true amplitude ≈ 0.55 D, and subjective amplitude = 2.50 D. (Adapted from Hamasaki D, Ong J, Marg E: The amplitude of accommodation in presbyopia. Am J Optom Arch Am Acad Optom 1956; 33:3–14.)

variations. For a summary of these effects, see Table 5-5.

Table 5-5 indicates that the data on factors influencing accommodative amplitude and presbyopia onset are inconsistent, and furthermore, some of these variations may be explained by factors other than ambient temperature and geographic latitude. For example, Kragha[61] noted that many investigations failed to adopt a standard definition of clinical presbyopia. Some have defined presbyopia in terms of the age at which a reading addition was first prescribed. However, such a definition depends upon factors such as the near visual demands (e.g., working distance, target size, and task duration), social and economic factors (e.g., access to and affordability of treatment and how an individual society accepts the wearing of spectacles), and the level of general health. Accordingly, better controlled studies are required before the hypothesis that the onset of presbyopia varies with geographic location or other related factors can be accepted.

# Assessment of the Accommodative Response

· · · · · · · · · · · · · · · · · · · · · · · · · · ·

The assessment of the accommodative response to a range of stimuli represents an important part of the clinical optometric examination. Measurement of the accommodative amplitude alone provides information only about the maximum potential accommodative response, rather than the actual response to a submaximal stimulus. Patients' symptoms frequently relate to near visual activities. Inappropriate responses, such as whether the patient underaccommodates or overaccommodates relative to the plane of the object of regard, are a frequent cause of asthenopia.[62] Accordingly, the clinician must determine the actual accommodative response to the specific stimulus demand for which the patient is reporting difficulty. Furthermore, in some cases a more complete examination of a range of responses may be appropriate, and this can be achieved by plotting an accommodative stimulus-response curve.[63, 64] An example of such a plot is shown in Figure 5-13. Only for a single stimulus level (the so-called cross-over point) are the accommodative stimulus and response equal.

While the plot illustrated in Figure 5-13 represents an average finding, patients presenting with symptoms relating to near visual activities may exhibit different results.[62] For example, some patients may show a tendency to overaccommodate for near targets, rather than exhibiting the more typical lag of accommodation.[63-66] Although the object of regard may remain clear (provided that the accommodative error does not exceed the

**TABLE 5–5** Comparison of the Age of Onset of Presbyopia
with Mean Annual High Temperature and Latitude*

| Study | Location | Temperature (°C) | Latitude (deg) | Age of Onset of Presbyopia (years) |
|---|---|---|---|---|
| Duane[45, 46] | New York, USA | 16 | 43–44 | 42 |
| Ayrshire study[179] | United Kingdom | 14 | 51–54 | 40.5 |
| Schapero and Nadell[36] | Los Angeles, USA | 23 | 34 | 39 |
| Kajiura[180] | Japan | 19 | 36–44 | 39 |
| Turner[181] | United Kingdom | 14 | 51–54 | 39 |
| Donders[44] | Netherlands | 12 | 51–53 | 39 |
| Bergman[182] | South Africa† | 21 | 26–29 | 39 |
| Coates[28] | South Africa‡ | 21 | 26–29 | 39 |
| Litsinger[183] | Chicago, USA | 14 | 42 | 39 |
| Kragha[61] | Nigeria | 31 | 4–13 | 38 |
| Coates[28] | South Africa§ | 21 | 26–29 | 37 |
| Miranda[54–55] | Puerto Rico | 28 | 18–18.5 | 36 |
| Coates[28] | South Africa¶ | 21 | 26–29 | 36 |

*Defined as an amplitude of accommodation of 5.00. In all cases in which a method of measurement was indicated, the push-up
procedure was used with the exception of the investigations by Miranda,[54–55] which used the minus lens technique.
†Afrikaans
‡Mixed race
§Bantu
¶Europeans
Adapted from Kragha IKOK: Amplitude of accommodation: Population and methodological differences. Ophthal Physiol Optom
1986; 6:75–80; Miranda MN: The geographic factor in the onset of presbyopia. Trans Am Ophthalmol Assoc 1979; 77:603–621;
Miranda MN: The environmental factor in the onset of presbyopia. *In* Stark L, Obrecht G (eds): Presbyopia. New York, Professional
Press, 1987, pp 19–27.

depth of focus of the eye—typically around $\pm 0.40$ D[67]), such a patient may still experience asthenopic symptoms, possibly due to the effect of accommodative convergence. Additionally, there is some suggestion that this tendency

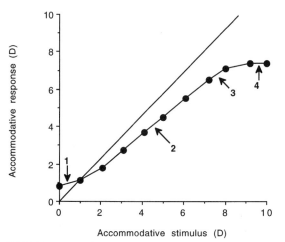

**FIGURE 5–13** Static accommodative stimulus-response curve for a normal subject. 1 = initial non-linear region, 2 = linear region, 3 = transitional soft saturation region, 4 = hard saturation presbyopic region. The diagonal line represents the unit ratio (or 1:1) line. (Redrawn from Ciuffreda KJ, Kenyon RV: Accommodative vergence and accommodation in normals, amblyopes and strabismics. *In* Schor CM, Ciuffreda KJ (eds): Vergence Eye Movements: Basic and Clinical Aspects. Boston, Butterworths, 1983, pp 101–173.)

to overaccommodate for near targets may be associated with the development of near work–induced myopia in certain predisposed individuals.[68, 69] An excessive lag, or underaccommodation, relative to the accommodative stimulus may also produce asthenopia. This is most typically found in early presbyopes but may also be associated with both systemic and ocular pathological conditions.[70, 71]

A number of techniques are available to the clinician for the assessment of the near accommodative response, and these are described below.

## DYNAMIC CROSSED CYLINDER

In this test, subjects view a pattern of intersecting horizontal and vertical lines through a crossed cylinder (typically $\pm 0.50$ D) to create mixed astigmatism, with the horizontal and vertical lines theoretically equidistant in front of and behind the retina (Fig. 5-14). The crossed cylinder is usually introduced before the eye with the negative cylinder axis vertical. This produces a myopic horizontal focal line and a hyperopic vertical focal line. The patient is directed to view the rectilinear target through the crossed cylinder and asked to indicate whether the vertical or horizontal lines are clearer.

If the patient is accommodating exactly in the plane of the target prior to the introduction of the crossed cylinder (Fig. 5-14A), then following the introduction of the crossed cylinder, the circle of least confusion lies on the retina, and the patient reports that both sets of lines (horizontal and vertical) are equally clear (or equally blurred). However, if the patient was initially underaccommodating for the target, that is, there was a lag of accommodation (Fig. 5-14B), then following the introduction of the crossed cylinder, the patient reports that the horizontal lines are clearer because the horizontal focal line is closer to the retina. Alternatively, if the patient was initially overaccommodating for the target (a lead of accommodation), then following the introduction of the crossed cylinder, the patient reports that the vertical lines are clearer (Fig. 5-14C). In the case of a lag of accommodation (horizontal lines clearer), plus spherical lenses are introduced until both sets of lines appear equally clear; for a lead of accommodation (vertical lines clearer), minus spheres are introduced. The lens power required to make the two sets of lines equally clear provides a measure of the accommodative error. For example, if the patient is viewing a target at 40 cm (accommodative stimulus = 2.50 D) and requires a +0.50 D lens to equalize the two sets of lines, there was a lag of accommodation of 0.50 D, and the initial accommodative response was 2.00 D.

This test is usually performed under dim illumi-

nation in order to minimize the depth of focus of the eye by achieving the largest pupillary diameter. However, sufficient illumination must be provided to allow the patient to see the target clearly. This low level of ambient illumination departs from the more typically recommended luminance levels for the performance of near vision tasks.

The test may be carried out under three different conditions, namely:

1. **Monocular.** This primarily assesses the blur-driven accommodative response, although there may also be a significant contribution from proximally-induced accommodation.
2. **Binocular fused.** Under this condition, the patient views the target binocularly, and crossed cylinders are introduced before each eye. Blur-driven, proximal, and convergent accommodation are stimulated. Thus the binocular response may differ from the monocular findings. The binocular fused test represents the most natural viewing condition.
3. **Binocular unfused.** Here, vertical prisms are introduced to induce vertical diplopia. Subjects view each of the vertically displaced targets in turn. Because the dissociation of the targets eliminates any requirement for disparity-vergence (i.e., opens the vergence loop), the response is the same as for the monocular condition.[72]

Unfortunately, a number of significant problems with the dynamic crossed cylinder test make it of limited value in pre-presbyopic patients with active accommodation. For example, it is assumed that a patient who accommodates accurately to a more conventional target produces an accommodative response to the dioptrically conflicting, rectilinear target that lies exactly midway between the two foci (i.e., places the circle of least confusion on the retina (Fig. 5-14A). However, little evidence supports this proposal. Both Rosenfield and Ciuffreda[73] and Adams and Johnson[74] demonstrated that the accommodative response to such a combination of targets varies widely between individuals. Some subjects accommodated accurately for the nearer target, others for the more distant target, and many focused between the two targets (but not necessarily at the midpoint). Thus, the assumption that the subject accommodates to place the circle of least confusion on the retina seems unfounded. Indeed, the rectilinear targets used are not conducive to maintaining the circle of least confusion on the retina owing to their horizontal and vertical orientations.[75] In addition, it

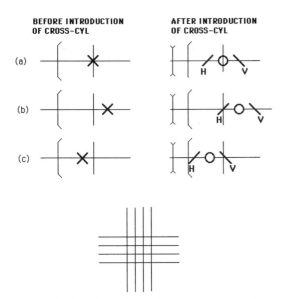

**FIGURE 5–14** Effect of introducing a crossed cylinder (negative axis vertical) in patients exhibiting (a) accurate accommodative responses, that is, response equals stimulus, (b) a lag of accommodation, that is, stimulus exceeds the response, and (c) a lead of accommodation, that is, response exceeds the stimulus. The rectilinear target typically used for this procedure is illustrated in the lower part of the figure.

seems questionable whether subjects would prefer to maintain the two sets of lines equally blurred by placing the circle of least confusion on the retina, or whether they would alter their accommodative response to improve the clarity of one set of lines at a time. This latter situation is frequently found in young patients, who often indicate that first the vertical lines are clearer, then the horizontal, then the vertical, and so on.

A technique that attempts to control these fluctuations of accommodation during the dynamic crossed cylinder test utilizes a +1.00 D spherical "fogging" lens.[76] This is introduced before the patient views the near target in order to stabilize the accommodative response. However, the introduction of such a lens only "fogs," that is, places the point conjugate with the object of regard in front of the retina, if the magnitude of the accommodative response remains unchanged. If the patient reduces his or her accommodation by an amount equal to the magnitude of the plus lens, then the point conjugate with the object of regard again coincides with the retina, and the position of the horizontal and vertical focal lines relative to the retina are the same as before the introduction of the +1.00 D lens.

The observation that the accommodative response changes following the introduction of lenses provides an additional difficulty with this test. If a lag of accommodation is observed (i.e., the subject indicates that the horizontal lines are clearer), then plus lenses are introduced to obtain the required end point. However, in a young patient with active accommodation, the introduction of additional plus power is likely to stimulate a reduction in the blur-driven accommodative response.[77, 78] If the reduction in accommodation is exactly equal to the magnitude of the plus lens, the response to the test remains unchanged. Thus a patient who initially indicates that the horizontal lines are clearer on the crossed cylinder target continues to make that same response after the introduction of plus lenses and the subsequent relaxation of accommodation. Accordingly, the observed end point of the dynamic crossed cylinder test is a function of the patient's ability to relax his or her accommodation under the test conditions. During monocular testing, this limit may be related to the output of proximally induced accommodation, that is, accommodation stimulated by knowledge of nearness of the object of regard. Because patients are fully aware of the relatively close testing distance, they are unlikely to reduce their accommodative response beyond the perceived target location.

Under binocular test conditions, the limit of the ability to reduce accommodation while maintaining single binocular vision is related to the necessity for an appropriate vergence response. Accordingly, one would predict a smaller lag of accommodation with the binocular dynamic crossed-cylinder test than with the monocular procedure. This was confirmed by Portello et al.[79]

## NEAR DUOCHROME

The duochrome (bichrome) test[80, 81] utilizes the chromatic aberration of the human eye[82, 83] to determine the locus of the point conjugate with the retina. However, it is unclear whether the use of the standard red and green filters is appropriate for near vision testing. Several investigators[84-86] have demonstrated that the wavelength conjugate with the retina changes from approximately 600 nm during distance fixation to approximately 530 nm when observing a target at a viewing distance of 40 cm. Indeed, Wilmut[87] suggested that blue (peak wavelength ≈495 nm) and yellow (peak wavelength ≈575 nm) filters should be used for near vision testing to account for this change in the location of the chromatic interval. However, a recent study demonstrated that the blue-yellow near duochrome does not provide an accurate estimation of the accommodative response.[79]

Probably the major reason why the duochrome test has not been used more widely for near examinations is the general unavailability of suitable near tests, particularly in the United States. However, units are commercially available, for example the near point analysis test produced by the Bernell Corporation (South Bend, IN), which also includes suppression and associated phoria tests. An example of an alternative near duochrome unit is shown in Figure 5-15.

The near duochrome test is performed in a similar manner to the distance test: Minus lenses are introduced if the patient indicates that the target on the red background appears clearer or darker or plus lenses if a green preference is indicated, until equality is achieved. When comparing the monocular lag of accommodation to a 2.50 D target using near duochrome, dynamic crossed cylinder, and an objective infrared optometer, Portello et al. observed significantly higher lags of accommodation with the two subjective methods.[79] This is illustrated in Figure 5-16. The near duochrome suffers from the same disadvantage as the fused crossed cylinder in that introduction of spherical lenses may themselves

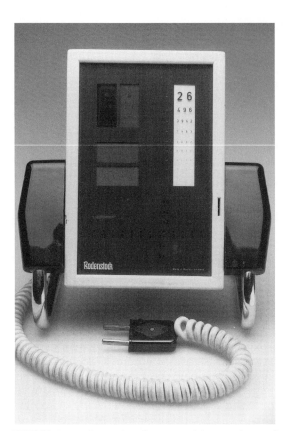

**FIGURE 5–15** Example of a near-vision testing unit which includes a near-duochrome test (*top left corner*). This particular instrument, the Rodenstock Nahprüfgerät Bestell-Nr 30 30.002 (Rodenstock, Germany), also contains near visual acuity, phoria, and suppression tests.

alter the magnitude of the accommodative response, thereby producing an apparently elevated lag of accommodation.

## DYNAMIC RETINOSCOPY

The principle of both static (i.e., with minimal accommodation) and dynamic (with a stimulated accommodative response) retinoscopy is that a neutral reflex is observed when the point conjugate with the retina coincides with the retinoscope peephole. Consider therefore a fully corrected patient viewing a target at a distance of 33 cm. If the patient exerts an accommodative response of 2.50 D, the point conjugate with the retina lies 40 cm in front of the principal point. Thus, a retinoscopist working at either 67 cm, 40 cm, or 33 cm observes an against, neutral, or with movement, respectively.

A number of variations on this technique exist, and these are detailed below.

## Cross-Nott Technique

This technique, initially devised by Cross[88] and then refined and clarified by Nott,[89, 90] does not require the use of supplementary lenses. The patient wears his or her full distance refractive correction and is directed to view a near target. If with motion is seen (reflecting the typical lag of accommodation), then the retinoscopist adjusts his or her working distance away from the patient, while the fixation target remains stationary. The reciprocal of the retinoscopic working distance (in meters) at which a neutral reflex is observed indicates the magnitude of the accommodative response.

## Sheard's Technique

Sheard was one of the earliest workers to note that a lag of accommodation to a near target was a normal finding.[91] Accordingly, he indicated that accommodative lag could be measured by placing a target attached to the retinoscope mirror at the patient's usual reading distance and performing retinoscopy through the patient's distance refraction. Appropriate spherical lenses are introduced until a neutral reflex is observed. Sheard stated that a range of neutrality is typically observed, and this range reflects the magnitude of negative relative accommodation.

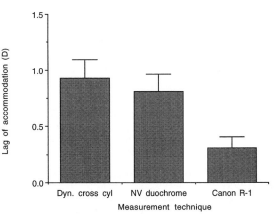

**FIGURE 5–16** Mean values of lag of accommodation for 15 subjects monocularly viewing a target at a distance of 40 cm (accommodative stimulus = 2.50 D). The accommodative response was assessed using dynamic crossed cylinder, near-duochrome, and an objective, open-field, infrared optometer (Canon Autoref R-1). The lag of accommodation recorded using the infrared optometer was significantly lower than the values observed with the two subjective techniques. Error bars indicate 1 SEM. (Data from Portello et al.[79])

## Monocular Estimate Method (MEM) Retinoscopy

It was discussed in the earlier section on the dynamic crossed cylinder test that the introduction of plus lenses during the course of an accommodation measurement procedure may themselves influence the accommodative response.[77, 78] The MEM procedure attempts to overcome this difficulty by interposing the lenses very briefly[92, 93] so that the subject does not have time to respond to the change in accommodative stimulus.[189] Furthermore, because the lens is introduced before only one eye, while the fellow eye continues to fixate the target, any lens-induced relaxation of accommodation may be minimized.

Rouse et al.[94] observed a high correlation between measurements of the accommodative response obtained using MEM retinoscopy and a Vernier optometer. However, they also observed that for all stimulus levels, the response determined using MEM retinoscopy was approximately 10% less than that found using the Vernier optometer. Thus, an increased lag of accommodation was found with MEM retinoscopy. This suggests that the introduction of the plus lenses in fact produces some relaxation of accommodation. Because the reaction time of accommodation is typically around 350 ms,[22, 95] it is essential that the lens be present for an interval shorter than this reaction time. This proposal was supported by Birnbaum,[62] who noted that the lens must be in front of the eye for no longer than one-fifth of a second. The degree of skill required to interpose a lens, assess the direction of motion of the retinoscopic reflex, and remove the lens in under 200 ms would seem to be extremely high. Interestingly, both Locke and Somers[189] and Jackson and Goss[96] observed no significant difference between dynamic retinoscopy measurements obtained using the MEM and Sheard techniques (Table 5–6). Thus, equivalent results were obtained whether the lenses were left in place

during the measurement procedure or introduced for only an extremely brief period. Accordingly, one must conclude that attempting to interpose the lenses for a period shorter than the typical accommodative response time ($\approx$ 350 ms) is either unnecessary and/or practically impossible.

### Bell Retinoscopy

In this technique (so called because it was originally carried out using a cat bell as the stimulus), the retinoscopic working distance is kept constant (usually at 50 cm) while a fixation target (generally a small chrome or lucite sphere) is slowly advanced toward the patient.[97] Typically, with motion is observed owing to the lag of accommodation, but as the target moves toward the patient, the motion of the retinoscopic reflex first changes to neutrality and then to against motion. The conventional procedure is to record the distance at which the reflex changes from with to against, and the distance at which the reflex changes from against to with. This is usually recorded as a fraction. Thus OD 41 cm/47 cm indicates that for the right eye, an initial with motion was seen which changed to against motion when the target was 41 cm from the patient, and that the against motion returned to with motion when the target was 47 cm from the patient. However, it would be more convenient if the mean of these positions was expressed in diopters; thus, in the example above, this would be recorded as 2.25 D (the reciprocal of 44 cm). This indicates that a 2.25-D stimulus produced the 2.00-D accommodative response. For a summary of the dynamic retinoscopy techniques and typical findings, see Figure 5–17 and Table 5–6.

## Autorefractors

. . . . . . . . . . . . . . . . . . . . . . . . .

Any commercial infrared autorefractor may be used to assess the accommodative response, pro-

| TABLE 5–6 Comparison of Mean Measurements of Lag of Accommodation to a 2.50 D Accommodative Stimulus* | | | | |
|---|---|---|---|---|
| | MEM | Cross/Nott | Sheard | DCC |
| Locke and Somers[189] (N = 10) | 0.50 (0.05) | 0.60† (0.05) | 0.61‡ (0.08) | 0.11 (0.14) |
| Jackson and Goss[96] (N = 244) | 0.23 (0.02) | 0.29§ (N/A) | 0.29¶ (0.02) | 0.72 (0.03) |

*Various dynamic retinoscopy techniques and dynamic fused crossed-cylinder (DCC) were used. In both studies, the dynamic crossed-cylinder finding differed significantly from the dynamic retinoscopy results. Figures in parentheses indicate ±1 SEM.
†Locke and Somers referred to this technique as Nott retinoscopy.
‡Locke and Somers referred to this technique as Cross retinoscopy.
§Jackson and Goss referred to this technique as Nott retinoscopy. However, they presented their results as the mean accommodative response so that the SEM of the lag was not provided.
¶Jackson and Goss referred to this technique as low neutral retinoscopy.

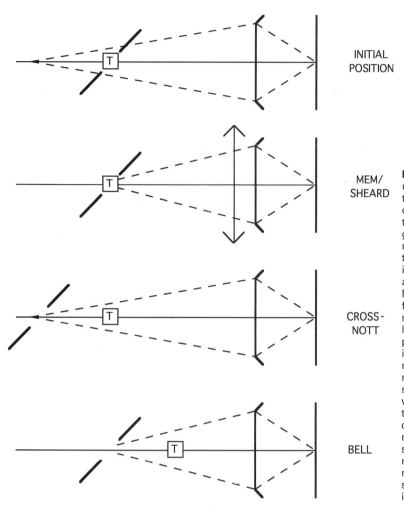

INITIAL
POSITION

MEM/
SHEARD

CROSS-
NOTT

BELL

**FIGURE 5–17**  Summary of the dynamic retinoscopy techniques. The top figure illustrates the initial condition for all procedures, namely that the subject fixates a near target (T) that is adjacent to the retinoscope. The broken lines indicate those rays conjugate with the retina, and, in this example, a lag of accommodation is observed. In the MEM/Sheard procedure, both the fixation target and retinoscope remain at this initial position, and lenses are introduced until the point conjugate with the retina coincides with the plane of the retinoscope. In the Cross-Nott technique, the fixation target remains stationary, but the retinoscopy working distance is adjusted until the point conjugate with the retina coincides with the plane of the retinoscope (i.e., a neutral reflex is observed). In Bell retinoscopy, the retinoscopy working distance remains constant, and the target position is varied until a neutral reflex is observed.

vided that it allows near stimuli to be presented. These have the advantages of being objective, taking measurements extremely quickly (typically in less than 0.2 second), and being relatively easy to operate. Ideally, a range of near dioptric stimuli should be available. One instrument that has been widely used for research purposes has been the Canon Autoref R-1 autorefractor.[98-100] This instrument is no longer manufactured, but its unique feature is an open field of view, which allows presentation of near targets at a wide range of physical viewing distances.

# Photorefraction

. . . . . . . . . . . . . . . . . . . . . . . . . . . .

Photorefractive techniques may be used for the assessment of accommodation in infants, young children, and handicapped patients who may not be able to cooperate with the requirements of the procedures previously described. Both or-

thogonal and eccentric (or paraxial) photorefractive procedures may be used to assess accommodation, although the eccentric technique is currently used more widely. The optical principles of these procedures have been fully described previously.[101-105] For a review of the clinical procedures, see Duckman.[106]

## ORTHOGONAL PHOTOREFRACTION

In this technique, a fiber-optic bundle delivers a point of light to the center of a 35-mm camera lens, and a photograph is obtained after refraction at the eye through an array of four 1.50 D cylindrical lenses that surround the fiber-optic bundle. The cylindrical lenses therefore produce a star pattern, with the length of the cross arms being proportional to the refractive power of the respective meridian. This is illustrated in Figure 5–18.

It should be noted that this procedure does

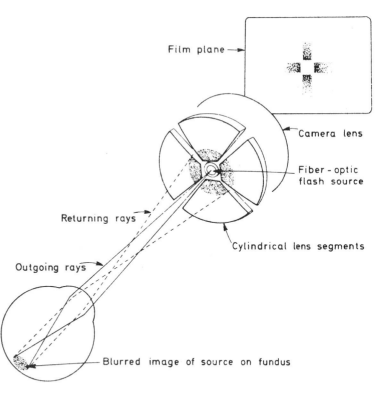

**FIGURE 5–18** Optics of orthogonal photorefraction. Light from a fiber-optic centered within an array of four cylinder lenses is focused on the retina of the subject who is myopic with respect to the camera. Light returning from the retina to the camera falls on the cylinder lens segments and is focused into a cross-shaped pattern, with the length of the cross arms being directly proportional to the degree of defocus in the corresponding meridian. (From Braddick O, Atkinson J, French J, Howland HC: A photorefractive study of infant accommodation. Vision Res 1979; 19:1319–1330.)

not provide any indication of the sign (i.e., whether myopic or hyperopic) of the defocus, and thus Howland and Sayles[107] used both orthogonal and isotropic photorefraction to determine the direction of accommodative change.[104, 105]

Braddick et al.[108] used orthogonal photorefraction to examine accommodative responsivity in infants as young as 1 day old and observed consistent and appropriate responses to targets located at a viewing distance of 75 cm in approximately 50% of infants between 1 and 9 days of age. Later, Howland et al. used a video camera photorefractive procedure to measure accommodation in infants and observed velocities of accommodation comparable to those of adults.[109]

### ECCENTRIC (PARAXIAL) PHOTOREFRACTION

This technique, also referred to as static photographic skiascopy or photoretinoscopy, may also be used for the assessment of accommodation. Unlike orthogonal photorefraction, the light source is not centered in the camera aperture. Thus, in the presence of ametropia, only a portion of the subject's pupil is illuminated by the reflected light, and the size and location of the illuminated crescent provide an indication of the refractive state. This is illustrated in Figure 5–19.

In the case of a myopic patient (Fig. 5–19*A*), the far point is located in front of the principal point of the eye. Thus, light reflected from the patient's retina is brought to a focus in the far point plane. It may be observed from Figure 5–19*A* that only those rays passing through the inferior portion of the pupil pass through the camera aperture. Conversely, in the case of a hyperopic patient (Fig. 5–19*B*), only those rays emerging through the superior pupil pass through the camera aperture (Fig. 5–20). With increasing refractive error, the size of the crescent imaged at the pupil plane increases. Several investigators have adopted this technique for the assessment of accommodation in infants.[110-112]

# Other Accommodative Parameters

### POSITIVE AND NEGATIVE RELATIVE ACCOMMODATION (PRA AND NRA)

Positive and negative relative accommodation represent changes in accommodation that can be elicited while the stimulus for vergence is held constant. These parameters are measured clinically by introducing increasing minus (for PRA)

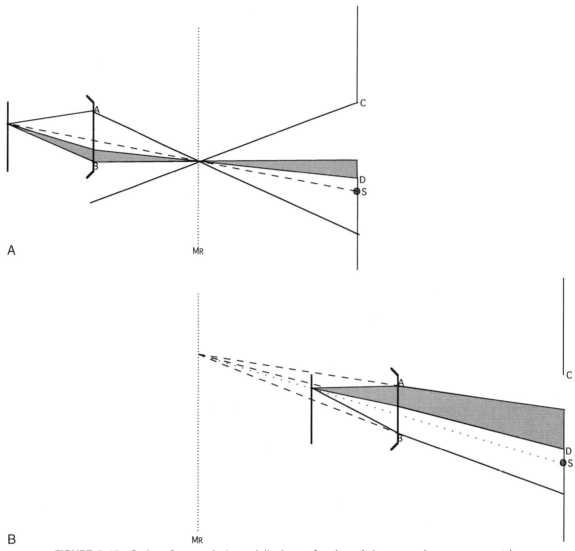

**FIGURE 5–19** Optics of eccentric (paraxial) photorefraction. *A,* In a myopic eye an eccentric light source (S) illuminates the retina. Light is reflected back from the retina through the patient's pupil (AB) to be imaged at the far point plane (M$_R$). Only those rays within the shaded ray bundle pass through both the patient's pupil and the camera aperture (CD). Thus, only the lower portion of the subject's pupil appears illuminated. *B,* In a hyperopic eye, the far point plane lies behind the principal point of the eye, and thus the upper portion of the subject's pupil appears illuminated.

or plus (for NRA) lenses while the patient views a near target, typically located at a viewing distance of 40 cm (2.50 D). The end point is taken when the patient reports the **first, slight, sustained blur.** As with the amplitude of accommodation, the patient should always be encouraged to try and clear the target. Particularly when introducing minus lenses (i.e., PRA), care must be taken to allow the patient adequate time to clear the image, especially at the higher accommodative stimulus levels. The amount of spherical power added to the original prescription represents the magnitude of relative accommodation. For pre-presbyopic patients, this test should be carried out with their distance prescription in place. For early presbyopic patients, the procedure should be performed through the appropriate near prescription.

Measurements of relative accommodation do not test the accommodative system in isolation but rather examine the interaction between accommodation and vergence. The changes that occur during PRA and NRA testing are shown in Table 5-7. In PRA, the minus lenses increase

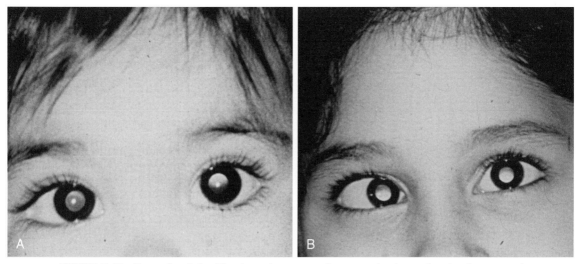

**FIGURE 5–20** Example of the illuminated crescents in eccentric photorefraction in cases of hyperopia with right esotropia (*A*) and bilateral myopia (*B*). (Courtesy of Dr. Robert Duckman.)

the demand for blur-driven accommodation. This change is necessarily accompanied by an increase in accommodative convergence. However, this increased vergence response would result in the subject overconverging for the object of regard, with resultant diplopia, unless compensated for by a reduction in an alternative vergence component. The most likely compensation for the increase in accommodative convergence is a concurrent decrease in the output of disparity-vergence. However, such a reduction is

accompanied by a decreased convergent accommodation response. This reduction in convergent accommodation must again be compensated for to prevent the target becoming blurred, and this probably occurs via an increase in blur-driven accommodation. This latter change causes the cycle to begin repeating itself, and this continues until an equilibrium is reached. Accordingly, it is clearly a gross oversimplification to state that PRA requires an increase in accommodation without any accompanying change in vergence. Although the latter approximates the ultimate changes in the aggregate accommodation and vergence responses, it fails to indicate the changes in component contributions from both oculomotor systems that must occur during this test. In fact, during PRA testing, the compensatory decrease in disparity-vergence is frequently less than the increase in accommodative convergence, resulting in an esophoric shift in fixation disparity. Conversely, an exophoric shift in fixation disparity is typically observed during NRA testing.

Because PRA requires an individual to shift accommodation closer than convergence, Birnbaum[62] has suggested that low PRA values may be an early sign of near point stress and characteristic of incipient and progressing myopia. The concept of balancing PRA and NRA findings, such as when determining a near vision addition, is analogous to the middle third technique for prescribing prism, that is, to provide maximum flexibility between the two oculomotor components.

Normal values in a pre-presbyopic patient for NRA and PRA are approximately +2.00 D and −2.50 D, respectively.

---

**TABLE 5–7** Component Changes in Accommodation and Vergence That Take Place During Assessment of Positive and Negative Relative Accommodation (PRA and NRA)

*Positive Relative Accommodation (PRA)*

(1) Increased blur-driven accommodation
↓
(2) Increased accommodative convergence
↓
(3) Decreased disparity-vergence
↓
(4) Decreased convergent accommodation
↓
(5) Increased blur-driven accommodation

*Negative Relative Accommodation (NRA)*

(1) Decreased blur-driven accommodation
↓
(2) Decreased accommodative convergence
↓
(3) Increased disparity-vergence
↓
(4) Increased convergent accommodation
↓
(5) Decreased blur-driven accommodation

## ACCOMMODATIVE FACILITY (OR ACCOMMODATIVE ROCK)

This test examines the ability to make rapid step changes in accommodation. The test may be performed using one of four procedures: (1) monocularly using "flipper" lenses, (2) binocularly using "flipper" lenses, (3) monocularly with distance-near alternate fixation, and (4) binocularly with distance-near alternate fixation.

### Monocularly Using "Flipper" Lenses

In this procedure, the patient monocularly views a line of fine print (20/25 or 20/30 Snellen equivalent letters) at a distance of 40 cm (2.50 D) through his or her optimum distance refractive correction. This correction should be either in the form of the patient's own spectacles (or contact lenses) or alternatively set up in a trial frame. The use of a phoropter is not suitable for this test. The examiner introduces $\pm 2.00$ D lenses alternatively before the viewing eye, and the patient indicates when the target becomes "absolutely clear," at which point the alternate lens is flipped in front of the eye as rapidly as possible. This procedure therefore provides accommodative stimuli of 0.50 and 4.50 D. Although these are the most commonly used stimulus levels, other values may be adopted if desired, such as the use of $\pm 1.00$ D lenses or a different working distance. This procedure tests the patient's ability to vary the blur-driven accommodative response rapidly and is quantified in terms of the number of cycles (i.e., clearing both the plus and minus lenses) completed in 60 seconds. The full 60-second test period should always be used to check for variations due to fatigue of accommodation.[113] However, care must be taken to note whether any asymmetry exists between the time taken to clear the plus and minus lenses.

### Binocularly Using "Flipper" Lenses

Here the same procedure is used except that the patient views the target binocularly. This tests the patient's ability to increase and decrease his or her accommodative response appropriately while maintaining the vergence response relatively constant (at approximately 2.5 MA; see the previous section on relative accommodation). Thus, it assesses the dynamics of PRA and NRA. Suppression tests should always be used to ensure binocularity, either by using polaroid filters and targets or more simply by introducing an additional target such as a pencil in the midline halfway between the patient and the object of regard. The patient should ensure that this supplementary stimulus is seen in physiological diplopia and is instructed to report if it becomes single at any time during the test. Both Burge[114] and Griffin[113] (Table 5–8) noted significantly elevated binocular findings when a suppression check was not used.

### Expected Findings in Young Adults

A summary of mean monocular and binocular findings obtained using the flipper technique in young adults is shown in Table 5–8. Accordingly, several studies[115-118] have suggested "clinical pass" criteria of 11 cycles per minute (cpm) for monocular testing and 8 cpm for binocular assessment. Hoffman and Rouse[119] also noted that a difference of more than 2 cpm between the two eyes should be regarded as a possible indicator of accommodative difficulties when accompanied by near visual symptoms.

### Expected Findings in Children

Scheiman et al.[120] examined accommodative facility in children between 6 and 12 years of age using $\pm 2.00$ D flippers. Their results are illustrated in Figure 5–21, and it may be observed from these data that the mean facility rates were considerably lower than those found in young adults (Table 5–8). Using a passing criterion of 1 standard deviation below the mean,[116] Scheiman et al.[120] proposed monocular pass rates for children as shown in Table 5–9.

### Monocularly with Distance-Near Alternate Fixation

This procedure was outlined by Haynes[121] and Haynes and McWilliams.[122] Here the patient is

---

**TABLE 5–8** Summary of Mean Accommodative Facility Findings (Cycles per Minute) in Young Adults Recorded Using $\pm 2.00$ D Flippers

| | Mean Monocular* | Mean Binocular* | Comments |
|---|---|---|---|
| Burge[114] | 12.6 (1.68) | 7.1 (1.55) | Binoc. without suppression check = 9.45 (1.53) |
| Zellers et al[115] | 11.6 (0.50) | 7.72 (0.51) | |
| Hennessy et al[116] | 11.8 (0.91) | 7.8 (1.13) | |
| McKenzie et al[117] | 13.2 | 10.64 | Data from first of three trials |
| Griffin[113] | 17 | 6 | Binoc. without suppression check = 13 |

*Numbers in parentheses indicate $\pm 1$ SEM.

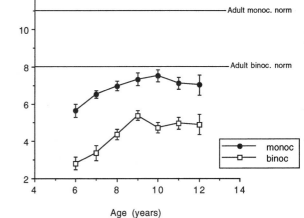

**FIGURE 5–21** Mean monocular and binocular accommodative facility findings (cycles per minute) as a function of age for children between 6 and 12 years of age. Error bars indicate ±1 SEM. (Data from Scheiman et al.[120]) For comparison, the adult monocular and binocular norms of 11 and 8 cpm, respectively, are also shown.

required to alternate fixation between a target at a viewing distance of 6 meters (0.17 D) and a target at 0.40 meter (2.50 D), and to indicate when each target becomes "absolutely clear." This procedure stimulates changes in both blur-driven and proximally induced accommodation. Furthermore, it represents a more natural setting than the use of flipper lenses. Introduction of a plus lens magnifies the retinal image, making the target appear to be closer, while actually decreasing the blur-driven accommodative stimulus. This ambiguity is eliminated with the distance-near alternate fixation technique because it does not require the use of lenses to vary the accommodative stimulus. Rosenfeld and Gatto (unpublished findings) observed mean monocular facility rates (N = 28) with the flipper and distance-near fixation techniques of 16.2 cpm and 30.2 cpm, respectively.

## Binocularly with Distance-Near Alternate Fixation

This is the most natural test condition, but it does not represent a pure test of accommodation because the patient is required to alter both the vergence and accommodative responses simultaneously. Thus, a patient may perform poorly on this test because of either accommodation or vergence difficulties. Suppression checks, such as polaroid charts or awareness of physiological diplopia, should be used.

## Clinical Implications of Accommodative Facility

In a comparison of accommodative facility findings in patients with and without near vision symptoms, Hennessy et al[116] reported significantly lower accommodative facility rates (for both monocular and binocular testing) in the symptomatic group. Although this difference in mean rates was not reproduced in a study by Levine et al., they observed greater variability in facility rates in symptomatic subjects tested repeatedly, compared with asymptomatic patients.[118] Additionally, Bobier and Sivak noted that an improvement in accommodative facility following vision training was associated with an improvement in the dynamically measured temporal characteristics (i.e., latency, movement time, response time) of the accommodative re-

**TABLE 5–9** Summary of Expected Findings, Standard Deviations (SD) and Pass Rates for Monocular and Binocular Accommodative Facility in Children

| | Monocular | | | Binocular | | |
|---|---|---|---|---|---|---|
| Age | Mean | SD | Pass Rate | Mean | SD | Pass Rate |
| 6 | 5.5 | 2.5 | 3.0 | 3 | 2.5 | 0.5* |
| 7 | 6.5 | 2 | 4.5 | 3.5 | 2.5 | 1.0* |
| 8–12 | 7 | 2.5 | 5.0 | 5 | 2.5 | 2.5* |

*Because these passing levels are so low, the value of the binocular test in children is questionable.
From Scheiman M, Herzberg H, Frantz K, Margolies M: Normative study of accommodative facility in elementary schoolchildren. Am J Optom Physiol Opt 1988; 65:127–134.

sponse.[30] These findings indicate that clinical accommodative facility testing is a valuable tool when screening patients for accommodative dysfunction and infacility.

# CONVERGENT ACCOMMODATION

Although the accommodative convergence/accommodation (AC/A) ratio is measured routinely in the clinical setting, the convergent accommodation/convergence (CA/C) ratio has received relatively little attention outside the research laboratory, primarily because of the difficulty in measuring this parameter. However, Schor and Horner[123] demonstrated that near vision disorders could be categorized using this parameter. For example, patients with convergence insufficiency and convergence excess had mean CA/C ratios of 0.75 D/MA and 0.05 D/MA, respectively. In addition, this parameter is clinically important where spherical lenses are used to treat vergence problems, e.g., in treating exophoria with minus lenses.[124]

A clinical procedure for measuring the CA/C ratio was described by Tsuetaki and Schor.[125] Here, the subject views a low spatial frequency (approximately 0.1 cpd) difference of Gaussian (DOG) target.[126] This target is illustrated in Figure 5–22. The accommodative response to this target may be assessed using the Sheard dynamic retinoscopy technique or any subjective or objective optometer. If the stimulus to disparity vergence is then changed by the introduction of ophthalmic prisms (e.g., 6Δ base-in, 6Δ base-out, 12Δ base-out) while the subject continues to view the DOG target, the resulting change in accommodative response reflects the output of convergent accommodation. The CA/C ratio may be quantified as the change in accommodative response divided by the change in vergence stimulus.

## Expected Values

Rosenfield and Gilmartin[127] observed mean CA/C ratios in young adults of approximately 0.4 D/MA. However, this ratio declines with age,[124, 128, 129] presumably owing to the loss of accommodative responsivity, and reaches a value of zero around 55 years of age. Rosenfield et al.[129] observed a weak negative correlation ($r = -0.37$; $p = 0.06$) between the response AC/A and CA/C ratios. However, these ratios are not reciprocals of one another.

# TONIC ACCOMMODATION

In the absence of an adequate visual stimulus, the accommodative response adopts an intermediate dioptric position of the order of 0.50 to 1.00 D.[130] This so-called stimulus-free response has been termed tonic accommodation (TA), although it has also been referred to as dark accommodation or dark focus to reflect the most common method of assessment. Both baseline measurements of this parameter and the transient changes that occur following sustained near vision tasks (also referred to as accommodative adaptation) have been suggested to be associated with refractive error development.[130, 131] However, this parameter may have other clinical implications; it has previously been associated with night, space, and instrument myopia.

A number of clinical techniques may be used to assess TA. These vary with the methodology used to measure the accommodative response and to open the accommodative loop, that is, to eliminate the effects of blur-driven, convergent, and proximally induced accommodation. In the clinical assessment of TA, the accommodative response may be measured using either an infrared autorefractor, if available, or dynamic retinoscopy. The most common procedure adopted in the research laboratory for opening the accommodation loop has been to place the subject in total darkness. However, this protocol is generally impractical in the clinical setting. Two alternative techniques that may be more practical for the clinician are the use of either the DOG target or the retinoscope beam itself to open the accommodative loop.

The DOG target illustrated in Figure 5–22 has been demonstrated to be a poor stimulus for blur-driven accommodation. Accordingly, if a subject views such a target monocularly, the effects of blur-driven and convergent accommodation are eliminated. Although the presence of the near target stimulates proximally induced accommodation and therefore prevents the precise quantification of TA, it still allows some assessment of this parameter, for example, into low (<1.00 D), medium (1.00 to 2.00 D), or high (>2.00 D) values.

An alternative procedure uses the technique of near retinoscopy. Owens et al.[132] reported that a retinoscope beam did not constitute a stimulus to accommodation. Accordingly, they adopted the method of near retinoscopy described by Mohindra[133] to measure TA. Here, the subject views the retinoscope beam monocularly while retinoscopy is performed in a darkened room. However, several studies suggested that viewing the illuminated retinoscope may stimulate both

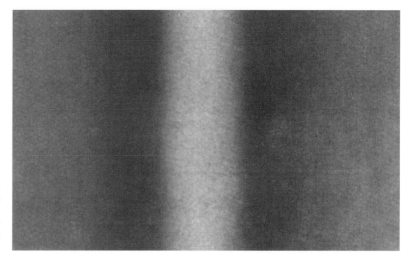

**FIGURE 5–22** A low center spatial frequency (≈0.1 cpd) difference of Gaussian (DOG) grating. This is taken from the reverse side of a Wesson fixation disparity card.[187]

blur and proximally induced accommodation and therefore is unlikely to provide a veridical estimate of TA.[134-136] Accordingly, the use of the DOG target seems to be the most appropriate technique for the clinical assessment of this parameter.

## Expected Findings

As previously indicated, laboratory measurements of TA in children and young adults[130, 131] are typically between 0.50 and 1.00 D. Clinical assessment using the DOG/dynamic retinoscopy technique may give slightly higher values (1.00 to 1.50 D) owing to the effects of proximal accommodation. Furthermore, it should be noted that TA declines with age[130] and the development of presbyopia owing to the age-related changes and limitations of the accommodative system.

## PROXIMAL ACCOMMODATION

This accommodative component has received very little attention in the clinical field, although recent reseach has indicated that its contribution to the overall accommodative response may be substantial, particularly under certain degraded stimulus conditions.[29, 34, 137] Furthermore, its relative importance may vary between symptomatic and asymptomatic individuals and, accordingly, should be measured in those patients presenting with near vision asthenopia that appears to be accommodative in origin.

In order to assess proximal accommodation, the output of both blur-driven and convergent accommodation must be minimized. This may be

achieved by having subjects monocularly view a DOG target (Fig. 5-22). A DOG target is placed at three or four near distances (e.g., 50 cm, 33 cm, 25 cm, 20 cm) and the accommodative response measured using the Sheard dynamic retinoscopy technique or any subjective or objective optometer for these target locations. The gradient of these measurements represents the proximal accommodation/accommodative stimulus (PA/AS) ratio.

## Expected Findings

For a population of young adults, Rosenfield et al.[34] reported a mean PA/AS ratio of 0.45 D/D. However, this ratio would also be predicted to decline with age owing to the loss of accommodative responsivity concurrent with the development of presbyopia.

# Anomalies of Accommodation

· · · · · · · · · · · · · · · · · · · · · · · · · ·

An anomaly of accommodation exists when the accommodative response is inappropriate for the magnitude of the stimulus. This may result from a failure either to initiate, maintain, or produce sufficiently rapidly a change in the dioptric power of the crystalline lens. These anomalies may be classified into five categories (based upon Duke-Elder and Abrams[2]): (1) fatigue of accommodation, (2) failure of accommodation, (3) accommodative inertia, (4) paralysis of accommodation, and (5) accommodative excess. However, it should be noted that these are not distinct conditions, and some degree of overlap exists between the categories.

## FATIGUE OF ACCOMMODATION

Accommodative fatigue has been defined as the inability of the ciliary muscle to maintain contraction while viewing a near object, with a resultant decrease in the accommodative response.[138] Lancaster and Williams[139] were the first workers to attempt to produce this condition experimentally. They used techniques such as reading of fine print at or near the near point of accommodation for up to 1 hour, sustained focusing at the near point of accommodation, fixating a test object placed slightly closer than the near point until it became clear, and focusing upon a test object that moved rhythmically forward and backward over the range of accommodation in an attempt to produce fatigue. They observed that, in many cases, the near point actually moved closer (i.e., increased its dioptric value) following these demanding near tasks. Furthermore, they noted that the subjective reports of fatigue were "surprisingly small." Subsequently, Howe[140] described an ophthalmic ergograph in which similar techniques to those of Lancaster and Williams could be used to examine accommodative fatigue. Using a modified version of an ophthalmic ergograph, Berens and Stark[141] reported approximately equal proportions of subjects ($\approx$30%) exhibiting increased and decreased amplitudes of accommodation, with the remaining 40% showing a relatively constant near point during the study.

Several studies confirmed that it is extremely difficult to fatigue the accommodative system,[2, 141] although Berens and Stark[143] demonstrated that a reduction in oxygen tension produced a more rapid recession of the near point. Earlier, Donders[44] had suggested that asthenopia was "the tendency to fatigue in looking at near objects" and resulted from "fatigue of the muscular system of accommodation." However, Donders's description of muscle fatigue seems to be more appropriate for striated muscle than for the ciliary smooth muscle responsible for accommodation. Nevertheless, Duke-Elder and Abrams[2] suggested that accommodative fatigue may be more commonly found in hyperopes (due to the increased accommodative demand when viewing a near object of regard) and in those individuals with low PRA. Several more recent studies have used the term *accommodative fatigue* while failing to demonstrate the pres ence of an inappropriate accommodative response.[144-146] If the definition of accommodative fatigue provided

above is adopted, then reports of asthenopia or other subjective symptoms in association ith near work are not necessarily indicative of accommodative fatigue. Rather, an increased lag of accommodation must be demonstrated to meet this definition.

## FAILURE OF ACCOMMODATION

Failure of accommodation is the inability to produce or maintain an appropriate accommodative response. It may be due to failure of the lens to change shape or loss of ciliary muscle function. The most common cause of failure of accommodation is presbyopia, which is discussed in a subsequent section of this chapter.

This category may be further subdivided into **accommodative insufficiency,** in which the accommodative response is consistently reduced, and **ill-sustained accommodation,** in which the response may initially be normal but cannot be maintained over time.

### Accommodative Insufficiency

Cline et al.[147] defined this condition as "insufficient amplitude of accommodation to afford clear imagery of a stimulus object at a specified distance, usually the normal or desired reading distance." Hofstetter's equation (see earlier section on age-related changes in the amplitude of accommodation) may be valuable in specifying an abnormally low amplitude, that is, [minimum amplitude = 15 − (0.25 × age in years)].[47] Scheiman and Wick[124] proposed that an amplitude of 2.00 D or more below the level specified by this equation should be considered abnormal. This is frequently accompanied by poor accommodative facility findings, low (less than −1.50 D) PRA, and a large lag of accommodation as assessed by either dynamic retinoscopy or dynamic crossed cylinder testing.[124, 148] Cooper[148] observed that these patients may, on occasion, be able to make appropriate accommodative changes but require such effort to do so that asthenopia results almost immediately. Amblyopic eyes typically fit into this category, demonstrating increased accommodative error and lag of accommodation.[149]

### Ill-Sustained Accommodation

Duke-Elder and Abrams[2] stated that this is essentially the same condition as accommodative insufficiency but of a lesser degree. Furthermore, it may also be a precursor to the former condition. The amplitude of accommodation appears to be normal but deteriorates over time,[1, 124] sometimes within 1 minute.[113] Accordingly, accommodative facility testing must be carried out for a period of at least 60 seconds in order to detect this condition.[113]

## ACCOMMODATIVE INERTIA

Duke-Elder[2] defined this as a rare condition in which the patient has difficulty in altering his or her accommodative response. Normally, the stimulus-driven change in accommodation is completed within approximately 1 second.[22] However, some individuals may demonstrate an increase in both the latency and time constant of the accommodative response,[30, 150, 151] although these temporal variations may be improved following orthoptic training.[151] Cooper[148] suggested that accommodative inertia is a common clinical problem in individuals who spend substantial periods of time at near vision tasks. An informal survey (Rosenfield and Chiu, unpublished data) of optometry students supports Cooper's observations. Eighty-three subjects were questioned as to whether they ever experienced blurred distance vision following periods of reading. Forty-five percent of the respondents reported that this occurred occasionally (i.e., approximately 25% of the time), and 26% of the individuals indicated that this occurred often (i.e., at least 50% of the time).

The relatively prolonged relaxation of accommodation following a period of sustained near vision has also been associated with near work–induced myopia.[152] For example, investigators have demonstrated transient, yet statistically significant myopic shifts in the far point of accommodation immediately following sustained near tasks.[145, 152] This is illustrated in Figure 5–23. However, when the within-task accommodative stimulus was reduced by the use of either plus lenses or pinholes, this post-task shift was attenuated.[152] Accordingly, this shift does appear to be produced by a slower than normal relaxation of the accommodative response. However, the proposal that this delay may be a precursor to the development of more permanent myopia is as yet unproven. This increased accommodative response following near work may also fall under the heading of accommodative excess.

## PARALYSIS OF ACCOMMODATION

Both Duane[153] and Prangen[154] noted that there is no clear division between paralysis and insuffi-

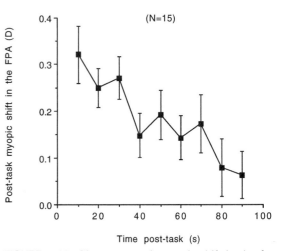

**FIGURE 5–23** Mean post-task myopic shift in the far point of accommodation (FPA), measured with respect to the pre-task level, during the 90-second period immediately following completion of a 10-minute near-vision task performed at a viewing distance of 20 cm (5.00 D) in 15 visually normal subjects. Error bars indicate ±1 SEM. (Data from Blustein et al., from Rosenfield M: Accommodation and myopia. Are they really related? J Behav Optom 1994; 5:3–11, 25.)

ciency of accommodation and that the only distinction between these two categories is one of degree. Duke-Elder and Abrams[2] observed that accommodative paralysis may be unilateral or bilateral, may be of sudden or insidious onset, and either can represent an isolated finding or may be accompanied by other oculomotor restrictions (which may also produce diplopia). It is frequently associated with pupillary mydriasis and micropsia (due to the effort of accommodation).

## ACCOMMODATIVE EXCESS

This general heading includes such conditions as accommodative spasm, ciliary spasm, pseudomyopia, hyperaccommodation, hypertonic accommodation, and tonic "cramp" of accommodation.[153] Suchoff and Petito[155] defined accommodative spasm as a condition in which a greater accommodative response than is considered normal is observed for a given accommodative stimulus. However, because a lead of accommodation (i.e., accommodative response exceeding the magnitude of the dioptric stimulus) is a normal finding when viewing distant objects of regard, and occasionally when viewing near objects, accommodative excess should be restricted to those conditions in which the accommodative response exceeds the stimulus by an amount greater than the depth of focus of the eye (typically of the order of ±0.40 D).[67, 156]

Duke-Elder and Abrams[2] indicated that this condition was first described adequately by von Graefe in 1856 and is generally produced by increased parasympathetic innervation to the ciliary muscle. Symptoms may include asthenopia, headaches, ocular fatigue, blurred vision, diplopia (from excessive accommodative convergence), and a requirement to perform near work at abnormally close distances.[1-2, 113, 151, 157] Its origin may be organic or functional, although the organic type is relatively rare.[2]

Functional accommodative excess most frequently occurs immediately following periods of prolonged near work. Other factors such as poor illumination, glare, stress, and general debility have also been associated with this condition. Although it has been described as resembling the fatigue cramps of other muscles,[2] it must be noted that accommodation is produced by contraction of the ciliary smooth muscle, which has different physiological properties from striated muscle. Indeed, Guyton[158] indicated that under normal functioning conditions, fatigue at the neural–smooth muscle junction probably occurs only at the most exhausting levels of muscular activity. This is consistent with the difficulty in producing accommodative fatigue.

Accommodative excess is demonstrated by a significant difference in refractive error under cycloplegic and non-cycloplegic conditions.[159-161] It should be suspected if a significantly greater amount (more than 1.00 D) of plus power (i.e., more hyperopia or less myopia) is found with retinoscopy than with subjective refraction findings, if the patient appears to have an abnormally low amplitude of accommodation for his or her age, or increases in esophoric posture are observed,[162] particularly toward the end of a working day. In addition, subjects may have difficulty in clearing the blur introduced by plus lenses during accommodative facility and NRA testing.[124]

The anomalous myopias (e.g., night, space, instrument, and empty field myopia) may also be said to fit into this category because they are caused by an excessive accommodative response with respect to the dioptric stimulus. They are produced by a composite accommodative response stimulated by a number of factors, including tonic accommodation, proximally induced accommodation, surround propinquity, and cognitive demand.[130, 131]

## PREVALENCE OF ACCOMMODATIVE ANOMALIES

Hokoda[163] reported the prevalence of accommodative dysfunction in an urban optometry clinic

to be 16.8% (n = 119). In a study of patients (n = 129) who had been selected for vision training, Hoffman et al.[164] indicated that 62% had anomalies of accommodation. The prevalence of individual categories of accommodative anomalies observed in Hokoda's study, and in an earlier investigation by Daum,[165] is shown in Table 5-10.

## CAUSES OF ACCOMMODATIVE ANOMALIES

Causes of accommodative anomalies have been fully reviewed,[2, 71, 154, 159, 165, 166] and the following list (which is not intended to be exhaustive) is compiled from these sources. Accommodative anomalies have been associated with a wide range of ocular and systemic conditions that may be classified under the following broad headings:

1. **Following trauma.** Accommodative failure or paralysis has been reported following these traumatic incidents: contusion of the eye, lens subluxation, trauma to the ciliary ganglion or oculomotor nerve, cryosurgery of a peripheral retinal tear, perforating injury of the ciliary region, and concussion of the eye with traumatic mydriasis. Accommodative excess has been reported following a road traffic accident with hematoma, dental extraction, and other head injuries.
2. **Inflammatory.** Accommodative failure or paralysis may be associated with syphilis, diphtheria, neurasthenia, tuberculosis, influenza, pertussis, measles, dental infections, arteriosclerosis, tonsilitis, infectious mononucleosis, encephalitis, malaria, viral ciliary ganglionitis, scarlatina, mumps, typhoid, toxemia, poliomyelitis, cyclitis, sympathetic ophthalmitis, nasal sinusitis, and inflammation of the superior orbital fissure. Accommodative excess has been reported following diphtheria, meningitis, rheuma-

**TABLE 5–10** Prevalence of Accommodative Anomalies Observed by Daum and Hokoda*

| | Daum[165] | Hokoda[163] |
|---|---|---|
| Accommodative insufficiency | 84% | 55% |
| Accommodative inertia/infacility | 12% | 30% |
| Accommodative spasm | 3% | 15% |
| Accommodative fatigue | 1% | N/A |

*Daum reported only on patients who had been diagnosed as having accommodative dysfunction. Hokoda examined the records of 119 patients, of whom 20 (16.8%) had accommodative dysfunction. Hokoda did not include a test for accommodative fatigue in his protocol.

tism, neurasthenia, tuberculosis, appendicitis, and dental sepsis.

3. **Toxic.** Accommodative failure or paralysis may be associated with lead poisoning, chronic alcoholism, botulism B, ergot, snake venom, bee stings, arsenic, and several forms of food poisoning.

4. **Metabolic.** Accommodative failure or paralysis may be associated with diabetes, anoxia, Graves' disease, and metabolic toxemias.

5. **Degenerative.** Accommodative failure or paralysis may be associated with lens sclerosis and cataract formation, Wilson's disease, myotonic dystrophy, degenerative conditions affecting the brain stem, tabes dorsalis, and myasthenia gravis.

6. **Neoplastic.** Accommodative failure may be associated with pineal tumors and neoplasia at the base of the skull.

7. **Vascular.** Accommodative failure may be associated with hemorrhages in the brain stem, aneurysms, cavernous sinus thromboses, and arteriovenous fistulas.

8. **Psychogenic.** Both accommodative paralysis and accommodative excess have been associated with psychogenic disorders.

9. **Iatrogenic/pharmacological.** The administration of both ocular and systemic pharmacological agents probably represents the most frequent cause of accommodative anomalies.[167-169]

# Assessment and Correction of Presbyopia

Presbyopia refers to the decline in accommodative responsivity with age (see Fig. 5-10). Although this typically does not present clinical difficulties until an individual reaches his or her early 40s, Donders[44] noted that the loss of amplitude actually begins around (or even slightly before) puberty. Many theories have been proposed relating to the cause of this condition, which may be divided into extralenticular and lenticular according to the locus of the age-related changes.

The **Duane-Fincham** theory of presbyopia proposes that the age-related decline in accommodative ability results from weakening of the ciliary muscle. This theory indicates that the maximum ciliary muscle contraction produces the maximum accommodative response independent of age. Accordingly, one unit of ciliary muscle contraction produces less dioptric change in an older eye than in a younger one. However,

impedance cyclography studies[170, 171] and investigations of isolated lens-zonule preparations[172] have demonstrated that the power of the ciliary muscle actually increases up to approximately 45 years of age. Thus, weakening of the ciliary muscle does not appear to be a factor in presbyopia.[173]

The **Hess-Gullstrand** theory of presbyopia proposed that this condition develops from changes in the lens and lens capsule alone while the ciliary muscle retains its ability to contract.[174] Accordingly, the amount of ciliary muscle force required to produce a 1.00 D change in accommodation remains constant with age.[71] It is likely that these lenticular changes are related to age-related processes, including an anterior shift in the position of the equatorial zonular insertions,[175] a change in the thickness of the lens capsule due to the alteration of the zonular insertions,[173] continued growth of the lens with age,[176] decreased lens capsule modulus of elasticity,[177] increased lens substance elasticity,[178] and changed lens shape with age.[177]

## CORRECTION OF PRESBYOPIA

Presbyopia may be corrected by using supplementary convex lenses (in addition to any correction for distance refractive error) to allow diverging rays from near objects of regard to be focused upon the retina. Seven standard clinical techniques are available for determining the appropriate near vision addition: (1) fused crossed cylinder, (2) plus "build up," (3) add based on patient's age, (4) proportion of amplitude, (5) dynamic retinoscopy, (6) NRA/PRA balance, and (7) near duochrome.

The first three techniques represent the most commonly used clinical procedures. Regardless of the technique used, it is essential that a careful case history be taken to determine the patient's visual requirements. For example, the patient should be questioned in detail about his or her visual activities, both during and outside work time. Special requirements such as VDT operation, musical instrument playing, or machine operation must be considered. A common error is to assume falsely that patients perform all (or any) of their near work at 40 cm (16 inches).

It should also be noted that each of the techniques described below represents only the first step in determining the appropriate near addition. The patient's actual reading performance through the add must always be checked. Both the level of visual acuity and the range of clear vision through the add should be examined. Increasing the near addition both decreases the available range of clear vision and moves it closer to the patient. For example, with an absolute presbyope (assuming a depth of focus of $\pm 0.40$ D), the range of clear vision through a $+2.00$ D add is 20.9 cm, that is, 41.6 to 62.5 cm, whereas through a $+3.00$ D add it is only 9.0 cm, that is, 29.4 to 38.4 cm. It is valuable to record the range of clear vision for a particular lens, for example, ADD $+2.00$, 20/20, range 22 to 41 cm, and to try and ensure that the patient's preferred (or required) working distance lies in the middle of the range. If practical, the patient should be encouraged to bring his or her particular near visual material to the examination (e.g., music, sewing, or unusual sized text). The near add should be assessed using a trial frame and lenses while viewing this material.

## Fused Crossed Cylinder

This test provides an indication of the accommodative error (lag of accommodation for a presbyope). It should be noted that many of the difficulties associated with this test in younger patients (e.g., large fluctuations of accommodation) disappear in the presbyopic individual. If the patient cannot initially see the target clearly, then sufficient plus power is introduced until the lines can be recognized. The binocular measurement is generally used as the tentative near addition, although monocular findings may be recorded, particularly if the binocular balance is in doubt. The binocular lag of accommodation is sometimes less than the monocular findings owing to the introduction of convergent accommodation under binocular viewing conditions.

## Plus Build-up

Plus spherical power is added to the distance refraction (in 0.25-D steps) until the patient is able to achieve optimal near visual acuity at the appropriate working distance. The minimum plus power consistent with comfortable vision at this near distance reflects the appropriate addition. This test is generally performed binocularly, but again may be done monocularly, particularly if the binocular balance is in doubt. The minimum plus power that gives clear vision at near places the proximal end of the depth-of-field coincident with the object of regard. Thus, additional plus power will be needed to place the preferred reading position in the center of the range of clear vision.

## Add Based on Patient's Age

The tentative add may simply be based on the patient's age. However, the required addition may need to be adjusted appropriately owing to variations in the required working distance or if the amplitude of accommodation differs significantly from the average for the patient's age. Typical adds for a Caucasian population are shown in Table 5–11. The required add may vary in other racial groups.

## Proportion of Amplitude

One rule-of-thumb is that a patient should be able to sustain one-half of his or her accommodative amplitude. Accordingly, the near add corresponds to the difference between the required working distance (in diopters) and one-half of the accommodative amplitude.

> **EXAMPLE**
> A patient has an amplitude of accommodation of 3.00 D and requires a working distance of 40 cm.
>
> ADD = working distance $-$ one-half amplitude
>     = 2.50 $-$ 1.50 D
>     = $+1.00$ D
>
> Note. Some practitioners advocate that this rule should indicate that a patient can maintain 67% of his or her accommodative amplitude rather than 50%.

## Dynamic Retinoscopy

Dynamic retinoscopy can be used to determine the accommodative response to a given stimulus. Plus lenses can then be introduced over the distance prescription until an appropriate response is obtained. It is usual to leave the patient with a small (0.25 to 0.50 D) lag of accommodation

**TABLE 5–11** Typical Near Vision Add Based Upon the Patient's Age for a Viewing Distance of 40 cm (2.50 D) in a Caucasian Population

| Age (years) | Near Add (D) |
|---|---|
| 40 | 0 |
| 45 | $+1.00$ |
| 48 | $+1.25$ |
| 50 | $+1.50$ |
| 52 | $+1.75$ |
| 55 | $+2.00$ |
| 60 | $+2.25$ |
| 63 | $+2.50$ |

because this is the typical response for a pre-presbyopic patient.

## NRA/PRA Balance

Having determined a tentative add using one of the techniques described above, NRA and PRA are measured through this preliminary add. The add is then modified so that PRA and NRA are balanced.

### EXAMPLE

A preliminary add of +1.00 D is determined on an emmetropic patient. Through this add, the NRA and PRA are measured. If the patient reports first blur (NRA) through a +2.00 D add [i.e., NRA = +1.00 D] and first blur (PRA) through a +0.50 D add [i.e., PRA = −0.50 D], the add should be modified to lie in the middle of the PRA/NRA range, that is, +1.25 D. Through this lens the patient will have PRA = NRA = 0.75 D.

## Near Duochrome

This test may be performed at near using a near duochrome unit placed at the appropriate working distance. The principles of the test are exactly the same as for the distance test. Appropriate lenses are added until a "balance point" is achieved.

### ACKNOWLEDGMENT

I would like to thank Nancy Chiu, M.S., Andrea Cohen, B.S., and Irene Vito for their assistance in obtaining many of the references cited.

# References

1. Borish IM: Clinical Refraction, 3rd ed. Chicago: Professional Press, 1970.
2. Duke-Elder S, Abrams D: System of Ophthalmology. Vol. V, Ophthalmic Optics and Refraction. St. Louis, CV Mosby, 1970.
3. Porterfield: A Treatise on the Eye. Vol. 1. Edinburgh, 1759, p 410 (cited in Donders, 1864).
4. Young: Phil Trans 1801; 91:23 (cited in Duke-Elder and Abrams[2]).
5. Southall JPC: Helmholtz's Treatise on Physiological Optics. New York: Dover Publications, 1962.
6. Fincham EF: The mechanism of accommodation. Br J Ophthalmol 1938; Monograph Suppl. VIII.
7. Alpern M: Accommodation. *In* Davson H (ed): The Eye, 2nd ed., Vol. III. New York: Academic Press, 1969, pp 217-254.
8. Weale RA: Presbyopia. Br J Ophthalmol 1962; 46:660-668.
9. Kikkawa Y, Sato T: Elastic properties of the lens. Exp Eye Res 1963; 2:210-215.
10. Warwick R: The ocular parasympathetic nerve supply and its mesencephalic sources. J Anat 1954; 88:71-93.
11. Ruskell GL, Griffiths T: Peripheral nerve pathway to the ciliary muscle. Exp Eye Res 1979; 28:277-284.
12. Westheimer G, Blair SM: The parasympathetic pathways to the internal eye muscles. Invest Ophthalmol 1973; 1:193-197.
13. O'Connor Davies PH: The Actions and Uses of Ophthalmic Drugs, 2nd ed. London: Butterworths, 1981.
14. Gilmartin B: A review of the role of sympathetic innervation of the ciliary muscle in ocular accommodation. Ophthalmic Physiol Opt 1986; 6:23-37.
15. Morgan MW: The nervous control of accommodation. Am J Optom Arch Am Acad Optom 1944; 21:87-93.
16. Wolff E: Anatomy of the Eye and Orbit, 7th ed. London: H. K. Lewis & Co., 1976.
17. Lograno MD, Reibaldi A: Receptor-responses of fresh human ciliary muscle. Br J Pharmacol 1986; 87:379-385.
18. Wax M, Molinoff PB: Distribution and properties of β-adrenergic receptors in human iris/ciliary body. Invest Ophthalmol Vis Sci 1987; 28:420-430.
19. Törnqvist G: The relative importance of the parasympathetic and sympathetic nervous systems for accommodation in monkeys. Invest Ophthalmol 1967; 6:612-617.
20. Törnqvist G: Effect of cervical sympathetic stimulation on accommodation in monkeys. Acta Physiol Scand 1966; 67:363-372.
21. Rosenfield M, Gilmartin B: Temporal aspects of accommodative adaptation. Optom Vis Sci 1989; 66:229-234.
22. Campbell FW, Westheimer G: Dynamics of the accommodation response of the human eye. J Physiol (London) 1960; 151:285-295.
23. Hurwitz BS, Davidowitz J, Chin NB, Breinin GB: The effects of the sympathetic nervous system on accommodation: 1. Beta sympathetic nervous system. Arch Ophthalmol 1972; 87:668-674.
24. Hurwitz BS, Davidowitz J, Pachter BR, Breinin GB: The effects of the sympathetic nervous system on accommodation: 2. Alpha sympathetic nervous system. Arch Ophthalmol 1972; 87:675-678.
25. Gilmartin B, Hogan RE, Thompson SM: The effect of timolol maleate on tonic accommodation, tonic vergence and pupil diameter. Invest Ophthalmol Vis Sci 1984; 25:763-770.
26. Gilmartin B, Bullimore MA: Sustained near-vision augments sympathetic innervation of the ciliary muscle. Clin Vis Sci 1987; 1:197-208.
27. Fitch RC: Procedural effects on the manifest human amplitude of accommodation. Am J Optom Arch Am Acad Optom 1971; 48:918-926.
28. Coates WR: Amplitudes of accommodation in South Africa. Br J Phys Opt 1955; 12:76-81,86.
29. Rosenfield M, Gilmartin B: Effect of target proximity on the open-loop accommodative response. Optom Vis Sci 1990; 67:74-79.
30. Bobier WR, Sivak JG: Orthoptic treatment of subjects showing slow accommodative responses. Am J Optom Physiol Opt 1983; 60:678-687.
31. Ogle KN, Martens TG, Dyer JA: Oculomotor Imbalance in Binocular Vision and Fixation Disparity. Philadelphia: Lea & Febiger, 1967, pp 165-166.
32. Hokoda SC, Ciuffreda KJ: Measurement of accommodative amplitude in amblyopia. Ophthalmic Physiol Opt 1982; 2:205-212.
33. Wold RM: The spectacle amplitude of accommodation of children aged six to ten. Am J Optom Arch Am Acad Optom 1967; 44:642-664.

34. Rosenfield M, Ciuffreda KJ, Hung GK: The linearity of proximally-induced accommodation and vergence. Invest Ophthalmol Vis Sci 1991; 32:2985-2991.

35. Duane A: Studies in monocular and binocular accommodation with their clinical applications. Am J Ophthalmol 1922; 5:865-877.

36. Schapero M, Nadell M: Accommodation and convergence responses in beginning and absolute presbyopes. Am J Optom Arch Am Acad Optom 1957; 34:606-622.

37. Otake Y, Miyao, M, Ishihara S, et al.: An experimental study on the objective measurement of accommodative amplitude under binocular and natural viewing conditions. Tohoku J Exp Med 1993; 170:93-102.

38. Ripple PH: Variation of accommodation in vertical directions of gaze. Am J Ophthalmol 1952; 35:1630-1634.

39. Knoll HA: The relationship between accommodation and convergence and the elevation of the plane of regard. Am J Optom Arch Am Acad Optom 1962; 39:130-134.

40. Takeda T, Neveu C, Stark L: Accommodation on downward gaze. Optom Vis Sci 1992; 69:556-561.

41. Somers WW, Ford CA: Effect of relative distance magnification on the monocular amplitude of accommodation. Am J Optom Physiol Opt 1983; 60:920-924.

42. Rosenfield M, Cohen AS: Push-up amplitude of accommodation and letter size. Ophthalmic Physiol Opt 1995; 15:231-232.

43. Berens C, Fonda G: A Spanish-English accommodation and near-test card using photoreduced type. Am J Ophthalmol 1950; 33:1788-1792.

44. Donders FC: On the Anomalies of Accommodation and Refraction of the Eye. (Trans. by WD Moore). London: The New Sydenham Society, 1864.

45. Duane A: The accommodation and Donders' curve and the need of revising our ideas regarding them. JAMA 1909; 52:1992-1996.

46. Duane A: Normal values of the accommodation at all ages. JAMA 1912; 59:1010-1013.

47. Hofstetter HW: A comparison of Duane's and Donders' table of the amplitude of accommodation. Am J Optom Arch Am Acad Optom 1944; 21:345-363.

48. Hamasaki D, Ong J, Marg E: The amplitude of accommodation in presbyopia. Am J Optom Arch Am Acad Optom 1956; 33:3-14.

49. Fledelius HC: Accommodation and juvenile myopia. Doc Ophthal Proc Series 1981; 28:103-108.

50. Maddock RJ, Millodot M, Leat S, Johnson CA: Accommodation responses and refractive error. Invest Ophthalmol Vis Sci 1981; 20:387-391.

51. McBrien NA, Millodot M: Amplitude of accommodation and refractive error. Invest Ophthalmol Vis Sci 1986; 27:1187-1190.

52. Fisher SK, Ciuffreda, KJ, Levine S: Tonic accommodation, accommodative hysteresis, and refractive error. Am J Optom Physiol Opt 1987; 64:799-809.

53. Weale RA: The Senescence of Human Vision. Oxford: Oxford University Press, 1992, pp 59-61.

54. Miranda MN: The geographic factor in the onset of presbyopia. Trans Am Ophthalmol Assoc 1979; 77:603-621.

55. Miranda MN: The environmental factor in the onset of presbyopia. In Stark L, Obrecht G (eds): Presbyopia. New York: Professional Press, 1987, pp 19-27.

56. Rambo VC: The first graph of accommodation of the people of India. All India Ophth Soc 1957; 5:51-54.

57. Rambo VC, Sangal SP: Study of the accommodation of the people of India. Am J Ophthalmol 1960; 49:993-1004.

58. Covell LL: Presbyopia. Comparative of white and negro populations. Am J Ophthalmol 1950; 33:1275-1276.

59. Weale RA: Human ocular aging and ambient temperature. Br J Ophthalmol 1981; 65:869-870.

60. Bamba M: Particular Features of the Correction of Presbyopia in Africa. In Stark L, Obrecht G (eds): Presbyopia. New York: Professional Press, 1987, pp 30-31.

61. Kragha IKOK: Amplitude of accommodation: Population and methodological differences. Ophthalmic Physiol Opt 1986; 6:75-80.

62. Birnbaum MH: Optometric Management of Nearpoint Vision Disorders. Boston: Butterworth-Heinemann, 1993, pp 53-71, 161-92.

63. Morgan MW: Accommodation and its relationship to convergence. Am J Optom Arch Am Acad Optom 1944; 21:83-195.

64. Ciuffreda KJ, Kenyon RV: Accommodative vergence and accommodation in normals, amblyopes and strabismics. In Schor CM, Ciuffreda KJ (eds): Vergence Eye Movements: Basic and Clinical Aspects. Boston: Butterworths, 1983, pp 101-173.

65. Heath GG: Components of accommodation. Am J Optom Arch Am Acad Optom 1956; 33:569-579.

66. Charman WN: The accommodative resting point and refractive error. Ophthalmic Optician 1982; 21:469-473.

67. Campbell FW: The depth of field of the human eye. Optica Acta 1957; 4:157-164.

68. Goss DA: Clinical accommodation and heterophoria findings preceding juvenile onset of myopia. Optom Vis Sci 1991; 68:110-116.

69. Goss DA, Grosvenor TP: Rates of childhood myopia progression with bifocals as a function of nearpoint phoria: Consistency of three studies. Optom Vis Sci 1990; 67:637-640.

70. Hofstetter HW: Factors involved in low amplitude cases. Am J Optom Arch Am Acad Optom 1942; 19:279-289.

71. Ciuffreda, KJ: Accommodation and its anomalies. In Charman WN (ed): Vision and Visual Dysfunction. Vol. 1. Visual Optics and Instrumentation. Boca Raton, FL: CRC Press, 1991, pp 231-279.

72. Ong J, Schuchert J: Dissociated versus monocular cross-cylinder method. Am J Optom Arch Am Acad Optom 1972; 49:762-764.

73. Rosenfield M, Ciuffreda KJ: Accommodative responses to conflicting stimuli. J Opt Soc Am A 1991; 8:422-427.

74. Adams CW, Johnson CA: Steady-state and dynamic response properties of the Mandelbaum effect. Vision Res 1991; 31:751-760.

75. Williamson-Noble FA: A possible fallacy in the use of the cross-cylinder. Br J Ophthalmol 1943; 27:1-12.

76. Grosvenor TP: Primary Care Optometry, 2nd ed. New York: Professional Press, 1989.

77. Fry GA: Significance of fused cross cylinder test. Optom Weekly 1940; 31:16-19.

78. Goodson RA, Afanador AJ: The accommodative response to the near point crossed cylinder test. Optom Weekly 1974; 65:1138-1140.

79. Portello JK, Rosenfield M, Blustein GH, Jang C: Comparison of clinical techniques to assess the near accommodative response. Optom Vis Sci (suppl) 1995; 72:195.

80. Bennett AG: The theory of bichromatic tests. Optician 1963; 146:291-296.

81. O'Connor Davies PH: A critical analysis of bichromatic tests used in clinical refraction. Br J Phys Opt 1957; 14:170-182, 213.

82. Bedford RE, Wyszecki G: Axial chromatic aberration of the human eye. J Opt Soc Am 1957; 47:564-566.

83. Charman WN, Jennings JAM: Objective measurements of the longitudinal chromatic aberration of the human eye. Vision Res 1976; 16:999-1005.

84. Ivanoff A: Les Aberrations de l'Oeil. Leur role dans

l'accommodation. Éditions de la revue d'optique théorique et instrumentale. Paris, 1953.

85. Jenkins TCA: Aberrations of the eye and their effects on vision. Part II. Br J Physiol Opt 1963; 20:161-201.

86. Millodot M, Sivak J: Influence of accommodation on the chromatic aberration of the eye. Br J Physiol Opt 1973; 28:169-174.

87. Wilmut EB: Chromatic selectivity of the eye in near vision. Optician 1958; 135:185-187.

88. Cross AJ: Dynamic Skiametry in Theory and Practice. New York: AJ Cross Optical Co., 1911.

89. Nott IS: Dynamic skiametry, accommodation and convergence. Am J Physiol Opt 1925; 6:490-503.

90. Nott IS: Dynamic skiametry. Accommodative convergence and fusion convergence. Am J Physiol Opt 1926; 7:366-374.

91. Sheard C: Dynamic skiametry. Am J Optom 1929; 6:609-623.

92. Haynes HM: Clinical observations with dynamic retinoscopy. Optom Weekly 1960; 51:2243-2246, 2306-2309.

93. Valenti CA: The Full Scope of Retinoscopy. Santa Ana, CA: Optometric Extension Program, 1990.

94. Rouse MW, London R, Allen DC: An evaluation of the monocular estimate method of dynamic retinoscopy. Am J Optom Physiol Opt 1982; 59:234-239.

95. Hogan RE, Gilmartin B: The choice of laser speckle exposure duration in the measurement of tonic accommodation. Ophthalmic Physiol Opt 1984; 4:365-368.

96. Jackson TW, Goss DA: Variation and correlation of clinical tests of accommodative function in a sample of school-age children. J Am Optom Assoc 1991; 62:857-866.

97. Apell RJ: Clinical application of bell retinoscopy. J Am Optom Assoc 1975; 46:1023-1027.

98. Matsumura I, Maruyama S, Ishikawa Y, et al.: The design of an open view autorefractor. In Breinin GM, Siegel IM (eds): Advances in Diagnostic Visual Optics. Berlin: Springer-Verlag, 1983, pp 36-42.

99. Berman M, Nelson P, Caden B: Objective refraction: Comparison of retinoscopy and automated techniques. Am J Optom Physiol Opt 1984; 61:203-209.

100. McBrien NA, Millodot M: Clinical evaluation of the Canon Autoref R-1. Am J Optom Physiol Opt 1985; 62:786-792.

101. Howland HC, Howland B: Photorefraction: A technique for study of refractive state at a distance. J Opt Soc Am 1974; 64:240-249.

102. Howland HC: Optics of photoretinoscopy: Results from ray tracing. Am J Optom Physiol Opt 1985; 62:621-625.

103. Bobier WR, Braddick OJ: Eccentric photorefraction: Optical analysis and empirical measures. Am J Optom Physiol Opt 1985; 62:614-620.

104. Bennett AG, Rabbetts RB: Clinical Visual Optics, 2nd ed. London: Butterworths, 1989.

105. Howland HC: Determination of ocular refraction. In Charman WN (ed): Vision and Visual Dysfunction. Vol. 1. Visual Optics and Instrumentation. Boca Raton, FL: CRC Press, 1991, pp 399-414.

106. Duckman R: Using photorefraction to evaluate refractive error, ocular alignment, and accommodation in infants, toddlers, and multiply handicapped children. Pediatr Optom 1990; 2:333-353.

107. Howland HC, Sayles N: A photorefractive characterization of focusing ability of infants and young children. Invest Ophthalmol Vis Sci 1987; 28:1005-1015.

108. Braddick O, Atkinson J, French J, Howland HC: A photorefractive study of infant accommodation. Vision Res 1979; 19:1319-1330.

109. Howland HC, Dobson V, Sayles N: Accommodation in infants as measured by photorefraction. Vision Res 1987; 27:2141-2152.

110. Abramov I, Hainline L, Duckman RH: Screening infant vision with paraxial photorefraction. Optom Vis Sci 1990; 67:538-545.

111. Hainline L, Riddell P, Grose-Fifer J, Abramov I: Development of accommodation and convergence in infancy. Behav Brain Res 1992; 49:33-50.

112. Hamer RD, Norcia AM, Day SH, et al.: Comparison of on- and off-axis photorefraction with cycloplegic retinoscopy in infants. J Pediatr Ophthalmol Strab 1992; 29:232-239.

113. Griffin JR: Binocular anomalies. In Procedures for Vision Therapy, 2nd ed. New York: Professional Press, 1988.

114. Burge S: Suppression during binocular accommodative rock. Optom Monthly 1979; 70:867-880.

115. Zellers JA, Alpert TL, Rouse MW: A review of the literature and a normative study of accommodative facility. J Am Optom Assoc 1984; 55:31-37.

116. Hennessy D, Iosue RA, Rouse MW: Relation of symptoms to accommodative infacility of school-aged children. Am J Optom Physiol Opt 1984; 61:177-183.

117. McKenzie KM, Kerr SR, Rouse MW, DeLand PN: Study of accommodative facility testing reliability. Am J Optom Physiol Opt 1987; 64:186-194.

118. Levine S, Ciuffreda KJ, Selenow A, Flax N: Clinical assessment of accommodative facility in symptomatic and asymptomatic individuals. J Am Optom Assoc 1985; 56:286-290.

119. Hoffman L, Rouse M: Referral recommendations for binocular function and/or developmental perceptual deficiencies. J Am Optom Assoc 1980; 51:119-125.

120. Scheiman M, Herzberg H, Frantz K, Margolies M: Normative study of accommodative facility in elementary schoolchildren. Am J Optom Physiol Opt 1988; 65:127-134.

121. Haynes HM: The distance rock test—a preliminary report. J Am Optom Assoc 1979; 50:707-713.

122. Haynes HM, McWilliams LG: Effects of training on near-far response time as measured by the distance rock test. J Am Optom Assoc 1979; 50:715-718.

123. Schor C, Horner D: Adaptive disorders of accommodation and vergence in binocular dysfunction. Ophthalmic Physiol Opt 1989; 9:264-268.

124. Scheiman M, Wick B: Clinical Management of Binocular Vision. Philadelphia: JB Lippincott, 1994.

125. Tsuetaki TK, Schor CM: Clinical method for measuring adaptation of tonic accommodation and vergence accommodation. Am J Optom Physiol Opt 1987; 64:437-449.

126. Kotulak, JC, Schor CM: The effects of optical vergence, contrast, and luminance on the accommodative response to spatially bandpass filtered targets. Vision Res 1987; 27:1797-1806.

127. Rosenfield M, Gilmartin B: Assessment of the CA/C ratio in a myopic population. Am J Optom Physiol Opt 1988; 65:168-173.

128. Fincham EF, Walton J: The reciprocal actions of accommodation and convergence. J Physiol (London) 1957; 137:488-508.

129. Rosenfield M, Ciuffreda KJ, Chen HW: Effect of age on the interaction between the AC/A and CA/C ratios. Ophthalmic Physiol Opt 1995; 15:451-455.

130. Rosenfield M, Ciuffreda KJ, Hung GK, Gilmartin B: Tonic accommodation: A review. I. Basic aspects. Ophthalmic Physiol Opt 1993; 13:266-284.

131. Rosenfield M, Ciuffreda KJ, Hung GK, Gilmartin B: Tonic accommodation: A review. II. Accommodative adaptation and clinical aspects. Ophthalmic Physiol Opt 1994; 14:265-277.

132. Owens DA, Mohindra I, Held R: The effectiveness of a retinoscope beam as an accommodative stimulus. Invest Ophthalmol Vis Sci 1980; 19:942-949.

133. Mohindra I: A non-cycloplegic refraction technique for infants and young children. J Am Optom Assoc 1977; 48:518-523.

134. Rosenfield M: Evaluation of clinical techniques to measure tonic accommodation. Optom Vis Sci 1989; 66:809-814.

135. Miller RJ: Ocular vergence-induced accommodation and its relation to dark focus. Percept Psychophys 1980; 28:125-132.

136. Rosenfield M, Chiu N, Ciuffreda KJ, Duckman R: Accommodative adaptation in children. Optom Vis Sci 1994; 71:246-249.

137. Hung GK, Ciuffreda KJ, Rosenfield M: Proximal contribution to a linear static model of accommodation and vergence. Opthalmic Physiol Opt 1995; 16:31-41.

138. Pigion RG, Miller RJ. Fatigue of accommodation: Changes in accommodation after visual work. Am J Optom Physiol Opt 1985; 62:853-863.

139. Lancaster WB, Williams ER: New light on the theory of accommodation, with practical applications. Trans Am Acad Ophthalmol Otolaryngol 1914; 19:170-195.

140. Howe L: The fatigue of accommodation. JAMA 1916; 67:100-104.

141. Berens C, Stark EK: Studies in ocular fatigue. IV. Fatigue of accommodation, experimental and clinical observations. Am J Ophthalmol 1932; 15:527-542.

142. Kurtz JI: An experimental study of ocular fatigue. I. General fatigue. Am J Optom 1938; 15:86-117.

143. Berens C, Stark EK: Studies in ocular fatigue. I11. Fatigue of accommodation. History, apparatus and methods of graphic study. Am J Ophthalmol 1932; 15:216-223.

144. Miller RJ, Pigion RG, Wesner MF, Patterson JG: Accommodation fatigue and dark focus: The effects of accommodation-free visual work as assessed by two psychophysical methods. Percept Psychophys 1983; 34:532-540.

145. Ehrlich DL: Near vision stress: Vergence adaptation and accommodative fatigue. Ophthalmic Physiol Opt 1987; 7:353-357.

146. Schor CM, Tsuetaki TK: Fatigue of accommodation and vergence modifies their mutual interactions. Invest Ophthalmol Vis Sci 1987; 28:1250-1259.

147. Cline D, Hofstetter HW, Griffin JR: Dictionary of Visual Science, 4th ed. Radnor, PA: Chilton, 1989.

148. Cooper J: Accommodative dysfunction. In Amos JF (ed): Diagnosis and Management in Vision Care. Boston: Butterworths, 1987, pp 431-459.

149. Ciuffreda KC, Levi DM, Selenow A: Amblyopia: Basic and Clinical Aspects. Boston: Butterworth-Heinemann, 1991.

150. Tucker J, Tomlinson A: An investigation of persistent paresis of accommodation. Am J Optom Physiol Opt 1974; 51:3-11.

151. Liu JS, Lee M, Jang J, et al.: Objective assessment of accommodation orthoptics. I. Dynamic insufficiency. Am J Optom Physiol Opt 1979; 56:285-294.

152. Rosenfield M: Accommodation and myopia: Are they really related? J Behav Optom 1994; 5:3-11, 25.

153. Duane A: Anomalies of accommodation clinically considered. Arch Ophthalmol 1916; 45:124-136.

154. Prangen AD: Subnormal accommodation. Arch Ophthalmol 1931; 6:906-918.

155. Suchoff IB, Petito GT: The efficacy of visual therapy: Accommodative disorders and non-strabismic anomalies of binocular vision. J Am Optom Assoc 1986; 57:119-125.

156. Charman WN, Whitefoot H: Pupil diameter and the depth-of-field of the human eye as measured by laser speckle. Optica Acta 1977; 24:1211-1216.

157. Rutstein RP, Daum KM, Amos JF: Accommodative spasm: A study of 17 cases. J Am Optom Assoc 1988; 59:527-538.

158. Guyton AC: Textbook of Medical Physiology, 7th ed. Philadelphia: WB Saunders, 1986, p 138.

159. Prangen AD: Spasm of the accommodation. In Transactions of the Section on Ophthalmology. Chicago: AMA Press, 1922, pp 282-292.

160. Alexander GF: Spasm of accommodation. Trans Oph Soc UK 1940; 60:207-212.

161. Sollom AW: Unilateral spasm of accommodation and transient convergent squint due to an anxiety neurosis. Br Orthop J 1966; 23:118-119.

162. Irvine G: A survey of esophoria and ciliary spasm. Br J Ophthalmol 1947; 31:289-304.

163. Hokoda SC: General binocular dysfunctions in an urban optometry clinic. J Am Optom Assoc 1985; 56:560-562.

164. Hoffman L, Cohen AH, Feuer G: Effectiveness of non-strabismus optometric vision training in a private practice. Am J Optom Arch Am Acad Optom 1973; 50:813-816.

165. Daum KM: Accommodative dysfunctions. Doc Ophthalmol 1983; 55:177-198.

166. London R: Accommodation. In Barresi BJ (ed): Ocular Assessment. The Manual of Diagnosis for Office Practice. Boston: Butterworths, 1984, pp 123-130.

167. Fraunfelder FT: Drug-Induced Ocular Side Effects and Drug Interactions, 2nd ed. Philadelphia: Lea & Febiger, 1982.

168. Jaanus SD, Bartlett JD: Adverse ocular effects of systemic drug therapy. In Bartlett JD, Jaanus SD (eds): Clinical Ocular Pharmacology. Boston: Butterworths, 1984, pp 917-939.

169. Gilmartin B: Ocular manifestations of systemic medication. Ophthalmic Physiol Opt 1987; 7:449-459.

170. Swegmark G: Studies with impedance cyclography on human ocular accommodation at different ages. Acta Ophthalmol 1969; 47:1186-1206.

171. Saladin JJ, Stark L: Presbyopia: New evidence from impedance cyclography supporting the Hess-Gullstrand theory. Vision Res 1975; 15:537-541.

172. Fisher RF: The force of contraction of the human ciliary muscle during accommodation. J Physiol (London) 1977; 270:51-74.

173. Adler-Grinberg D: Questioning our classical understanding of accommodation and presbyopia. In Stark L, Obrecht G (eds): Presbyopia. New York, Professional Press, 1987, pp 250-257.

174. Stark L: Presbyopia in light of accommodation. Am J Optom Physiol Opt 1988; 65:407-416.

175. Farnsworth PN, Shyne SE: Anterior zonular shifts with age. Exp Eye Res 1979; 28:291-297.

176. Weale RA: A Biography of the Eye. London: HK Lewis & Co., 1982, pp 185-237.

177. Fisher RF: The significance of the shape of the lens and capsular energy changes in accommodation. J Physiol (London) 1969; 201:21-47.

178. Fisher RF: Presbyopia and the changes with age in the human crystalline lens. J Physiol (London) 1973; 228:765-779.

179. Ayshire Study Circle: An investigation into accommodation. Br J Physiol Opt 1964; 21:31-35.

180. Kajiura M: Studies of presbyopia. Jpn J Ophthalmol 1965; 9:85-92.

181. Turner MJ: Observations on the normal subjective amplitude of accommodation. Br J Physiol Opt 1958; 15:70-100.

182. Bergman S: Research into the amplitudes of accommodation of Afrikaans groups. Br J Physiol Opt 1957; 14:59-64.

183. Litsinger GG: Amplitude of accommodation. Optom Monthly 1981; 72 (4):42-44.

184. Daum KM: Accommodative facility. *In* Eskridge JB, Amos JF, Bartlett JD (eds): Clinical Procedures in Optometry. Philadelphia: JB Lippincott, 1991, pp 687–697.

185. Jackson E: A Manual of the Diagnosis and Treatment of the Diseases of the Eye. Philadelphia: WB Saunders, 1900, p 126.

186. Sheard C: Dynamic Skiametry and Methods of Testing the Accommodation and Convergence of the Eyes. Chicago: Cleveland Press, 1920.

187. Wesson MD, Koenig R: A new clinical method for direct measurement of fixation disparity. South J Optom 1983; 1:48–52.

188. Blustein GH, Rosenfield M, Ciuffreda KJ: Effect of target illumination on task-induced shifts in the far point of accommodation. Invest Ophthalmol Vis Sci (Suppl) 1993; 34:1312.

189. Locke LC, Somers W: A comparison study of dynamic retinoscopy techniques. Optom Vis Sci 1989; 66:540–544.

**6**

*Ruth E. Manny, OD, PhD*
*Karen D. Fern, OD*

# Binocular Function

As you read this chapter, the words on the page are focused on the retina of each eye. If your binocular system is functioning normally, the two separate images formed in each eye are combined into a single image. This process involves two major elements—a motor component and a sensory component.

The motor component simultaneously directs your two foveas to the same word on the page. There are six extraocular muscles controlled by three cranial nerves (III, IV, and VI) which move each eye. Accurate control and coordination of these muscles are required for the motor component of the binocular system to function normally.

The sensory component combines the two images into a single percept through a process termed "fusion" (specifically, second-degree fusion). Before the two images of the word can be combined or fused, the images must be similar in size and clarity. Thus, a proper refraction with the best correction in place is required prior to the assessment of binocular function (see Chapter 4).

To be fused, the image from each eye must also fall on corresponding retinal areas within Panum's fusional area. Normally, the foveas are corresponding points, and the locus of all points in space with images that fall on corresponding points is the **horopter**. Objects located off the horopter are viewed from slightly different perspectives owing to the horizontal separation between the two eyes. The images of these objects do not fall on corresponding retinal areas and are disparate. This horizontal disparity between the two retinal images gives rise to the sensation of depth or space between objects located on the horopter and objects off the horopter. This depth sensation is termed **stereopsis** and provides extremely accurate localization of objects in space.

If the binocular system is functioning normally, both the motor and sensory components occur reflexively, operate efficiently, and are not associated with eye strain (asthenopia). However, if the binocular system fails to function normally, the motor and/or sensory components of the binocular system may be compromised. An eye turn may be present so that the two eyes do not align on the same object at the same time (strabismus, tropia, or squint), or the two eyes may be inefficient at maintaining alignment on a target requiring effort to avoid diplopia or double vision (i.e., poorly compensated heterophoria). If the images between the two eyes are too dissimilar (in size or clarity, for example), the sensory components may be compromised. Stereoacuity may be reduced or absent, or fusion may

not occur because one of the two images is ignored or suppressed.

Anomalies of binocular vision lie on a continuum that stretches from no binocular vision, as seen in patients with only a single functioning eye, to an inefficient binocular system that may produce a variety of symptoms (Table 6-1). In a recent study by Scheiman and co-workers, 26.4% of pediatric patients presenting to a primary care eye practice had either strabismus or other binocular disorders,[1] not including patients with amblyopia or accommodative disorders. A 1963–1965 survey of noninstitutionalized children in the United States found a prevalence of strabismus and other oculomotor problems to be 6.72% for 6- to 11-year-old children[2] and 5.28% for 12- to 17-year-old children.[3] Many of these patients[4] can be helped through lenses, prisms, or therapy. Although the treatment of binocular anomalies is beyond the scope of this chapter,[4-6] the first step in treatment is a proper diagnosis. This chapter presents a variety of methods to examine the integrity of the motor and sensory aspects of binocular function. The assessment techniques are divided into objective techniques, which require very little cooperation or response on the part of the patient, and subjective methods, which depend on the patient's active participation and response. These different approaches are often helpful when the clinician is faced with conflicting results or with a patient whose young age or cognitive ability precludes complex subjective responses.

# Ocular Motility

The movements of the eye are primarily rotary in nature. These movements occur around a cen-

---

**TABLE 6-1** Symptoms of Binocular Dysfunction

Asthenopia
Avoidance of near work
Blurred vision
Car sickness
Covering or closing an eye in bright sunlight
Dizziness
Double vision
Excessive tearing
Eye strain
Headache
Inability to attend and/or concentrate when detailed
  vision is required
Light sensitivity or photophobia
Loss of place while reading
Nausea
Print "swimming" or moving on the page
Pulling sensation
Sleepiness while reading
Use of finger as a pointer while reading

**TABLE 6–2** Monocular Eye Movements

| Type of Duction | Axis of Rotation | Direction of Movement | Agonist | Antagonist | Figure |
|---|---|---|---|---|---|
| Abduction | Vertical | Temporal | LR | MR | 6–1*B* |
| Adduction | Vertical | Nasal | MR | LR | 6–1*H* |
| Supraduction (sursumduction) | Horizontal | Up | SR | IR | 6–1*D* |
| | | | IO | SO | |
| Infraduction (deorsumduction) | Horizontal | Down | IR | SR | 6–1*F* |
| | | | SO | IO | |
| Incycloduction | Anteroposterior | Upper pole* nasal | SO | IO | |
| | | | SR | IR | |
| Excycloduction | Anteroposterior | Upper pole* temporal | IO | SO | |
| | | | IR | SR | |

*Upper pole refers to the upper pole of the vertical meridian of the eye.
LR = lateral rectus; MR = medial rectus; SR = superior rectus; IR = inferior rectus; IO = inferior oblique; SO = superior oblique.

ter of rotation and are produced by the movement of the eye around one of three axes. The anteroposterior axis of the eye is coincident with the line of sight. The vertical and horizontal axes are perpendicular to the line of sight. From the straight-ahead or primary position, rotation of the eye around one of these axes places the eye in a secondary position.

## MONOCULAR EYE MOVEMENTS

Monocular rotations of the eye are termed ductions. The muscle or muscles that contract to produce the movement are the agonist(s). When two muscles move the eye in the same direction, the muscles are synergists. For each agonist that contracts to move the eye, an antagonist muscle, which produces movement in the direction opposite the agonist, relaxes. Table 6-2 lists each type of duction and shows the axis of rotation, direction of movement, the agonist and antagonist muscles, and the reference to a photograph in Figure 6-1 which illustrates the movement.

## BINOCULAR EYE MOVEMENTS

Binocular eye movements maintain alignment of the eyes and move the object of regard onto the

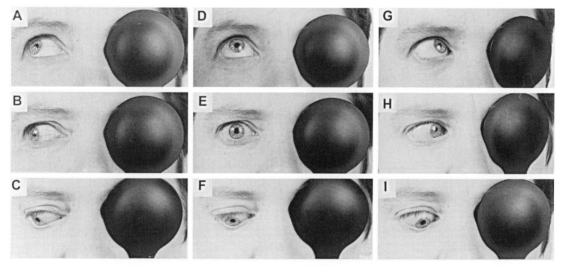

**FIGURE 6–1** Ductions, monocular eye movements of the right eye from the primary position. *A*, The right eye is moved to a tertiary position, up and right. It is also extorted. *B*, The right eye is moved to a secondary position. It is in abduction. *C*, The right eye is moved to a tertiary position, down and right. It is also intorted. *D*, The right eye is moved to a secondary position. It is in supraduction or sursumduction. *E*, The right eye is in the primary position. *F*, The right eye is moved to a secondary position. It is in infraduction or deorsumduction. *G*, The right eye is moved to a tertiary position, up and left. It is also intorted. *H*, The right eye is moved to a secondary position. It is in adduction. *I*, The right eye is moved to a tertiary position, down and left. It is also extorted.

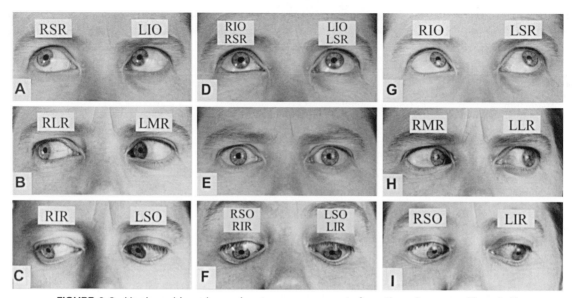

**FIGURE 6–2** Versions, binocular conjugate eye movements from the primary position. *A, B, C, E, G, H,* and *I* are known as the diagnostic action fields. The extraocular muscles that exert their primary action in the each of the action fields are also shown (see Table 6–7 for the abbreviations.) *D* and *F* are useful in the diagnosis of "A" and "V" patterns, but because more than one muscle has a major action, they are not considered diagnostic action fields. *A,* Up and right. *B,* Dextroversion. *C,* Down and right. *D,* Supraversion, elevation, or sursumversion. *E,* Primary position. *F,* Infraversion, depression, or deorsumversion. *G,* Up and left. *H,* Levoversion. *I,* Down and left.

fovea. The two types of binocular movements are termed versions and vergences. Versions are simultaneous and synchronous (conjunctive) movements of the two eyes in the same direction whereas vergences are movements in the opposite direction (disjunctive).

Both version and vergence require the contraction of one or more agonists in each of the eyes and the relaxation of the antagonist to each agonist. The muscles, one from each eye, that move the eyes in the same direction are yoke muscles. Whereas synergistic muscles from each eye are involved in all binocular movements, yoke muscles are typically designated only for horizontal and vertical versions and horizontal vergences owing to the clinical significance of these eye movements.[6] More than one pair of yoke muscles may contribute to the movement of the eyes to a direction of gaze, and the yoking of muscles may change depending upon the type of eye movement. For each type of version and vergence, Table 6-3 lists the direction of movement, the yoke muscles when applicable, and reference to photographs in Figures 6-2 through 6-4 that illustrate the movement.

## Extraocular Muscles

Each eye has six extraocular muscles. Each muscle has an origin and insertion within the orbit. The recti muscles originate at the annulus of Zinn and insert onto the globe at 5.5 to 7.7 mm

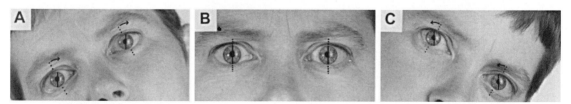

**FIGURE 6–3** Versions around the anteroposterior axis in response to vestibular stimulation via head tilt. The vertical meridian of the eye is shown as the solid line. The dotted line references the position of the vertical meridian for the eye in primary position. *A,* Levocyclover-sion (right eye incyclotorsion, left eye excyclotorsion). *B,* Eyes in primary position. *C,* Dextro-cycloversion (right eye excyclotorsion, left eye incyclotorsion).

**TABLE 6–3** Binocular Eye Movements

| Type | Direction of Movement | Yoke Muscle(s) | Figure |
|---|---|---|---|
| **Versions** | | | |
| Dextroversion | Right | RLR & LMR | 6–2B |
| Levoversion | Left | RMR & LLR | 6–2H |
| Supraversion (sursumversion) | Up | RSR & LIO LSR & RIO | 6–2D |
| Infraversion (deorsumversion) | Down | RSO & LIR LSO & RIR | 6–2F |
| Levocycloversion | Right upper pole* nasal Left upper pole* temporal | | 6–3A |
| Dextrocycloversion | Left upper pole* nasal Right upper pole* temporal | | 6–3C |
| **Vergences** | | | |
| Convergence | Nasal | RMR & LMR | 6–4A |
| Divergence | Temporal | RLR & LLR | 6–4B |
| Right supravergence (right sursumvergence) | Up | | |
| Left infravergence (left deorsumvergence) | Down | | 6–4C |
| Left supravergence (left sursumvergence) | Up | | |
| Right infravergence (right deorsumvergence) | Down | | 6–4D |
| Incyclovergence | Upper pole* nasal | | |
| Excyclovergence | Upper pole* temporal | | |

*Upper pole refers to the upper pole of the vertical meridian of the eye.
LIR = left inferior rectus; LIO = left inferior oblique; LLR = left lateral rectus; LMR = left medial rectus; LSO = left superior oblique; LSR = left superior rectus; RIR = right inferior rectus; RIO = right inferior oblique; RLR = right lateral rectus; RMR = right medial rectus; RSO = right superior oblique; RSR = right superior rectus.

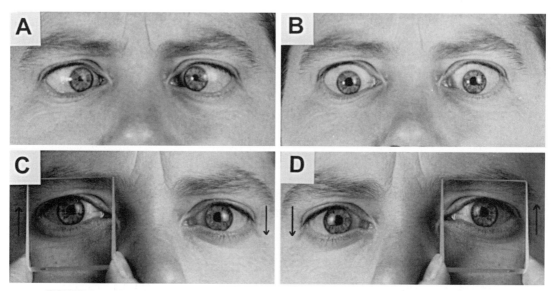

**FIGURE 6–4** Vergences, the binocular disjunctive eye movements. A, Convergence. B, Divergence. C, Vertical fusional vergence. Right supravergence (right sursumvergence) or left infravergence (left deorsumvergence). D, Vertical fusional vergence. Left supravergence (left sursumvergence) or right infravergence (right deorsumvergence).

from the corneal limbus, with the insertion of the medial rectus closest and the superior rectus farthest from the limbus. The origin of the superior oblique is the small wing of the sphenoid, but the trochlea is considered its physiological origin. The insertion is located behind the equator of the eye. The inferior oblique originates from the anterior floor of the orbit near the lacrimal fossa and inserts behind the equator just below the insertion of the lateral rectus.

Table 6-4 lists the muscles, the cranial nerve that innervates each muscle, and their actions. The action exhibited by a muscle is influenced by the position of the eye. To understand how eye position influences the action of a muscle, the muscle planes that are formed by joining the midpoint of the origin with the midpoint of insertion must be considered.

The plane for the horizontal recti lies in the horizontal plane of the eye and the axis of rotation is coincident with the vertical axis of the eye. As a result, contraction of these muscles produces only horizontal movement in primary position but also contributes to elevation and depression in extreme elevation and depression, respectively.

The muscle plane for the vertical recti is shown in Figure 6-5. This plane forms an angle of 23° temporal to the line of sight and does not coincide with any of the axes of the eye in primary position.[6] Therefore, the action produced by the vertical recti is not singular; it is a combination of the primary and secondary actions. As the eye moves away from primary position, the actions of the vertical recti change. With abduction the muscle plane of the vertical recti approaches the horizontal axis of the eye. The vertical action (elevation or depression) is maximized, and the muscles are pure vertical movers when the eye is abducted 23°. Adduction of the eye from primary position increases the torsional effect of the vertical recti muscles. If the eye could be adducted 67°, the recti would produce pure torsional action.

The muscle planes of the oblique muscles are also shown in Figure 6-5. The plane of the infe-

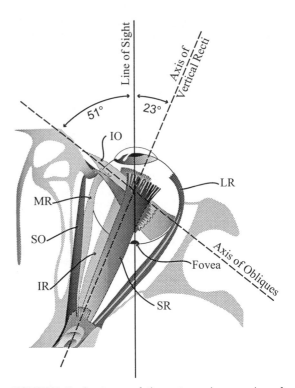

**FIGURE 6-5** Anatomy of the extraocular muscles of the right eye as viewed from above. The inferior rectus and inferior oblique muscles are shaded lighter to indicate their position under the globe. The axes of the vertical and oblique muscles are shown in relation to the line of sight to aid in the understanding of the muscles' actions (see text and Table 6-4 for additional details). (Modified from Pernkopf A: Atlas of Topographical and Applied Human Anatomy. Philadelphia: WB Saunders Co, 1963.)

rior oblique forms an angle of 51° nasal to the line of sight and the superior oblique an angle of 54°. The muscle planes of the oblique muscle are not coincident with any axes of the eye in primary position. As a result, the obliques, like the vertical recti, have both primary and secondary actions. With adduction the vertical action of the inferior oblique increases, and with the eye adducted 51° the inferior oblique becomes a pure elevator. Similarly, when the eye is adducted

| | | | | |
|---|---|---|---|---|
| **TABLE 6-4**  Extraocular Muscles | | | | |
| **Muscle** | **Cranial Nerve** | **Primary Action** | **Secondary Action** | |
| Medial rectus | III | Adduction | | |
| Lateral rectus | VI | Abduction | | |
| Inferior rectus | III | Depression | Extorsion, adduction | |
| Superior rectus | III | Elevation | Intorsion, adduction | |
| Inferior oblique | III | Extorsion | Elevation, abduction | |
| Superior oblique | IV | Intorsion | Depression, abduction | |

54°, the superior oblique becomes a pure depressor. Abduction from primary position increases the torsional action of the muscles, with the maximum incyclotorsion produced when the eye is abducted 36° (superior oblique) and maximum excyclotorsion with 39° of abduction (inferior oblique). The changes of the muscle actions with position of gaze are used in the diagnosis of underactions and overactions of muscles and are discussed in the following section.

## Eye Alignment

· · · · · · · · · · · · · · · · · · · · · · · · ·

An evaluation of the motor components of binocular function begins with an assessment of eye alignment. Individuals with normal eye alignment are able to direct the foveas of both eyes toward the object of interest so that an image of the object is formed on the fovea of each eye. Their eyes appear straight, and they are able to maintain this bifoveal alignment as the eyes move into any position of gaze (see Figs. 6-2 to 6-4).

Many individuals who demonstrate normal eye alignment when both eyes are open have a latent deviation or phoria. A **phoria** or heterophoria is a deviation that is kept latent by fusional vergence and manifests itself only when fusion is disrupted. As seen in Figure 6-6, when both eyes are open, both eyes are aligned. When fusion is disrupted by the infrared occluder, the eye behind the occluder goes to the phoria position, as seen through the filter by an infrared camera. If a phoria is present, the clinician must determine the direction of the phoria (inward toward the nose—esophoria [as in Fig. 6-6]; outward toward the ear—exophoria; up—hyperphoria; down—hypophoria; rotated toward the nose—incyclophoria; rotated toward the ear—excyclophoria), the magnitude of the phoria (measured in prism diopters), and whether the magnitude of the phoria is the same in all directions of gaze (comitant) or varies with eye position (noncomitant).

When both eyes are open but the two foveas do not align with the object of interest, an eye turn or **strabismus** is present. Figure 6-7 shows a left exotropia combined with a left hypotropia. When the left eye is covered, the right eye continues to fixate and the left eye remains in the deviated position behind the occluder. When the right eye is covered, the left eye takes up fixation, and the right eye assumes the deviated position behind the occluder. Other terms synonymous with strabismus include tropia, heterotropia, and squint. If a strabismus is present, the clinician must determine the frequency of the

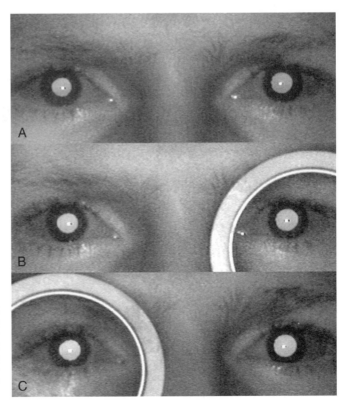

**FIGURE 6–6** *A*, Eyes in primary position viewing a target binocularly. The eyes are aligned, and the line of sight of each eye is directed toward the target. There is no strabismus. *B* and *C*, When fusion is disrupted by an infrared occluder, the eye under the cover (as seen by the infrared camera) goes to the phoric position (esophoria in this case) and the corneal reflex is decentered temporally.

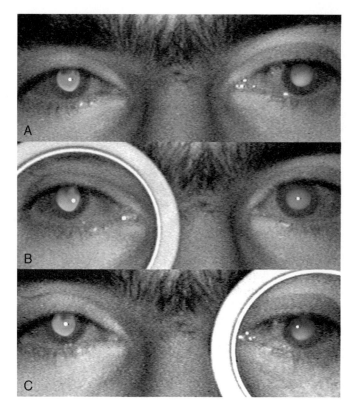

**FIGURE 6–7** *A,* Eyes in primary position viewing a target binocularly. The right eye is fixating the target, but the line of sight of the left eye is deviated outward (exotropia) and downward (hypotropia). The patient has a strabismus. *B,* When the right eye is occluded, the left eye moves in to pick up fixation while the right eye assumes the deviated position (out and up) behind the occluder. *C,* When the left eye is occluded, the right eye fixates and the left eye assumes its deviated position behind the occluder.

eye turn (constant or occasional), which eye is deviated (laterality), the direction of the eye turn (inward toward the nose—esotropia; outward toward the ear—exotropia; up—hypertropia; down—hypotropia; rotated toward the nose—incyclotropia; rotated toward the ear—excyclotropia), the magnitude of the deviation (measured in prism diopters), and whether the strabismus is the same in all directions of gaze (comitant) or the eye turn varies with eye position (noncomitant). Horizontal and vertical deviations can be measured by both objective and subjective techniques; however, torsional deviations can be measured only by subjective methods.

# Interpupillary Distance (PD)

. . . . . . . . . . . . . . . . . . . . . . . . . . .

The interpupillary distance is a useful measurement that can provide information ranging from the detection or monitoring of craniofacial disorders[7] to the proper positioning of corrective lenses.[8] In the context of evaluating a patient's binocular status, the PD is used to accurately position the optical centers of instruments and lenses along the patient's line of sight to avoid induced prism or peripheral aberrations. Because distance and/or near viewing may be required, a distance and near PD are typically measured. The distance PD is also used to compute the calculated accommodative convergence/accommodation ratio. The underlying assumption is that the distance between the centers of rotation (a theoretical construct because the eyes do not rotate around a single point) of the two eyes when the lines of sight are parallel is equal to the distance PD.

A 15- to 18-mm rule and penlight or transilluminator are used to determine the patient's PD.

1. The examiner is positioned directly in front of the patient at a distance of 40 cm. The patient and examiner should be on the same vertical plane.
2. The millimeter rule is placed on the bridge of the patient's nose (in the spectacle plane) with the millimeter scale positioned under both the right and left eyes.
3. The transilluminator or penlight is placed under the examiner's left eye and directed toward the patient's right eye. The patient is told to look directly at the light. The examiner closes his or her right eye and positions his or her left eye directly in front of the patient's right eye. The "zero" on the millimeter rule is then aligned with the

corneal light reflex in the patient's right eye. Once the zero has been aligned with the patient's right eye, the rule is not moved until the PD measurement is complete.

4. While the examiner's right eye is closed and the patient is fixating the light under the examiner's open left eye, the examiner notes the position of the corneal light reflex in the patient's left eye on the millimeter rule as viewed by the examiner's left eye. The *near* PD is the value in millimeters aligned with the position of the corneal light reflex in the patient's left eye.

5. Without moving the millimeter rule, the examiner opens his or her right eye and closes his or her left eye. The transilluminator is moved and positioned under the examiner's open right eye, which should be positioned directly in front of the patient's left eye. Again, the patient is instructed to look at the light. The position of the corneal light reflex in the patient's left eye is noted on the millimeter rule. The PD for *distance* viewing is the value in millimeters aligned with the position of the corneal light reflex in the patient's left eye while viewing the light under the examiner's right eye.

The PD is recorded in millimeters. The distance PD is traditionally recorded first followed by a "/" and then the near PD.

**EXAMPLE**
PD 63/60

When a light is used as the fixation target and the corneal light reflex is used to measure the PD, the PD measurement is referenced to a line that closely approximates the visual axis.[9] Some clinicians prefer to use the center of the pupil (or more correctly, the center of the entrance pupil, the image of the pupil as viewed through the cornea) to measure the distance and near PD. When the center of the entrance pupil is the measurement landmark, the PD is referenced to the line of sight. PDs referenced to the line of sight are typically 1 to 2 mm greater than those obtained using the corneal light reflex method described above.[9] Some clinicians believe that the line of sight provides the most appropriate reference for aligning optical devices in front of the eyes.[9] However, others believe that the ease with which the corneal light reflex is located, combined with the difficulties often encountered in locating the center of the pupil (particularly in dark irises), compensates for referencing the PD to the visual axis rather than the line of sight.

The distance and near PD referenced to the line of sight may also be estimated using the limbus rather than the center of the pupil as the measurement landmark. With this modification, the near PD is measured from the temporal limbus of the patient's right eye (step 3) to the nasal limbus of the patient's left eye (step 4) while the patient views the examiner's left eye. The distance PD is measured from the temporal limbus of the patient's right eye with the patient viewing the examiner's left eye (step 3) to the nasal limbus of the patient's left eye while the patient views the examiner's right eye (step 5).

Many commercial pupillometers are available to measure PD. Some of the pupillometers use the corneal reflections, whereas others rely on the center of the pupil. When precise positioning of lenses is critical (i.e., progressive addition lenses), these commercial instruments may aid in the accurate measurement of the PD in cooperative patients.

Measuring the PD in patients with strabismus requires modification of the techniques described above. The examiner must have the patient cover the eye not being aligned with the light or millimeter rule to ensure that the eye being measured is fixating the light. For example, in step 3 of the PD measurement, when the penlight or transilluminator is positioned below the examiner's left eye and the patient is directed to look at the light, the patient must cover his or her left eye to be sure that the right eye is fixating the light. Then in step 4, the patient's right eye is occluded and the location of the reflex in the patient's left eye is noted for the near PD. For the distance PD, the light is moved below the examiner's right eye (step 5), and the patient is directed to fixate the light. The patient's right eye remains covered to ensure that the patient is fixating the light with his or her left eye.

When measuring the PD on an infant or preschool child, limited cooperation may preclude the accurate fixation and alignment required to obtain an accurate PD by traditional measurement techniques. Hence, the distance PD is often estimated by measuring the distance of the outer canthus of the patient's right eye to the inner canthus of the left eye. (The inner canthus of the right eye to the outer canthus of the left eye may also be used). The near PD is often arbitrarily assigned a value of 3 mm less than this estimated distance PD.

For many patients, the eyes are not symmetrically located about the midline. Occasionally, when precise positioning of a lens or optical device is required (e.g., high correcting lenses, multifocal prescriptions, progressive addition lenses, or low vision devices), it becomes important to determine the patient's monocular PD. The monocular PD is the distance between the visual axis (or the line of sight) and the patient's midline. With the zero of the millimeter rule aligned with the corneal light reflex (or center of the pupil) in the patient's right eye as the patient views the examiner's left eye (examiner's right eye closed), note the mark on the millimeter rule that is positioned in the center of the patient's bridge. This measure is the distance, monocular, right eye PD. To measure the distance, monocular, left PD, align a centimeter mark on the millimeter rule with the patient's midline for an easy reference. The examiner opens his or her right eye, moves the penlight to his or her right eye, and closes his or her left eye. The examiner then directs the patient to look at the light. The mark on the millimeter rule which is aligned with the corneal light reflex (or center of the pupil) in the patient's left eye is noted. The difference between this measure and the centimeter value positioned on the patient's midline is the distance, monocular, left PD.

Monocular near PDs require a slightly different procedure. The examiner closes his or her non-dominant eye and aligns his or her open, dominant eye with the patient's midline. The light is positioned below the examiner's open, dominant eye, and the patient is asked to fixate the light. The millimeter rule is positioned in the spectacle plane on the bridge of the patient's nose with the zero aligned with the corneal light reflex (or the center of the pupil) in the patient's right eye. The near, monocular, right PD is the mark on the millimeter rule which is aligned with the middle of the patient's bridge. To measure the near, monocular, left PD, align a centimeter mark on the millimeter rule with the patient's midline for an easy reference. The patient continues to fixate the light below the examiner's open dominant eye while the examiner's nondominant eye remains closed. The mark on the millimeter rule which is aligned with the corneal light reflex (or center of the pupil) in the patient's left eye is noted. The difference between this measure and the centimeter value positioned on the patient's midline is the near, monocular, left PD.

Most pupillometers are designed to accurately measure distance and near monocular PDs. Monocular PDs may be recorded by specifying the distance PD/near PD for each eye.

**EXAMPLE**

PD   R 30/28.5 or OD 30/28.5
     L 31/29.5 or OS 31/29.5

The near PD varies as a function of the near working distance. If the working distance is sub-

stantially different from the conventional 40 cm, the examiner should be positioned at the near working distance to obtain the near PD. Alternatively, the PD for any near distance can be calculated from the PD measured at 40 cm using similar triangles.[9]

# Objective Measurements of Eye Alignment

## GROSS OBSERVATION

It is important to observe the patient's head posture. An abnormal head posture is often associated with a noncomitant, periodic strabismus (an occasional strabismus that occurs only under certain very predictable viewing conditions, in this case, one that is present only in a particular direction of gaze) or occasionally in cases of noncomitant phoria.[10] The abnormal head posture is adopted to move the eyes to a position where the deviation is minimized and kept latent by fusional vergence. An abnormal head posture that results from a muscle paresis or paralysis usually suggests that binocular vision is present and that the head is positioned toward the field of action of the paretic muscle. With the head positioned toward the field of action of the involved muscle, the eyes are moved in the opposite direction to where the deviation is minimized and fusion is promoted.

1. Observe the patient's normal head posture. A good time to make this observation is during the case history.
2. Three aspects of the head position are observed: face turn, head tilt, and chin position.

Table 6–5 shows the theoretical adaptive head postures in cases of a single isolated muscle paresis.[11] As seen in the table, the specific muscle cannot be determined by head posture alone, but often the choice may be reduced from 12 muscles to 2 yoked muscles, one in each eye.

However, this theoretical approach is often limited in actual clinical practice.[10, 12] For example, in cases of the vertical recti, the torsion action is relatively weak and often only a chin elevation or depression is present. Owing to the innervation of the inferior oblique (see Table 6–4), it is very rare that the inferior oblique is affected in isolation. However, in this rare case, the patient often manifests only a chin elevation to compensate for the increased diplopia on elevation. Thus, a chin elevation can compensate for a paresis of the superior rectus, inferior

| | **TABLE 6–5** Theoretical Head Postures in Cases of a Single Muscle Paresis | | | |
|---|---|---|---|---|
| **Face Turn** | **Chin Elevation** | **Head Tilt** | **Possible Muscles** | |
| Right | | | RLR, LMR | |
| Left | | | RMR, LLR | |
| Right | Up | Left | RSR, LIO | |
| Right | Down | Right | RIR, LSO | |
| Left | Up | Right | RIO, LSR | |
| Left | Down | Left | RSO, LIR | |

LIR = left inferior rectus; LIO = left inferior oblique; LLR = left lateral rectus; LMR = left medial rectus; LSO = left superior oblique; LSR = left superior rectus; RIR = right inferior rectus; RIO = right inferior oblique; RLR = right lateral rectus; RMR = right medial rectus; RSO = right superior oblique; RSR = right superior rectus.

oblique, or medial rectus (due to the greater convergence in downgaze). A chin depression may compensate for a paralysis of a lateral rectus and sometimes an inferior rectus or superior oblique.

Two head postures are characteristic and thus deserve special attention.[10] A face turn to the right or left without a head tilt or a chin elevation or depression typically indicates a paralysis of the lateral rectus because an isolated paralysis of the medial rectus is very rare. The second posture is a head tilt to the left and a face turn to the left with a chin elevation or depression. This posture suggests a paralysis of the right superior oblique. The chin is lowered (as predicted from the muscle actions, see Table 6-4) if there is no secondary spasm of the right inferior oblique. However, in a longstanding paralysis the chin may be elevated to avoid the field of action of the spastic right inferior oblique. A similar appearance is seen in a left superior oblique paralysis, where the head tilt is to the right and the face is turned to the right with the chin elevated or depressed, depending on the state of the left inferior oblique.

In summary, if the chin is elevated or depressed, a vertical rectus muscle is involved. If the head is tilted, an oblique muscle is involved. If a face turn is seen in isolation, it is usually the lateral rectus. However, the involved muscle may not be the primary problem because of secondary adaptations that occur as a result of a muscle paresis or paralysis. Although it may be difficult to determine the affected muscle by observation of the head posture alone, an abnormal head posture is usually associated with a muscle paresis or paralysis and indicates that binocular vision is or was present in a particular direction of gaze. Thus, an abnormal head posture is clinically significant and should be observed and recorded.

Note any abnormal head posture in the patient's record, such as "Face turn to the right" or "Face turn right, chin depression, and right head tilt."

It is often useful to ask for old photographs of the patient. The photographs can be reviewed for the abnormal head posture, and the time of onset of the problem may be roughly determined. Determining the time of onset provides important diagnostic and prognostic information.

Occasionally a patient adopts an abnormal head posture that makes a target visible to only one eye. This head posture eliminates diplopia and may be opposite to that adopted to obtain fusion.

Patients with nystagmus often adopt an abnormal head posture if the nystagmus is reduced in frequency or amplitude in a particular direction of gaze.[10] This point is called the **null point**.

## DIAGNOSTIC FIELDS OF ACTION

The integrity of the oculomotor system should be investigated. By positioning the eye in the six diagnostic fields of action, each muscle may be assessed with minimal influence from the other muscles. The six diagnostic fields of action are up and right, right, down and right, up and left, left, and down and left. As discussed in the extraocular muscle section (see Fig. 6-5), the superior and inferior recti are the primary vertical movers when the eye is abducted by about 23°. The vertical action of the superior and inferior oblique muscles is greatest when the eye is adducted by about 51°. The lateral recti may be evaluated by moving the eyes horizontally, in a plane parallel to the floor. Figure 6-2A to C and G to I shows the eyes in the six diagnostic fields of action. The muscles evaluated in each position are also shown in Figure 6-2.

Because the extraocular muscles are controlled by three different cranial nerves (see Table 6-4), abnormalities uncovered by the ocular motility assessment could result from a lesion anywhere along the motor pathway, beginning with supranuclear control of cranial nerves III, IV, or VI and extending to the nucleus of these three nerves, the nerves themselves, or the muscles. Determining the location of the lesion in the oculomotor pathway is beyond the scope of this chapter. However, loss of bilateral conjugate movements is associated with supranuclear lesions.

As shown in Figure 6-2, it is also important to evaluate the eyes in up and down fields of gaze. Although the up and down fields of gaze are not considered diagnostic action fields because the action of a single muscle is not isolated in each

| TABLE 6-6 Possible Causes of A and V Patterns | | |
|---|---|---|
| | Overaction | Underaction |
| **V pattern** | | |
| Esotropia is greater in downgaze than in up gaze | Inferior rectus<br>Inferior oblique | Superior oblique<br>Superior rectus |
| or | | |
| Exotropia is greater in upgaze than in downgaze | Inferior oblique<br>Inferior rectus | Superior rectus<br>Superior oblique |
| **A pattern** | | |
| Esotropia is greater in upgaze than in downgaze | Superior rectus<br>Superior oblique | Inferior oblique<br>Inferior rectus |
| or | | |
| Exotropia is greater in downgaze than in upgaze | Superior oblique<br>Superior rectus | Inferior rectus<br>Inferior oblique |

eye, these two positions are important in evaluating A and V patterns. If a strabismus is present, the deviation in upgaze must be at least 10 prism diopters more eso or less exo than in downgaze before it is classified as an A pattern. In a V pattern strabismus, the deviation in upgaze must be at least 15 prism diopters or more exo or less eso than in downgaze.[12, 13] A and V patterns are quite common in strabismus, and the difference in the magnitude of the deviation as a function of the vertical gaze results in a noncomitant strabismus. A and V patterns are most often associated with overactions or underactions of the oblique muscles but the vertical recti muscles have also been implicated. Table 6-6 summarizes the suspected roles of the vertical acting muscles in A and V patterns.[13] A and V patterns are also seen in patients with phorias, but the difference in upgaze and downgaze is considerably less than that found in strabismus.[14, 15] In patients with phorias, these patterns are seen more often with near fixation and usually require 20 to 40° elevation or depression before the noncomitancy is apparent.

1. The patient is seated comfortably facing the examiner and directed to view a hand-held target. At this point the habitual head posture should again be noted. If the head is not in the straight-ahead position, the patient must be directed to position his or her head straight and to look straight ahead (see Fig. 6-2E), or in the case of a young child, the head may be positioned by the examiner.
2. Testing is typically performed without spectacle correction, but if the patient presents with contact lenses, testing may be performed with the contact lenses in place. High-powered spectacles of unequal power between the two eyes can induce prism in

extreme positions of gaze, which could lead to misinterpretation. In addition, spectacles may make the observation of the eyes more difficult, and the frame may prevent the eyes from viewing the test target in the diagnostic action fields.

3. The target used for this test is not critical but must be within the resolving power of the patient's visual acuity. Many examiners prefer a penlight or transillumilluator so that the corneal light reflex may be observed.[16] The penlight or transilluminator is particularly useful when comparisons between the two eyes are made in the binocular assessment of versions. For young children, a small finger puppet, interesting picture, sticker on a popsicle stick, or Lang fixation stick or cube[17, 18] may be used to help maintain attention (Fig. 6-8).
4. Like the test target, the distance the target is held from the patient is not critical. Most

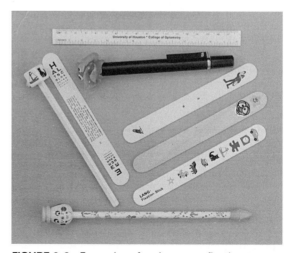

**FIGURE 6-8** Examples of various near-fixation targets.

examiners hold the target in their dominant hand between 30 and 50 cm from the patient. This distance allows the examiner to elevate the lids or control the head posture with his or her nondominant hand for better observation of the eyes in downgaze.

5. The eye movements are assessed under both binocular (see Fig. 6-2) and monocular (see Fig. 6-1) conditions. Binocular assessment of versions is typically performed before the monocular assessment of ductions. For the binocular version assessment, the examiner directs the patient to follow the target with his or her eyes while keeping his or her head in the primary position and to report any discomfort or doubling of the target. The examiner then slowly moves the target in an "H" pattern or a "figure 8" pattern while carefully observing the patient's eyes (Fig. 6-9). Although the field of fixation is roughly circular with a radius of 40 to 50° from the primary position,[19, 20] a 25° excursion is usually sufficient to isolate the muscles without interference from the cheek ligaments and thus to detect most abnormalities.[13] Therefore, if the target is positioned 40 cm from the patient, a 20-cm excursion from the primary position would be sufficient to uncover most overactions or underactions.

6. Monocular testing of ductions is similar to binocular version testing except that one eye is occluded. Because monocular assessment is used to determine if an underaction detected during version testing is due to a mechanical restriction, if no problems are observed under careful binocular testing, monocular evaluation is often omitted. If monocular testing is done, convention dictates that the right eye is tested first. The examiner again directs the patient to follow the target and report any discomfort as the examiner slowly moves the target in an "H" pattern or a "figure 8." With one eye occluded, diplopia should not be reported by the patient even if the motor system is compromised.

During version testing, the examiner must carefully observe the position of both eyes and the relationship of each eye to the other. The movement of the eyes should be smooth and symmetrical. The patient should not report any pain or double vision. If the full range of fixation is evaluated and the limit of excursion is reached, a small end point nystagmus is often visible.[19]

In assessing binocular versions, a lag (underaction) or an overshoot (overaction) of one eye is abnormal. Underactions or overactions in the version movements may be detected by observing the relative relationship of the two eyes and by observing the cornea and its relationship to the punctum and lateral canthus. Figure 6-10 schematically demonstrates the expected normal position of the eyes in levoversion as well as underactions and overactions. If a penlight or transilluminator is used, underactions and overactions may be observed as a change in the position of the corneal light reflex. When an underaction or overaction is detected, the field of action and the suspected eye must be noted and recorded. In addition, the patient's subjective responses of diplopia or pain are noted and recorded.

During monocular duction testing, each eye should track the target smoothly into the diagnostic action fields without evidence of an underaction, overaction, or pain on movement. The guidelines shown in Figure 6-10 for underactions and overactions of versions apply to ductions as well. Often an underaction due to paresis seen on version testing may be less apparent when the suspected eye is tested monocularly. Similarly, an overaction seen on version testing is not present when tested monocularly. This pattern suggests an innervational problem or muscle paresis. An underaction that is about equally apparent both binocularly and monocularly is suggestive of a

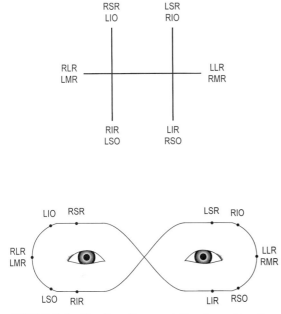

**FIGURE 6–9** The H pattern and the figure-8 pattern used to test the extraocular muscles. The fixation target is moved through space in one of these patterns and the patient follows the target with his or her eyes, without moving the head. The examiner observes the pursuit eye movements and the eyes in the diagnostic action fields.

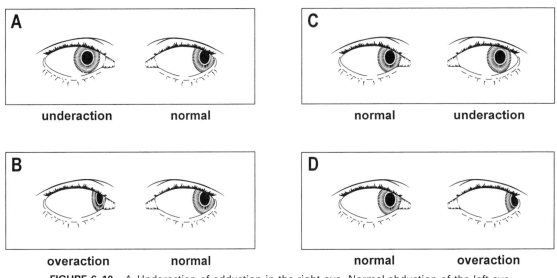

FIGURE 6–10  *A*, Underaction of adduction in the right eye. Normal abduction of the left eye. *B*, Overaction of adduction in the right eye. Normal abduction of the left eye. *C*, Underaction of abduction in the left eye. Normal adduction of the right eye. *D*, Overaction of abduction in the left eye. Normal adduction of the right eye.

mechanical restriction and may require forced duction testing for a more definitive diagnosis.

Several different methods have been proposed for recording the results of version and duction testing.

## Abbreviations

Extraocular muscle evaluation is frequently recorded using abbreviations. If the versions are symmetrical, smooth, and without overactions or underactions, SAFE or FESA is sometimes used to indicate (S) smooth, (A) accurate, (F) full, and (E) extensive ocular motility. A list of abbreviations commonly used in binocular vision assessment is found in Table 6-7. Some practitioners record normal versions simply as unrestricted.

EXAMPLES
EOM: SAFE
EOM: Unrestricted
EOM: Diplopia on gaze down and right with OD underaction
EOM: Unrestricted, pain on right gaze

## Grading Scales

If an abnormality is detected, additional information may be recorded using a grading scale. Several grading scales have been developed, but none is universally accepted. One scale popularized by Jampolsky[21] utilizes a 4-point scale to quantify the magnitude of an underaction or

overaction, with "0" indicating normal movement. Underactions are recorded with negative integers (−1 through −4), whereas overactions are scored with positive numbers (+1 through +4). Using abduction as an example, a −1 indicates a slight reduction in abduction while a −4 indicates that the eye would not move past the midline. Often this scale is placed on a sketch of the diagnostic action fields, as illustrated in Figure 6–11.

With young patients, it may be easier to move the patient's head to position the eyes into the desired diagnostic action field (Fig. 6–12). By controlling the patient's head, better control and attention are often achieved with the infant or young pre-school child.

Children less than 1 year of age may be more interested in the examiner's face than in any conventional fixation target. The diagnostic fields can be explored by the examiner moving his or her face into the diagnostic fields while stabilizing/maintaining the infant's head in the straight-ahead position with his or her hand.

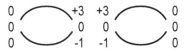

FIGURE 6–11  Grading scale and recording method for versions popularized by Jampolsky (1971).[21] Normal function is indicated by a zero. Overactions are designated with positive numbers (1 to 4) and underactions with negative numbers (1 to 4). This example illustrates a significant overaction of the inferior obliques and a bilateral underaction of the superior obliques.

**TABLE 6–7** Abbreviations Used in the Assessment of Binocular Function

| | | | |
|---|---|---|---|
| abnormal or anomalous retinal correspondence | ARC | Maddox rod | MR |
| | | meter | m |
| accommodative convergence/ accommodation ratio | AC/A | millimeter | mm |
| | | nasal | N |
| alternate cover test | ACT | near point of convergence | NPC |
| base down | BD | normal retinal correspondence | NRC |
| base in | BI | occasional or intermittent esotropia at distance | E(T) |
| base out | BO | | |
| base up | BU | occasional or intermittent esotropia at near | E(T)′ |
| binocular vision | BV | | |
| both eyes (oculi unitas or uterque) | OU | occasional or intermittent exotropia at distance | X(T) |
| centimeter | cm | | |
| cover test | CT | occasional or intermittent exotropia at near | X(T)′ |
| cycle | cy | | |
| diopter | D | orthophoria | ∅ |
| diopter sphere | DS | plano | pl |
| dissociated vertical deviation | DVD | prism diopter (Δ) | pd |
| eccentric fixation | EF | punctum proximum of convergence | PPC |
| esophoria at distance | E or EP | pupillary distance | PD |
| esophoria at near | E′ or EP′ | refraction providing the best visual acuity | BVA |
| esotropia at distance | ET | right | R |
| esotropia at near | ET′ | right eye (oculus dexter) | OD or RE |
| exophoria at distance | X or XP | right inferior rectus | RIR |
| exophoria at near | X′ or XP′ | right inferior oblique | RIO |
| exotropia at distance | XT | right lateral rectus | RLR |
| exotropia at near | XT′ | right medial rectus | RMR |
| extraocular muscles | EOM | right superior rectus | RSR |
| fixation disparity | FD | right superior oblique | RSO |
| headache | HA | second | sec |
| hypertropia | HT | single binocular vision | SBV |
| left | L | smooth, accurate, full, and extensive ocular motility | SAFE or FESA |
| left eye (oculus sinister) | OS or LE | | |
| left inferior rectus | LIR | temporal | T |
| left inferior oblique | LIO | to the nose (in NPC) | TTN |
| left lateral rectus | LLR | unilateral cover test | UCT |
| left medial rectus | LMR | vergence facility | VF |
| left superior rectus | LSR | with correction (cum correction) | c.c. |
| left superior oblique | LSO | without correction (sine correction) | s.c. |

Patients with esotropia often have trouble abducting the deviating eye. In these cases, moving the head to position the eyes in the diagnostic fields is also useful during monocular duction testing and may demonstrate abduction when the patient appears to be unable to abduct the deviating eye. For example, if a constant unilateral right esotropia is present, it may be difficult

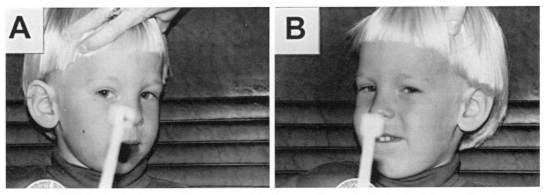

**FIGURE 6–12** *A*, Dextroversion assessed by turning the patient's head while keeping the fixation target in the primary position. *B*, Levoversion assessed by turning the patient's head while keeping the fixation target in the primary position.

to get the right eye to abduct or move temporally. If the patient maintains fixation on an object located directly in front of him or her and then his or her head is turned to the left by the examiner, an abduction may occur.

The patient's ability to fixate and follow an object is sometimes used as an indirect measure of acuity if the patient is very young (typically less than 1 year of age), nonverbal, or cognitively challenged. During testing of ductions, a qualitative impression of each eye's ability to fixate and follow the object may be made. If differences between the two eyes are noted, a difference in acuity between the eyes may be present. Several grading scales and notations have been suggested.[22-24] In addition, the child's reaction to occlusion may be observed during the evaluation of the ductions to provide additional information about the vision in each eye.[25] For additional information on visual acuity assessment in the young child, see Chapter 2.

Abnormal versions and ductions occur more frequently in strabismus. If the strabismus is paralytic, the magnitude of the strabismic deviation varies with the direction of gaze, and the deviation is noncomitant. In cases of strabismus, it is important to identify and record the fixating eye during version testing. When a muscle paresis results in a secondary strabismus, the deviating eye is usually the eye with the paretic muscle. As the eyes are moved in the direction of the palsied muscle, an underaction of the affected eye is noted. However, when the fixating eye is occluded for duction testing, motility is usually normal, suggesting a palsy rather than a mechanical restriction. If the affected eye fixates during version testing, an overaction of the noninvolved eye is observed in the field of action of the affected muscle. As with the underaction, the overaction is not apparent upon the evaluation of ductions.

## Brückner Test

The Brückner test[26, 27] offers an assessment of eye alignment in young patients or multiply challenged individuals whose eye alignment may be impossible to assess using the subjective methods described below and whose limited cooperation and fixation prevent an accurate assessment by the cover test.

1. The child is situated in a parent's lap watching the examiner positioned about 1 meter from the child. The room illumination is dim to help focus the child's attention on the examiner's light and to aid the examiner's observations.

2. Because the test is influenced by asymmetrical refractive errors, the habitual refraction should be worn if the test is used specifically for the detection of eye misalignment.[28] However, the sensitivity for detecting deviations of 2° or less is decreased with correction.[29] If the patient presents without correction, the refractive error must be known before an accurate interpretation of the results can be made. Testing is done with natural pupils before dilation or cycloplegia.

3. The examiner directs the light from a direct ophthalmoscope at the patient so that both eyes are simultaneously illuminated. Often singing, animal sounds, or other unusual noises are necessary to maintain the child's attention on the light.

4. The examiner then focuses the ophthalmoscope so that the pupil and red reflexes are in sharp focus for optimal observation. The brightnesses of the two red reflexes are compared.

If the red fundus reflexes are of equal brightness in the two eyes, normal eye alignment is present. The corneal light reflex (Hirschberg test, see below) may also be observed and should appear symmetrical in the two eyes when no strabismus is present.

If one reflex is brighter than the other, a problem is suspected in the eye with the brighter reflex. In patients with strabismus, the deviating eye has the brighter reflex. Figure 6–13 shows a patient whose Brückner reflex in the left eye is brighter than that in the right. The corneal light reflex in the left eye is decentered nasally relative to the fixating right eye, suggesting a left exotropia (see Hirschberg test, below).

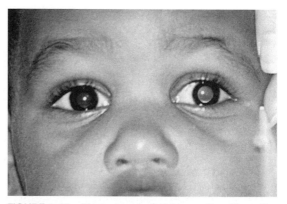

**FIGURE 6–13** Photographic Brückner reflex. The reflex in the left eye is brighter than in the right, suggesting a problem with the left eye. As seen by gross observation and the position of the corneal light reflexes, the left eye is exotropic.

The magnitude of the deviation cannot be determined by the Brückner test. However, if the deviation is greater than about 5° or 10 prism diopters, the magnitude may be estimated by the Hirschberg test, which relies on the location of the corneal light reflex.

The advantage of the Brückner test is its ability to detect deviations smaller than the lower limit of the Hirschberg test (about 0.5 mm or 10 prism diopters). As reported by Kaakinen,[26] and later by Tongue and Cibis,[27] Brückner suggested that a deviation of 1.5° (about 3 prism diopters) induced an observable change in the red reflex of the deviating eye. The experience of Kaakinen[26] confirms this sensitivity originally reported by Brückner and suggests that a small deviation missed by the Hirschberg or Krimsky test may be detected by the Brückner test.

There is no established method to record the results of the Brückner test. The test results should be recorded along with other binocular findings. The record should reflect what the examiner actually observes. Because the eye with the brighter reflex is more often the abnormal eye, noting the eye with the brighter reflex may be preferable to noting the eye with the dimmer reflex.

EXAMPLES

Brückner: Equal reflexes
Brückner: OD brighter than OS

The Brückner test is not specific for strabismus. Unequal refractive errors in the two eyes, media opacities, anisocoria, or abnormalities of the posterior pole may all induce a difference in the red fundus reflex.[27] In cases of retinal abnormalities, the nature of the abnormality determines which eye has the brighter reflex. In anisometropia, the viewing distance, the patient's accommodative state, and the direction and magnitude of the anisometropia determine the eye with the brighter reflex. Griffin and colleagues[30] have reported that a simulated anisometropia of 2.00 D or greater is detectable when a photographic Brückner test is used.

There is some indication in the literature that the Brückner test may not be appropriate for infants under 8 months of age.[31] Most normal infants under 2 months of age and many normal infants 2 to 8 months of age show an asymmetrical Brückner reflex, which suggests caution when applying this test to infants under 8 months of age.

The test, as described by Tongue and Cibis[27] from the original work of Brückner, was administered with an ophthalmoscope. Kaakinen, who replaced the ophthalmoscope with a conventional camera and flash, found that a deviation of 1° (about 2 prism diopters) was sufficient to induce an observable change in the red reflex of the deviating eye.[26]

The work of Roe and Guyton[32] suggests that the Brückner test may also be performed with a transilluminator or penlight as long as the examiner places his or her eye as close to the light source as possible to observe the light reflected from the patient's fundus.

The mechanism by which the difference in the brightness of the two reflexes occurs is still debated. One theory[27] suggests that the brighter reflex of the deviating eye is the result of the greater reflectance that occurs outside the macular area, where the macular pigment is absent. However, this hypothesis does not explain the difference in brightness that occurs with unequal refractive errors. Roe and Guyton[32] have suggested that the asymmetrical brightness in the red reflex is due to the deviating eye's loss of conjugacy with the light source. This lack of conjugacy causes the light from the retina to "spill" past the light source, creating a brighter red reflex.

Using a limited sample of patients with inexperienced observers, Griffin and Cotter[28] found the Brückner test to yield an unacceptable number of false positives. They suggest caution in applying the Brückner test as the sole screening test to detect strabismus.

In cases of nystagmus, where the cover test may not be useful in establishing the patient's eye alignment, the Brückner test may offer an additional tool to evaluate the patient's ocular alignment.

## Hirschberg and Krimsky Modification

The Hirschberg test, also known as the corneal light reflex test, is used to detect the presence of strabismus. If a strabismus is detected, many of the characteristics of the deviation may also be determined using the Hirschberg test. The laterality of the strabismus (unilateral or alternating), the direction of the deviation (esotropia, exotropia, vertical tropia), the magnitude of the deviation, an estimation of comitancy (whether the deviation is the same in all directions of gaze), and some estimate of the frequency of the deviation (constant or occasional) can all be made with the Hirschberg test. However, the Hirschberg test is typically limited to measurement of the deviation at the near point because physical limitations make this test impractical for measuring the deviation at the far point without considerable modification.[33]

The Krimsky modification of the Hirschberg test (Krimsky's prism reflex test) uses a prism to improve the estimate of the magnitude of deviation at near. However, even with the Krimsky modification, the test is considerably less accurate than the cover test and need **not** be performed routinely on all patients. This test is most useful in infants and young pre-schoolers because it is entirely objective and requires only momentary fixation.

1. The patient is seated facing the examiner wearing his or her habitual prescription in moderate room illumination.
2. The light from a transilluminator or small penlight is directed toward the midline of the patient from a distance of 30 cm to 1 meter. The distance is determined by the position in space at which the information about deviation is desired. Traditionally, near point testing is done at 40 cm; thus 40 cm is often selected. Both eyes are illuminated simultaneously. Because the size and quality of the corneal light reflex de-

pend on the source, a small bright light should be used.
3. The patient must fixate the light with both eyes open. If the patient is too young to understand these instructions, dimming the room lights and making interesting sounds or blinking the light on and off may help secure the patient's fixation on the light long enough to make the measurements.
4. The examiner must sight monocularly, directly over the light source, and note the position of the corneal light reflex in the pupil of each eye. Proper sighting directly over the light is critical to avoid inducing errors. If the reflex is displaced nasally relative to the center of the pupil, positive values are assigned to the displacement. For reflexes displaced temporally from the center of the pupil, negative values are assigned to the displacement. In the Hirschberg test, the examiner estimates, in millimeters, the displacement of the corneal reflex from the center of the pupil.

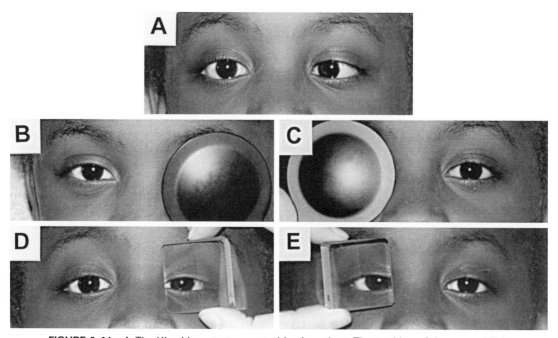

**FIGURE 6–14** *A,* The Hirschberg test on a strabismic patient. The position of the corneal light reflex in the right eye is +0.5 mm nasal. The position of the corneal light reflex in the left eye is −1.0 mm. A left esotropia is suspected. *B,* Angle kappa of the right eye. Note that the reflex in the right eye is in the same position as that seen under binocular viewing (+0.5 mm). *C,* Angle kappa of the left eye. The reflex in the left eye when viewing monocularly is also +0.5 mm nasally, confirming that the left eye is the deviating eye. The estimated angle of deviation is about 33 prism diopters. *D,* A base out prism is placed over the deviating left eye to move the temporally displaced corneal reflex (seen in *A* above) nasally so it appears in the same position as angle kappa in the left eye. This is the prism reflex test or the Krimsky modification of the Hirschberg test. *E,* A base out prism is placed over the fixating right eye. A levoversion occurs (both eyes move to the left) and the temporally displaced reflex in the left eye (seen in *A* above) now appears nasally, in the same position as angle kappa in the left eye. This is the modified Krimsky version of the Hirschberg test.

5. Following observation of the position of the corneal light reflex in each eye when both eyes of the patient are open, the observation is repeated with only one eye viewing the fixation light. This monocular observation of the corneal light reflex is clinically referred to as **angle kappa**. Although the correct term for this angle, the angle formed at the center of the entrance pupil by the intersection of the line of sight and the pupillary axis, is angle lambda, the misnomer is so widespread that it has become the accepted. In practice, the monocular assessment of angle kappa (lambda) is really necessary only if an asymmetry in the corneal light reflexes is noted when the patient views the light with both eyes open. This monocular assessment allows the examiner to determine the fixating eye in cases of strabismus.

6. In the Krimsky modification[33] of the Hirschberg test, a prism is placed before the nonfixating eye (usually the eye with the reflex that is most displaced from the center of the pupil). The apex of the prism points in the direction the reflex must move in order to be symmetrical with the reflex in the fixating eye (e.g., in the direction opposite to the displacement of the corneal light reflex). For example, if the reflex in the right eye is located 0.5 mm nasally but the reflex in the left eye is displaced more temporally, the patient has a left esotropia. Base out prism is then placed in front of the left eye (Fig. 6-14*D*). The power of the prism is increased until the reflex in the deviating eye is in the same relative position as the corneal light reflex in the fixating eye—in this example, 0.5 mm nasally.

Some examiners prefer to place the prism before the fixating eye, believing that the reflex in the deviating eye is easier to observe (Fig. 6-14*E*). This variant of the test has been referred to as the modified Krimsky by Lennarson.[34]

The corneal light reflex should appear in the same relative location within the pupil of each eye in the normal patient. The most usual position is 0.5 mm nasally (Fig. 6-15).

If the corneal light reflex does not appear in the same relative location in the pupil of each eye when both eyes are simultaneously illuminated, a strabismus may be present (Fig. 6-14*A*). Angle kappa must then be measured in each eye to determine the fixating eye and laterality of the deviation. Most often the eye with the reflex located closer to the center of the pupil (usually

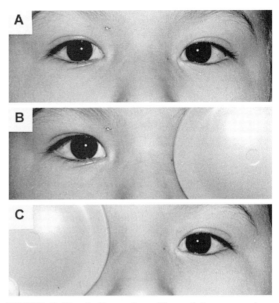

**FIGURE 6–15** *A*, Normal position of the corneal reflexes as seen during the Hirschberg test. The reflexes are symmetrical in each eye and are 0.5 mm nasally, or +0.5 mm. *B* and *C*, The corneal reflexes remain in the same position when angle kappa is evaluated monocularly.

0.5 mm nasally) is the fixating eye. To measure angle kappa and verify the fixating eye, the suspected deviating eye is covered while the position of the corneal light reflex is carefully observed (Fig. 6-14*B*). The position of the corneal light reflex in the patient's fixating eye does not move when the nonfixating eye is covered (Fig. 6-14*C*). The position of the corneal light reflex is then observed in the deviating eye as the fixating eye is covered. The position of the corneal light reflex moves as the deviating eye picks up fixation. The position of the corneal light reflex in each eye, referenced to the center of the pupil, is estimated in millimeters and recorded as angle kappa.

Once the fixating eye has been identified, the position of the corneal light reflex in the deviating eye during monocular viewing (angle kappa) is compared with that observed under binocular conditions. The displacement is estimated in millimeters and is a measure of the magnitude of the strabismus. An estimation of the magnitude of the deviation in prism diopters may be obtained using the conversion (Hirschberg ratio) of 1 mm ≈ 22 prism diopters. Other conversions have been proposed in the literature and are summarized in Table 6-8.

The direction of the deviation is determined by the direction of displacement of the binocular reflex in the deviating eye. If the reflex is displaced temporally, an esotropia is present. Exo-

| TABLE 6–8  Hirschberg Ratio | | |
|---|---|---|
| **Reference** | **Hirschberg Ratio** | **Method** |
| Hirschberg (1885) as cited by Krimsky (1948)[35] | about 7 deg/mm. | Calculation based on corneal radius of curvature of 8 mm. |
| Wheeler (1943)[46] | 8 deg/mm | Based on standard that was accepted at the time, Wheeler compared the Hirschberg to the screen test (cover test) in strabismic patients. The Hirschberg test underestimated the deviation in 66% of 25 patients by an average of 11 deg. |
| Flom (1956)[36] | Deviation in pd = (11 + X)/X where X = the difference in the position of the reflected image for the deviating eye compared with that for the fixating eye. | |
| Jones and Eskridge (1970)[37] | Method 1<br>21.6 pd/mm<br>Method 2<br>12 deg/mm (up to 20 deg)<br><br>22 pd/mm (to approximate any magnitude) | Mathematical model.<br><br>Photographic displacement of reflex from center of entrance pupil in four normal observers.<br>Extrapolation based on data of du Bois-Reymond. |
| Griffin and Boyer (1974)[38] | Method 1<br>24.66 pd/mm<br>(SD 17)<br>ET (n = 18)<br>23.3 pd/mm<br>XT (n = 4)<br>30.76 pd/mm<br>Method 2<br>20.75 pd/mm<br>(SD 8.57)<br>ET (n = 21)<br>20 pd/mm<br>XT (n = 4)<br>24.67 pd/mm<br>Recommendation<br>22 pd/mm | Photographic method. Reflex referenced to center of entrance pupil compared with alternate cover test in 22 strabismic patients.<br><br><br><br>Photographic method. Reflex referenced to center of cornea compared with alternate cover test in 25 strabismic patients. |
| Carter and Roth (1978)[39] | 13.6 deg<br>(SD 3.8 deg) | Photographic method. Reflex referenced to nearest limbus using 15 normal subjects. |
| Brodie (1987)[40] | approximately<br>21 pd/mm | Photographic method. Reflex referenced to midpoint between nasal and temporal limbus in three normal observers. |
| Eskridge et al. (1988)[41] | Method 1<br>22.94 pd/mm<br>Method 2<br>21.7 pd/mm | Photographic method with normal observer, slope of best fit line.<br>Empirical masked comparison of photographic method with alternate cover test in 15 strabismic patients based on slope of best fit line. |
| DeRespinis et al. (1989)[42] | 20.89 pd/mm<br>(SD about regression line 6.58 pd) | Photographic method with strabismic patients, referenced to the center of the cornea compared with prism neutralization with alternate cover test. |

ET = esotropia; deg = degree; mm = millimeters; n = number in sample; pd = prism diopters; SD = standard deviation; XT = exotropia.

tropia presents with a nasal displacement of the corneal light reflex. If the reflex is positioned below the center of the cornea, a hypertropia is present. In hypotropia the reflex is positioned above the center of the cornea.

The test distance at which the deviation is measured should be noted.

**EXAMPLES**

*Symmetrical reflexes*

Hirschberg @ 40 cm: aligned

Hirschberg @ 40 cm: ortho

Hirschberg @ 40 cm: OD +0.5 mm; OS +0.5 mm

*Asymmetrical reflexes*

Angle kappa: OD +0.5 mm, OS +0.5 mm

Hirschberg @ 40 cm: OD +0.5 mm; OS −1.5 mm

The notation above suggests a left esotropia of about 44 prism diopters (1.5 + 0.5 = 2; 2 × 22 = 44).

If the Krimsky modification is used, the deviation should be recorded in prism diopters and the fixating eye and the eye with the measuring prism should be noted:

Krimsky (prism OD): 25 pd right esotropia

Both the Hirschberg and the Krimsky modification use a light as a fixation target. However, a small light does not serve as an adequate stimulus to accommodation.[43, 44] Because the deviation is measured at near where accommodation should be active, a strabismus, particularly a convergence excess associated with a high accommodative convergence/accommodation ratio, may be missed (Fig. 6–16). Further, if the deviation is detected, the magnitude of esotropic deviations may be underestimated, whereas exotropic deviations may be overestimated. Aouchiche and Dankner[45] found that the Krimsky test underestimated the deviation in 16 of 19 patients (17 of whom were esotropic) compared with prism neutralization with the alternate cover test. The magnitude of the underestimation varied between the two examiners (6.3 to 11.2 prism diopters). In addition to differences in the accommodative demand, they suggest that fusion is not disrupted to the same degree with the Hirschberg and alternative cover tests.

Under the best conditions, the sensitivity of the Hirschberg test has been estimated to be on the order of 0.5 mm, or about 11 prism diopters.[46, 47] Thus, strabismic deviations less than about 10 prism diopters may be missed by the Hirschberg test. Griffin and colleagues,[30] using a photographic Hirschberg test, reported an improved sensitivity. When strabismic deviations were simulated via asymmetrical vergence, devia-

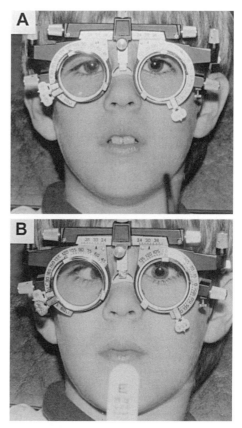

**FIGURE 6–16** *A,* Patient viewing a light at near. The eyes are aligned; no strabismus is present. *B,* The same patient viewing a 20/20 letter at near. With the proper stimulus to accommodation, a right esotropia is manifested.

tions of 8.5 prism diopters were detected 80% of the time, and deviations of 4.5 prism diopters were detected about 78% of the time. The Krimsky modification of the Hirschberg test may improve the estimates of the magnitude of the deviations through bracketing.

The limitations of the Hirschberg test, discussed above, suggest that the test should *not* be performed routinely on all patients. However, the Hirschberg test can be very useful in a number of patients who cannot muster the cooperation required for cover testing. Patients less that 18 months of age, whose limited attention may preclude the accurate fixation required to perform a cover test, are good candidates for the Hirschberg test. The Hirschberg test is also useful to rule out pseudostrabismus caused by unequal epicanthal folds, often present in infants. Patients with very poor vision or no vision in the deviating eye are also good candidates for the Hirschberg test because the deviating eye is not able to accurately take up fixation during cover testing. The eye alignment of patients with manifest or latent nystagmus may also be more easily evaluated with the Hirschberg test than with the cover test.

The magnitude of strabismus depends on the accommodative state of the patient. Thus, the deviation should be measured with the best "sensory" prescription in place. If the refraction differs significantly from the patient's habitual prescription, the magnitude of the deviation should be remeasured with the best sensory prescription. It is also sometimes useful to measure the deviation unaided to determine the presence of any accommodative component. However, as explained above, the Hirschberg test is limited in this regard because a light is not an adequate stimulus to accommodation.

The Hirschberg test can also be used to estimate the comitancy of the deviation. As the fixation light is moved into the diagnostic action fields, the patient is asked to follow the light with his or her eyes only, keeping his or her head in the straight-ahead position. The examiner must move with the light and continue to sight monocularly directly above the light to avoid errors of parallax. The position of the corneal light reflexes is observed in each of the diagnostic action fields. If the position of the corneal light reflexes does not remain constant in the different fields of gaze, the deviation is non-comitant. The magnitude of the non-comitancy can be quantified by estimating the magnitude of the deviation in each field of gaze.

Occasionally an asymmetrical angle kappa gives a false impression of a strabismus. In these cases the position of the corneal light reflex, although asymmetrical, is the same in each eye under monocular and binocular conditions. Although these patients may appear strabismic, no strabismus is usually found with additional testing.

Often a patient who remains attentive for the Krimsky modification of the Hirschberg test and allows prisms to be placed in front of his or her eyes will allow the more accurate assessment of eye alignment with the cover test. However, the Krimsky or Hirschberg test may allow the less experienced examiner to estimate the magnitude of the prism needed to neutralize the deviation with the cover test. This increased efficiency may be sufficient enough to allow verification of the estimated magnitude through more accurate cover testing in a young pre-school patient with limited attention.

## Unilateral Cover Test

The unilateral and alternate cover tests are among the most simple and elegant tests available to evaluate a patient's eye alignment. Although these tests are objective and very simple to perform, they are often confusing for the beginning practitioner to understand and interpret. If the tests are thought of as two separate entities, performed sequentially, with the unilateral cover test preceding the alternate cover test, much of the confusion is eliminated.

The unilateral cover test is used to establish the presence of a phoria or a tropia. If the patient has a strabismus, the laterality (unilateral or alternating) of the squint is also determined with the unilateral cover test. The direction of the phoria or tropia may also be ascertained with the unilateral cover test, but it is easier for the less experienced examiner to determine the direction of the phoria or tropia during the alternate cover test described below.

1. The patient is seated facing the examiner in full room illumination. Auxiliary indirect illumination directed on the patient's face via an overhead lamp (usually available on the phoroptor stand) is advisable to ensure a good view of the patient's eyes.
2. The cover test is performed at two different test distances—traditionally 6 meters (20 ft) and 40 cm (16 in). During near point testing, the examiner is positioned directly in front of the patient on the patient's eye level. During far point testing, the examiner must be positioned slightly below the patient's line of sight to avoid obstructing the patient's view of the distance fixation target.
3. The patient's eye alignment can be influenced by the patient's accommodative state. The true distance deviation is obtained when accommodation is relaxed, and thus it is measured with the patient's refractive error fully corrected. The true near deviation is typically measured at 40 cm, where the stimulus to accommodation is 2.50 D when the patient is fully corrected for distance. However, in cases of presbyopia, the near deviation should be measured through the most appropriate near add.
4. Careful attention to the test target is also necessary to ensure accurate results. For adults and school-age children, the distance measurement is made with the patient viewing an isolated letter close to the acuity threshold. For young children, pictures or actual objects of interest (e.g., a puppet with detail or a mechanical toy) make it easier to ensure the patient's attention by

engaging in conversations about the objects.

For near point testing, adults and older school-age children should fixate a single letter close to threshold on a reduced Snellen chart. Pictures, finger puppets, or numbers on a ruler (equivalent to the child's age) may ensure better cooperation from the pre-school patient (see Fig. 6–8). However, the child's attention is directed at the small details in these targets to ensure accurate and stable accommodation during the measurements.

If the vision is not equal in the two eyes, the acuity of the poorer eye is used to guide the target selection. Because reduced vision in one eye with the best correction in place (amblyopia) is often associated with unilateral strabismus, this becomes an important consideration.

5. Once the target is selected and the patient and examiner are properly positioned, the patient's fixation is directed at the distance target and the right eye is covered with an occluder (Fig. 6–17). The examiner carefully observes the left eye for any movement as the right eye is occluded. The oc-

cluder is left in place only briefly, no longer than 1 second. The right eye is then uncovered while the left eye is again observed for any movement. The procedure should be repeated several times to be sure no small movement of the left eye upon occlusion of the right eye or upon removal of the cover from the right eye is missed.

The right eye is now carefully observed for any movement as the left eye is covered for about 1 second and then uncovered (Fig. 6–17). Again, the procedure is repeated several times to ensure that no small movement is overlooked. The examiner's attention is always focused on the unoccluded eye.

6. The same procedure is repeated with the patient fixating a near target.

Three key concepts are used to interpret the unilateral cover test:

1. In patients with a phoria, both eyes fixate the target when the target is viewed binocularly.
2. In patients with strabismus, only one eye fixates the target when the target is viewed binocularly; the line of sight of the deviating eye is directed somewhere else.
3. When one eye is covered, the remaining open eye fixates the target with the fovea unless eccentric fixation is present.

Putting the direction of the deviation aside and limiting the discussion to constant strabismus, there are four broad categories of eye alignment: a phoria (including orthophoria), a unilateral right eye strabismus, a unilateral left eye strabismus, and an alternating strabismus. By carefully observing the eye that is not covered during the unilateral cover test and applying the three concepts described above, the examiner can determine which of these conditions is present (Table 6–9).

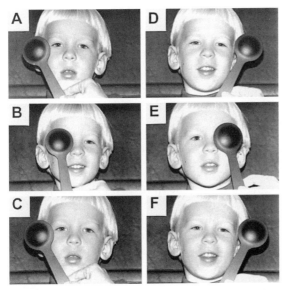

**FIGURE 6–17** Unilateral cover test. *A,* The patient views an accommodative target with his head straight and his eyes in the primary position. *B,* The right eye is covered while the examiner carefully observes the patient's left eye for any movement. *C,* The right eye is uncovered while the examiner carefully observes the patient's left eye for any movement. *D,* The occluder is switched to the left side and the patient continues to view the fixation target. *E,* The left eye is covered while the examiner carefully observes the right eye for any movement. *F,* The left eye is uncovered while the examiner carefully observes the right eye for any movement.

### Phoria, No Strabismus

In this case, both eyes fixate the target under binocular conditions. When the right eye is covered, the left eye does not move to pick up fixation because it was already fixating the target when both eyes were open. There is also no movement of the left eye as the right eye is uncovered because under binocular conditions both eyes continue to fixate the target. Similarly, when the left eye is covered, the right eye does not move to pick up fixation because it, like the left eye, was already fixating the target when both eyes were open. Again, when the left eye

| Procedure | Phoria | Constant Unilateral OD Tropia | Constant Unilateral OS Tropia | Constant Alternating Tropia† OS Initially Fixating | Constant Alternating Tropia† OD Initially Fixating |
|---|---|---|---|---|---|
| Cover OD Watch OS | No motion OS | No motion OS | OS moves in = XT out = ET | No motion OS OS fixating eye | OS moves in = XT out = ET |
| Uncover OD Watch OS | No motion OS | No motion OS | OS moves in = ET out = XT | No motion OS OS still the fixating eye | No motion OS OS now the fixating eye |
| Cover OS Watch OD | No motion OD | OD moves in = XT out = ET | No motion OD | OD moves in = XT out = ET | OD moves in = XT out = ET |
| Uncover OS Watch OD | No motion OD | OD moves in = ET out = ET | No motion OD | No motion OD OD now the fixating eye | No motion OD OD now the fixating eye |

**TABLE 6–9** Unilateral Cover Test

OD = right eye, OS = left eye, XT = exotropia, ET = esotropia
†The movements described for the constant alternating strabismus are based on performing the unilateral cover test in the order listed under the procedure column (from top to bottom).

is uncovered, no movement of the right eye is seen, as it continues to maintain fixation under binocular conditions. If there is central fixation in each eye (the visual acuity is equal in each eye and should be 20/20 [6/6] or better if fixation is central) and neither the right eye nor the left eye moved when the opposite eye was covered, no strabismus is present. However, the patient may have a phoria or latent deviation, which is measured with the alternate cover test, as described in the next section.

### Unilateral Right Eye Strabismus

In this case the left eye is fixating the target when both eyes are open but the line of sight of the right eye is not directed toward the target. When the right eye is covered, no movement of the left eye is seen because the left eye is fixating the target when both eyes are open while the right eye is deviated. When the right eye is uncovered, no movement of the left eye is observed because it remained fixated on the target when the right eye was covered. However, when the left eye is covered, the right eye must move to pick up fixation with the fovea of the right eye. If you could see behind the occluder, the left eye would no longer be aligned with the target. When the left eye is uncovered, the right eye moves back to its originally deviated position while the left eye moves to pick up fixation.

### Unilateral Left Eye Strabismus

In this case, the right eye fixates the target when both eyes are open, but the line of sight of the left eye is not directed toward the target. When the right eye is covered, the left eye must move

from its deviating position to pick up fixation. If you could see behind the occluder, the right eye would no longer be aligned with the target (Fig. 6-7). When the right eye is uncovered, the left eye moves back to its original deviated position while the right eye moves to fixate the target. When the left eye is covered and then uncovered, the right eye does not move because it was already fixating the target when both eyes were open.

### Alternating Strabismus

In an alternating strabismus, one eye is always deviated, but which eye is deviating and which eye is fixating the target varies with the viewing conditions. There are also degrees of alternation, but for this discussion the assumption is that the patient is freely alternating; the patient is able to fixate equally well with the right or the left eye. An additional assumption is that the patient is fixating the target with the left eye (i.e., the right eye is deviated) when the unilateral cover test begins. In this case, when the right eye is covered, there is no movement of the left eye because when both eyes are open the line of sight of the left eye is directed toward the target. When the right eye is uncovered, there is still no movement of the left eye because it continues to view the target when both eyes are open. As the occluder is placed over the left eye, the right eye moves to pick up fixation. Up to this point, the observations are the same as they were for a unilateral right strabismus. However, as the cover is removed from the left eye, the right eye does not move but continues to fixate the target. The patient has changed fixation. The patient was initially fixating the target with the left eye, but when the left eye was covered the patient took up fixation with the right eye. As the left eye is uncovered, the patient continues to fixate with the right eye.

If the test is repeated and the right eye is again covered, the left eye (which is now the deviating eye) moves to pick up fixation. As the cover is removed from the right eye, no movement of the left eye is seen because the left eye has become the fixating eye. If, however, the left eye is now covered, the right eye moves to pick up fixation. As the left eye is uncovered, no movement of the right eye is seen.

No method of recording the results of the unilateral cover test is universally accepted. If no tropia is detected, many practitioners make no notation of the results and record only the magnitude of the phoria as measured by the alternate cover test. However, if a strabismus is detected, the beginning practitioner may find it easiest to record what was observed and hold the interpretation of the results for the assessment section of the record, where the complete binocular status of the patient is summarized.

When the results are recorded, it is imperative that the test conditions be clearly specified. The test distance and the correction worn during the testing must be included. The abbreviation "c.c." is used to indicate that the test was performed with correction; "s.c." indicates no correction was in place when the test was performed. (See Table 6-7 for additional abbreviations pertinent to the binocular vision assessment.) If the test was done with correction, the correction must be specified.

**EXAMPLES**

| UCT @ 6 m c.c. | cover OD: no movement OS |
|---|---|
| OD −0.50 −1.00 × 180 | cover OS: OD moves in |
| OS −1.00 −0.75 × 175 | |
| UCT @ 40 cm c.c. | cover OD: no movement OS |
| OD −0.50 −1.00 × 180 | cover OS: OD moves in |
| OS −1.00 −0.75 × 175 +1.50 add | |

If this prescription was the patient's habitual correction noted somewhere else in the record, the following is sufficient:

| UCT @ 6 m c.c. (habitual) | cover OD: no movement OS cover OS: OD moves in |
|---|---|

| UCT @ 40 cm c.c. (habitual) | cover OD: no movement OS cover OS: OD moves in |
|---|---|

More experienced practitioners often record the interpretation of the test. In the example above, the following would be noted in the chart.

| UCT @ 6 m c.c. (habitual) | constant right exotropia |
|---|---|
| UCT @ 40 cm c.c. (habitual) | constant right exotropia |

When the vision is very poor in the deviating eye, the deviating eye may not pick up fixation when the normally fixating eye is occluded. Hence, no movement of either eye is observed, and the examiner may falsely conclude that no strabismus is present. However, most of these patients have large deviations that are apparent upon casual observation of the patient. In addition, making sure the target is visible to the deviating eye helps the patient fixate with the deviating eye when the normally fixating eye is covered. It is also helpful to give the patient additional time to fixate and to provide an auditory cue as the normally fixating eye is covered. The examiner may say "ready, set, now look" and occlude the fixating eye as he or she says the work "look."

Up until this point, central fixation was assumed. Central fixation refers to the normal condition where, under monocular conditions, the eye fixates the target so that the image of the target falls on the fovea. In some patients with abnormal binocular vision (most frequently seen in cases of strabismus with amblyopia), when the fixating eye is covered, the deviating eye fixates the target eccentricity. Under monocular viewing conditions, the image of the target does not fall on the fovea but on some eccentric, non-foveal retinal area. Because the magnitude of eccentric fixation is typically small (usually less than 3 prism diopters),[48] it has little impact on the examiner's ability to detect large angles of strabismus. However, when the eccentric fixation is in the same direction as the deviation (i.e., nasal eccentric fixation and esotropia or temporal eccentric fixation and exotropia) and the magnitude of the strabismus is equal to the amount of eccentric fixation, no movement of the deviating eye is seen when the fixating eye is covered. In these rare cases, the results of the unilateral cover test suggest normal eye alignment, and the strabismus is missed. Thus, the examiner must know the monocular fixation characteristics of the patient before the cover test can be properly interpreted. A reduction in vision in one eye alerts the examiner to the possibility of eccentric fixation.

Latent nystagmus, or nystagmus present only when one eye is occluded, is often present in patients with infantile esotropia and makes the assessment of binocular function with the cover test very difficult. Using a high plus lens instead of an occluder may dissociate the patient enough to prevent that eye from maintaining fixation without inducing a nystagmus. Other possibilities include the use of the Hirschberg, Krimsky, or Brückner test to assess the binocular status of patients with latent nystagmus.

In addition to the standard test conditions (6 meters and 40 cm with the refractive error fully corrected), it is often useful to perform the unilateral cover test with the patient's habitual correction to determine his or her presenting binocular status. Some examiners also like to perform the cover test unaided to determine how much of the deviation is due to accommodation. To avoid confusion, the test distance and the correction used during the cover test must be clearly indicated in the record.

Not all patients with an alternating strabismus freely alternate, showing no preference for fixation with either eye. Some patients with alternating strabismus have a fixation preference for one eye over the other. The strength of the fixation preference can be estimated during the unilateral cover test by observing how easy it is for the patient to hold and maintain fixation with either eye.

Not all patients with a strabismus manifest the strabismus all the time. Part of the time these patients are able to overcome the deviation through motor fusion, manifesting the strabismus only occasionally when fusion is lost. Upon initial evaluation with the unilateral cover test, no strabismus may be detected. However, through repeated disruptions of fusion during the cover test or perhaps later in the examination, the strabismus may become manifest. A careful case history may also alert the examiner.

An additional cue that may alert the more experienced examiner to the possibility of an occasional strabismus is the quality of re-fusion once the occluder is removed. If no movement of either eye is seen as the fellow eye is occluded, a constant strabismus is ruled out (with the exception noted above for eccentric fixation), and thus a phoria or an occasional strabismus may be present. If the eye that is occluded is observed as the occluder is removed, the speed at which fusion is regained may be observed. If recovery is almost instantaneous, fusion is strong and an occasional strabismus is unlikely. However, if re-covery of fusion is slow or the patient shows evidence of effort (blinking, wrinkling of the brow, report of diplopia), the possibility of an occasional strabismus or poor binocular function must be explored in greater detail.

Children less than about 2 years of age are often apprehensive of the occluder. In these young patients, the examiner may use his or her thumb to occlude the patient's eyes. By placing his or her dominant hand on the child's head (palm down, fingers away from the face), the thumb is free to occlude the eyes. However, the examiner must be sure to fully occlude the child's eye to avoid misinterpretation.

## Alternate Cover Test

The alternate cover test follows the unilateral cover test and is used to determine the direction of the phoria or tropia and the magnitude of the latent (phoria) or manifest (tropia) deviation. If the alternate cover test is performed without the unilateral cover test, the examiner can determine the direction and magnitude of the deviation but is not able to state if the deviation is a phoria or tropia.

The first four points are the same for both the unilateral and alternate cover test.

1. The patient is seated facing the examiner in full room illumination. Auxiliary indirect illumination directed on the patient's face via an overhead lamp (usually available on the phoroptor stand) is advisable to ensure a good view of the patient's eyes.
2. The cover test is performed at two different test distances; traditionally 6 meters (20 ft) and 40 cm (16 in). During near point testing, the examiner is positioned directly in front of the patient on the patient's eye level. During far point testing, the examiner must be positioned slightly below the patient's line of sight to avoid obstructing the patient's view of the distance fixation target.
3. The patient's eye alignment can be influenced by the patient's accommodative state. The true distance deviation is obtained when accommodation is relaxed and thus is measured with the patient's refractive error fully corrected. The true near deviation is typically measured at 40 cm, where the stimulus to accommodation is 2.50 D when the patient is fully corrected for distance. However, in cases of presbyopia, the near deviation should be measured through the most appropriate near add.

4. Careful attention to the test target is also necessary to ensure accurate results. For adults and school-age children, the distance measurement is made with the patient viewing an isolated letter close to the acuity threshold. For young children, pictures or actual objects of interest (e.g., a puppet with detail or a mechanical toy) make it easier to ensure the patient's attention by engaging in conversations about the objects.

For near point testing, adults and older school-age children should fixate a single letter close to threshold on a reduced Snellen chart. Pictures, finger puppets, or numbers on a ruler (equivalent to the child's age) may ensure better cooperation from pre-school patients (see Fig. 6–8). However, the child's attention is directed at the small details in these targets to ensure accurate and stable accommodation during the measurements.

If the vision is not equal in the two eyes, the acuity of the poorer eye is used to guide the target selection. Because reduced vision in one eye with the best correction in place (amblyopia) is often associated with unilateral strabismus, this becomes an important consideration.

5. Once the target is selected and the patient and examiner are properly positioned, the patient's fixation is directed at the distance target and the right eye is covered with an occluder (Fig. 6–18). The examiner then moves the occluder to the left eye while observing the right eye as it is uncovered. The occluder is then moved back to the right eye while the examiner observes the left eye as it is uncovered. The examiner notes the direction and the amount of movement of the eye as it is uncovered. This alternate occlusion continues for at least 30 seconds. The examiner is always watching the eye being uncovered.

It is very important that fusion be completely disrupted so that the maximum deviation is uncovered. The cover must be moved rapidly between the eyes so that one eye is always occluded and fusion is prevented. However, the occluder can remain in front of each eye for several seconds to ensure complete dissociation. Failure to completely dissociate is one of the most common errors.

6. The direction of the deviation is determined by the direction the eye moves as the cover is removed. If the eye was turned in behind the occluder (esophoria or eso-

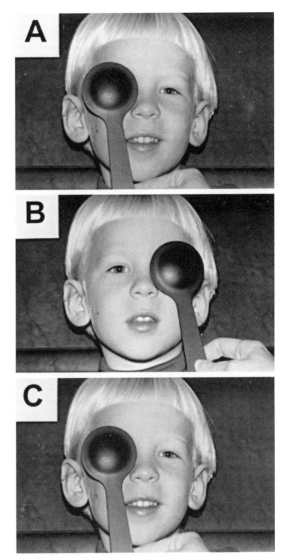

**FIGURE 6–18** Alternate cover test. *A*, The right eye is occluded as the patient views an accommodative target in primary gaze. *B*, The occluder is moved to the left eye as the examiner observes the right eye for any movement as the occluder is removed. *C*, The occluder is moved back to the right eye as the examiner observes the left eye for any movement as the occluder is removed. The patient must be completely dissociated for the full deviation to be manifested. The alternate cover test must be repeated and continued for at least 30 seconds so that dissociation is complete.

tropia), the examiner sees the eye move out to pick up fixation when the occluder is moved to the other eye. If the right eye was down (right hypophoria, or right hypotropia) when it was occluded, the right eye must move up to pick up fixation when the occluder is moved to the left eye. Table 6–10 summarizes the primary directions of movement seen as the eye is uncovered

| | | | | | | |
|---|---|---|---|---|---|---|
| **TABLE 6–10** Alternate Cover Test | | | | | | |
| Phoria by UCT<br>Tropia by UCT† | Hypophoria*<br>Hypotropia‡ | Hyperphoria*<br>Hypertropia‡ | Exophoria<br>Exotropia | Esophoria<br>Esotropia | Encyclophoria<br>Encyclotropia | Excyclophoria<br>Excyclotropia |
| Position of the deviated eye (tropia) or eye under cover (phoria) | Down | Up | Out | In | Upper pole of vertical meridian rotated nasally | Upper pole of vertical meridian rotated temporally |
| Direction eye moves as occluder is removed | Up | Down | In | Out | Upper pole of vertical meridian rotated temporally | Upper pole of vertical meridian rotated nasally |
| Prism to neutralize | Base up | Base down | Base in | Base out | | |

*Vertical phorias describe the relative position of the two eyes when fusion is disrupted. A right hypophoria is equivalent to a left hyperphoria. Therefore, in cases of vertical phoria, an eye must be specified so that the relative position of each eye is clear.
†For a complete assessment of a strabismus, the frequency, deviating eye, magnitude, direction, and comitancy must be specified.
‡In cases of vertical tropia or a vertical component of a tropia, the deviating eye must be specified.
UCT = unilateral cover test.

and the phoric or strabismic posture these movements represent. Some patients may show a diagonal eye movement as the occluder is moved to the other eye. These patients have both a horizontal and vertical component to the deviation, and both components must be specified and measured.

7. The magnitude of the deviation can be estimated based on the amount of movement. A millimeter of limbal shift corresponds to about 8 prism diopters.[49] However, a much more accurate measure of the deviation is obtained through prism neutralization.

If the unilateral cover test revealed no strabismus, the prism may be placed in front of either eye during the alternate cover test. The base of the prism is placed in the same direction as the eye movement observed during the alternate cover test. If the eye moves out as the occluder is moved to the other eye, the patient is esophoric and the deviation is neutralized with base out prism. Table 6–10 indicates the direction of the neutralizing prism based on the direction of the observed eye movement. The prism is placed in front of the eye in the proper orientation, and the occluder is then placed in front of the prism. The eye is observed through the prism as the occluder is moved to the other eye. The power of the prism is adjusted until no movement of the eye behind the prism is seen as the occluder is removed from this eye and placed over the fellow eye.

If the unilateral cover test indicated a unilateral strabismus, the magnitude of the primary and secondary deviation should be

measured. The primary deviation is the deviation when the normally fixating eye is fixating. The deviation is measured as described above with the neutralizing prism in front of the deviating eye (Fig. 6-19). As in the case of a phoria, the base of the prism is placed in the direction of the observed eye movement. The power of the prism is adjusted until no movement of the eye is seen through the prism as the occluder is moved to the other eye. The secondary deviation is the deviation when the normally deviating eye is fixating. It is measured by placing the prism (base placed in the direction of the observed movement) in front of the normally fixating eye (Fig. 6-20).

It is important to keep the patient dissociated during the measurement. Therefore, the examiner should continue to occlude an eye between measurements while the prism power is adjusted.

8. The same procedures used to determine the direction and magnitude of the deviation at distance must be repeated with the patient fixating a near target. In cases of strabismus, the secondary deviation needs to be measured at only one viewing distance (far or near). However, the primary deviation must be measured at both distance and near.

Only the direction and magnitude of the deviation are measured with the alternate cover test. This information must be combined with the results of the unilateral cover test to determine the patient's binocular status (tropia versus phoria).

In patients with phorias, the magnitude of the phoria measured with the alternate cover test should be very similar to that obtained subjectively by the von Graefe method. Thus, the "expected" values listed in Table 6–11 apply to phorias measured with the alternate cover test when the refractive error is fully corrected.

Measurement of the primary and secondary deviations yields a preliminary estimation of the comitancy of the deviation. If the primary and

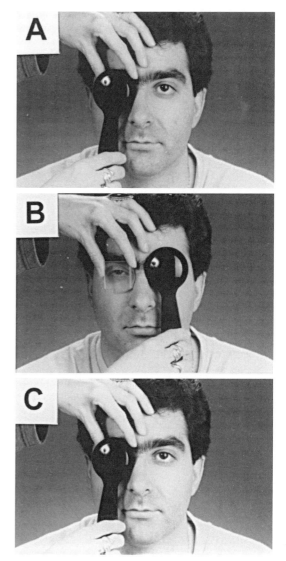

**FIGURE 6–20** Prism neutralization of the secondary deviation. The patient has a left exotropia and left hypotropia (as seen in Figures 6–7 and 6–19). *A*, The prism is placed behind the occluder in front of the fixating right eye. *B*, The occluder is moved to the left eye as the examiner observes the right eye through the prism for movement. *C*, The occluder is returned to the right eye. The magnitude of the prism is adjusted based on the movement of the right eye (seen in *B*) as the occluder is moved to the left eye.

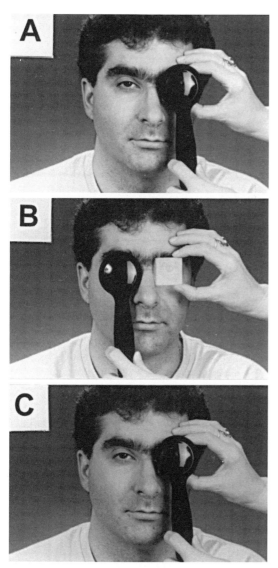

**FIGURE 6–19** Prism neutralization of the primary deviation. The patient has a left exotropia and left hypotropia (as seen in Figure 6–7). *A*, The prism is placed behind the occluder in front of the deviating left eye. *B*, The occluder is moved to the right eye as the examiner observes the left eye through the prism for movement. *C*, The occluder is returned to the left eye. The magnitude of the prism is adjusted based on the movement of the left eye (seen in *B*) as the occluder is moved to the right eye.

secondary deviations are significantly different (one author recommends a difference of more than 5 prism diopters,[11]) the deviation is noncomitant and a muscle paresis or paralysis should be suspected. The examiner should carefully watch for an underaction when versions are tested in a patient with a difference in the magnitude of the primary and secondary deviations.

If the patient is not strabismic, only the magnitude and direction of the phoria are required.

**TABLE 6–11** Expected Values for Phorias and Vergences

| Finding | Morgan[70] Mean | Morgan[70] SD | OEP[55] |
|---|---|---|---|
| **Phorias** | | | |
| horizontal @ 6 m | 1ΔXP | 2Δ | 0.5ΔXP |
| horizontal @ 40 cm | 3ΔXP′ | 5Δ | 6ΔXP′ |
| vertical | | | φ |
| **Vergences** | | | |
| vertical | | | equal |
| BO @ 6 m | | | |
| blur | 9Δ | 4Δ | ≥7Δ |
| break | 19Δ | 8Δ | ≥19Δ |
| recovery | 10Δ | 4Δ | ≥10Δ |
| BI @ 6 m | | | |
| break | 7Δ | 3Δ | ≥9Δ |
| recovery | 4Δ | 2Δ | ≥5Δ |
| BO @ 40 cm | | | |
| blur | 17Δ | 5Δ | ≥ 15Δ |
| break | 21Δ | 6Δ | ≥ 21Δ |
| recovery | 11Δ | 7Δ | ≥ 15Δ |
| BI @ 40 cm | | | |
| blur | 13Δ | 4Δ | ≥ 14Δ |
| break | 21Δ | 4Δ | ≥ 22Δ |
| recovery | 13Δ | 5Δ | ≥ 18Δ |

OEP = Optometric Extension Program; Δ = prism diopters; BO = base-out prism; BI = base-in prism.

**EXAMPLES**

| | |
|---|---|
| ACT @ 6 m c.c. (habitual): | orthophoria (or φ) |
| ACT @ 40 cm c.c. (habitual): | 5Δ exophoria (or 5Δ XP′) |

In cases of strabismus, the primary angle of deviation should be recorded for both fixation distances, but the secondary deviation needs to be measured and recorded at only one of the fixation distances:

| | |
|---|---|
| ACT @ 6 m c.c. (BVA) | OD fixating: 20Δ BO OS OS fixating: 25Δ BO OD |
| ACT @ 40 cm c.c. (BVA) | OD fixating: 30Δ BO OS |

The magnitude of a strabismic deviation measured by the alternate cover test is affected by the presence of eccentric fixation. If the eccentric fixation and the strabismus are in the same direction (i.e., exotropia and temporal eccentric fixation), the measured deviation is less than the true deviation by the amount of the eccentric fixation. If the eccentric fixation and the strabismus are in opposite directions (i.e., exotropia and nasal eccentric fixation), the measured deviation is greater than the true deviation by the amount of the eccentric fixation. The true deviation may be obtained by the following formula:

$$H(T) = H(M) + EF$$

*where*

H(T)  is the true strabismic deviation in prism diopters, esotropia is plus (+), and exotropia is minus (−)

H(M)  is the deviation measured in prism diopters by the alternate cover test, esotropia is plus (+), and exotropia is minus (−)

EF  is the magnitude of eccentric fixation in prism diopters, nasal EF is plus (+), and temporal EF is minus (−)

In cases of nystagmus, neutralization of the eye movement during the alternate cover test may be extremely difficult or impossible. The Hirschberg, Krimsky, Brückner, or subjective methods described below may prove more useful to ascertain the direction and magnitude of the deviation.

In addition to the standard test conditions (6 meters and 40 cm with the refractive error fully corrected), it is often useful to perform the alternate cover test with the patient's habitual correction to determine his or her presenting binocular status. Some examiners also like to perform the alternate cover test through added lenses at near to more closely evaluate the accommodation and convergence relationship. To avoid confusion, the test distance and the correction used during the alternate cover test must be clearly indicated in the record.

If a noncomitant deviation is suspected (based on history, the version assessment, the head posture, or a difference in the primary and secondary deviations), the magnitude of the deviation should be measured using the alternate cover test in the nine diagnostic positions of gaze. The results are often recorded on a chart as shown in Figure 6–21.

When neutralizing the deviation, accurate fixation on the target by the eye as it is uncovered is essential to minimize measurement error. Giving the patient additional time to fixate and providing an auditory cue as the occluder is moved to the other eye may help improve attention and fixation. The examiner may say "ready, set, now look" as the occluder is moved to the other eye.

If no strabismus was detected during the unilateral cover test but a large movement is seen on the alternate cover test, fusion may not always be sufficient to keep the large deviation latent. After neutralizing the deviation with a prism, the occluder and the prism are removed and the patient is carefully observed to see if fusion is regained. It may also be advantageous to repeat the unilateral cover test to see if an occasional strabismus has now become manifest.

Occasionally, only a small movement is seen on the unilateral cover test, but a much larger movement is seen on the alternate cover test. These strabismic patients are able to use peripheral fusion to reduce the magnitude of the deviation when both eyes are open, but a residual deviation remains uncompensated. Some examiners measure the full deviation with the alternate cover test but also like to estimate the smaller deviation seen during the unilateral cover test. The smaller deviation is neutralized by simultaneously covering the normally fixating eye and introducing a neutralizing prism in front of the normally deviating eye. The power of the prism that produces no movement of the deviating eye when it is placed in front of the deviating eye at the same time the fixating eye is covered provides an estimate of the smaller deviation seen on the unilateral cover test. This test has been termed the simultaneous prism cover test.[50]

If a diagonal movement is observed as the eye is uncovered, both horizontal and vertical deviations are present. The horizontal deviation is neutralized first. With the prism that neutralized the horizontal deviation in place, a vertical prism is then added until the vertical movement is neutralized. The horizontal movement should be checked again after the vertical is neutralized. If the horizontal deviation is no longer neutralized, the horizontal prism is adjusted with the vertical prism in place until the horizontal movement is again neutralized, and then the vertical is rechecked. This process is repeated until both the horizontal and vertical movements are neutralized by the appropriate prism.

In cases of strabismus, particularly infantile esotropia,[51, 52] an unusual vertical eye movement may be seen during the alternate cover test. As the occluder is removed from each eye in turn, the eye moves down. This condition is most frequently termed a dissociated vertical deviation. Other terms for this condition include alternating sursumduction, double hyperphoria, intermittent hyperphoria, and occlusion hypertropia. When both eyes are open, no vertical deviation is present; the vertical deviation is easily manifested by occlusion. The vertical movement seen with dissociated vertical deviations on alternate cover testing differs from the movement of a typical vertical phoria or tropia, where one eye moves down but the other eye moves up as the occluder is alternated between the two eyes.

## Cover Test in Diagnostic Positions of Gaze

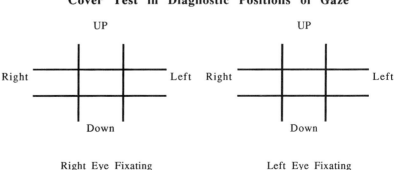

**FIGURE 6–21** Format used to record the magnitude of the deviation measured with the alternate cover test in the diagnostic fields of gaze. The perspective is from the examiner as he or she views the patient.

# Subjective Measurements of Eye Alignment

. . . . . . . . . . . . . . . . . . . . . . . . .

Subjective measures of eye alignment differ from objective measures in two ways. First, subjective methods require a verbal response from the patient. As a result, the application of these tests in the pre-school population and older, mentally challenged patients is limited by their verbal capabilities and understanding of the task. Older pre-school children may be capable of responding to some of the less complex tests. Second, subjective and objective measures may be used interchangeably to describe the phoria in nonstrabismic patients, but these tests do not always measure the same attribute in strabismus. The magnitude of the deviation measured with prism neutralization on the cover test is the objective angle of strabismus. The magnitude of the deviation measured subjectively is the subjective angle of directionalization, or subjective angle.

When the magnitudes of the subjective and objective angles are equal, the strabismic patient has normal binocular correspondence. The two foveas correspond or have the same binocular visual direction. When the subjective and objective angles differ, the patient's binocular correspondence is diagnosed as anomalous.[53] **Anomalous retinal correspondence** (ARC) is a term frequently used to describe this sensory adaptation to the strabismus.[11] When ARC is present, the patient's two foveas no longer give rise to the same binocular visual direction. The foveas in the two eyes no longer correspond; the fovea in one eye has the same binocular visual direction as a nonfoveal point in the fellow eye. ARC is considered a sensory adaptation to strabismus and is important in determining the prognosis for obtaining binocular function in strabismic patients.[54] Further discussion of this topic is beyond the scope of this book but may be found in books dedicated to the topic of strabismus or binocular vision. The issue is that in cases of phoria and strabismus with normal correspondence, the objective and subjective measures are the same. However, in cases of strabismus with ARC, the objective and subjective angles are not the same. To be certain you are describing the magnitude of deviation in strabismus, use only the objective measure until the type of correspondence is established.

## VON GRAEFE METHOD

The von Graefe method is frequently used for the assessment of horizontal and vertical phorias.

The eyes are dissociated, and diplopia is produced with a prism. The magnitude and direction of the prism necessary to align the diplopic images indicates the magnitude and direction of the phoria. The technique may also be used to determine the subjective angle of strabismus. Owing to the complexity of the task, this test is used primarily in school-age children and adults.

1. The phoria is measured at distance (6 meters) and near (40 cm).
2. The target is placed at the appropriate test distance. Dim the room illumination slightly for the distance measure, and illuminate the near target with the reading light. A single letter, a block of letters, or a row of letters is used as the target. If a row of letters is used, the letters are oriented vertically to measure the horizontal phoria and horizontally for the vertical phoria assessment. These orientations aid the patient in accurately judging the target alignment. Select a letter size at or near the patient's acuity threshold to aid in the control of accommodation. Instruct the patient to keep the letters clear throughout testing.
3. The patient is seated behind the phoropter with the distance interpupillary distance and subjective refraction in the phoropter for the distance measure and the near interpupillary distance for the near phoria. Appropriate added plus lenses are necessary for the near measurement in presbyopic patients.
4. Instruct the patient to close his or her eyes; 12 prism diopters base in is placed in the Risley prism over the right eye and 6 prism diopters base up over the left eye. The prisms may be reversed with prism diopters base up over the right and 12 prism diopters base in over the left. The Risley prism arrangements are shown in Figure 6–22.
5. Ask the patient to open his or her eyes and indicate how many targets he or she sees. Two targets should be visible simultaneously. The upper target should be to the right of the lower target when base in prism is in front of the right eye. The upper target should be to the left when base in prism is in front of the left eye. If the targets are not in the expected locations, increase the amount of base in prism until the targets are appropriately arranged.

### Horizontal Deviation

6. Instruct the patient to look at the lower target, keep the letters clear, and report

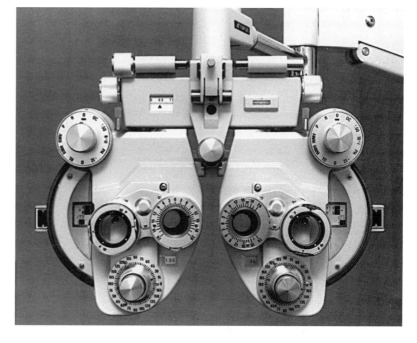

FIGURE 6-22 Phoroptor arrangement for measuring horizontal and vertical phorias or the subjective angle of strabismus using the von Graefe method. In this example the measuring prism for a horizontal deviation is in front of the right eye and the prism used to measure the vertical deviation is in front of the left eye.

when the two targets are aligned vertically.

7. Occlude the eye behind the measuring prism (horizontal) with a hand-held occluder, and decrease the prism by several prism diopters. The prism amount is changed only when the eye is occluded. Remove the occluder for 1 second and then reocclude the eye. Ask the patient to report the location of the upper target as it appears relative to the lower target. As the targets approach alignment, smaller changes (i.e., 1 prism diopter) are made while the eye is occluded. Continue this process of "flashing" the target until the targets are aligned. Note the amount and direction of the measuring prism.

8. The phoria measurement may be bracketed. After the patient reports that the targets are aligned, continue to change the prism in the same direction for several additional prism diopters. The upper target appears on the opposite side as the aligned position is passed. Now change the prism in the opposite direction, and flash the target until the patient again reports alignment of the targets. Note the amount and direction of the measuring prism each time alignment is reported. If they are not the same, record the average values.

## Vertical Deviation

9. The patient is instructed to view the upper target, keep the target clear, and re-

port when the two targets are aligned horizontally.

10. Occlude the eye behind the measuring prism (vertical) with a hand-held occluder and decrease the prism by 1 or 2 prism diopters. The prism amount is changed only when the eye is occluded. Remove the occluder for 1 second and then reocclude the eye. Ask the patient to report the location (up, down, or aligned) of the right target as it appears relative to the left target. As the targets approach alignment, smaller changes (i.e., 0.5 prism diopter) are made. Continue this process of "flashing" the target until the targets are aligned. Note the amount and direction of the measuring prism. After the patient reports that the targets are aligned, continue to change the prism in the same direction for several additional prism diopters. The upper target becomes the lower target as the alignment position is passed.

11. Now change the prism in the opposite direction until the patient again reports alignment of the two targets. Note the amount and direction of the measuring prism that aligns the targets.

Phorias may also be measured while viewing the targets simultaneously throughout testing (no flashing is used), but this method is less desirable. When targets are viewed simultaneously, fluctuations in accommodation and the effects of fusional vergence may influence the measured phoria. If flashing is omitted, the same set-up is used with the following modification to the procedure:

1. Slowly decrease the amount of the measuring prism by 2 to 3 prism diopters/second for the horizontal phoria and by 1 prism diopter/second for the vertical phoria. Note the amount and direction of the measuring prism that aligns the targets.

3. Continue to change the prism in the same direction for several additional prism diopters. The target locations will reverse.

4. Now change the prism in the opposite direction until the patient again reports alignment of the two targets. Note the amount and direction of the measuring prism that aligns the targets.

If the patient demonstrates motor alignment (absence of strabismus) on the unilateral cover test, the von Graefe results are a measure of the phoria. The direction of the phoria is determined by the direction of the measuring (neutralizing) prism. Table 6-10 shows the relationship between the phoria direction and the neutralizing prism. The magnitude of the phoria is the amount of measuring prism required to align the targets. Population norms for distance and near phorias are shown in Table 6-11. Other authors have reported norms similar to those listed in the table.[56-69] Individuals with phorias falling outside this range may be considered abnormal. However, for the diagnosis of binocular vision anomalies, phoria measures are typically considered in conjunction with fusional reserves and symptomology rather than in isolation.

In patients with strabismus, the von Graefe technique yields a measure of the subjective angle of deviation; it is *not* a measure of the phoria. The subjective angle is compared with the objective angle to determine if the patient has ARC.

Suppression may be present if only one target is seen. Procedures to elicit diplopia are outlined below. If suppression persists, the von Graefe technique cannot be used, and an alternative method to assess the phoria or the subjective angle of strabismus must be used (i.e., cover test or Maddox rod). Suppression is characteristic of a binocular vision anomaly.

The test distance, magnitude, and direction of the phoria or subjective angle are recorded. A vertical measure is recorded with reference to the "hyper" eye.

**EXAMPLES**

| | |
|---|---|
| von Graefe @ 6 m c.c. (habitual): | 2 prism diopters exophoria (or 2Δ XP), 4 prism diopters left |

hyperphoria (or 4Δ LHP)

| | |
|---|---|
| von Graefe @ 40 cm c.c. (habitual): | 3 prism diopters esophoria (or 3Δ EP'), 4 prism diopters left hyperphoria (or 4Δ LHP') |
| von Graefe @ 6 m c.c. (BVA): | subjective angle 25 prism diopters esotropia (or ⊰5 = 25Δ ET) |

Information regarding the frequency and laterality of the strabismus is not available from the von Graefe method. Record "suppression" if suppression precludes the use of the von Graefe method.

The comitancy of a phoria may not be determined using the von Graefe method. Measurement through the phoroptor limits assessment to the primary position only; the phoria in other positions of gaze cannot be assessed with this method. Suspect a noncomitant phoria when an abnormal head posture is present or when symptoms of a binocular vision anomaly are reported (see Table 6-1) and no binocular anomaly is apparent in primary position. To assess comitancy, use an alternative technique outside the phoroptor and measure the phoria in the six diagnostic positions (see Fig. 6-2) and in the up and down fields of gaze. If a particular direction of gaze is suspected based on the history, it may not be necessary to explore all the diagnostic positions.

If the patient sees only one target, attempt the following to elicit diplopia.

1. Check the phoroptor, as one eye may be occluded.

2. Alternately occlude the eyes so that each eye's target is shown. This often aids the patient in locating both targets or in eliminating suppression.

3. Increase the amount of vertical prism in front of the left eye; 6 prism diopters may not be adequate to dissociate the patient.

The distance and near vertical phorias should be equal because the vertical deviation is not influenced by changes in accommodation and the von Graefe phorias are measured in primary position. Thus, any difference in distance and near vertical phorias should be attributed to measurement error. Potential sources of error and solutions are outlined below:

1. The error may be induced by the vertical prismatic effect that occurs when the patient views off the optical centers of lenses that differ by 1.00 D or more in the vertical

meridians of the two eyes. This effect is governed by Prentice's rule and increases with increasing dioptric difference between the two eyes. This off-axis viewing may be caused by a tilted phoroptor and/or a head tilt. To ensure that the patient is viewing through the optical centers, select the pinhole for both eyes. If the patient can see the right and left eye targets simultaneously, he or she is viewing through the optical centers. The pinholes are then removed to measure the phoria.

2. A head tilt may also mask a vertical phoria during the von Graefe measure. Even when the head is straightened, the head tilt may reappear during testing. Carefully watch the patient's head posture during testing to ensure that the head remains straight. You may wish to assess the vertical phoria with an alternative technique in free space where head posture is more easily monitored.

3. The accuracy of the patient's response is critical. Because small amounts of vertical phoria (0.5 or 1 prism diopter) may produce symptoms, small inaccuracies in the patient's responses may influence the diagnosis and management of vertical phorias. Small inaccuracies in horizontal phoria assessment have less impact on diagnosis and management. Objective tests may be used when the patient's response is suspect.

## MADDOX ROD

The Maddox rod test is an alternative procedure to assess horizontal and vertical phorias or the subjective angle of strabismus and may be used in older pre-school children as well as school-age children and adults. The Maddox rod is a clear or red lens composed of a series of parallel plano-convex cylinders. The rod is available in the phoroptor, as a trial lens, and hand-held on an occluder. A light source (i.e., a penlight, a transilluminator, or a muscle light) is viewed binocularly, with the eye behind the rod perceiving the light as a narrow streak of light while the fellow eye sees the light unaltered. The streak seen by the patient is oriented perpendicular to the Maddox rod grooves. These dissimilar images (streak and spot of light) are dissociative and cannot be fused. The resultant separation of the two images is a measure of the patient's phoria or subjective angle of strabismus.

The Maddox rod is unique relative to the other subjective measures of eye alignment. It is the only method discussed in this chapter capable of quantifying a cyclodeviation. This double Maddox rod procedure is described later.

1. The phoria is measured at distance (6 meters) and near (40 cm).
2. The room illumination is dimmed. A light is used as the fixation target—a white muscle light for the distance measure and a penlight or a transilluminator for near fixation.
3. The phoria may be assessed using the phoroptor or in free space. If the phoroptor is used, the patient is seated behind the phoroptor with the distance interpupillary distance and subjective refraction in the phoroptor for the distance measure and the near interpupillary distance for the near phoria. Appropriate added plus lenses are necessary for the near measurement in presbyopic patients. If the measurement is made in free space, the patient wears the appropriate lens powers at the appropriate interpupillary distance in a trial frame, or the habitual spectacle or contact lenses may be worn if the prescription is similar to the subjective refraction.

## Horizontal Deviation

4. The Maddox rod (either red or white) is placed in front of one eye with the axis at 180° (grooves horizontal). If measurements are made through the phoroptor, 12 prism diopters base in is placed in the measuring (Risley) prism over the fellow eye. The phoroptor set-up is shown in Figure 6–23A. For testing in free space, either a horizontal prism bar or a loose prism is used over the eye without the Maddox rod.
5. Instruct the patient to look at the light. Ask the patient if he or she sees both a vertical streak (seen by the eye with the Maddox rod) and a spot of light (seen by the eye with the prism). The streak and the light should be separated in space and perceived simultaneously. The streak should appear on the same side as the eye with the Maddox rod. For example, for the set-up in Figure 6–23 the streak should appear to the left of the light. If the streak is not in this location, add additional base in prism.
6. The base in prism is decreased until the streak and light are superimposed. Note the magnitude and the direction of the prism that results in superimposition of the streak and light.

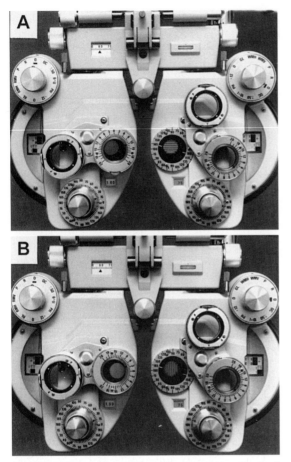

**FIGURE 6–23** *A,* Arrangement for measuring the horizontal deviation (phoria or subjective angle of strabismus) using the Maddox rod in the phoroptor. The Maddox rod is oriented horizontally and placed in front of the left eye in this example. The measuring prism is in front of the right eye. *B,* Arrangement for measuring the vertical deviation (phoria or subjective angle of strabismus) using the Maddox rod in the phoroptor. The Maddox rod is oriented vertically and placed in front of the left eye in this example. The measuring prism is in front of the right eye.

## Vertical Deviation

7.  The Maddox rod (either red or white) is placed in front of one eye with the axis at 90° (grooves vertical). If the measurements are made through the phoroptor, 6 prism diopters base up is placed in the measuring (Risley) prism over the fellow eye. The phoroptor arrangement is shown in Figure 6–23B. For testing in free space, either a vertical prism bar or a loose prism is used over the eye without the rod. Careful attention to head posture is required to avoid measurment error.

8.  Instruct the patient to look at the light. Ask

the patient if he or she sees both a horizontal streak (seen by the eye with the Maddox rod) and a spot of light (seen by the eye with the prism) and to report the location of the vertical streak relative to the light. The streak and light should be perceived simultaneously with the streak above the light. If the streak is not in this location, add additional base up prism.

9.  The base up prism is decreased until the streak and light are superimposed. Note the magnitude and the direction of the prism that results in superimposition of the streak and light.

## Torsion—Double Maddox Rod Test

The assessment of the torsion of the eye differs from the horizontal or vertical measurement. Two Maddox rods, preferably one red and one white, are used. The technique requires a phoroptor with rods that may be rotated. If such a phoroptor set-up is not available, the rods (usually a part of a complete trial lens kit) are placed in a trial frame.

1.  A rod is placed in front of each of the patient's eyes with the axes at 180°. (Axis 90° orientation may also be used.) The orientation of the axes must be precise.

2.  Instruct the patient to look at the light. He or she should see two streaks simultaneously. If the streaks are superimposed, horizontal prism is placed in front of one eye to separate the streaks. (Vertical prism is used with axis 90°.)

3.  Ask the patient if the streaks are parallel to each other. If the streaks are not parallel, the patient rotates the lens producing the tilted streak until the streaks appear parallel.

4.  The number of degrees that the Maddox rod is rotated is the magnitude of the torsion. Note the new axis location.

If the patient demonstrates motor alignment (absence of strabismus) on the unilateral cover test, the Maddox rod results are a measure of the phoria.

The direction of the phoria is determined by the direction of the measuring (neutralizing) prism. Table 6-10 shows the relationship between the phoria direction and the neutralizing prism. The direction of the phoria may also be determined by the location of the light and the streak relative to the rod location. When the targets are uncrossed (i.e., the streak is on the same side of the light as the rod), esophoria is present; when the targets are crossed (i.e., the streak is on the opposite side of the light from the rod), exophoria is present. The streak is located below the light with hyperphoria of the eye behind the rod and above the light in hyperphoria of the eye without the rod.

The magnitude of the phoria is the amount of measuring prism that superimposes the targets. Population norms for distance and near phorias are shown in Table 6-11. Other authors have reported norms similar to those listed in the table.[56-69] Individuals with phorias falling outside of this range may be considered abnormal. However, for the diagnosis of binocular vision anomalies, the phoria is considered in conjunction with fusional reserves and symptomatology (see Table 6-1) rather than in isolation.

In patients with strabismus, the Maddox rod provides a measure of the subjective angle of deviation; it is *not* a measure of the phoria. The subjective angle is compared with the objective angle to determine if the patient has ARC.

The orientation of the tilted streak indicates the direction of the cyclodeviation. With the Maddox rod at axis 180° (vertical streak), an excyclophoria is present when the top of the streak is rotated nasally relative to the eye perceiving the streak. An encyclophoria is present when the top of the streak is rotated temporally. Figure 6-24 demonstrates the effect of torsion on the perceived position of the streak. The magnitude of a cyclodeviation is equal to the number of degrees that the Maddox rod was rotated to make the streaks appear parallel.

Suppression is present when only one target is seen. Procedures to elicit diplopia are outlined below. If suppression persists, the Maddox rod technique cannot be used, and an alternative method to assess the phoria or subjective angle must be used. Suppression is characteristic of a binocular vision anomaly.

The test distance, test, refractive correction, and magnitude and direction of the phoria or subjective angle are recorded. A vertical measure is recorded with reference to the hyperphoric eye.

**EXAMPLES**

| | |
|---|---|
| Maddox rod (or MR) @ 6 m c.c. (BVA): | orthophoria (or φ) |
| Maddox rod (or MR) @ 40 cm c.c. (BVA): | 3 prism diopters exophoria (or 3Δ XP′), 2 prism diopters right hyperphoria (or 2Δ RHP) |
| Maddox rod (or MR) @ 40 cm c.c. (habitual): | subjective angle 35 prism diopters esotropia (or ⊲S = 35Δ ET′) |
| Double Maddox rod @ 6 m c.c. (BVA): | 5° R excyclotropia |

Information regarding the frequency and laterality of the strabismus cannot be obtained with the Maddox rod. Record "suppression" if suppression precludes the use of the Maddox rod.

Some controversy exists surrounding the use of the Maddox rod to measure horizontal phorias, particularly at near. It is unclear whether the test stimuli produce an excessive, reduced, or appropriate accommodative response at the near test distance. The fixation target, a light, is not considered an appropriate stimulus to accommodation.[43] Typically, a light generates significantly less accommodative response than expected for the test distance. This decrease in accommodation would underestimate an esophoria and overestimate an exophoria owing to a reduction in the associated accommodative con-

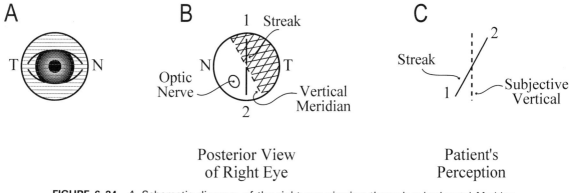

Posterior View
of Right Eye

Patient's
Perception

**FIGURE 6–24** *A*, Schematic diagram of the right eye viewing through a horizontal Maddox rod. *B*, Posterior view of the right eye (standing behind the eye and looking through the back of the eye), which is intorted. *C*, Patient's perception of the streak formed by the Maddox rod when the right eye is intorted.

vergence. However, the patient usually perceives the streak located between himself or herself and the fixation target. Morgan[70] suggests that the accommodative response exerted is excessive, as the patient focuses for the perceived distance of the streak rather than the light. This response overestimates an esophoria and underestimates an exophoria. Results comparing the phoria measured with the Maddox rod to the von Graefe method are mixed. Scobee and Green[56] reported a mean value of exophoria with the Maddox rod that was 3 prism diopters greater than the mean von Graefe value. However, other reports suggest that similar but slightly *less* exophoria is found with the Maddox rod.[68, 71] Although the Maddox rod and von Graefe results do not differ dramatically in groups of patients with presumably diverse phorias and accommodative convergence/ accommodation (AC/A) ratios, it is possible that Maddox rod results may not correlate as well in specific groups of patients, such as those with high AC/A ratios. Until it is known whether Maddox rod phorias correlate well in all patients, regardless of accommodative vergence or phoria, a horizontal phoria measured with the Maddox rod should be viewed with caution, or a detailed target should be incorporated into the near measure.

The Thorington card, by incorporating a row of small numbers or letters, contains a detailed target that is used with the Maddox rod to provide an appropriate stimulus to accommodation. Phorias measured with the modified Thorington technique are similar to those found with the von Graefe method.[66, 73] To measure the phoria, the fixation light is projected through a small hole centered in the card. The patient is instructed to keep the scale clear and to report the location of the streak on the scale. Each division on the scale typically corresponds to 1 prism diopter at 40 cm, but to be certain of the scale it should be measured. A 4-mm separation is equal to 1 prism diopter at a 40-cm viewing distance. The value read from the card is recorded as the magnitude of the phoria. The direction of the phoria is determined by the location of the streak; a streak located on the same side of the light as the rod (uncrossed diplopia) indicates esophoria, and a streak on the opposite side of the light from the rod (crossed diplopia) indicates exophoria. Figure 6–25 demonstrates the use of the Thorington card or a modification of this card.

If the patient does not see the light and the streak simultaneously, attempt the following to elicit diplopia:

1. If using the phoropter, make sure both eyes are unoccluded.

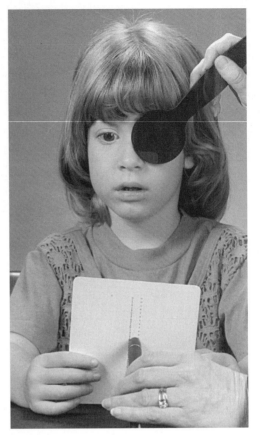

**FIGURE 6–25** The modified Thorington card. The patient is viewing a penlight through a hole in the card. A hand-held Maddox rod is over the patient's left eye. The patient reports over which letter or number the streak (created by viewing the light through the Maddox rod) appears. The letters and numbers provide an accommodative stimulus.

2. Alternately occlude the eyes so that each eye's target is shown. This often aids the patient in locating both targets or eliminating suppression.
3. Dim the room illumination or extinguish the room lights completely.
4. If the suppressed eye is habitually suppressed (i.e., deviating eye in strabismus), placing the rod on the fellow eye may eliminate the suppression.

The comitancy of a phoria or tropia with normal correspondence may be assessed when the Maddox rod is used in free space. The phoria or tropia is assessed in the six diagnostic action fields. The measurements are also made in upgaze and downgaze to diagnose an A or V pattern. The A pattern exo and V pattern eso (phoria or tropia is greatest in downgaze) often produce near point problems, particularly in bifocal wearers or other patients who turn their eyes downward to view at near. Anisometropic lens prescriptions (vertical power at least 1.00 D different between eyes) may induce significant vertical prism when the patient views away from the optical centers of the lens. The vertical prism induced in the reading position (downgaze) may interfere with comfortable and efficient binocular function. Assess the vertical phoria in downgaze whenever a significant vertical anisometropia is present and the patient turns his or her eyes downward at the near point.

## ASSOCIATED PHORIA AND FIXATION DISPARITY

The previously discussed techniques assess eye alignment when fusion is disrupted (i.e., von Graefe method and Maddox rod). The associated phoria and fixation disparity are measures of eye alignment under binocular conditions. This evaluation of eye alignment and vergence under the presumably more natural conditions of binocular viewing provides additional information regarding binocular interactions which is not obtained when fusion is disrupted.

In the absence of a fixation disparity, it is presumed that the binocularly fixated objects fall on exactly corresponding retinal points in the two eyes. A slight misalignment of the eyes, or fixation disparity, causes the images to fall on points in the two eyes that do not precisely correspond but are within Panum's fusional area.[74] Therefore, a fixation disparity does not preclude single binocular vision. Fusion may occur as long as the vergence error does not exceed Panum's fusional limit.[75] The associated phoria is the amount of prism necessary to reduce the fixation disparity to zero.[76]

The fixation disparity is quantified in minutes of arc and measured through a range of prism or lens powers producing various demands on fusional vergence. A forced fixation disparity curve is generated by plotting these findings,[74] and the curve reveals how the eye alignment changes with binocular vergence stimulation. The various attributes of this curve are used in conjunction with dissociated phoria and vergence measures to make diagnostic and management decisions regarding binocular vision.[77-80]

A number of tests are available to assess the fixation disparity and/or associated phoria. Two examples of fixation disparity tests are shown in Figure 6–26. The various fixation disparity and associated phoria tests are listed in Table 6–12. The associated phoria can be determined with any of these tests. The choice of tests for quantifying the fixation disparity is more limited. The

| Test | Associated Phoria | Fixation Disparity |
|---|---|---|
| **TABLE 6–12** Associated Phoria and Fixation Disparity Tests | | |
| **Distance** | | |
| Mentor BVAT II BVS | √ | √ |
| Woolf card* | √ | √ |
| Bernell lantern slides | √ | |
| Mallet unit | √ | |
| Reichert (AO) vectographic slide (adult and child versions) | √ | |
| Stereo optical vectographic slide (adult and child versions) | √ | |
| **Near** | | |
| Bernell fixation disparity card | √ | √ |
| Disparometer | √ | √ |
| Wesson fixation disparity card | √ | √ |
| Bernell lantern slides | √ | |
| Mallet unit | √ | |
| Stereo optical nearpoint vectographic acuity card | √ | |

*Instructions for its production may be obtained from Dr. Bruce Wick, College of Optometry, University of Houston, Houston, TX 77204–6052.

various tests are not identical, but all of the tests have two or more oppositely polarized lines (one line seen by each eye) and a fusion lock (seen by both eyes) and should provide an appropriate stimulus to accommodation (i.e., small letters).

It may be desirable to make the horizontal measures with and without the vertical prism in place when the patient has a vertical associated phoria.[81] Therefore, the vertical assessment is typically made before the horizontal measure. Careful attention to head posture is required to avoid measurement error. The test procedures for the Wesson card and the disparometer, which are near point tests, are described below. Administration of other fixation disparity and associated phoria tests may be adapted from these instructions.

1. The associated phoria and fixation disparity are measured at 6 meters and 40 cm.
2. The target is placed at the appropriate test distance. Dim the room illumination slightly for the distance measure, and illuminate the near target with the reading light.
3. The associated phoria may be assessed using the phoropter or in free space. An example of free space testing is shown in Figure 6–27. If the phoropter is used, the patient is seated behind the phoropter

**A**

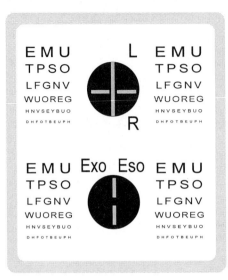

**B**

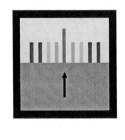

**FIGURE 6–26** *A,* A close-up view of the fixation disparity targets on the disparometer. The patient views these targets through Polaroid lenses to isolate the images to the two eyes. *B,* The Wesson card used to measure the fixation disparity or associated phoria. The patient views the card through Polaroid lenses to isolate the images to the two eyes.

with the distance interpupillary distance and subjective refraction in the phoroptor for the distance measure and the near interpupillary distance for the near associated phoria. Appropriate added plus lenses are necessary for the near measurement in presbyopic patients. For measurements in free space, the patient wears the appropriate lens powers at the appropriate interpupillary distance in a trial frame. The habitual spectacle correction or contact lenses may be worn if the prescription is similar to the subjective refraction. Polaroid analyzers are worn by the patient. They are placed over the trial frame or habitual spectacles or worn behind the phoroptor, or analyzers in the phoroptor may be used when available.

4. If measurements are made through the phoroptor, the measuring (Risley) prisms are placed over each eye. They are set at zero and placed so that horizontal or vertical prism may be added, depending upon the measure being made. (See Figure 6–22, except set both the prisms to zero.)
5. Ask the patient if he or she sees all the components of the target simultaneously. (These vary with the test used.)

**Wesson Fixation Disparity Card**

6. Place the card with the scale and arrow (seen by the right eye) oriented horizontally for vertical measures. The scale and

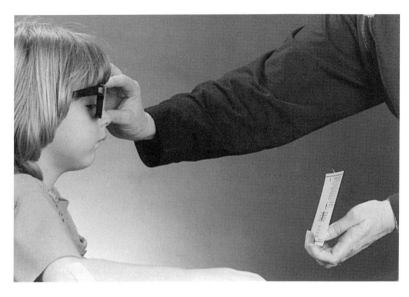

**FIGURE 6–27** The Wesson card. Polaroid glasses are worn to isolate the images to the two eyes. The fixation disparity is measured in free space and in the normal reading position.

arrow are oriented vertically for the horizontal measures; note that the arrow is now seen by the left eye.

7. Instruct the patient to keep the words clear and to report the relative location of the arrow and central red line.

### Associated Phoria

8. If the arrow does not point to the central red line, a fixation disparity is present and prism is added to determine the magnitude of the associated phoria.

   **Vertical** A left hyper associated phoria is present if the arrow is higher than the central red line and a right hyper if the arrow is lower. Add base down prism (Risley, prism bar, or loose prism) in front of the hyper eye until the patient reports that the arrow points to the central red line; this prism value is the magnitude of the associated phoria.

   **Horizontal** An eso associated phoria is present when the arrow is to the left of the central red line, and an exo associated phoria is present when the arrow is to the right of the red line. Add prism (Risley, prism bar, or loose prism)—base out for an esophoria and base in for an exophoria—over one eye until the patient reports that the arrow points at the red line; the prism value is the magnitude of the associated phoria. Note the magnitude and direction.

### Fixation Disparity

9. The magnitude is zero when the arrow points to the central red line. If the patient reports that the arrow points to any other colored line or between lines, the magnitude is read from a chart on the card. Note the magnitude. The direction is determined in the same manner as for the associated phoria.

## Disparometer

### Associated Phoria

6. Set the knob on the back of the disparometer to position the lines at the zero fixation disparity setting (lines physically aligned). To back-illuminate the target via a fiber-optic system, shine a penlight on the transparent area on the front of the disparometer.

7. Instruct the patient to keep the letters clear and report the relative location of the two horizontal lines for assessment of the vertical associated phoria. The right line should be seen by the right eye. To assess the horizontal phoria, the patient reports the relative location of the two vertical lines. The upper line should be seen by the right eye.

8. Prism is added to align the lines.

   **Vertical** A left hyper associated phoria is present if the right line is higher than the left, and a right hyper associated phoria is present if the left line is higher than the right. Add base down prism (Risley, prism bar, or loose prism) in front of the hyper eye until the patient reports alignment. This prism value is the magnitude of the associated phoria.

**Horizontal**  An eso associated phoria is present if the upper line is to right of the lower line, and an exo associated phoria is present if the upper line is to the left of the lower. Add prism (Risley, prism bar or loose prism)—base out for an esophoria and base in for an exophoria—over one eye until the patient reports alignment. This prism value is the magnitude of the associated phoria. Note the magnitude and direction. The associated phoria may also be neutralized with added lenses (plus for eso; minus for exo) in pre-presbyopic patients.

## Fixation Disparity

9. The lines are presented physically misaligned. For the horizontal measure, set the knob by positioning the knob to one of the fixed settings at 10 minutes of exo fixation disparity. If the patient reports that the top line is to the left of the bottom line, increase the misalignment until the patient reports that the top line is to the right of the bottom line. Then decrease the misalignment by changing the setting until the patient reports alignment of the vertical lines. The viewing time should be limited to a few seconds at each setting. If longer viewing time is necessary, have the patient close his or her eyes and view the targets again. Continue to change the setting in the same direction until the patient reports misalignment in the opposite direction. The midpoint of the aligned range is the magnitude of the fixation disparity.

## Forced Fixation Disparity (Wesson and Disparometer)

10. To generate a near horizontal forced fixation disparity curve, the fixation disparity measure is repeated with the patient viewing through prisms presented in the following order: 3 prism diopters base in, 3 prism diopters base out, 6 prism diopters base in, 6 prism diopters base out, and so on.[82, 83] Base in prism is introduced in 2 prism diopter steps instead of 3 prism diopter steps when generating the distance curve.

11. Occlude one eye, or have the patient close his or her eyes, between each fixation disparity measure. He or she should report the relative location of the lines within the first few seconds of viewing.

12. Testing is complete when both a base out and a base in prism power is reached that produces diplopia or suppression. Diplopia frequently occurs with lesser amounts of base in than base out prism. If the base in end point is reached before the base out end point, continue to alternate base in and base out prism, but use the maximum base in prism the patient can fuse. The fixation disparity plotted for this base in prism value is the first one that is measured. This procedure may also be used if the base out end point is reached before the base in end point.

The associated phoria and fixation disparity results are plotted to produce a forced fixation disparity curve. The associated phoria is the x-intercept; the point is plotted to the right of the y-axis if base out prism neutralized the phoria and to the left if it was neutralized with base in prism. The fixation disparity without added prism or lenses is the y-intercept of the curve; eso is plotted above the x-axis and exo below the x-axis. The midpoint and the range of alignment are plotted when the measurements are made with the disparometer. The remaining fixation disparity measures are plotted with regard to the prism or lens power through which they were measured; base in prism or minus lenses to the left of the y-axis and base out prism or plus lenses to the right of the y-axis.

The slope of the curve from 3 prism diopters base in to 3 prism diopters base out may be calculated.[77] The type of curve and the slope of the curve may be used to predict binocular anomalies. The four types of horizontal fixation disparity curves[76] are shown in Figure 6–28. Individuals with type I curves are frequently asymptomatic. However, if the slope is steep, greater than 0.77 minute/prism diopter in esophoria and 1.06 minutes/prism diopter in exophoria, it is a predictor of asthenopia.[77] A type II curve is often associated with high esophoria and a type III with high exophoria. Type II and III curves frequently do not intersect the x-axis. In these patients, the associated phoria cannot be measured. Unstable binocularity is associated with a type IV curve. Individuals with type II, III, and IV curves are frequently symptomatic.[77-80] The frequency of occurrence of the curves differs, with type I found most frequently, followed by types II, III, and IV.[69, 76]

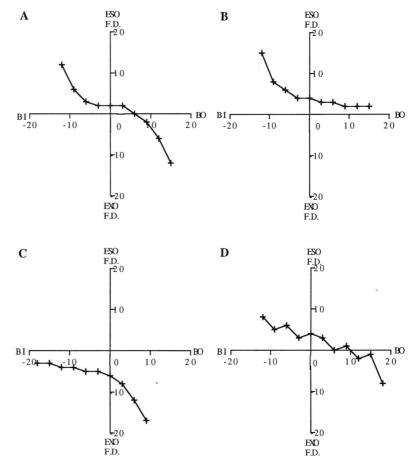

**FIGURE 6–28** The four types of fixation disparity curves. *A*, Type I. *B*, Type II. *C*, Type III. *D*, Type IV.

The flattest portion of the curve (center of symmetry) represents the conditions under which the most rapid adaptation to the vergence stimuli occurs.[84] It is desirable to allow the patient to operate at this point on the curve, as asthenopic symptoms are reduced or eliminated.[79, 80] A prism prescription that incorporates the least amount of prism necessary to shift the curve and place the flattest portion of the curve (center of symmetry) at the *y*-axis allows the patient to operate in this region of rapid adaptation. The prism power is read from the *x*-axis and is the point where the flat portion of the curve begins. The prism prescription based on the center of symmetry approximates the associated phoria in a type I curve with a steep slope; however, in type I curves with a flatter slope and in type II and III curves, the associated phoria may overestimate the minimum prism necessary for improved binocular function. Because it is desirable to prescribe the minimum amount of prism necessary to improve binocular function, prescribing prism from the associated phoria alone can result in an excessive prism prescription in some patients.[79, 80]

Vision therapy may also be considered and frequently eliminates symptoms by flattening the central portion of the steep type I curves.[76, 79, 80] Vision therapy may also be utilized for some patients with type II and III curves that do not cross the *x*-axis.[5]

The associated vertical phoria finding typically yields an appropriate prism prescription for symptomatic patients. Therefore, it is rarely necessary to generate a vertical forced fixation disparity curve. If the vertical prism determined by a vertical associated phoria measure flattens the slope of a type I curve, this vertical prism alone may alleviate the symptoms.[81]

Associated phoria and fixation disparity may be measured in patients with an occasional strabismus when fusion is present. Diagnostic and management decisions are based on the same criteria used in patients with phorias.

The test distance, test, refractive correction, magnitude, and direction of the associated phoria and fixation disparity are recorded.

Disparometer @ 40 cm c.c. (habitual): 4 prism diopters eso-phoria (or 4Δ EP′); 3 min fixation dispar-ity (3 min E′ FD)

Wesson Card @ 40 cm c.c. (BVA): 2 prism diopters eso-phoria (or 2Δ EP′), 2 prism diopters right hyperphoria (or 2Δ RHP′); 2.5 min of arc exo fixa-tion disparity (or 2.5 min X′FD)

The forced fixation disparity results, along with the associated phoria and fixation disparity, are plotted as described above and are included in the patient's chart.

Associated phoria and fixation disparities are not measured in constant strabismics or in occasional strabismics when fusion is absent.

The testing time required to generate a horizontal forced fixation disparity curve can be shortened by modifying the procedure. Testing with zero, 3 prism diopters, 6 prism diopters, and 12 prism diopters base in and base out may provide adequate information to determine the prism correction needed.[5]

Vergence (prism) adaptation influences the fixation disparity measure.[84, 85] Therefore, the viewing time is limited to a few seconds, the eyes are closed between presentations, and base in and base out prisms are alternated. Failure to alternate prism base may change the shape of the fixation disparity curve.

The forced fixation disparity at near may also be assessed using the lens method in pre-presbyopic patients. The fixation disparity is measured while the patient views through added lenses instead of prism. The lens power is increased in 0.50 D or 1.00 D steps up to +2.00 D and −3.00 D unless diplopia or suppression occurs before the end points are reached. Measurements should first be taken through plus power and then through minus power lenses.

Near point measurements may be made to determine if the vertical or horizontal associated phoria is noncomitant (varies with position of gaze) and increases in downgaze. This is particularly useful in bifocal wearers or other patients who turn their eyes downward to view at near.

Anisometropic lens prescriptions (vertical power at least 1.00 D difference between eyes) may induce significant vertical prism when the patient views away from the optical centers of the lens. The vertical prism induced in the reading position (downgaze) may interfere with comfortable and efficient binocular function. Vertical

associated phoria measurements should be made in downgaze whenever a significant vertical anisometropia is present, and the patient turns his or her eyes downward at the near point.

# Vergence Amplitude

· · · · · · · · · · · · · · · · · · · · · · · · ·

There are four types of vergence movements: convergence, divergence, vertical vergence, and cyclovergence. Compared with versions, vergence movements are slow, on the order of 8 to 25°/second, and are almost entirely reflexive. However, most individuals can learn to voluntarily converge. Voluntary divergence does not occur and can only be accomplished indirectly through relaxation of convergence. Clinically, convergence, divergence, and vertical vergences are typically assessed, with the greatest emphasis placed on the horizontal vergences.

## OBJECTIVE MEASUREMENTS OF VERGENCE AMPLITUDE

### Near Point of Convergence (NPC)

Objects approaching the eyes serve as a fusional stimulus to convergence. Convergence is almost always initiated reflexively but is also influenced by the patient's cooperation, the effort he or she makes to converge (voluntary convergence), the level of accommodation exerted (accommodative vergence), the acuity in each eye, and the test target. Some of these variables are difficult to control or measure in the clinical setting, making a precise and repeatable measure of the NPC difficult. These variables may also be partially responsible for the wide range of values accepted as normal. Despite these obstacles, a reduced or receded NPC has been consistently associated with convergence insufficiency[86] and is useful in the diagnosis of this condition.

1. The patient should be seated facing the examiner with his or her habitual near correction in place. Normal room illumination is used.
2. No single target has been recommended to measure the near point of convergence. The selection of the target depends in part on whether the examiner wishes to measure the near point of accommodation or the push-up amplitude of accommodation (see Chapter 5) at the same time. If a measure of accommodation is desired, the target must contain detail to stimulate the ac-

commodative system (e.g., reduced Snellen chart, Lang fixation cube; see Fig. 6–8), and the instructions to the patient must emphasize keeping the target clear and reporting when the target blurs. If, however, the maximum amount of convergence, irrespective of the accommodative state, is desired, the target may be devoid of detail (i.e., a penlight, a transilluminator, or a pencil eraser). Other considerations in target selection include the patient's age because the measurement of the NPC is influenced by the patient's interest and cooperation. In this chapter the emphasis is on convergence without accommodative control.

3. The target is placed on the patient's visual midline, 30 to 40 cm from the patient. The target is then moved slowly toward the patient on midline, and the patient is asked to report when the target doubles (Fig. 6–29). The examiner also observes the patient's eyes and notes when the patient can no longer maintain fusion through convergence. At this point, one or both eyes swing out, and if the patient does not suppress, he or she should report that the target doubles. If a penlight or transilluminator is used and one eye swings out, the corneal light reflexes no longer appear symmetrical; the reflex in the eye that fails to converge is displaced nasally.

4. The NPC is the distance from the centers of rotation to the point where fusion is lost. The average distance from the center of rotation to the corneal plane is 1.35 cm.

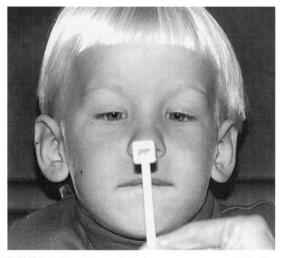

**FIGURE 6–29** Near point of convergence, or NPC. The NPC is being measured with the Lang fixation cube.[17, 18] The limit of convergence has not yet been reached, as convergence is present and the corneal reflexes in the two eyes are symmetrical.

Clinically, the NPC should be measured by placing a ruler on the temporal bony margin of the orbit near the outer canthus, which approximates the plane containing the centers of rotation.

5. The point at which fusion recovers is then measured by moving the target away from the patient and noting when both eyes are again converged on the target. If the patient reported the target doubled when fusion was lost, he or she should be asked to report when the target becomes single again. The distance in centimeters from the temporal bony orbital rim to the point of recovery is recorded.

6. As described above, the NPC can be measured objectively by observing the patient's loss of fusion and subsequent recovery or subjectively by asking the patient to report when the target doubles and then when it becomes single again. If the patient is old enough, both procedures should be used simultaneously.

Normal values for the NPC vary in the literature. Duane[20, 86] suggests that the NPC should be 5.5 cm or less except in presbyopia, in which 8 or 9 cm is considered normal. Krimsky's expected values are similar and also change as a function of age, with 5.4 cm expected at age 20, 7 cm at age 30, and 8 cm over the age of 40.[35] Hoffman and Rouse[60] suggest that the break should be less than or equal to 5 cm, with a recovery at no more than 8 cm. The patient should report diplopia at the point that fusion is lost.

If fusion is lost at a greater distance from the patient than is considered normal, the patient is said to have a receded NPC. A receded NPC is most often suggestive of convergence insufficiency.[86] If no diplopia is reported when fusion is lost, the patient is suppressing the image from the deviating eye. While the expected result is diplopia, suppression may not be significant unless the NPC is receded. In these cases, the clinician must be especially concerned with monitoring suppression if a treatment plan is pursued.

The point at which fusion is lost and the point at which fusion recovers are typically recorded. This point is measured in centimeters from the temporal bony rim of the orbit. Other notations include the eye which loses fixation and whether diplopia was reported. It is also helpful to record if tested with correction (c.c.) or without correction (s.c.). Additional notation should include a description of the target. A common abbreviation used if the patient maintained convergence to his or her nose is TTN (to the nose).

**EXAMPLES**

| NPC c.c. light: (habitual) | 8 cm, OS out, diplopia/12 cm |
| NPC s.c. letters: (habitual) | 12 cm, OD out, suppression/18 cm |
| NPC c.c. light: (habitual) | TTN |

When fusion is lost and only one eye swings out, the eye that fails to converge is the nondominant eye and the eye that remains fixed on the target is the dominant eye.[6]

If there are problems or concerns about binocular performance at the near point, the NPC should be done in the primary position as described above and in upgaze and downgaze. Grigorieva[87] has shown that the NPC in normal patients is greater in downgaze than in upgaze. Because most near work is done in downgaze, assessment under conditions in which the problem occurs appears to be a prudent approach.

**EXAMPLES**

| Up | 8 cm OS out, suppression/10 cm |
| NPC Primary | 5 cm OS out, diplopia/7 cm |
| Down | 4 cm OS out, diplopia/8 cm |

The examiner also observes the patient for signs of strain or stress during the NPC assessment. Signs of stress or strain include wrinkling of the brow or forehead, tearing, excessive blinking, or backing away from the target as the target approaches the patient. These behaviors should be noted in the record and serve to alert the examiner to potential near point problems requiring further investigation.

Davies[88] suggested a modification to evaluate fatigue. He proposed moving the target from 20 to 16 inches rapidly and repeatedly just before testing the NPC. Mohindra and Molinari[89] suggested repeating the NPC four to five times to induce fatigue. In cases of convergence insufficiency, a sluggish or reduced NPC that is not apparent during the initial assessment will often be uncovered with repeated testing. Therefore, repeated measures of NPC may be useful in young patients who are unable to articulate the symptoms often associated with convergence insufficiency or in patients who may avoid near work and thus report no symptoms.

In cases of exotropia, it is often useful to determine if the patient can exert voluntary convergence. Although not strictly a measure of the near point of convergence, the information often helps direct the treatment strategy.[4] To demonstrate voluntary convergence, the patient closes his or her eyes and is asked to imagine something very close. The target is then positioned on the midline about 5 to 8 cm from the patient. It is sometimes helpful to have the patient hold the test target to enlist proximal convergence. The patient is then asked to open his or her eyes, and the examiner, positioned directly in front of the patient, observes the patient's eyes for any signs of convergence immediately upon eye opening.

## Loose Prism Vergence

Assessment of fusional vergence with loose prisms provides an objective evaluation of the patient's ability to maintain motor and sensory fusion, as the vergence demand changes abruptly through the introduction of prisms. This objective technique is often used with children or patients with symptoms of binocular dysfunction (see Table 6–1). It differs from the subjective techniques described below in that the vergence demand is changed in discrete increments or steps and the examiner observes the patient's eyes to determine if fusion is present. Vergence facility qualitatively evaluates the response latency, velocity, and accuracy of the vergence response and quantitatively evaluates the magnitude and fatigue of the vergence response.

1. The patient is comfortably seated facing the examiner. Full room illumination with auxiliary light from the overhead lamp illuminating the patient's eyes aids in the observation of the patient's eye movements. The examiner is positioned as close to the patient's eye level as possible without blocking the patient's view of the fixation target.
2. This test is performed with the refractive error fully corrected. If the refractive error correction is significantly different from the habitual prescription, the full refractive correction is placed in a trial frame.
3. The assessment is done at the two standard viewing distances, 6 meters (distance) and 40 cm (near).
4. The distance fixation target is a single letter or a vertical row of letters near the patient's acuity threshold. For young children, a picture or symbol near the acuity threshold holds their interest and attention throughout the test. The near fixation target should also be close to the acuity threshold, with sufficient detail to ensure accurate accommodation. For adults, a reduced Snellen chart on a fixation stick or a single letter is suggested. For children, a small picture, number, or finger puppet like that used

for cover testing is recommended (see Fig. 6-8). The patient is instructed to keep the target clear.

5. Two different procedures have been proposed. In the first procedure, reported by Hoffman and Rouse,[60] prism flippers similar to those used to test accommodative facility (see Chapter 5) are employed. Base in prism is placed in one side of the flipper and base out prism in the other. The patient views a row of 20/30 letters and tries to maintain fusion as base in prism is introduced. Once fusion is observed, the flippers are switched so that the patient is now trying to fuse base out prism. Fusing the base in and then the base out prism constitutes a cycle. Christenson and Winkelstein[90] have reported that normal young adults can fuse only about five cycles of 4 prism diopters base in to 8 prism diopters base out at distance. However, Buzzelli[91] has confirmed that children 5 to 13 years of age can fuse 8 to 10 cycles per minute at the near point if slightly different prism values (4 prism diopters base in to 16 prism diopters base out) are used. The fusion response can be determined objectively during the prism flipper test by observing the patient's eyes; however, all the reports cited above relied on the patient's subjective report of fusion.

Duane[20, 86] was one of the first to mention the second procedure, which has received new interest by contemporary clinicians in the assessment of children.[92] In this procedure, loose prisms are used in place of prism flippers. The examiner introduces the prism and observes the eyes for a fusion response. Once fusion is obtained, the prism is removed and the eyes are again observed for the fusion response (Fig. 6-30). Fusion to the introduction and removal of the prism is considered one cycle. The process is repeated for 30 seconds or until three cycles are completed. When testing at 6 meters, completing three cycles in 30 seconds with a 6 prism diopter base in prism and 12 prism diopter base out prism is considered normal. For near point testing, three cycles in 30 seconds with a 12 prism diopter base in prism and a 14 prism diopter base out prism is considered normal. If the patient is unable to successfully fuse these prism values, the magnitude of the prism is decreased until three cycles can be fused in 30 seconds. If the patient can easily fuse these values with time to spare, the prism power is increased until the patient fails to fuse three cycles in 30 seconds. Both objective and subjective responses are used to assess the patient's fusional vergence ability.

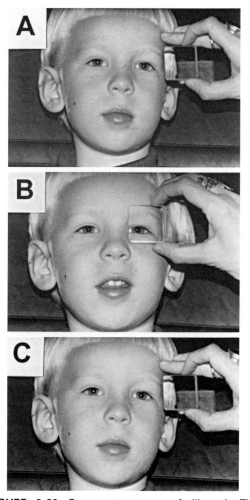

**FIGURE 6-30** Base out vergence facility. *A,* The patient's head is straight, his eyes are in the primary position, and he is fixating an appropriate target. *B,* A base out prism is introduced in front of the left eye and fusion is apparent. *C,* The prism is removed and fusion is again noted. This sequence constitutes a cycle. The patient is timed to determine the number of cycles that can be fused in 30 seconds or 1 minute.

In patients less than 3 years of age, the examiner must rely on the objective observation of the patient's eye movements to determine if fusion has been obtained. When base out prism is introduced, a convergence movement should be observed. If fusion is not obtained, the patient may alternate fixation between the diplopic images. Divergence is often harder to observe, but steady fixation without alternation is suggestive of fusion.

The examiner may also use the corneal light reflex (Hirschberg) to determine if fusion is present.[33] The reflexes appear symmetrical in the presence of fusion. However, the light should not be used as the target but in conjunction with an accommodative target. The examiner must sight directly over the light to avoid misinterpretation.

The unilateral cover test can also be used to determine if fusion has been obtained. With the prism in question in front of the patient, the examiner occludes one eye at a time, watching for a movement of the unoccluded eye. Any movement of the unoccluded eye suggests that fusion was not present. Care must be taken to make the occlusion as brief as possible to avoid disrupting the fragile fusion that may be present and interfering with the timed aspects of the testing procedure.

The report of a single image can be used in older patients, but the examiner must still observe the patient's eyes to be certain that fusion, not suppression, is responsible for the single image.

EXAMPLES

VF @ 6 m c.c. (BVA)
  4 BI/8 BO 5 cy/min
VF @ 40 cm c.c. (BVA)
  4 BI/16 BO 8 cy/min

VF @ 6 m c.c. (habitual)
  12 BO; 3 cy/30 sec
  6 BI; 3 cy/30 sec
VF @ 40 cm c.c. (habitual)
  14 BO; 3 cy/30 sec
  12 BI; 3 cy/30 sec

Although loose prism vergence testing is easy to perform, no universally accepted standard has been established. As seen in Table 6-13, the amount of prism and the number of times the prism should be fused vary considerably in the literature. Support for these values is limited, with few investigations offered to support their selection.

Steadying the patient's head, holding the prism and the near fixation target, and maintaining a hand free to verify fusion with the unilateral cover test usually require the assistance of a second person. In a young child, the parent can be enlisted to hold the near point target and/or to stabilize the child's head. The older patient can be asked to hold the near fixation target. In patients under 18 months of age, it may not be possible to evaluate motor fusion at distance owing to their limited attention.

While the information is limited for horizontal jump vergences, no proposed standards are available for vertical jump vergences.

Loose prism vergence can also be done through added lens ($+/-1.00$ D) at near to investigate the effect of accommodation on the vergence ranges.

## Prism Bar Vergence

Another assessment of fusional vergence can be made with a prism bar. Like the loose prism fusional vergence described above, the technique is often used with infants and young children or in patients with symptoms of binocular dysfunction. Although the fusional demand is changed in discrete increments as in the loose prism vergence assessment, prism bar vergence is similar to the subjective techniques described below in that the vergence demand is changed in smaller increments, and loss of fusion and recovery of fusion are both ascertained. In addition, prism bar vergence testing is not timed and not repeated, so flexibility and fatigue are not typically assessed.

The first four points of the prism bar vergence procedure are the same as those described above for the loose prism vergence.

1. The patient is comfortably seated facing the examiner. Full room illumination with auxiliary light from the overhead lamp illuminating the patient's eyes aids in the observation of the patient's eye movements. The examiner is positioned as close to the patient's eye level as possible without blocking the patient's view of the fixation target.
2. This test is performed with the refractive error fully corrected. If the refractive error correction is significantly different from the habitual prescription, the full refractive correction is placed in a trial frame.
3. The assessment is done at the two standard viewing distances, 6 meters (distance) and 40 cm (near).
4. The distance fixation target is a single letter or a row of vertical letters near the patient's acuity threshold. For young children a picture or symbol near the acuity threshold may hold their interest and attention throughout the test. The near fixation target should also be close to the acuity threshold with sufficient detail to ensure accurate accommodation. For adults, a reduced Snellen chart on a fixation stick or a single letter is suggested. For children, a small picture, number, or finger puppet like that used for cover testing is recommended (see Fig. 6-8).
5. The patient is directed to look at the fixation target as the examiner introduces the smallest prism power (base out or base in) in front of one of the patient's eyes (Fig. 6-31). The prism power is then slowly increased as the examiner observes the

| TABLE 6–13 Vergence Facility | | |
|---|---|---|
| | **Test Distance** | |
| **Reference** | **Distance (6 m)** | **Near (40 cm)** |
| Duane (1914)[86] | Repeated trials of 12 or 15 prism deg BO<br>Repeated trials of 3 to 8 prism deg BI | Repeated trials of 12 or 15 prism deg BO<br>Usually done at distance but may be done at near |
| Rosner (1979)[147] | | n = 34; 3 to 6.5 yrs<br>average = 4.75 yrs<br>8.1$\Delta$ BI<br>11.4$\Delta$ BO<br>RDE at 40 cm not timed |
| Hoffman and Rouse (1980)[60] | 4$\Delta$ BI/8$\Delta$ BO<br>8–10 cy/min<br>20/30 letters | 8$\Delta$ BI/12$\Delta$ BO<br>8–10 cy/min<br>20/30 letters |
| Griffin (1982)[11] | 5$\Delta$ BI/15$\Delta$ BO<br>20 cy/min | 5$\Delta$ BI/15$\Delta$ BO<br>20 cy/min |
| Rosner (1982)[92]<br>Rosner and Rosner (1990)[148] | 6$\Delta$ BI/pl<br>3 cy/30 sec<br>12$\Delta$ BO/pl<br>3 cy/30 sec | 12$\Delta$ BI/pl<br>3 cy/30 sec<br>14$\Delta$ BO/pl<br>3 cy/30 sec<br>20/30 vertical row of letters |
| Grisham (1983)[149] | | 6$\Delta$ BI/pl<br>6$\Delta$ BO/pl<br>Qualitative, not quantitative; judge if response is slow, moderate, or fast |
| Buzzelli (1986)[91] | | n = 310;<br>5 to 13 yrs<br>16$\Delta$ BO/4$\Delta$ BI<br>5 to 8 yrs<br>8.2 cy/min<br>9 to 13 yrs<br>11.6 cy/min<br>Anaglyph figures; subjective patient response |
| Christenson and Winkelstein (1988)[90] | 4$\Delta$ BI/8$\Delta$ BO<br>5.59 cy/min<br>(SD = 4.16)<br>n = 54<br>non-athletes average age =<br>19.7 (male)<br>18.7 (female) | |
| Scheiman and Wick (1994)[5] | | 4$\Delta$ BI/16$\Delta$ BO<br>5–7 yrs<br>2.5 cy/min<br>8–10 yrs<br>5.5 cy/min<br>11–13 yrs<br>6 cy/min<br>8$\Delta$ BI/8$\Delta$ BO<br>7 cy/min |

BI = base in; BO = base out; cm = centimeters; cy = cycles; deg = degrees; m = meters; min = minute; n = number in sample; pl = plano; RDE = Random Dot E stereo test; yrs = years; $\Delta$ = prism diopters.

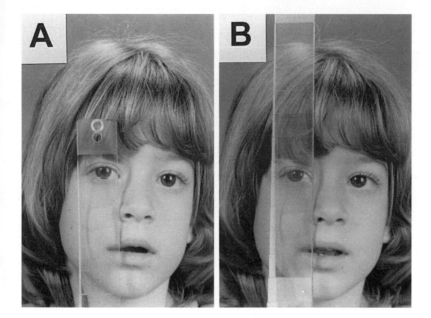

**FIGURE 6-31** Base-out fusional vergence with a prism bar. *A,* The test begins with the introduction of the smallest amount of prism. *B,* The prism is increased and the point at which fusion is lost is noted. The prism is then decreased until fusion is regained.

patient's eyes for a loss of fusion. The prism power where fusion is first lost is noted and recorded as the break.

6. Once fusion is lost, the prism power is reduced until the examiner observes that the patient has regained fusion. The prism where fusion is first regained is noted and recorded as the recovery.

When convergence is lost as the base out prism is increased, the patient's eyes fail to converge further and often assume a more divergent position. The break point may also be seen as an alternation in fixation when the patient switches fixation between the diplopic images. The loss of divergence is often harder to observe. It may be seen as no further increase in divergence as the base in prism is increased or an alternation of fixation between the diplopic images.

If the examiner is not certain whether fusion has been lost, a unilateral cover test can be performed. With the prism in question in front of the patient, the examiner occludes one eye at a time, watching for a movement of the unoccluded eye. Any movement of the unoccluded eye suggests that fusion has been lost. Care must be taken to make the occlusion as brief as possible to avoid disrupting the fragile fusion that may be present.

Recovery of fusion during base out testing is usually seen as a convergence movement. Recovery during divergence may be seen as a small divergence movement or loss of alternation of fixation. The unilateral cover test can again be used to verify that fusion is present. No movement of either eye, as the fellow eye is occluded, is observed if fusion is present.

The results expected for normal individuals vary but are similar to those found subjectively with the von Graefe technique. Table 6-14 summarizes some of the values reported in the literature.

**EXAMPLES**
Prism bar @ 6 m c.c. (BVA)
  BO 10/8
  BI 6/4
Prism bar @ 40 cm c.c. (BVA)
  BO 16/12
  BI 10/8

Although useful in young patients because no subjective response is required, the prism bar can be more threatening to the apprehensive pre-schooler than the single loose prisms.

Steadying the patient's head, holding the prism bar, and the near fixation target and maintaining a hand free to verify the break and recovery with the unilateral cover test usually require the assistance of a second person. In a young child, the parent can be enlisted to hold the near point target and/or to stabilize the child's head. The older patient can be asked to hold the near fixation target. In patients under 18 months of age, it may not be possible to evaluate motor fusion at distance owing to their limited attention.

Although both horizontal and vertical prism bars are available, prism bar vergences are usually limited to the break and recovery of convergence and divergence at 6 meters and 40 cm.

School-age patients may be asked to report

| TABLE 6–14 Prism Bar Vergence | | |
|---|---|---|
| | Wesson (1982)[150] | Scheiman et al. (1989)[151] |
| Age | 4 to 70 yrs<br>n = 79 | 6 to 12 yrs<br>n = 386 |
| BO @ 6 m | | |
| break | 11Δ<br>(SD = 7Δ) | |
| recovery | 7Δ<br>(SD = 6Δ) | |
| BI @ 6 m | | |
| break | 7Δ<br>(SD = 3Δ) | |
| recovery | 4Δ<br>(SD = 2Δ) | |
| BO @ 40 cm | | Vertical line 20/30 suppression check; child's subjective report |
| break | 19Δ<br>(SD = 9Δ) | 6 yrs (n = 45)<br>19Δ<br>(SD = 7Δ)<br>7 to 12 yrs<br>23Δ<br>(SD = 8Δ) |
| recovery | 14Δ<br>(SD = 7Δ) | 6 yrs (n = 45)<br>10Δ<br>(SD = 5Δ)<br>7 to 12 yrs<br>16Δ<br>(SD = 6Δ) |
| BI @ 40 cm | | |
| break | 13Δ<br>(SD = 6Δ) | 6 yrs (n = 45)<br>12Δ<br>(SD = 5Δ)<br>7 to 12 yrs<br>12Δ<br>(SD = 5Δ) |
| recovery | 10Δ<br>(SD = 5Δ) | 6 yrs (n = 45)<br>6Δ<br>(SD = 4Δ)<br>7 to 12 yrs<br>7Δ<br>(SD = 4Δ) |

BI = base in; BO = base out; cm = centimeters; m = meters; n = number in sample; SD = standard deviation; yrs = years; Δ = prism diopters.

when the image doubles and then when it returns to one. If there is no suppression, the patient should report diplopia when the examiner notes that fusion has been lost. The object should return to single when fusion is regained. However, the younger the child, the less reliable these subjective reports may be, and the examiner should carefully observe the eye movements for the objective signs of loss of fusion and recovery of fusion.

Prism bar vergence can also be done through added lens (+/−1.00 D) at near to investigate the effect of accommodation on the vergence ranges. The test can be performed quickly and thus may be used to assess the vergence ability of infants at the near point. Prism bar vergence testing can also be used with strabismic patients to determine the range of fusion around the objective angle of deviation. In this case, testing is begun with the prism needed to neutralize the angle of deviation. Base out and base in prisms are then introduced from this point. For example, a patient with a 25 prism diopter constant unilateral right esotropia would be tested with 25 prism diopter base out in front of the right eye. The base out prism bar is then increased to ascertain the base out vergence and decreased from 25 prism diopters to measure the base in range.

## SUBJECTIVE MEASUREMENTS OF VERGENCE AMPLITUDE

### Risley Prism Vergences ("Ductions")

Risley prism vergences provide a measure of the ability to use fusional vergence to maintain motor and sensory fusion. Negative relative vergence is assessed with base in prism, positive relative vergence with base out prism, and supravergence and infravergence with vertical prism. The amplitude is measured through a smooth gradual increase in prism power rather than discrete increases, as with jump vergences. As the prism is increased, the eyes move toward the apex of the prism, maintaining fusion until a blur of the target or two targets are reported by the patient. The blur, or the break in the absence of a blur finding, is a measure of the limit of the patient's fusional vergence and is designated positive (base out prism) or negative (base in prism) relative convergence. The blur finding indicates that the limit of fusional vergence has been reached, and accommodation is no longer held at the target. This change in the accommodative response may occur through a change in either vergence accommodation or accommodative vergence. If vergence accommodation is responsible for the blur, the convergence (base out) or divergence (base in) that is used to maintain fusion produces either additional accommodation (base out) or relaxation of accommodation (base in). If accommodative vergence produces the blur, the accommodative response is either increased (base out) or decreased (base in) to provide the additional convergence or divergence necessary to maintain single binocular vision. The break, obtained with or without blur, is the limit of the patient's vergence amplitude.

1. Horizontal vergences are measured at distance (6 meters) and near (40 cm). Verti-

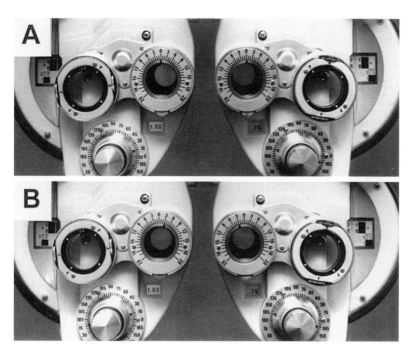

**FIGURE 6–32**  Base in, negative fusional vergence, or divergence. *A,* The initial phoroptor arrangement set-up to measure negative fusional vergence. Both prisms are set to introduce lateral prism but are set to zero. *B,* Base in prism is slowly and simultaneously increased in front of the right and left eyes. The magnitude of each prism resulting in a loss of fusion is noted and the prisms are then reduced until fusion is regained.

cal vergences are not always routinely assessed.

2. The target is placed at the appropriate test distance. Dim the room illumination slightly for the distance measure, and illuminate the near target with the reading light. A single letter, a block of letters, or a row of letters is used as the target. A vertical row of letters is appropriate for the horizontal vergence and a horizontal row for the vertical vergence. Select a letter size at or near the patient's acuity threshold to aid in the control of accommodation. Instruct the patient to keep the letters clear throughout testing.

3. The patient is seated behind the phoroptor with the distance interpupillary distance and subjective refraction in the phoroptor for the distance measure and the near interpupillary distance for the near assessment. Appropriate added plus lenses are necessary for the near measurement in presbyopic patients.

### *Horizontal*

4. Instruct the patient to close his or her eyes. Place the Risley prisms in front of both eyes set at zero, so that horizontal prism may be added (Fig. 6–32*A*).

5. Ask the patient to open his or her eyes. He or she should see one clear target. The patient is instructed to report if the target

blurs, when he or she sees two targets, or if the target moves to the left or right.

6. Base in prism is slowly (1 to 3 prism diopters/second) and equally introduced in front of each eye (Fig. 6–32*B*). Note the prism power over each eye if the patient reports that the target blurs. The total power (right plus left eye prism) is the "blur" finding. Continue to increase the prism power until the patient reports two targets. Note the prism power over each eye. The total power is the "break" finding.

7. Add several additional prism diopters of base in prism in front of each eye. Instruct the patient to report when he or she sees one target again. Now decrease the prism power until one target is reported. Note the prism power over each eye. The total power is the "recovery."

8. Have the patient close his or her eyes. Return the prism power to zero.

9. Ask the patient to open his or her eyes. Base out vergences are measured by adding base out prism following the base in vergence procedure (Fig. 6–33*A* and *C*).

### *Vertical*

### **Right Supra**

4. Instruct the patient to close his or her eyes. Place the Risley prisms in front of both eyes set at zero so that vertical prism may be added (Fig. 6–34*A*).

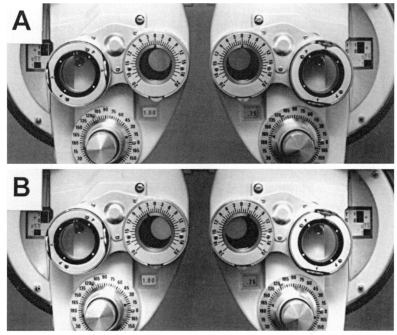

**FIGURE 6–33** Base out, positive fusional vergence, or convergence. *A*, The initial phoroptor arrangement to measure positive fusional vergence. Both prisms are set to introduce lateral prism but are set to zero. Note that the initial arrangement for base in and base out vergence is the same. *B*, Base out prism is slowly and simultaneously increased in front of the right and left eyes. The magnitude of each prism resulting in a loss of fusion is noted, and the prisms are then reduced until fusion is regained.

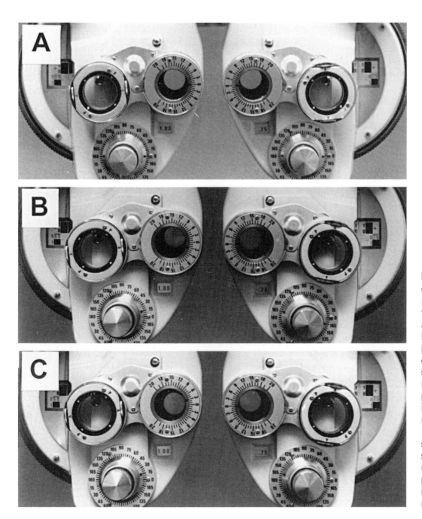

**FIGURE 6–34** Vertical vergences. *A*, The initial phoroptor arrangement to measure vertical fusional vergence. Both prisms are set to introduce vertical prism but are set to zero. *B*, Right supravergence (right sursumvergence). A base down prism is slowly increased in front of the right eye. The magnitude of the prism resulting in a loss of fusion is noted and the prism is then reduced until fusion is regained. *C*, Right infravergence/right deorsumvergence. A base up prism is slowly increased in front of the right eye. The magnitude of the prism resulting in a loss of fusion is noted, and the prism is then reduced until fusion is regained.

5. Ask the patient to open his or her eyes. He or she should see one clear target. The patient is instructed to report when he or she sees two targets and when the targets are single again.
6. Slowly introduce base down prism at 0.5 to 1 prism diopter/second in front of the right eye (Fig. 6-34B). Note the prism power over the right eye when the patient reports two targets. This power is the "break."
7. Add several additional prism diopters of base down in front of the right eye. Instruct the patient to report when he or she sees one target again. Decrease the prism power until one target is reported. Note the prism power over the right eye. This power is the "recovery."
8. Have the patient close his or her eyes. Return the prism power to zero.

**Right Infra**

9. Introduce base up prism over the right eye, measure the break and recovery (Fig. 6-34A and C).

**Left Supra**

10. Introduce base down prism over the left eye, and measure the break and recovery (Fig. 6-35A and B).

**Left Infra**

11. Introduce base up prism over the left eye, and measure the break and recovery (Fig. 6-35A and C).

Norms for base out and base in vergences at distance and near are given in Table 6–11. Other authors have reported norms similar to those listed in the table.[57, 58, 60-62, 65, 69, 93, 94] Vergences are rarely evaluated in isolation; they are considered in conjunction with the phoria and patient symptomatology (see Table 6–1) in the diagnosis and management of binocular vision.

Sheard[95] proposed that the compensating vergence blur finding should be twice the magnitude of the phoria to ensure comfortable binocular vision. (Base in is the compensating vergence for esophoria and base out for exophoria.) Therefore, a patient with a 6 prism diopter esophoria should have a base in blur finding of at least 12 prism diopters. If the base in blur is less than 12 prism diopters, Sheard's criterion suggests that a base out prism prescription may be necessary for comfortable binocular vision. The power of the prism prescription may be calculated with the equation

$$prism = \frac{(2)(phoria) - compensating\ vergence}{3}$$

where a positive value indicates a need for the prism value calculated and a negative or zero value that no prism is necessary.[96] Data suggest that this criterion may be more effective at identifying exophoric patients with asthenopia than esophoric patients.[77, 78]

Another guideline for identifying binocular anomalies has been proposed by Percival.[97] He suggested that a patient should function in the middle third of his or her binocular zone; if the magnitude of the larger of the horizontal vergences is more than double the smaller, the criterion suggests that prism may be needed to improve binocular function. The equation

$$prism = \frac{greater\ vergence\ range - (2)(lesser\ vergence\ range)}{3}$$

is used to evaluate the need for prism.[96] A positive value suggests a prism prescription of the amount calculated. A negative value or zero indicates no need for prism. Percival's criterion may be more effective at identifying esophoric than exophoric patients with asthenopia.[77, 78]

The supravergences and infravergences are equal when the patient does not have a vertical phoria. An asymmetry of the supravergences and infravergences within an eye suggests a vertical phoria. The vertical vergence findings may be used to determine the vertical prism prescription. The prism power is the amount needed to equalize the vertical vergences. The amount is determined with the equation

$$prism = \frac{base\ down\ to\ break - base\ up\ to\ break}{2}$$

where a plus value indicates a base down prism and a minus value a base up prism prescription for the eye over which the vergences were measured.[98]

If the patient reports a target moving horizontally (horizontal vergence) or vertically (vertical vergence), suppression is present. The suppressing eye can be identified by noting the direction of movement of the target. The target moves in the direction of the apex of the prism in front of the non-suppressing eye. When suppression occurs, vergence ranges cannot be measured with a subjective technique. An objective method is necessary.

For horizontal measures, indicate the test distance, direction of prism, and refractive correction, and blur, break, and recovery prism values. The value recorded is the sum of the right and left prism powers. A recovery that requires prism of the opposite base as the vergence measured (i.e., recovery is base in on base out vergences) is

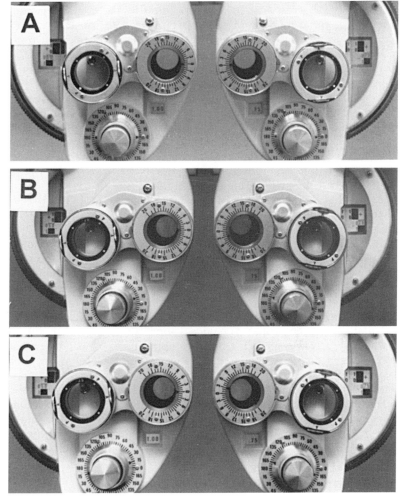

**FIGURE 6–35** Vertical vergences. *A,* The initial phoroptor arrangement to measure vertical fusional vergence. Both prisms are set to introduce vertical prism but are set to zero. *B,* Left supravergence/left sursumvergence. A base down prism is slowly increased in front of the left eye. The magnitude of the prism resulting in a loss of fusion is noted, and the prism is then reduced until fusion is regained. *C,* Left infravergence/left deorsumvergence. A base up prism is slowly increased in front of the left eye. The magnitude of the prism resulting in a loss of fusion is noted, and the prism is then reduced until fusion is regained.

recorded as a minus value. If no blur is reported, record an "X."

**EXAMPLES**

BI vergences @ 6 m c.c. (habitual): X/11/7
BO vergences @ 6 m c.c. (habitual): 6/10/−1

For vertical measures, indicate the test distance, eye the prism was placed over, refractive correction, and break and recovery prism values. The direction of the vergence may be indicated by recording supra or infra or the direction of the prism base (i.e., base up). A recovery that requires prism of the opposite base as the vergence measured is recorded as a minus value.

**EXAMPLES**

OS supra @ 6 m c.c. (BVA): 4/2
OS infra @ 6 m c.c. (BVA): 2/−1
or
BD OS @ 6 m c.c. (BVA): 4/2
BU OS @ 6 m c.c. (BVA): 2/−1

If suppression occurs, note the suppressing eye.

Risley prism vergences are rarely attempted in pre-school children owing to a limited language ability and the difficulty of the task. This technique is used in school-age children and adults.

The patient's eye cannot be viewed during testing. If you are not certain that the patient understands the task or the responses are questionable, use an objective measure of vergence. Objective measures are also preferred in patients with intermittent strabismus. It is necessary to observe the patient's eyes to be certain that the strabismus is not manifest during testing.

No blur point is expected for the base in vergence at distance. Relaxation of accommodation at distance as indicated by blur suggests that the patient has not been properly refracted. The subjective refraction needs additional plus power or less minus power. No blur finding is expected during the vertical vergence measure, as accommodation should not change.

Traditionally, it is recommended that base in vergences be measured before base out vergences.[99, 100] This test sequence is supported by the finding of an increase in esophoria and decrease in exophoria found after vergences were assessed (base out vergence tested before base in) compared with the phoria found prior to the vergence measure.[100, 101] The prism adaptation produced by base out prism appeared greater than that created by base in prism, producing a reduction in the measured base in vergences if assessed after rather than before base out vergences. More recently, Schor[84] reported that prism adaptation is not always greater for base out than base in prism. This suggests that the traditional recommendation for measuring base in before base out vergences may not apply to all patients.

Vertical vergences are normally measured over only one eye. Prism should be introduced more slowly for vertical vergence measures than for horizontal measures because vertical vergences are much slower than horizontal vergences.[103] Vertical vergences may be influenced by prism adaptation.[102] The initial vergence amplitude measured may be greater than the opposing vergence measured second. This prism adaptation may make the patient appear to have a vertical phoria when none is present or might mask a true asymmetry of vertical vergence ranges.

# Accommodative Convergence to Accommodation (AC/A) Ratio

. . . . . . . . . . . . . . . . . . . . . . . . .

Accommodative vergence is the alteration in horizontal eye alignment that occurs with a change in accommodation. When an increase in accommodation occurs, an increase in convergence also occurs; when the accommodative response decreases, a decrease in convergence takes place. The comparison of the change in horizontal eye alignment produced by a unit change in accommodation is termed the AC/A ratio. The value of this ratio varies within the population. Morgan[70] reported a mean AC/A ratio of 4 prism diopters/D with a standard deviation of 2 prism diopters/D.

Clinically, the AC/A ratio is determined by measuring the magnitude of the horizontal phoria or strabismus under two or more conditions that produce a different stimulus to accommodation. The stimulus is altered either by changing test distance (calculated AC/A) or through the introduction of plus or minus lenses at a fixed test distance (gradient AC/A). The eye alignment is assessed with dissociative methods such as the cover test, von Graefe method, or Maddox rod method.

The patient's refractive error must be corrected during these measurements to eliminate its effect on the accommodative demand of the task. For example, if an uncorrected $-1.00$ D myope's phoria is measured at 40 cm, the demand on accommodation for this patient is 1.50 D rather than 2.50 D.

## STIMULUS VERSUS RESPONSE AC/A RATIO

Clinically, the AC/A ratio is determined by assuming that the response of accommodation is equal to the stimulus to accommodation. (The stimulus or demand on accommodation is the inverse of the test distance in meters.) Use of the stimulus value provides a measure of the stimulus AC/A.[104] However, the accommodative response is typically greater than the stimulus when the target is located at optical infinity (accommodation is not completely relaxed), and the response is less than the accommodative stimulus at 40 cm (lag of accommodation). This stimulus-response curve is shown in Chapter 5. The response AC/A considers the patient's actual accommodative response rather than the stimulus and is about 8% higher than the stimulus AC/A.[104] Clinically, it is difficult to monitor the accommodative response; hence the stimulus AC/A is the accepted method.

## CALCULATED AC/A RATIO

The calculated method is frequently used to determine the AC/A ratio. The magnitude of the phoria or strabismus is measured at distance (6 meters) and at near (40 cm). The phoria may be determined by objective or subjective means, but the angle of strabismus is measured with the cover test. The equation is

$$\text{AC/A ratio} = \text{PD}_{cm} + \frac{(\text{H}_N - \text{H}_D)}{\text{A}_N - \text{A}_D}$$

where $\text{PD}_{cm}$ = distance interpupillary distance in centimeters, $\text{H}_N$ = near phoria or tropia (eso is plus and exo is minus), $\text{H}_D$ = distance phoria or tropia (eso is plus and exo is minus), $\text{A}_N$ = the accommodative stimulus at near, and $\text{A}_D$ = the accommodative stimulus at distance.[105] For example, in a patient with an interpupillary distance of 6.2 cm, 1 prism diopter exophoria at 6 meters and 6 prism diopters exophoria at 40 cm, the calculated AC/A ratio is

$$AC/A \text{ ratio} = 6.2 + \frac{(-6 - (-1))}{2.50 - 0}$$
$$= 4.2 \text{ prism diopters/D}$$

## GRADIENT AC/A RATIO

To determine the AC/A ratio by the gradient method, the phoria or tropia is measured through the refractive error correction with and without added lenses at a fixed test distance. Hence, proximal convergence does not influence the gradient AC/A ratio measure because its effect is constant for both phoria measures. The phoria measurements may be made with the target located at distance or at near. At distance, $-1.00$ or $-2.00$ D is added over the refractive correction, and at near either plus or minus lenses may be used, although Ogle and Martens[106] suggest that minus lenses yield more reliable results than plus lenses.

The gradient AC/A ratio is equal to the change in phoria divided by the added lens power. For example, a patient with a 12 prism diopter esophoria at 40 cm through the subjective refraction and a 1 prism diopter esophoria through the subjective refraction and $+2.00$ D added lenses has a gradient AC/A of 5.5 prism diopters/D or

$$\frac{12 - 1}{2.00} = 5.5.$$

Although both the calculated and gradient AC/A ratios are used and accepted clinically, the calculated and gradient AC/A ratios often differ.[106] The difference in the AC/A ratios is attributed to the effects of proximal vergence, which is convergence produced by the awareness of nearness of the target. Although proximal vergence is constant for the phorias used to determine the gradient AC/A ratio, only the near phoria, not the distance, is influenced in the calculated AC/A ratio.

## APPLICATION

The AC/A ratio is used clinically in two ways. First, the ratio may be used in the diagnosis of binocular anomalies. For example, esophoria at near associated with a high AC/A ratio is diagnosed as convergence excess.[107] Second, the management of binocular anomalies is influenced by the AC/A ratio. Added lenses are of limited usefulness when the AC/A ratio is low, compared with a high or moderate AC/A ratio. For example, if the AC/A ratio is 2 prism diopters/D, 2.00 D of added lenses alters the phoria by only 4 prism diopters. However, when the AC/A is 6 prism diopters/D, a 2.00 D change in lens power produces a change of 12 prism diopters. Whereas added lenses might produce a dramatic improvement in binocular function in the latter patient, the lenses would have little influence on the binocularity of the former. Prism would generally be preferred to added lenses in a patient with a low AC/A ratio.

# Sensory Fusion

## STEREOPSIS (THIRD-DEGREE FUSION)

There are many cues to the relative position of objects in space: overlay, perspective, aerial perspective, shadows, parallax, height, accommodation, convergence, and stereopsis.[108, 109] Among these cues to depth, stereopsis is unique in that it relies on binocular viewing. Stereopsis results in the perception of an empty space between objects which is experienced only through binocular viewing. The horizontal separation between the two eyes which permits objects off the horopter to be viewed from slightly different perspectives produces the horizontal retinal disparity that gives rise to stereopsis.

Although binocular viewing is required for stereopsis, stereopsis can occur when Panum's fusional areas are exceeded and objects are seen as double.[110, 111] Under certain viewing conditions, both stereopsis and binocular rivalry can be perceived simultaneously.[112, 113] Stereopsis can also occur under some conditions of suppression.[112, 114, 115] Thus, the mere presence of stereopsis does not ensure normal sensory and motor fusion. However, when clinical measures of stereopsis are in the range of expected thresholds, normal sensory fusion and motor alignment at the time of testing can be assumed.

## Methods of Evaluating Stereopsis

Tests currently available for the clinical assessment of stereopsis can be divided into three categories: local stereograms, random dot stereograms, and real depth tests. Local stereograms are sometimes termed linear or contour stereograms. Depth is created by introducing a horizontal disparity between corresponding edges or boundaries in the picture seen by each eye. The depth is associated with small individual features. The most common form of image separation used

| | | | | | TABLE 6-15  Stereoacuity Tests |
|---|---|---|---|---|---|

| Stereo Test | Manufacturer | Test Distance | Test Design | Image Dissociation | Range of Stereoacuity (sec of arc) |
|---|---|---|---|---|---|
| **A. At Near** | | | | | |
| Frisby* | Clement Clarke | variable | Real depth | Real depth | @ 40 cm  @ 60 cm<br>6 mm 340 sec  150 sec<br>3 mm 170 sec  75 sec<br>1 mm 55 sec  25 sec |
| Lang I† | Lang-Stereotest (Clement Clarke) | 40 cm | Random dot | Panography | Cat = 1200 sec<br>Star = 600 sec<br>Car = 550 sec |
| Lang II† | Lang-Stereotest (Clement Clarke) | 40 cm | Random dot | Panography | Star<br>  monocular = 0 sec<br>  binocular = 200 sec<br>Elephant = 600 sec<br>Moon = 200 sec<br>Car = 400 sec |
| Random dot‡ | Stereo Optical Co., Inc | 40 cm | Random dot and Local | Polaroid | Forms (RD) 500 & 250 sec<br>Circles (L) 400–20 sec<br>Animals (L) 400–100 sec |
| Random dot E* | Stereo Optical Co., Inc. | variable | Random dot | Polaroid | @ 50 cm = 504 sec<br>@ 1 m = 252 sec<br>@ 1.5 m = 168 sec<br>@ 2 m = 126 sec |
| Stero butterfly‡ | Stereo Optical Co., Inc. | 40 cm | Random dot and Local | Polaroid | Butterfly (RD)<br>  Upper wings 2000 sec<br>  Lower wings 1150 sec<br>  Body 700 sec<br>Circles (L) 800–40 sec<br>Animals (L) 400–100 sec |
| Stereo fly‡ | Stereo Optical Co., Inc. | 40 cm | Local | Polaroid | Fly wings = 3552 sec<br>Circles = 800–40 sec<br>Animals = 400–100 sec |
| Stereo reindeer‡ | Stereo Optical Co., Inc. | 35.56 cm | Local | Polaroid | Approximately 10% (600 sec) to 85% (30 sec) |
| TNO‡ | Lameris Instrumenten b.v. (Clement Clarke) | 40 cm | Random dot | Anaglyph | Screening<br>  1980 sec<br>Plates V-VII<br>  480–15 sec |
| Viewer-free random-dot circle, square, E† | Synthetic Optics Corp. | 40 cm | Random dot | Prismatic printing process based on panography | Square = 850 sec<br>Circle = 650 sec<br>"E" = 450 sec |
| Viewer-free random dot figures† | Synthetic Optics Corp. | 39.88 cm | Random dot and Local | Prismatic printing process based on panography | Figures (RD) 170–85 sec<br>Circles (L) 526–28 sec |
| Viewer-free stereo butterfly† | Synthetic Optics Corp. | Butterfly 30.48 cm<br>Circles and animals 33.78 cm | Random dot and Local | Prismatic printing process based on panography | Butterfly (RD)<br>  Top of upper wings<br>    2350 sec<br>  Tip of botton wing<br>    1350 sec<br>  Body/antenna 820 sec<br>Circles (L) 800–40 sec<br>Animals (L) 400–100 sec |
| **B. At Distance** | | | | | |
| Adult vectograph slide (#9300)‡ | Stereo Optical Co., Inc. | 3 or 6 m projector slide | Local | Polaroid | 255–90 |
| AO vectograph adult slide (#11895)† | Reichert | 6 m projector slide | Local | Polaroid | 240–30 |
| AO vectograph child slide (#11896)‡ | Reichert | 6 m projector slide | Local | Polaroid | 285–45 |
| B-VAT II†<br>  Stereo test 5<br>  Stereo test 6 | Mentor | 3 to 6 m | Random dot<br><br>Local | Liquid crystal shutter | 20/320 E with variable orientation disparities of 240–15 sec<br>1 of 4 circles in depth 240–15 sec |
| Child vectograph slide (#9400)‡ | Stereo Optical Co., Inc | 3 or 6 m projector slide | Local | Polaroid | 215–40 |

*Crossed or uncrossed disparity depending on the test orientation.
†Crossed disparity only.
‡Typically crossed disparity; disparity may be changed to uncrossed by changing the filters or rotating the test plate 180°.
RD = Random dot; L = Local.

for local stereograms is polarization, although a prismatic printing process based on panography appears to be gaining in popularity.[116] The biggest disadvantage of this form of stereo test is the presence of monocular cues for the patient. Parallax or an offset can often be used by the astute observer to locate the correct choice in the absence of stereopsis.[117]

Random dot stereograms differ from local stereograms in that no monocular contours are available. Stereopsis is created by a horizontal displacement of a group of elements in a random array. This form of stereopsis has been termed global stereopsis and was popularized by Julesz.[118] The elements used for the background and figure can be almost anything (e.g., dots, lines, patterns), but dots or squares are used for all clinical tests currently available. Any figure can be created by selective displacement of corresponding elements in the random background. Image isolation between the two eyes is most commonly done through polarization, but anaglyphics and panography have also been used.[116] The advantages of testing global stereopsis in a clinical setting are the lack of monocular cues and the poor or absent stereoacuity typically present in patients without bifoveal fixation.[119-123]

The last group of stereo tests is based on real depth. This group includes some of the first tests of stereopsis, the Howard-Dolman and Verhoeff stereoptor.[108, 124] These classic tests are no longer employed in routine clinical practice, but the Howard-Dolman test is still used in the laboratory. The Frisby stereo test is currently the most widely used clinical test of stereopsis based upon real depth. The depth is created by an actual physical separation, and hence no filters are required to isolate the images seen by the two eyes. However, like tests of local stereopsis using contour stereograms, monocular cues such as parallax and shadows can give a false impression of stereopsis.[125-127]

Table 6–15 summarizes the characteristics of the most popular tests of stereopsis currently available. Table 6–16 lists the manufacturers of these tests.

## Clinical Considerations

### *Approaches to Stereo Testing*

Because normal levels of stereopsis cannot occur without accurate motor alignment and because similar images in the two eyes are required to promote sensory fusion, there are two different approaches to the clinical assessment of stereopsis. The first approach uses stereopsis as a screen-

| TABLE 6–16 Manufacturers of Stereoacuity Tests | |
|---|---|
| **Manufacturer and Address** | **Phone and FAX** |
| Clement Clarke Inc.<br>3128 East 17th Avenue,<br>  Suite D<br>Columbus, OH 43219 | Phone: (800) 848-8923<br>FAX: (614) 478-2622 |
| Lameris Optech<br>P.O. Box 9<br>3737 ZJ Groenekan<br>The Netherlands | Phone: +31/3461-4114<br>FAX: +31/3461-4015 |
| Lang-Stereotest<br>P.O. Box CH-8127 Forch<br>Zurich Switzerland | |
| Mentor O & O<br>5425 Hollister Drive<br>Santa Barbara, CA 93111 | Phone: (800) 992-7557<br>FAX: (805) 681-6182 |
| Reichert Ophthalmic<br>  Instruments (Leica Inc.)<br>(American Optical)<br>P.O. Box 123<br>Buffalo, NY 14240 | Phone: (716) 686-4500<br>FAX: (716) 686-4555 |
| Stereo Optical Co., Inc.<br>3539 N. Kenton Avenue<br>Chicago, IL 60641 | Phone: (800) 344-9500<br>FAX: (312) 777-4985 |
| Synthetic Optics Corp.<br>903 Mohawk Road<br>Franklin Lakes, NJ 07417 | Phone: (201) 847-0007 |

ing tool, evaluating stereoacuity early in the examination sequence, often as one of the preliminary assessments. The rationale behind this approach is that if the patient demonstrates *normal* stereopsis, the prerequisites required for normal stereoacuity must have been met. Thus, a constant strabismus cannot be present. In addition, the vision in each eye should be normal or nearly normal without a large difference in the clarity or size of the image in each eye.[128-130] If stereopsis is absent or poorer than expected, the examiner is alerted to a potential problem with acuity, refraction, and/or ocular alignment and the need to carefully evaluate these functions in detail. Once the problem is uncovered and corrected, stereoacuity is then remeasured.

The second approach evaluates stereopsis later in the examination sequence, after motor alignment, refraction, and visual acuity have been assessed. In adult patients with normal alignment and without significant changes in refractive error or acuity, the stereoacuity will not be significantly altered by a modest change in refraction. Thus, patients with normal binocular vision and normal habitual acuities require only one measure of stereoacuity with either approach. However, patients with problems uncovered and corrected prior to the stereoacuity assessment would require only one assessment of stereopsis rather than two using this second approach. This difference is usually not significant in adults and older children. However, when examining infants and pre-school children, whose attention and interest are often limited to a single presentation of a particular test, the examiner may get only one opportunity to evaluate stereoacuity. It is prudent to maximize the chances of a successful stereoacuity assessment in these young patients by ruling out oculomotor disorders and uncorrected refractive errors prior to the administration of the stereopsis test.

Regardless of the approach taken, the examiner must remember that normal stereopsis can be measured in patients with an intermittent strabismus if motor alignment is present at the time of testing. Symptomatic patients with inefficient binocular systems may also demonstrate normal stereopsis. Thus, normal stereopsis does not mean that the binocular assessment is complete and no other binocular testing is necessary, particularly if symptoms of a binocular problem are uncovered during the case history (see Table 6-1). Motor components such as the recovery of fusion, flexibility, and reserves must still be evaluated.

### Selection of the Stereoacuity Test

The selection of the most appropriate stereoacuity test depends on the age of the patient and the examiner's approach to stereoacuity testing. In testing adults as part of the preliminary assessment, a stereoacuity test containing global stereopsis to rule out a constant strabismus is preferred to a local test with the potential of monocular cues. The test should also contain disparities as close to absolute threshold as possible to maximize the ability to detect small differences between the two eyes. However, if stereopsis is tested after ruling out the presence of strabismus and the acuity has been optimized by careful refraction and is normal in each eye, stereoacuity is expected to be normal. Although selecting a stereoacuity test with disparities approaching threshold would confirm this expectation, demonstrating the presence of global stereopsis may be all that is required in the normal patient.

When testing infants or young pre-school children, tests that allow a forced choice or pointing response and do not require filters improve testability. Tests of global stereopsis are useful to rule out small eye alignment errors that may escape detection in an active pre-school child. However, both the test selected and the age of

the child influence the expected result.[131, 132] Thus, determining the stereothreshold of a young child may not be very useful, and tests with disparities approaching adult threshold may not be necessary for this population.[133]

The specific protocol varies with the test selected, but the examiner should carefully follow the instructions included with the test. The general points discussed below apply to all tests of stereopsis.

1. The patient is comfortably seated facing the examiner in normal room illumination. Additional illumination from the overhead light on the stand should also be directed at those tests of near point stereopsis. However, care must be taken to avoid glare and shadows falling on the test materials.
2. The patient is tested with correction if any significant refractive error is present unless the stereo test is used as a preliminary screening, as discussed above. In this case, the patient's habitual correction is used.
3. The examiner must present the test directly in front of the patient. To avoid introducing monocular cues such as parallax, the test must be held still and the patient must not be permitted to move his or her head.

Individuals with normal vision have stereothresholds better than 10 seconds of arc.[134-136] Because the smallest disparity available on clinical tests of stereopsis is considerably larger (see Table 6-15), adults and older children with normal eye alignment and normal visual acuity in each eye should correctly identify the smallest disparity offered by the test. Von Noorden suggests that 15 to 30 seconds be considered normal.[6] Parks and Eustis[50] found stereoacuities of 40 seconds or better on clinical tests of stereopsis in patients with bifixation. Similarly, Scott and Mash[137] considered a stereoacuity of at least 40 seconds to be normal. Based on the work of Hofstetter,[138] Reading[139] has estimated the adult mean threshold to be 14.45 seconds. However, different tests of stereopsis provide different stereoacuity thresholds, further complicating the guidelines for normal stereoacuity.[135]

Unfortunately, the picture is less clear for infants and pre-school children. Several investigators report an improvement in stereoacuity as a function of age.[132, 140] However, it is not clear how much of the improvement is due to an actual improvement in stereothreshold because infants 5 months of age have demonstrated stereopsis of 60 seconds of arc,[141] much better than that reported in many clinical studies of pre-school children. The picture is further complicated by the fact that stereothreshold varies considerably with the clinical test selected.[131, 132, 140, 142] Tables 6-17 through 6-19 summarize some of the norms for children found in the literature for the most popular clinical stereoacuity tests.

Authorities vary as to what should be considered abnormal stereoacuity in adults and school-age children. One approach is to consider any patient with stereopsis poorer than 30 seconds as abnormal. However, not all clinical tests have disparities as small as 30 seconds, and the patient's threshold depends on the stereoacuity test selected.[135, 143] Tillson[144] has suggested that

100 seconds or better on the Titmus test and 120 seconds or better on the TNO test is the generally accepted dividing line between normal and abnormal binocular function, particularly when used in screening. Based on the work of Hofstetter,[138] Reading[139] has argued that 97.5% of the population have thresholds between about 2 and 38 seconds of arc, and hence, persons with stereoacuity poorer than 38 seconds would be considered abnormal.

Another approach is to measure stereopsis in patients with known binocular abnormalities. Patients with small misalignments (strabismus less

## TABLE 6-17  Stereoacuity Norms for Local Stereopsis

### A. Stereo Fly (sec of arc)

| Age (yrs) | Tatsumi and Tahira (1972) (reported by Simons, 1981)[131]* | Amigo (1973)[152] | Scott and Mash (1974)[137] | Romano et al. (1975) (reported by Simons, 1981)[131]* | Cooper et al. (1979)[140]† | Marsh et al. (1980)[142]‡ | Heron et al. (1985)[132]§ | Zhou et al. (1988)[153]‡ |
|---|---|---|---|---|---|---|---|---|
| 3 | 200 | 200¶ (300**) | | 200 | 140 | | 57.5 | |
| 4 | 100 | 100¶ (173**) | | 140 | 95 | | 61.5 | |
| 5 | 100 | 100* (167**) | | 100 | 102 | | 30.5 | |
| 6 | | | | | 94 | | 29.5 | |
| 7 | | | | | 42 | | 26.5 | |
| 8 | | | | | 41 | | | |
| 9 | | | | | 41 | | | |
| 10 | | | | | 42 | | | |
| 2–7 | | | | | | 80 (63.1**) | | |
| 6–14 | | | | | | | | 50 |
| 9–13 | | | 40 | | | | | |
| adults | | | | | | | 18 | |

*At least 75% of children had this level of stereoacuity or better.
†Median stereoacuity.
‡82% at this level of stereoacuity or better; excludes patients whose stereoacuity was extrapolated.
§Median stereoacuity, altered test distance to approach threshold.
¶At least 70% of children had this level of stereoacuity or better.
**Average stereoacuity.

### B. Randot Test (sec of arc)

| Age (yrs) | Simons (1981)[131]* | Heron et al. (1985)[132]† | Zhou et al. (1988)[153]‡ |
|---|---|---|---|
| 3 | 70 | 47.5 | |
| 4 | 70 | 44.5 | |
| 5 | 70 | 30.5 | |
| 6 | | 23.5 | |
| 7 | | 22.5 | |
| 11 | | | |
| 6–12 | | | 40 |
| adults | | 20 | |

*At least 75% of children had this level of stereoacuity or better.
†Median stereoacuity, altered test distance to approach threshold.
‡At least 81% of children had this level of stereoacuity or better.

### TABLE 6–18  Stereoacuity Norms for Real Depth

| Age (yrs) | Simons (1981)[131]* | Simmerman (1984)[127]† | Heron et al. (1985)[132]‡ | Zhou et al. (1988)[153]§ |
|---|---|---|---|---|
| 3 | 250 | | 27.5 | |
| 4 | 250 | | 29.5 | |
| 5 | 250 | | 19.5 | |
| 6 | | | 17.5 | |
| 7 | | | 16.5 | |
| 6–14 | | | | 40 |
| adults | | 11.86 (3.6–29.5)¶ | 8 | |

*At least 75% of children had this level of stereoacuity or better.
†Average stereothreshold in 20 adults with normal vision.
‡Median stereoacuity, altered test distance to approach threshold.
§At least 87% of children had this level of stereoacuity or better.
¶Range of stereoacuity.

than 10 prism diopters) or central suppression but no manifest deviation might be missed during a cursory assessment. The stereoacuity achieved by these abnormal patients could serve as guidelines to abnormal stereoacuity. Table 6–20A summarizes several investigations of patients with small angle strabismus (less than 10 prism diopters) or monofixation syndrome.[115] Table 6–20B summarizes the results of normal and abnormal children tested with fixed random dot stereo tests. Considering the results presented in Table 6–20, stereoacuity poorer than 200 seconds on a random dot test or 50 seconds on a test of local stereopsis should be considered abnormal when obtained at near.

Because the guidelines for infants and preschool children are less clear than those for adults and older children, the prudent approach is to apply the values obtained from studies on adults with abnormal vision. However, the stereoacuity of most normal pre-school children is poorer than the 50-second cut-off for local stereograms based on recommendations from older children and adults (see Table 6–17). The picture is a bit clearer for random dot tests. Most normal pre-school children above age 4 achieve better

### TABLE 6–19  Stereoacuity Norms for Random Dots

*A. TNO (sec of arc)*

| Age (yrs) | Cooper et al. (1979)[140]* | Marsh et al. (1980)[142]† | Simons (1981)[125]‡ | Heron et al. (1985)[132]§ | Zhou et al. (1988)[153]¶ | Williams et al. (1988)[154]† |
|---|---|---|---|---|---|---|
| 3 | 390 | | 120 | 64.5 | | |
| 4 | 90 | | 120 | 47 | | |
| 5 | 72 | | 120 | 35.5 | | |
| 6 | 120 | | | 36.5 | | |
| 7 | 60 | | | 26.5 | | 480 |
| 8 | 58 | | | | | |
| 9 | 120 | | | | | 60 |
| 10 | 108 | | | | | |
| 11 | | | | | | 60 |
| 2–7 | | 120 (113.4**) | | | | |
| 6–12 | | | | | 60 | |
| adults | | | | 32 | | |

*Median stereoacuity.
†At least 82% of children had this level of stereoacuity or better.
‡At least 75% of children had this level of stereoacuity or better.
§Median stereoacuity, altered test distance to approach threshold.
¶At least 90% of children had this level of stereoacuity of better.
**Average.

*B. Random Dot E (sec of arc)*

| Age (yrs) | Reinecke and Simons (1974) (reported by Simons 1981)[125]* | Marsh, et al. (1980)[142]† | Simons (1981)[125]* |
|---|---|---|---|
| 3 | 138 | | 168 |
| 4 | 110 | | 126 |
| 5 | 138 | | 126 |
| 2–7 | | 123 (126.3‡) | |

*At least 75% of children had this level of stereoacuity or better.
†72% of children had this level of stereoacuity of better; excludes patients whose stereoacuity was extrapolated.
‡Average stereoacuity.

than 200 seconds of stereopsis when tested with random dot stereograms. However, considerable variability is found in younger children across the random dot stereo tests. Because these random dot tests are generally devoid of monocular cues and the stereopsis can only rarely be appreciated without normal eye alignment,[121, 122, 145] random dot stereo tests may provide more useful information about the binocular status of these young patients. If an infant or pre-school child demonstrates even gross levels of stereopsis on a properly administered random dot test, it should be viewed as an indication of normal eye alignment at the time of testing.[133] Ciner and colleagues,[146] using a new random dot test, suggest children up to 24 months of age should demonstrate at least 300 seconds of stereopsis, and those older than 24 months are expected to have a stereoacuity of at least 100 seconds. If the child appears to understand the stereo test but fails to demonstrate stereopsis using a random dot test, the examiner must further consider the possibility of a small ocular misalignment.

Both the test and the stereoacuity should be recorded. Because stereoacuity is typically assessed with the refractive error fully corrected, the prescription need not be noted unless testing was done under non-standard conditions.

EXAMPLES

Lang stereo test:   550 sec
Stereo fly:   40 sec

If a strabismus is detected during cover testing and retinal correspondence is normal, stereopsis should be assessed with the refractive error fully corrected and with the prism that neutralizes the deviation in place. However, many of these patients have amblyopia and suppression that compromise the stereoacuity. Therefore, if the strabismus is associated with amblyopia of 20/50 or worse or marked suppression is present, testing stereopsis at the angle of deviation may not provide any useful additional information.

Patients with reduced stereopsis should be retested monocularly. If performance deteriorates under monocular testing, the stereoacuity measured binocularly was the result of binocular viewing. However, if the performance is unaffected by occlusion of one eye, the stereopsis was based on monocular cues and does not represent true stereopsis.

Stereopsis can be used to demonstrate the value of correcting a refractive error. This approach may be particularly useful for patients with myopic anisometropia or mild hyperopic anisometropia with only a small amblyopia. These patients are often asymptomatic but frequently have reduced stereopsis. Testing stereopsis with and without correction can demonstrate improved performance when the proper correction is applied.

## SECOND-DEGREE FUSION

### Worth Dot Test

Patients unable to demonstrate stereopsis are often strabismic or amblyopic or have unequal vision in the two eyes from some other cause. In these patients, an evaluation of second-degree fusion is useful. Second-degree fusion is sensory fusion of similar objects seen by each eye without disparity and, hence, without an appreciation of depth.

1. The patient is comfortably seated facing the examiner with the refractive error fully corrected. Red/green filters are placed over the spectacle correction.
2. The target for the Worth dot test consists of two green lights, one red light, and a white light, arranged in a diamond pattern (Fig. 6–36). The patient should not be permitted to view the target without the red/green filters in place.
3. The test is usually performed both at distance and near.
4. The examiner shows the patient the test lights and asks the patient to describe what he or she sees.

Patients with normal second-degree fusion report four lights when the Worth target is viewed

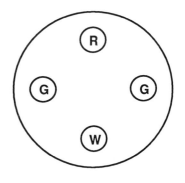

### Worth  Dot  Test

FIGURE 6–36 Schematic diagram of the Worth dot test to assess second-degree fusion. R = red light; G = green light; W = white light. The test target is viewed through red and green (anaglyphic) filters.

**TABLE 6–20** A. Stereoacuity in Monofixation Syndrome (as defined by Parks, 1971)[115] (sec of arc)

| Investigator | Wirt Circles (Stereo Fly) | | Frisby | | TNO | | Random Dot E | |
|---|---|---|---|---|---|---|---|---|
| | Best | Average* | Best | Average | Best | Average* | Best | Average* |
| Helveston and von Noorden (1967)[155] | 20 | 126 | | | | | | |
| Parks (1971)[115] | 67 | | | | | | | |
| Epstein and Tredici (1973)[156] | 40‡ | 203‡ | | | | | | |
| Frisby et al. (1975)[157] | 40 | 200 | 35 | 220.5 | 60 | 640 | | |
| Hill et al. (1976)[158] | 40 | 424 | | | 60 | 239.5 | 50 | 296.6 |
| Marsh et al. (1980)[142] | 40 | 272.5 | | | | | | |
| Rutstein and Eskridge (1984)[120] | 200 | 400 | | | 240 | 360 | 275 | 427 |
| | 50† | 253.6† | | | | | | |

*Average stereoacuity of those demonstrating stereopsis.
†Random dot test, local stereopsis.

Helveston and von Noorden (1967)[155]
n = 20; age: 9–34 years
1. No movement on cover test.
2. Eccentric fixation.
3. Positive on 4 prism test for scotoma.

Parks (1971)[115]
n = 100; age: not specified
1. Straight or nearly straight eyes, all deviations less than 8 prism diopters.
2. Peripheral fusion with fusional vergence amplitudes.
3. Absolute scotoma including the macular field of the nonfixating eye.
4. Gross stereopsis.

Epstein and Tredici (1973)[156]
n = 15; age: 18–43 years
1. Five of the 15 patients showed no tropia on cover test at near, and hence, excluded (n = 10). All deviations 1 to 6 prism diopters.
2. Of the 10 in the sample, all showed ARC by at least one test.
‡Includes only those six subjects with manifest tropia at near who responded to the stereo fly test.

Frisby et al. (1975)[157]
n = 14; age: 8–18 years
1. Includes only those patients with a diagnosis of microtropia or manifest deviation from Table 6–1.
2. Must have quantifiable stereoacuity.

Hill et al. (1976)[158]
n = 40; age: 7–33 years
1. Manifest deviation of up to 9 prism diopters or no detectable deviation on cover test.
2. Positive on 4 prism test for scotoma.
3. Some stereopsis with the stereo fly stereo test.

Marsh et al. (1980)[142]
n = 19; age: 4–7 years
1. From Table 6–2, includes only those with manifest deviation at near of less than 10 prism diopters.
2. Includes only those with actual measures of stereoacuity, no extrapolation or arbitrary values; number for individual stereo tests will vary.

Rutstein and Eskridge (1984)[120]
n = 28; age: 7–54 years
1. Deviation less than 10 prism diopters.
2. Peripheral fusion at near with the Worth dot test.
3. A positive result by the 4 prism test.

**TABLE 6–20** B. Random Dot Stereo Test Fixed Disparity (% of Normal and Abnormal Patients Passing)

| Investigator | Johnstone and Brown (1985)[121]* | | Lang and Lang (1988)[122]† | | Broadbent and Westall (1990)[159]‡ | Cooper and Feldman (1978)[123] | | |
|---|---|---|---|---|---|---|---|---|
| Test | Lang I 1200, 600, 550 seconds of arc | | Lang I 1200, 600, 550 seconds of arc | | Lang I 1200, 600, 550 seconds of arc | Custom made Polaroid projection 660 seconds of arc | | |
| Age | Normals Passing | Microtropias Passing | Normals Passing | Microtropias Passing | Normals Passing | Normals Passing | Microtropias Passing | Constant Strabismus Passing |
| 3–30 mos | 90 | | | | | | | |
| 6–12 mos | | | 42 | | 50 | | | |
| 12–18 mos | | | 75 | | 72 | | | |
| 18 mos–4 yrs | | | 90 | | 78 | | | |
| 3–11 yrs | 97 | 13 | | | | | | |
| 5–6 yrs | | | 93.5 | | | | | |
| unknown | | | | 11.5 | | 100 | 0 | 0 |

*Passing criterion—any objective or subjective response noted by the examiner.
†Passing criterion—not specified.
‡Passing criterion—only required to respond to one of the three figures.

through red/green filters. Two green lights, one red, and a yellow or red/green light are visible. The appearance of the white light as viewed through the red/green filters varies somewhat with the patient.

Abnormal responses include a report of two, three, or five lights. If two or three lights are reported, the patient is suppressing. A report of five lights indicates a lack of sensory fusion but no suppression.

If the patient reports three green lights, the eye behind the red filter is suppressing. The two green lights are visible to the eye behind the green filter and the white light also appears green.

If the patient reports two red lights, the eye behind the green filter is suppressing. The red light is seen by the eye behind the red filter and the white light also appears red.

If a strabismus is present and there is no suppression and no harmonious anomalous retinal correspondence, the patient reports five lights—two red and three green. The eye behind the red filter sees both the red and white lights as red. The eye behind the green filter sees the two green lights and the white light as green. Therefore, five lights are visible.

In cases of normal correspondence the red lights appear on the same side as the red filter in esotropia (uncrossed diplopia). In exotropia with normal correspondence, the red lights appear on the same side as the green filter (crossed diplopia).

The Worth dot test should be done both in normal room illumination and in the dark to eliminate or reduce peripheral fusion cues. If the patient is suppressing, the examiner should try switching filters. It has been reported that suppression is less likely to occur if the red filter is placed in front of the abnormal eye. In cases of strabismus without suppression, the separation between the red and green lights can be measured. When the test distance is known, the subjective angle of directionalization can be calculated. The subjective angle can also be measured by inserting prism until the red and green lights are fused and the patient reports four lights. When suppression is present, the size of the suppression zone can be determined by decreasing the viewing distance until four or five lights are seen by the patient. By knowing the size of the Worth target and the distance at which four or five lights are first seen, the size of the suppression zone can be calculated by simple trigonometry. If stereopsis is present and within the normal range, it is not necessary to test for second-degree fusion.

# Secondary Binocular Anomalies: Conditions Requiring Urgent Attention

Table 6–1 lists some of the presenting symptoms reported by patients with binocular vision disorders. Although this list should serve to alert the clinician to the possibility of a binocular vision disorder, none of these symptoms is specific or pathognomonic for a binocular vision anomaly. Many of these symptoms and the associated binocular disorders can signal a serious and even life-threatening underlying condition. Thus, it is imperative that the clinician be able to determine when a binocular problem is a sign of a secondary disorder rather than an isolated oculomotor problem. The differentiation is aided by a careful case history (see Chapter 1) of associated ocular and systemic symptoms and conditions. The guidelines that follow assist the clinician in this critical decision-making process.

## BLURRED OR REDUCED VISION: IS IT AMBLYOPIA OR SOMETHING ELSE?

1. Amblyopia is associated with amblyogenic factors. Table 6–21 lists the common conditions associated with amblyopia. If one or more of these conditions is *not* present,

| TABLE 6–21 Amblyogenic Factors |
|---|
| *Deprivation/degradation* |
| Ptosis |
| Unilateral |
| Asymmetrical bilateral |
| Covering visual axis |
| Therapeutic occlusion |
| Media opacities |
| Cornea |
| Lens |
| Vitreous |
| *Strabismus* |
| Constant unilateral |
| *Refractive error* |
| Anisometropic |
| Hyperopic |
| ≥3.50 D (100% amblyopic)[171] |
| Myopic |
| ≥5.50 D (100% amblyopic)[171] |
| Isometropic |
| Hyperopic |
| ≥5.00 D[172, 173] |
| Myopic |
| ≥10.00 D[174] |
| Meridional |
| 1.50 to 2.00 D[175] |

the reduction in vision is not likely to be amblyopia, and an organic cause must be explored.

2. Amblyopia is a developmental disorder and does not appear after the development of form vision is complete. Once the sensitive period for the development of form vision is complete, ages 8 to 10,[160-162] and normal acuity (20/20; 6/6) has been achieved, any subsequent decrease in vision cannot be attributed to amblyopia. If the factors listed in Table 6-21 present after 8 to 10 years of age, they do not produce an amblyopia.

3. The onset of amblyopia is *not* sudden. Amblyopia develops gradually over time. A rapid loss of vision is an ocular emergency and not amblyopia. However, the younger the patient, the more rapid the development of amblyopia, and it is often difficult to determine the history of vision loss in a young child.

4. Amblyopia is a diagnosis of exclusion. Uncorrected refractive error, organic causes, malingering, and a hysterical vision loss or conversion reaction must *all* be ruled out prior to the diagnosis of amblyopia. In addition, an amblyogenic factor (Table 6-21) must be present or must have been present during the development of spatial vision.

## SUDDEN ONSET OF DOUBLE VISION (DIPLOPIA): IS IT A PRIMARY OCULOMOTOR PROBLEM OR IS IT A SECONDARY CONDITION?

1. Monocular diplopia is not a binocular problem. If the diplopia remains when one eye

*Text continued on page 196*

---

**TABLE 6-22** Sudden Onset of Strabismus in Adult

| | |
|---|---|
| *Systemic Condition* | *Inflammatory* |
|   Coccidioidomycosis |   Cranial |
|   Diabetes mellitus |     Pseudotumor |
|   Graves' ophthalmopathy |     Meningitis |
|   Multiple sclerosis |   Orbital |
|   Myasthenia gravis |     Pseudotumor |
|   Sarcoid |     Optic neuritis |
|   Systemic lupus erythematosus |   Temporal arteritis |
|   Syphilis |   Tolosa-Hunt syndrome |
|   Tuberculosis |   Herpes zoster |
| *Vascular Conditions* | *Infections* |
|   Cavernous sinus |   Encephalitis |
|     Thrombosis |   Meningitis |
|     Carotid cavernous fistula |   Sinusitis/cellulitis |
|   Hypertension | *Toxic* |
|   Stroke |   Anticonvulsants |
|   Vascular spasm (migraine) |     Phenobarbital |
|   Vertebrobasilar insufficiency |     Phenytoin |
|     Emboli |   Arsenic |
|     Hemorrhage |   Beta blockers |
|     Aneurysm |     Acebutolol, atenolol |
| *Space-occupying Lesions* |     Metoprolol, pindolol |
|   Cranial |     Propranolol, sotalol |
|     Chordoma |     Timolol |
|     Craniopharyngioma |   Carbamazepine |
|     Glioma |   Carbon monoxide |
|     Hemangioma |   Cardiac glycosides |
|     Meningioma |     Digoxin, digitoxin |
|     Metastatic lesions |   Lead |
|     Nasopharyngeal carcinoma |   Lithium |
|     Pituitary adenoma |   Minocycline |
|   Orbital |   Vitamin A |
|     Glioma | |
|     Hemangioma | |
|     Meningioma | |
|     Metastatic lesions | |
| *Trauma* | |
|   Closed head | |
|     Subdural hematoma | |
|   Orbital edema | |
|   Orbital fracture | |
|   Orbital hematoma | |

**TABLE 6–23** Secondary Strabismus: Pediatric

| Condition | Description | Associated Signs and Symptoms | Diagnostic Tests | Referral | References |
|---|---|---|---|---|---|
| *Media opacities* | | | | | |
| Corneal | | | | | |
| Peter's anomaly (central anterior chamber cleavage abnormality or mesodermal dysgenesis of the iris and cornea) | Local attenuation or absence of endothelium and Descemet's membrane with central corneal stromal opacity | Iris-corneal or lens-corneal adhesions, peripheral cornea usually normal, glaucoma | Biomicroscopy, ultrasonography, tonometry | Corneal surgeon for penetrating keratoplasty | Reese and Ellsworth (1966)[176]; Waring et al. (1975)[177] |
| Birth trauma | Usually unilateral corneal edema localized to area surrounding breaks in Descemet's membrane | At onset: vertical corneal striae, conjunctival hemorrhage; later sequelae: corneal scars, high and/or irregular astigmatism | History, visual acuity, biomicroscopy, refraction, keratometry, corneal topography | Typically not required; treat refractive error, consider PMMA contact lenses | Hofmann et al. 1981[178] |
| Primary infantile glaucoma (congenital glaucoma) | Increased intraocular pressure with associated optic nerve sequelae due to aqueous outflow problem | Photophobia, epiphora, blepharospasm, horizontal corneal striae (Haab's striae), megalocornea, buphthalmos, corneal edema, conjunctival injection | Tonometry, horizontal corneal diameter >11.5 mm, gonioscopy, ophthalmoscopy, visual fields, refraction, A scan | Surgical treatment by pediatric ophthalmologist or anterior segment specialist | Barkan (1955)[179]; DeLuise and Anderson (1983)[180]; Wagner (1993)[181] |
| Lens | | | | | |
| Hereditary congenital | Opacification of the lens: zonular or lamellar, nuclear, anterior or posterior polar | Photophobia, leukokoria, posterior lenticonus, coloboma, microphthalmia, persistent hyperplastic primary vitreous | Visual acuity, birth history, familial history, biomicroscopy, ophthalmoscopy, blood work-up as indicated by history | Pediatrician to rule out intrauterine infections: toxoplasmosis, rubella, cytomegalic inclusion disease and herpes simplex; geneticist, ophthalmologist if lens removal is necessary | Lloyd et al.(1992)[182] |
| Metabolic | Opacification of the lens: lamellar, punctate cortical dots, posterior capsule | Leukokoria, galactosemia, hypoparathyroidism, diabetes, hypoglycemia, failure to thrive | Visual acuity, history, biomicroscopy, ophthalmoscopy, review of systems, blood work-up | Pediatrician, internist, or endocrinologist; ophthalmologist if lens removal is necessary | Endres and Shin (1990)[183]; Lloyd et al. (1992)[182] |

| | | | | |
|---|---|---|---|---|
| Traumatic | Opacification of the lens: anterior rosette cataract, total or localized opacification | Leukocoria, facial trauma, blow-out fracture, trauma to globe and retina, Vossius ring, subluxation of lens, glaucoma, child abuse | History, visual acuity, biomicroscopy, ophthalmoscopy, tonometry | Ophthalmologist, oculoplastic surgeon; imaging if foreign body suspected Child Protective Services if child abuse suspected | Jones (1991)[184]; Ajamian (1993)[185] |
| **Vitreous** | | | | | |
| Persistent hyperplastic primary vitreous (anterior and posterior) | Dense white vitreous band typically extending from disc to peripheral fundus or lens; failure of primary vitreous to regress | Leukocoria, retinal detachments, vitreoretinal traction, retinal folds, macular pigmentary degeneration, glaucoma, cataract, microphthalmos, shallow anterior chamber, engorged iris vessels | Ophthalmoscopy, biomicroscopy, ultrasonography | Retinal specialist for lensectomy and vitrectomy if severe | Pruett and Schepens (1970)[186] |
| **Retinal** | | | | | |
| Coats' disease | Retinal telangiectasia with secondary subretinal exudation appearing as a white or yellow mass; manifests more frequently in males | Telangiectatic retinal vessels, hemorrhage, retinal detachment, leukocoria, cataract, glaucoma | Ophthalmoscopy | Ophthalmologist (retinal) | Haik (1991)[187]; Kaur and Taylor (1992)[188] |
| Coloboma | Glistening white defect with distinct margins, irregular pigment clumping, includes but is not limited to inferior nasal retina; presumed etiology: incomplete closure of the embryonic fissure | Retinal detachment, retinal hemorrhage, iris and disc coloboma; microphthalmia; associated multisystemic disorders | Ophthalmoscopy | Low vision consult (visually impaired); pediatrician and genetics specialist if multisystem disorder suspected, case history (familial, teratogen) | Pagon (1981)[189], Warburg (1991)[190] |
| Leber's congenital amaurosis | Congenital retinal dystrophy with profound acuity loss in the first year of life which may precede retinal changes; frequently associated with systemic and neurological disorders; loss of acuity | Normal retina or a variety of pigmentary abnormalities (e.g., salt and pepper; retinitis pigmentosa-like; macular dysplasia) nystagmus, cataracts, keratoconus, abnormal pupillary light reflex, mental retardation, kidney disease, hearing loss | Ophthalmoscopy, electroretinogram | Low vision consult, pediatrician, school district (programs for visually impaired) | Schroeder et al. (1987)[191]; Lambert et al. (1989)[192]; Heher et al. (1992)[193] |

**TABLE 6–23** Secondary Strabismus: Pediatric *Continued*

| Condition | Description | Associated Signs and Symptoms | Diagnostic Tests | Referral | References |
|---|---|---|---|---|---|
| Retinoblastoma | Neoplasm of childhood. Endophytic: white or pink nodular mass extending into the vitreous Exophytic: mass behind the retina Diffuse infiltrative: cells in vitreous and infiltration into adjacent structures | Leukocoria, retinal detachment, dilated retinal vessels, vitreous seeds, glaucoma, pseudo-hypopyon (infiltrative), proptosis, metastasis | Ophthalmoscopy; case history (childhood cancer deaths or enucleation), ultrasonography, CT scan, MRI | Ophthalmologist (pediatric/retinal/oncology) | Abramson and Servodidio (1993)[194]; Abramson (1990)[195] |
| Toxocariasis | Infestation with *Toxocara canis*; larvae produce yellow-white or white mass (endophthalmitis) or white elevated ill-defined lesion resolving to a glistening white or gray lesion (granuloma) | Acute: vitritis, retinal detachment, anterior uveitis (keratic precipitates and posterior synechiae) Chronic: cyclitic membrane, leuko-coria, cataract, glau-coma (endophthal-mitis), traction bands (granuloma) | Ophthalmoscopy, biomicroscopy, enzyme-linked immunosorbent assay | Ophthalmologist if acute or glaucoma (depending on state laws) | Molk (1983)[196]; Shields (1984)[197] |
| Toxoplasmosis | Parasitic infestation with *Toxoplasma gondii*; congenital or acquired; yellow-white ill-defined, focal lesions resolving to white atrophic and pigmented scars; congenital may produce ocular and systemic disease at birth or later in life; ocular infestation may reactivate | Acute: edema, vasculitis, vitritis, floaters, anterior uveitis, glaucoma Congenital: cerebral calcification, hydro-cephalus, convulsions, hearing loss or asymptomatic (present at birth or later onset) | Ophthalmoscopy, biomicroscopy, IgG fluorescent antibody (IgG-IFA) test, enzyme-linked immunosorbent assay | Pediatrician if previously undiag-nosed; retinal ophthalmologist if acute; low vision consult for visually impaired | Rothova (1993)[198]; Primo (1994)[199]; Jabs (1990)[200] |
| Retinopathy of prematurity | At risk: premature infants < 1300 gm at birth or who received supplemental oxygen; abnormal retinal vessel growth at the junction of vascular and avascular retina which may produce retinal detachment | Fibrovascular proliferation into the vitreous, vitreous haze or hemorrhage, dilatation and tortuosity of retinal vessels, dilated iris vessels, pupillary rigidity (plus disease) | Ophthalmoscopy | Ophthalmologist (pediatric or retinal) if acute phase or detachment; low vision consult if visually impaired | Quinn et al. (1992)[201]; Kalina (1992)[202]; Phelps (1992)[203] |

| | | Clinical Findings | Diagnostic Methods | Management | References |
|---|---|---|---|---|---|
| **Trauma** Accidental | Birth process, head or direct ocular trauma, perforating ocular injury | Macular and vitreous hemorrhage, retinal detachment, chorioretinal scarring, optic atrophy, conjunctival ecchymosis, commotio retinae, choroidal rupture, lid ecchymosis, hyphema, cataract, lens dislocation, corneal opacity, or orbital fracture (direct trauma) | Ophthalmoscopy, biomicroscopy, ultrasonography (if fundus not visible) | Pediatrician, neurologist, ophthalmologist | Jain et al. (1980)[204]; Eagling (1974)[205] |
| Child abuse | Whiplash or shaken baby syndrome resulting from repeated rapid back and forth flexions of head; head trauma; or direct trauma to the eye | Preretinal, retinal and vitreous hemorrhage, retinal detachments and scarring, papilledema, optic atrophy, cortical blindness, conjunctival and lid ecchymosis, hyphema, cataract, lens dislocation (direct trauma), subdural hematoma, bruises, burns, bite marks, fractures of long bones | Ophthalmoscopy, fundus photography (documentation) | Pediatrician, neurologist, ophthalmologist, psychologist, psychiatrist report suspected abuse to appropriate agency and police | Harley (1980)[206]; Smith (1988)[207] |
| *Optic Nerve* Hypoplasia | Small grayish disc with retinal vessels entering and exiting centrally, double ring sign, tortuosity of vessels, tilting of optic nerve head, range of anomalies from subtle segmental changes to nerve one-half to one-third normal size | Afferent pupillary defect, nystagmus, myopia, colobomas, microphthalmos, optic atrophy, vascular tortuosity, fetal alcohol syndrome, endocrine disorders, delayed development | Visual acuity, ophthalmoscopy, pupil assessment, visual fields; consider CT scan depending on severity | Pediatrician, internist, or endocrinologist; consider neurologist; consider low vision consult if severe loss | Awan (1976)[208]; Francois and De Rouck (1976)[209]; Skarf and Hoyt (1984)[210]; Ouvrier and Billson (1986)[211]; Ouvrier (1990)[212] |

**TABLE 6–23** Secondary Strabismus: Pediatric *Continued*

| Condition | Description | Associated Signs and Symptoms | Diagnostic Tests | Referral | References |
|---|---|---|---|---|---|
| Coloboma | Glistening white enlargement of papillary area, partial/total excavation of the disc, retinal vessels enter and exit disc from coloboma border; presumed etiology is incomplete closure of embryonic fissure | Coloboma of retina and choroid and/or iris, retinal detachments, associated congenital forebrain anomalies (encephaloceles) | Ophthalmoscopy, visual fields, B-scan | Low vision consult or orientation and mobility, depending on extent of loss; consider genetic counseling, neurologist | Pagon (1981)[189]; Apple et al. (1982)[213] |
| Glioma | Benign pilocytic astrocytic proliferations—intraorbital, optic nerve, chiasmal, or cranial | Neurofibromatosis, nystagmus, proptosis, papilledema, optic atrophy, afferent pupillary defect, hydrocephalus, endocrine disorders | Visual acuity, pupil assessment, ophthalmoscopy, visual fields, CT scan; if chiasmal consider pituitary and hypothalmic function studies | Retinal specialist, neurologist, or endocrinologist, depending on location | Hoyt and Baghdassarian (1969)[214]; Eggers et al. (1976)[215]; Alvord and Lofton (1988)[216]; Dutton (1994)[217] |
| Optic atrophy | Usually a secondary condition; damage to optic nerve fibers resulting in pale, white optic nerve, loss of nerve fiber layer | Increased intracranial pressure, (hydrocephalus in children), optic nerve glioma, optic nerve hypoplasia, intracranial compressive lesion, trauma, heredodegenerative disorders, inflammatory, vascular | History, visual acuity, pupil assessment, ophthalmoscopy, visual fields, color vision, tonometry, imaging | Low vision specialist; neurologist if progressive or of unknown etiology | Sher (1985)[218]; Ouvrier (1990)[212] |
| *Cortical Trauma* Accidental | Blunt trauma to frontal area or any closed head trauma | Optic nerve trauma, loss of consciousness, relative afferent pupillary defect, IV nerve | History, visual acuity, pupils, ophthalmoscopy, biomicroscopy, visual fields, neurological assessment, imaging | Neurologist | Kline et al. (1984)[219]; Zimmerman and Bilaniuk (1994)[220] |

| Condition | Mechanism | Signs | Evaluation | Team | References |
|---|---|---|---|---|---|
| Whiplash or shaken baby syndrome (child abuse) | Repeated rapid back and forth flexions of head resulting in intracranial and intraocular hemorrhages | Subdural hematoma, retinal and vitreous hemorrhages, optic atrophy, retinal detachment, hyphemas, hydrocephalus, papilledema, cortical blindness, bruises, fracture of long bones, burns | History, visual acuity, ophthalmoscopy, biomicroscopy, X-rays, imaging | Pediatrician, neurologist, psychiatrist, psychologist, police, appropriate social service agency | Harley (1980)[206]; Smith (1988)[207]; Zimmerman and Bilaniuk (1994)[220]; Brown and Minns (1993)[221] |
| Hydrocephalus | Increased intracranial pressure | Headache, nausea and vomiting, transient visual obscurations, setting sun sign, nystagmus, papilledema, optic atrophy, VI nerve palsy, nonpatent shunt in previously controlled hydrocephalus may present with strabismus or a change in a pre-existing strabismus | Visual acuity, ophthalmoscopy, extraocular muscle assessment, pupil assessment, visual fields, spinal tap, imaging | Neurologist | France (1975)[222]; Wybar and Walker (1980)[223]; Holman and Merritt (1986)[224]; Hamed et al. (1993)[225] |

is covered, consider an optical or retinal cause rather than a binocular anomaly. Although not usually associated with a systemic disorder, some retinal disorders giving rise to monocular diplopia could require urgent attention.

Only patients under treatment for anomalous retinal correspondence or eccentric fixation might experience a monocular diplopia that is associated with a binocular problem. These cases are rare and, although disconcerting, are usually undergoing treatment and do not require immediate attention.

2. If the object fixated is single and objects not directly fixated are double, the diplopia is physiological. Occasionally the sudden onset of diplopia reported by a patient is nothing more than the discovery of physiological diplopia. Physiological diplopia is a normal phenomenon in which objects located off the horopter are seen as double. No strabismus is detected with the unilateral cover test. No further evaluation is required, but reassurance may be necessary.

3. If the object fixated is double, the diplopia is pathological and requires further evaluation. Pathological diplopia is associated with a strabismus detected by the unilateral cover test. However, not all individuals with strabismus have diplopia; some may suppress or have anomalous retinal correspondence. The cause of the strabismus associated with the pathological diplopia requires further evaluation. A complete case history with a review of systems (Chapter 1) is an invaluable tool in the differential diagnosis of pathological diplopia.

4. Sudden onset of strabismus or diplopia is an ocular urgency. A recent-onset strabismus, with or without diplopia, requires immediate evaluation to determine if the cause is secondary to an ocular or systemic condition. Because the vast majority of primary ocular deviations present by 7 years of age,[163-165] a recent-onset strabismus in an older patient is more likely secondary and requires urgent attention. Table 6–22 lists various systemic and ocular conditions that may present with sudden onset diplopia and/or strabismus. This list should serve as a guide, along with a complete history which includes a review of systems, when evaluating a patient with a sudden onset of diplopia.

Three ocular conditions may present with sudden-onset diplopia but are not ocular urgencies: a decompensated phoria, a decompensated small-angle strabismus (often with anomalous retinal correspondence), and a change in the fixation pattern or fixation switch in a unilateral strabismus patient.[166] However, a complete examination is necessary to arrive at the diagnosis and is often aided by reviewing the patient's previous ocular examination records.

## SUDDEN ONSET OF STRABISMUS IN A YOUNG CHILD: IS IT A PRIMARY OCULOMOTOR PROBLEM, OR IS IT SECONDARY TO A LOSS IN VISION?

1. If the strabismus is unilateral, consider the deviation as secondary to an organic vision loss. At onset, most infantile strabismus is alternating[167, 168] and not associated with amblyopia. If the strabismus is unilateral, a decrease in vision in the deviating eye may be present. Consider anisometropia, media opacities, retinal anomalies, optic nerve disorders, and cortical anomalies in the differential diagnosis. Table 6–23 presents some of the more common pathological entities that produce a unilateral decrease in vision. Often in the pediatric patient the first manifestation of this unilateral decrease in vision is a unilateral strabismus. Conditions that would present with a history suggesting a traumatic etiology (e.g., chemical burn, penetrating injury to the globe) are not included in Table 6–23.

2. If the vision in the deviating eye is severely reduced, consider that the deviation may be secondary to an organic vision loss. The vision in strabismic amblyopia is rarely worse than 20/200.[169, 170] If vision is poorer than 20/200, or "fix and follow" vision is compromised, an organic cause must be ruled out. In addition, the amblyopia that results in strabismus has a more gradual onset, rather than a rapid loss of vision.

# References

1. Scheiman M, Gallaway M, Coulter R, et al.: Prevalence of vision and ocular disease in a clinical pediatric population. Optom Vis Sci 1992; 69(Suppl):108.
2. Roberts J: Eye examination findings among children, United States. Vital and Health Statistics, series 11, no

115. Rockville, DHEW Publication (HSM) 72-1057, June 1972.

3. Roberts J: Eye examination findings among youths aged 12-17, United States. Vital and Health Statistics, series 11, no 155. Rockville, DHEW Publication (HRA) 76-1637, Nov 1975.

4. Caloroso EE, Rouse MW: Clinical Management of Strabismus. Boston: Butterworth-Heinemann, 1993; pp. 236-237.

5. Scheiman M, Wick B: Clinical Management of Binocular Vision. Heterophoric, Accommodative, and Eye Movement Disorders. Philadelphia, JB Lippincott, 1994; pp. 225-227, 451.

6. von Noorden GK: Binocular Vision and Ocular Motility. Theory and Management of Strabismus, 4th ed. St. Louis: CV Mosby, 1990; pp. 27, 189, 196.

7. Miller M, Pruzansky S: Craniofacial anomalies. In Peyman GA, Sanders DR, Goldberg MF (eds): Principles and Practice of Ophthalmology. Philadelphia: WB Saunders, 1980; pp. 2387-2395.

8. Stimson RL: Eye planes and interocular distance. In Ophthalmic Dispensing, 2nd ed. Springfield: Charles C Thomas, 1971; pp. 134-171.

9. Brown WL: Interpupillary distance. In Eskridge JB, Amos JF, Bartlett JD (eds): Clinical Procedures in Optometry. Philadelphia: JB Lippincott, 1991; pp. 39-52.

10. Hugonnier R, Clayette-Hugonnier S: Strabismus, heterophoria, and ocular motor paralysis. Clinical ocular muscle imbalance. In Veronneau-Troutman (ed). St. Louis: CV Mosby, 1969; pp. 278-285, 641.

11. Griffin JR: Binocular Anomalies. Procedures for Vision Therapy, 2nd ed. Chicago: Professional Press, 1982; pp. 5, 20.

12. Sugar HS: The Extrinsic Eye Muscles. A Manual Prepared for the use of Graduates in Medicine. Section on Instruction Home Study Courses. American Academy of Ophthalmology and Otolaryngology, 5th revision. Omaha: Douglas Printing Co., 1964.

13. Breinin GM: The physiopathology of the "A" and "V" patterns. Trans Am Acad Ophthalmol Otol 1964; 68:363-374.

14. Magee AJ: Minimal values for the A and V syndromes. Am J Ophthalmol 1960; 50:753-756.

15. Stuart JA, Burian HM: Changes in horizontal heterophoria with elevation and depression of gaze. Am J Ophthalmol 1962; 53:274-279.

16. Griffin JR, Boyer FM: Strabismus measurement with the Hirschberg test. Optometric Weekly 1974; 65:863-866.

17. Lang J: The two-pencil test and the new Lang stereotest. Br Orthoptic J 1984; 41:15-21.

18. Lang J: A new fixation device: The Lang Fixation Cube. Binocular Vision 1987; 2:157.

19. Landolt E: Examination of the Eyes. Facsimile of 1879 Edition. New York: Robert E. Krieger Publishing Company, 1979; pp. 47-48.

20. Duane A: A new classification of the motor anomalies of the eye, based upon physiologic principles. Ann Ophthalmol Otol 1896; 5:969-1008.

21. Jampolsky AA: Simplified approach to strabismus diagnosis. In Burian HM, Dunlap EA, Dyer JA, et al. (eds): Symposium on Strabismus, Transactions of the New Orleans Academy of Ophthalmology. St. Louis: CV Mosby, 1971; pp. 49-50.

22. Costenbader F, Bair D, McPhail A: Vision in strabismus: A preliminary report. Arch Ophthalmol 1948; 40:438-453.

23. Raab EL: Amblyopia. In Scott WE, D'Agostino DD, Lennarson LW (eds): Orthoptics and Ocular Examination Techniques. Baltimore: Williams & Wilkins, 1983; p. 77.

24. Day S: History, examination and further investigation. In Taylor D (ed): Pediatric Ophthalmology. Boston: Blackwell Scientific Publications, 1990; pp. 49-50.

25. Fern KD, Manny RE, Burghart C: Resistance to occlusion: Sensitivity to induced blur in 6- to 12-month-old infants. J Am Optom Assoc 1994; 65:651-659.

26. Kaakinen K: A simple method for screening of children with strabismus, anisometropia or ametropia by simultaneous photography of the corneal and the fundus reflexes. Acta Ophthalmol 1979; 57:161-171.

27. Tongue AC, Cibis GW: Bruckner test. Ophthalmology 1981; 88:1041-1044.

28. Griffin JR, Cotter SA: The Bruckner test: Evaluation of clinical usefulness. Am J Optom Physiol Opt 1986; 63:957-961.

29. Abrahamsson M, Fabian G, Sjostrand J: Photorefraction: A useful tool to detect small angle strabismus. Acta Ophthalmol (Copenh) 1986; 64:101-104.

30. Griffin JR, McLin LN, Schor CM: Photographic method for Brückner and Hirschberg testing. Optom Vis Sci 1989; 66:474-479.

31. Archer SM: Developmental aspects of the Bruckner test. Ophthalmology 1988; 95:1098-1101.

32. Roe LD, Guyton DL: The light that leaks: Bruckner and the red reflex. Surv Ophthalmol 1984; 28:665-670.

33. Krimsky E: Effect of a prism on the corneal light reflex. Arch Ophthalmol 1948; 39:351-370.

34. Lennarson LW: Basic examination. In Scott WE, D'Agostino DD, Lennarson LW (eds): Orthoptics and Ocular Examination Techniques. Baltimore: Williams & Wilkins, 1983; p. 228.

35. Krimsky E: The Mangement of Binocular Imbalance. Philadelphia: Lea & Febiger, 1948; pp. 23, 175-184.

36. Flom MC: A minimum strabismus examination. J Am Optom Assoc 1956; 27:642-649

37. Jones R, Eskridge JB: The Hirschberg test—A re-evaluation. Am J Optom Arch Am Acad Optom 1970; 47:105-114.

38. Griffin JR, Boyer FM: Strabismus measurement with the Hirschberg test. Optom Wkly 1974; 65:863-866.

39. Carter AJ, Roth N: Axial length and the Hirschberg test. Am J Optom Physiol Opt 1978; 55:361-364.

40. Brodie SE: Photographic calibration of the Hirschberg test. Invest Ophthalmol Vis Sci 1987; 28:736-742.

41. Eskridge JB, Wick B, Perrigin D: The Hirschberg test: A double-masked clinical evaluation. Am J Optom Physiol Opt 1988; 65:745-750.

42. DeRespinis PA, Naidu E, Brodie SE: Calibration of Hirschberg test photographs under clinical conditions. Ophthalmology 1989; 96:944-949.

43. Owens DA, Leibowitz HW: The fixation point as a stimulus for accommodation. Vision Res 1975; 15:1161-1163.

44. Owens DA, Mohindra I, Hild R: The effectiveness of a retinoscope beam as an accommodative stimulus. Invest Ophthalmol Vis Sci 1980; 19:942-949.

45. Aouchiche K, Dankner SR: What's the difference? Krimsky vs alternate cover testing. Am Orthoptic J 1988; 38:148-150.

46. Wheeler MC: Objective strabismometry in young children. Arch Ophthalmol 1943; 29:720-736.

47. Putnam OA, Quereau JVD: Precisional errors in measurement of squint and phoria. Arch Ophthalmol 1945; 34:7-15.

48. Kandel GL, Grattan PE, Bedell HE: Monocular fixation and acuity in amblyopia and normal eyes. Am J Optom Physiol Opt 1977; 54:598-608.

49. Paliaga GP, Ghisolfi A, Giunta G, et al.: Millimetric cover test—a linear strabismometic technique. J Pediatr Ophthalmol Strabismus 1980; 17:331-336.

50. Parks MM, Eustis AT: Small angle esodeviations. Am Orthoptic J 1962; 12:32-38.

51. Bielschowsky A: Disturbances of the vertical motor

muscles of the eyes. Arch Ophthalmol 1938; 20:175–200.

52. Helveston EM: Dissociated vertical deviation, a clinical and laboratory study. Trans Am Ophthalmol Soc 1981; 78:734–779.
53. Duke-Elder E: System of Ophthalmology. Vol VI, Ocular Motility and Strabismus. St. Louis: CV Mosby, 1973; p. 343–344.
54. Flom MC: Issues in the clinical management of binocular anomalies. In Rosenbloom AA, Morgan MW (eds): Principles and Practice of Pediatric Optometry. Philadelphia: JB Lippincott, 1990; pp. 227–230.
55. Margach CB: Introduction to functional optometry. In: Duncan OK. Optometric Extension Program Foundation, Inc, 1979; p 19.
56. Scobee RG, Green EL: Tests for heterophoria. Reliability of tests, comparisons between tests, and effect of changing testing conditions. Trans Am Acad Ophthalmol Otolaryng 1947; 51:436–451.
57. Amigo G: Signs of binocular inco-ordination. Aust J Optom 1974; 57:358–365.
58. Haines HF: Normal values of visual functions and their application in case analysis. The analysis of findings and determination of normals. Part IV. Am J Optom Arch Am Acad Optom 1941; 18:58–73.
59. Vaegan, Pye D: Independence of convergence and divergence: Norms, age trends, and potentiation in mechanized prism vergence tests. Am J Optom Physiol Opt 1979; 56:143–152.
60. Hoffman LG, Rouse M: Referral recommendations for binocular function and/or developmental perceptual deficiencies. J Am Optom Assoc 1980; 51:119–126.
61. Daum KM, Rutstein RP, Houston G, et al.: Evaluation of a new criterion of binocularity. Optom Vis Sci 1989; 66:218–228.
62. Jackson TW, Goss DA: Variation and correlation of standard clinical phoropter tests of phorias, vergence ranges, and relative accommodation in a sample of school-age children. J Am Optom Assoc 1991; 62:540–547.
63. Letourneau JE, Giroux R: Nongaussian distribution curve of heterophorias among children. Optom Vis Sci 1991; 68:132–137.
64. Betts EA, Austin AS: Seeing problems of school children. Optometric Weekly 1941; 32:369–371.
65. Shepard CF: The most probable "expecteds." Optometric Weekly 1941; 32:538–541.
66. Hirsch MJ: Clinical investigation of a method of testing phoria at forty centimeters. Am J Optom Arch Am Acad Opt 1948; 25:492–495.
67. Hirsch MJ, Alpern M, Schultz HL: The variation of phoria with age. Am J Optom Arch Am Acad Optom 1948; 25:535–541.
68. Soderberg DC: An evaluation in the use of the Maddox rod. J Am Optom Assoc 1968; 39:472–478.
69. Saladin JJ, Sheedy JE: Population study of fixation disparity, heterophoria, and vergence. Am J Optom Physiol Opt 1978; 55:744–750.
70. Morgan MW: The clinical aspects of accommodation and convergence. Am J Optom Arch Am Acad Optom 1944; 21:301–313.
71. Daum KM: Analysis of seven methods of measuring the angle of deviation. Am J Optom Physiol Opt 1983; 60:46–51.
72. Hirsch MJ, Bing LB: The effect of testing method on values obtained for phoria at forty centimeters. Am J Optom Arch Am Acad Optom 1948; 25:407–416.
73. Morris FM: The influence of kinesthesis upon near heterophoria measurements. Am J Optom Arch Am Acad Optom 1960; 37:327–351.
74. Ogle KN, Mussey F, Prangen AD: Fixation disparity and the fusional processes in binocular single vision. Am J Ophthalmol 1949; 32:1069–1087.
75. Schor CM: Fixation disparity and vergence adpatation. In Schor CM, Ciuffreda KJ (eds): Vergence Eye Movements. Basic and Clinical Aspects. Boston: Butterworths, 1983; pp. 465–466.
76. Ogle KN, Martens TG, Dyer JA: Oculomotor Imbalance in Binocular Vision and Fixation Disparity. Philadelphia: Lea & Febiger, 1967; pp. 41, 43, 75–93, 220–228.
77. Sheedy JE, Saladin JJ: Phoria, vergence, and fixation disparity in oculomotor problems. Am J Optom Physiol Opt 1977; 54:474–478.
78. Sheedy JE, Saladin JJ: Association of symptoms with measures of oculomotor deficiencies. Am J Optom Physiol Opt 1978; 55:670–676.
79. Sheedy JE: Fixation disparity analysis of oculomotor imbalance. Am J Optom Physiol Opt 1980; 57:632–639.
80. Sheedy JE: Actual measurement of fixation disparity and its use in diagnosis and treatment. J Am Optom Assoc 1980; 51:1079–1084.
81. London RF, Wick B: Vertical fixation disparity correction: Effect on the horizontal forced-vergence fixation disparity curve. Am J Optom Physiol Opt 1987; 64:653–656.
82. Ogle KN, Prangen AD: Further considerations of fixation disparity and the binocular fusional processes. Am J Ophthalmol 1951; 34:57–72.
83. Mitchell AM, Ellerbrock VJ: Fixational disparity and the maintenance of fusion in the horizontal meridian. Am J Optom Physiol Opt Arch Am Acad Optom 1955; 32:520–535.
84. Schor CM: The influence of rapid prism adaptation upon fixation disparity. Vis Res 1979; 19:757–765.
85. Schor CM: The relationship between fusional vergence eye movements and fixation disparity. Vis Res 1979; 19:1359–1367.
86. Duane A: Motor anomalies of the eye. The relative value of the tests used in diagnosing them. NY Med J 1914; 99(9):409–416.
87. Scobee RG: The Oculorotary Muscles, 2nd ed. Saint Louis: CV Mosby, 1952; pp. 348–352.
88. Davies CE: Etiology and management of convergence insufficiency. Am Orthoptic J 1956; 6:124–127.
89. Mohindra I, Molinari J: Convergence insufficiency: Its diagnosis and management. Part I. Optom Mon 1980; 73:155–160.
90. Christenson GN, Winkelstein AM: Visual skills of athletes versus nonathletes: Development of a sports vision testing battery. J Am Optom Assoc 1988; 59:666–675.
91. Buzzelli AR: Vergence facility: Developmental trends in a school age population. Am J Optom Physiol Opt 1986; 63:351–355.
92. Rosner J: Pediatric Optometry. Boston: Butterworth, 1982; pp. 264–266.
93. Giles GH: The principles and practice of refraction and its allied subjects, 2nd ed. Philadelphia: Chilton Co., 1965; p. 223.
94. Vaegan: Convergence and divergence show large and sustained improvement after short isometric exercise. Am J Optom Physiol Opt 1979; 56:23–33.
95. Sheard C: Zones of ocular comfort. Am J Optom 1930; 7:9–25.
96. Borish IM: Clinical Refraction, 3rd ed. Chicago: The Professional Press, 1975; p. 872.
97. Percival AS: The Prescribing of Spectacles. Bristol: John Wright & Sons, 1928; p. 125.
98. Tubis RA: An evaluation of vertical divergence tests on the basis of fixation disparity. Am J Optom Arch Am Acad Optom 1954; 31:624–635.
99. Crindland N: The measurement of heterophoria. Br J Ophthalmol 1941; 25:141–167.

100. Morgan MW: The direction of visual lines when fusion is broken as in duction tests. Am J Optom Arch Am Acad Optom 1947; 24:8-12.

101. Alpern M: The after effect of lateral duction testing on subsequent phoria measurements. Am J Optom Arch Am Acad Optom 1946; 23:442-447.

102. Ellerbrock VJ: Tonicity induced by fusional movements. Am J Optom Arch Am Acad Optom 1950; 27:8-20.

103. Houtman WA, Roze JH, Scheper W: Vertical vergence movements. Doc Ophthalmol 1981; 51:199-207.

104. Alpern M, Kincaid WM, Lubeck MJ: Vergence and accommodation: III. Proposed definitions of the AC/A ratios. Am J Ophthalmol 1959; 48:141-148.

105. Flom MC: Treatment of binocular anomalies of vision. *In* Hirsch MJ, Wick RE (eds): Vision of Children. Philadelphia: Chilton Co., 1963; p. 216.

106. Ogle KN, Martens TG: On the accommodative convergence and the proximal convergence. Arch Ophthalmol 1957; 57:702-715.

107. Tait EF: Accommodative convergence. Am J Ophthalmol 1951; 34:1093-1107.

108. Howard HJ: A test for the judgment of distance. Am J Ophthalmol 1919; 2:656-675.

109. Ogle KN: Researches in Binocular Vision. New York: Hafner Publishing, 1972; p. 134.

110. Ogle KN: On the limits of stereoscopic vision. J Exp Psychol 1952; 44:253-259.

111. Westheimer G, Tanzman IJ: Qualitative depth localization with diplopic images. J Opt Soc Am 1956; 46:116-117.

112. Asher H: Suppression theory of binocular vision. Br J Ophthalmol 1953; 37:37-39.

113. Wolfe JM: Stereopsis and binocular rivalry. Psychol Rev 1986; 93:269-282.

114. Kaufman L: On the nature of binocular disparity. Am J Psychol 1964; 77:393-402.

115. Parks MM: The monofixation syndrome. *In* Burian HM, Dunlap EA, Dyer JA, et al. (eds): Symposium on Strabismus. Transactions of the New Orleans Academy of Ophthalmology. St. Louis: CV Mosby, 1971; pp. 121-153.

116. Lang J: A new stereotest. J Pediatr Ophthalmol Strabismus 1983; 20:72-74.

117. Cooper J, Warshowsky J: Lateral displacement as a response cue in the Titmus Stereo Test. Am J Optom Physiol Opt 1977; 54:537-541.

118. Julesz B: Foundations of Cyclopean Perception. Chicago: University of Chicago Press, 1971.

119. Simons K, Reinecke RD: A reconsideration of amblyopia screening and stereopsis. Am J Ophthalmol 1974; 78:707-713.

120. Rutstein RP, Eskridge JB: Stereopsis in small-angle strabismus. Am J Optom Physiol Opt 1984; 61:491-498.

121. Johnstone R, Brown S: A comparative assessment of the Lang, T.N.O. and Titmus stereo tests. Aust Orthoptic J 1985; 22:27-30.

122. Lang JI, Lang TJ: Eye screening with the Lang Stereotest. Am Orthoptic J 1988; 38:48-50.

123. Cooper J, Feldman J: Random-Dot-Stereogram performance by strabismic, amblyopic, and ocular pathology patients in an operant-discrimination task. Am J Optom Physiol Opt 1978; 55:599-609.

124. Verhoeff FH: Simple quantitative test for acuity and reliability of binocular stereopsis. Arch Ophthalmol 1942; 28:1000-1019.

125. Simons K: A comparison of the Frisby, Random-Dot E, TNO and Randot Circles stereotests in screening and office use. Arch Ophthalmol 1981; 99:446-452.

126. Cooper J, Feldman J: Assessing the Frisby stereotest under monocular viewing conditions. J Am Optom Assoc 1979; 50:807-809.

127. Simmerman JS: Absolute threshold of stereopsis using the Frisby stereotest. J Am Optom Assoc 1984; 55:50-53.

128. Levy NS, Glick EB: Stereoscopic perception and Snellen visual acuity. Am J Ophthalmol 1974; 78:722-724.

129. Westheimer G, McKee SP: Stereoscopic acuity with defocused and spatially filtered retinal images. J Opt Soc Am 1980; 70:772-778.

130. Goodwin RT, Romano PE: Stereoacuity degradation by experimental and real monocular and binocular amblyopia. Invest Ophthalmol Vis Sci 1985; 26:917-923.

131. Simons K: Stereoacuity norms in young children. Arch Ophthalmol 1981; 99:439-445.

132. Heron G, Dholakia S, Collins DE, et al.: Stereoscopic threshold in children and adults. Am J Optom Physiol Opt 1985; 62:505-515.

133. Manny RE, Martinez AT, Fern KD: Testing stereopsis in the preschool child: Is it clinically useful? J Pediatr Ophthalmol Strabismus 1991; 28:223-231.

134. Hofstetter HW, Bertsch JD: Does stereopsis change with age? Am J Optom Physiol Opt 1976; 53:664-667.

135. Reading RW, Tanlamai T: Finely graded binocular disparities from random-dot stereograms. Ophthalmic Physiol Opt 1982; 2:47-56.

136. Fox R, Patterson R, Francis EL: Stereoacuity in young children. Invest Ophthalmol Vis Sci 1986; 27:598-600.

137. Scott WE, Mash J: Stereoacuity in normal individuals. Ann Ophthalmol 1974; 6:99-101.

138. Hofstetter HW: Absolute threshold measurements with the Diastereo test. Arch Soc Amer Oftal Optom 1968; 6:327-342.

139. Reading RW: Binocular Vision: Foundation and Applications. Boston: Butterworth-Heinemann, 1983; pp. 173-217.

140. Cooper J, Feldman J, Medlin D: Comparing stereoscopic performance of children using the Titmus, TNO, and Randot stereo tests. J Am Optom Assoc 1979; 50:821-825.

141. Birch EE, Gwiazda J, Held R: Stereoacuity development for crossed and uncrossed disparities in human infants. Vision Res 1982; 22:507-513.

142. Marsh WR, Rawlings SC, Mumma JV: Evaluation of clinical stereoacuity tests. Ophthalmology 1980; 87:1265-1272.

143. Hall C: The relationship between clinical stereotests. Ophthal Physiol Opt 1982; 2:135-143.

144. Tillson G: Two new clinical tests for stereopsis. Am Orthoptic J 1985; 35:126-134.

145. Garzia RP, Richman JE: Stereopsis in an amblyopic small angle esotrope. J Am Optom Assoc 1985; 56:400-404.

146. Ciner EB, Schanel-Klitsche E, Herzberg C: Stereoacuity development: 6 months to 5 years. A new tool for testing and screening. Optom Vis Sci 1996; 73:43-48.

147. Rosner J: A procedure for measuring the near-point fusional vergence reserves of young children. J Am Optom Assoc 1979; 50:473-474.

148. Rosner J, Rosner J: Pediatric Optometry. 2nd ed. Boston: Butterworth, 1990; pp. 269-271.

149. Grisham JD: Treatment of binocular dysfunctions. *In* Schor CM, Ciuffreda KJ (eds): Vergence eye movements: Basic and Clinical Aspects. Boston: Butterworth, 1983; pp. 610-612.

150. Wesson MD: Normalization of prism bar vergences. Am J Optom Physiol Opt 1982; 59:628-634.

151. Scheiman M, Herzberg H, Frantz K, et al.: A normative study of step vergence in elementary schoolchildren. J Am Optom Assoc 1989; 60:276-280.

152. Amigo G: Preschool vision study. Br J Ophthalmol 1973; 52:125-132.

153. Zhou Y, Yuan N, Li J, Liu M: Comparison of the stereovisual acuity, Randot stereotests, Frisby stereotest, Wirt test, TNO test of 442 normal children with stereovisual

test chart. Ye Ko Hsueh Pao [Eye Science] 1988; 4:60–64.

154. Williams S, Simpson A, Silva PA: Stereoacuity levels and vision problems in children from 7 to 11 years. Ophthalmic Physiol Opt 1988; 8:386–389.

155. Helveston EM, von Noorden GK: Microtropia: A newly defined entity. Arch Ophthalmol 1967; 78:272–281.

156. Epstein DL, Tredici TJ: Microtropia (monofixation syndrome) in flying personnel. Am J Ophthalmol 1973; 76:832–841.

157. Frisby JP, Mein J, Saye A, et al.: Use of random-dot stereograms in the clinical assessment of strabismic patients. Br J Ophthalmol 1975; 59:545–552.

158. Hill M, Perry J, Wood ICJ: Stereoacuity in microtropia. *In* Moore S, Mein J, Stockbridge L (eds): Orthoptics Past Present Future. Transactions of the Third International Orthoptic Congress, Boston, July 1–3, 1975, pp. 25–29. New York: Stratton Intercontinental Medical Book Corp., 1976.

159. Broadbent H, Westall C: An evaluation of techniques for measuring stereopsis in infants and young children. Ophthalmic Physiol Opt 1990; 10:3–7.

160. Harwerth RS, Smith EL III, Duncan GC, et al.: Multiple sensitive periods in the development of the primate visual system. Science 1986; 232:235–238.

161. Harwerth RS, Smith EL III, Crawford MLJ, von Noorden GK: Behavioral studies of the sensitive periods of development of visual functions in monkeys. Behav Brain Res 1990; 41:179–198.

162. Vaegan, Taylor D: Critical period for deprivation amblyopia in children. Trans Ophthalmol Soc UK 1979; 99:432–439.

163. Costenbader FD: The physiology and management of divergent strabismus. *In* Allen JH (ed): Strabismus, Ophthalmic Symposium. St. Louis: CV Mosby, 1950; p. 353.

164. Costenbader FD: The management of convergent strabismus. *In* Allen JH (ed): Strabismus, Ophthalmic Symposium. St. Louis: CV Mosby, 1950; p. 338.

165. Parks MM: Abnormal accommodative convergence in squint. Arch Ophthalmol 1958; 59:364–380.

166. Rutstein RP: Fixation switch: An unusual cause for adolescent and adult onset diplopia. J Am Optom Assoc 1985; 56:862–865.

167. von Noorden GK: Bowman lecture. Current concepts of infantile esotropia. Eye 1988; 2(Pt-4):343–357.

168. Helveston EM: 19th Annual Frank Costenbader Lecture: The origins of congenital esotropia. J Pediatr Ophthalmol Strab 1993; 30:215–232.

169. Brock FW: Visual Training. Optometric Weekly 1952; 43:1641–1645.

170. Flom MC, Bedell HE: Identifying amblyopia using associated conditions, acuity, and nonacuity features. Am J Optom Physiol Opt 1985; 62:153–160.

171. Tanlamai T, Goss DA: Prevalence of monocular amblyopia among anisometropes. Am J Optom Physiol Opt 1979; 56:704–715.

172. Abraham SV: Bilateral ametropic amblyopia. J Pediatr Ophthalmol 1964; 1:57–61.

173. Fern KD: Visual acuity outcome in isometropic hyperopia. Optom Vis Sci 1989; 66:649–658.

174. France TD: Amblyopia. *In* Isenberg SJ (ed): The Eye in Infancy. Chicago: Year Book Medical Publishers, 1989; p. 103.

175. Mitchell DE, Freeman R, Millodot M, Haegerstrom G: Meridional amblyopia: Evidence for modification of the human visual system by early visual experience. Vision Res 1973; 13:535–538.

176. Reese AB, Ellsworth RM: The anterior chamber cleavage syndrome. Arch Ophthalmol 1966; 75:307–318.

177. Waring GO, Rodrigues MM, Laibson PR: Anterior chamber cleavage syndrome. A stepladder classification. Surv Ophthalmol 1975; 20:3–27.

178. Hofmann RF, Paul TO, Pentelei-Molnar J: The management of corneal birth trauma. J Pediatr Ophthalmol Strab 1981; 18(1):45–47.

179. Barkan O: Pathogenesis of congenital glaucoma. Gonioscopic and anatomic observation of the angle of the anterior chamber in the normal eye and in congenital glaucoma. Am J Ophthalmol 1955; 40(1):1–11.

180. DeLuise VP, Anderson DR: Primary infantile glaucoma (congenital glaucoma). Surv Ophthalmol 1983; 28:1–19.

181. Wagner RS: Glaucoma in children. Pediatr Clin North Am 1993; 40:855–867.

182. Lloyd IC, Goss-Sampson M, Jeffrey BG, et al.: Neonatal cataract: Aetiology, pathogenesis and management. Eye 1992; 6(Pt-2):184–196.

183. Endres W, Shin YS: Cataract and metabolic disease. J Inher Metab Dis 1990; 13:509–516.

184. Jones WL: Traumatic injury to the lens. Optom Clin 1991; 1:125–142.

185. Ajamian PC: Traumatic cataract. Optom Clin 1993; 3:49–56.

186. Pruett RC, Schepens CL: Posterior hyperplastic primary vitreous. Am J Ophthalmol 1970; 69:534–543.

187. Haik BG: Advanced Coats' disease. Trans Am Ophthalmol Soc 1991; 89:371–476.

188. Kaur B, Taylor D: Fundus hemorrhages in infancy. Surv Ophthalmol 1992; 37:1–17.

189. Pagon RA: Ocular coloboma. Surv Ophthalmol 1981; 25:223–236.

190. Warburg M: An update on microphthalmos and coloboma. A brief survey of genetic disorders with microphthalmos and coloboma. Ophthal Paediatr Gen 1991; 12:57–63.

191. Schroeder R, Mets MB, Maumenee IH: Leber's congenital amaurosis. Retrospective review of 43 cases and a new fundus finding in two cases. Arch Ophthalmol 1987; 105:356–359.

192. Lambert SR, Taylor D, Kriss A: The infant with nystagmus, normal appearing fundi, but an abnormal ERG. Surv Ophthalmol 1989; 34:173–186.

193. Heher KL, Traboulsi EI, Maumenee IH: The natural history of Leber's congenital amaurosis. Age-related findings in 35 patients. Ophthalmology 1992; 9:241–245.

194. Abramson DH, Servodidio CA: Retinoblastoma. Optom Clin 1993; 3:49–61.

195. Abramson DH: Retinoblastoma 1990: Diagnosis, treatment and implications. Pediatr Ann 1990; 19:387–395.

196. Molk R: Ocular toxocariasis: A review of the literature. Ann Ophthalmol 1983; 15:216–219.

197. Shields JA: Ocular toxocariasis. A review. Surv Ophthalmol 1984; 28:361–381.

198. Rothova A: Ocular involvement in toxoplasmosis. Br J Ophthalmol 1993; 77:371–377.

199. Primo SA: Infectious and inflammatory diseases. Optom Clin 1994; 3:99–127.

200. Jabs DA: Ocular toxoplasmosis. Int Ophthalmol Clin 1990; 30:264–270.

201. Quinn GE: Retinopathy of prematurity: Natural history and classification. *In* Flynn JT, Tasman W (eds): Retinopathy of Prematurity. A Clinician's Guide. New York: Springer-Verlag, 1992; pp. 7–22.

202. Kalina RE: Nursery examination of the premature infant. *In* Flynn JT, Tasman W (eds): Retinopathy of Prematurity. A Clinician's Guide. New York: Springer-Verlag, 1992; pp. 37–43.

203. Phelps DL: Retinopathy of prematurity. Curr Prob Pediat 1992; 22:349–371.

204. Jain IS, Singh YP, Grupta SL, et al.: Ocular hazards during birth. J Pediatr Ophthalmol Strab 1980; 17:14–20.

205. Eagling EM: Ocular damage after blunt trauma to the eye. Its relationship to the nature of the injury. Br J Ophthalmol 1974; 58:126–140.

206. Harley RD: Ocular manifestations of child abuse. J Pediatr Ophthalmol Strab 1980; 17:5–13.

207. Smith SK: Child abuse and neglect: A diagnostic guide for the optometrist. J Am Optom Assoc 1988; 59:760–766.

208. Awan KJ: Ganglionic neuroretinal aplasia and hypoplasia: Aplasia and hypoplasia of optic nerve. Ann Ophthalmol 1976; 8:1193–1202.

209. Francois J, De Rouck A: Electroretinographical study of the hypoplasia of the optic nerve. Ophthalmologica 1976; 172:308–330.

210. Skarf B, Hoyt CS: Optic nerve hypoplasia in children. Association with anomalies of the endocrine and CNS. Arch Ophthalmol 1984; 102:62–67.

211. Ouvrier R, Billson F: Optic nerve hypoplasia: A review. J Child Neurol 1986; 1:181–188.

212. Ouvrier RA: Pallor of the optic disc in children. Aust NZ J Ophthalmol 1990; 18:375–379.

213. Apple DJ, Rabb MF, Walsh PM: Congenital anomalies of the optic disc. Surv Ophthalmol 1982; 27:3–41.

214. Hoyt WF, Baghdassarian SA: Optic glioma of childhood. Natural history and rationale for conservative management. Br J Ophthalmol 1969; 53:793–798.

215. Eggers H, Jakobiec FA, Jones IS: Tumors of the optic nerve. Doc Ophthalmol 1976; 41:43–128.

216. Alvord EC, Lofton S: Gliomas of the optic nerve or chiasm. Outcome by patients' age, tumor site, and treatment. J Neurosurg 1988; 68:85–98.

217. Dutton JJ: Gliomas of the anterior visual pathway. Surv Ophthalmol 1994; 38:427–452.

218. Sher PK: Neurologic disorders associated with visual loss in childhood. Neurol Clin 1985; 3:3–17.

219. Kline LB, Morawetz RB, Swaid SN: Indirect injury of the optic nerve. Neurosurg 1984; 14:756–764.

220. Zimmerman RA, Bilaniuk LT: Pediatric head trauma. Neuroimaging Clin North Am 1994; 4:349–366.

221. Brown JK, Minns RA: Non-accidental head injury, with particular reference to whiplash shaking injury and medico-legal aspects. Devel Med Child Neurol 1993; 35:849–869.

222. France TD: Strabismus in hydrocephalus. Am Orthopt J 1975; 25:101–105.

223. Wybar K, Walker J: Surgical management of strabismus in hydrocephalus. Trans Ophthalmol Soc UK 1980; 100:475–478.

224. Holman RE, Merritt JC: Infantile esotropia: Results in the neurologic impaired and "normal" child at NCMH (six years). J Pediatr Ophthalmol Strab 1986; 23:41–45.

225. Hamed LM, Fang EN, Fanous MM, et al.: The prevalence of neurologic dysfunction in children with strabismus who have superior oblique overaction. Ophthalmology 1993; 10:1483–1487.

*Joseph T. Barr, OD, MS*

7

# The Cornea

The cornea is the most important refractive element of the eye. A clear, regular cornea with a normal precorneal tear film is critical, not only for normal vision and eye health but to support contact lens wear. Therefore, examination of the cornea to identify normal variations and to diagnose, treat, and manage disease is a substantial portion of optometric practice. The purpose of this chapter is to completely describe the optometric examination, measurement, and documentation of the cornea.

## Corneal Physiology

The corneal endothelium receives its oxygen, glucose, and other important nutrients from the aqueous humor. The epithelium receives its oxygen from the tears and the air. Limbal blood vessels provide nutrients and oxygen only to the peripheral cornea. Carbon dioxide is vented from the epithelium into the tears, and lactate from the epithelium is released toward the endothelium. During contact lens wear, hypoxia causes anaerobic glycolysis, and excess lactate compromises the normal endothelial bicarbonate pump, which maintains normal corneal deturgescence.

Nearly similar indices of refraction and regular organization of the collagen lamellae in the stroma along with normal endothelial pump activity and the epithelial barrier function provide for corneal transparency. Corneal swelling or clouding may occur as a result of hypotonic tearing, exposure to water, or hypoxia.

After the epithelium is compromised, it may heal in minutes to hours or days, depending on the size of the abrasion caused by sliding of the epithelial cells and mitosis of the basal epithelium. This assumes that the limbal basal stem cells are viable because compromise of these cells or disease within the corneal anterior limiting (Bowman's) layer and stroma may result in corneal scarring.

The corneal endothelial cells do not divide in the adult and may become pleomorphic or demonstrate polymegethism after long-term use of relatively oxygen-impermeable contact lenses or in Fuchs' dystrophy.

Under closed-eye conditions, the tears become more acidic (below 7.3 or 7.4 pH), the tears and ocular surface are warmer, and the oxygen for the cornea is provided by the blood vessels in the palpebral conjunctiva. Only about one-third of the normal 21% oxygen (155 mm Hg) is available to the cornea during sleep. This results in about 4% overnight corneal swelling.[1]

## Overall or Gross Examination of the Cornea

Diffuse light from a source such as an overhead lamp, a penlight, a transilluminator, or—in an emergency—a flashlight, can be used to determine generally whether the cornea is clear, free of large scars, wet, clear (of debris, large foreign body, laceration, or exudate), and generally regular in shape. Angle kappa and Hirschberg results (see Chapter 6) can be determined with this type of illumination, and general observations such as large corneal leukomas, furrows, gross pannus, or Munson's sign of keratoconus are also possible with overall inspection with or without a magnifying lens or loupe.

The corneal diameter or horizontal visible iris diameter can be assessed with a ruler, and the relationship of the corneal vertical dimension to the upper and lower eyelid margins can also be observed and recorded. These last two observations may be helpful for the diagnosis of ptosis and in contact lens fitting for the selection of lens diameter and assessment of bifocal contact lens type. The clinician may draw a diagram of where the eyelid margins rest on the cornea in primary gaze. A reticule within the slit-lamp eyepiece may also be used for these measurement tasks.

## Precorneal Tear Film Examination and Measurement

The precorneal tear film forms the first refracting surface of the eye. Thus, its regularity and consistency are critical to normal visual function. The corneal epithelium and tear film depend on one another for normal function. The tear film is in intimate contact with the epithelial surface of the cornea except when the tear film ruptures and dry spots form on the epithelium. This tear film break-up can be observed *invasively*, after instilling fluorescein, or *noninvasively* with special illumination or with a keratometer. The Tear Scope (Keeler Instruments, Inc., Broomall, PA), which projects diffuse light on the cornea, noninvasively measures the tear break-up time over the entire corneal surface, whereas the keratometer is limited to the central cornea. After fluorescein instillation, the tear film break-up time can be determined with a Burton lamp or slit lamp using the cobalt filter:

□ Have the patient blink three times, then ask the patient to hold his or her eye open.
□ Measure the time in seconds until the first rupture in the tear film is seen (a black area if using fluorescein).
□ Repeat two times.
□ Record the median time in seconds.

Normal tear break-up time findings are 10 to 15 seconds. Lower values are highly predictive of dry eye (unless a contact lens has just been removed, then tear break-up time is always abnormally low), but normal values may or may not indicate the presence or absence of dry eye.[2]

Contact lens front surface break-up time can also be determined noninvasively. For soft contact lenses, a normal tear break-up time is 10 seconds or not more than 25% less than the pre–contact lens findings. Tear film debris, the height of the lower tear prism (normal is 0.22 mm or greater), and the tear lipid layer interference patterns can be observed with a slit lamp. Special instruments that create interference patterns on the cornea with specific wavelength light sources may be used to assess tear film break-up and thickness.[3]

## SCHIRMER TEST

Although the Schirmer test is advised for the comprehensive evaluation of a dry eye suspect, the test is highly unreliable. The Schirmer test is done without anesthetic and employs filter paper (commercially available with a notch where the filter paper should be folded), inserted behind the lower lateral eyelid margin while the patient fixates away from the strip. After five minutes, the distance from the fold to the end of wetting of the strip is measured. Dry eye patients wet less than 5 mm of the strip.[4] However, dry eye patients may have reflex tearing and wet *more* than 5 mm of the strip. The Schirmer Test II is performed after corneal anesthesia and is designed to test only basic tear secretion and not reflex secretion.

More recently, a phenol red, cotton thread test (Menicon, Clovis, CA) has improved upon the Schirmer test. A value of less than 9 mm of wetting is considered diagnostic of dry eye. The test takes only 15 seconds.[5]

## LACRIMAL LAKE TEST OR TEAR PRISM HEIGHT

Using the slit-lamp biomicroscope with a 1- to 2-mm wide beam and just enough illumination to

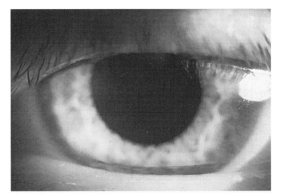

**FIGURE 7–1**  Tear prism along lower eyelid margin.

see the lacrimal lake well, the height from the top of the lower lid margin to the top of the lacrimal lake (tear prism) can be estimated (Fig. 7-1). This test can be performed with or without fluorescein. The practitioner is advised to use a precision reticule to learn what value is considered indicative of dry eye.[6]

# Keratometry

Measurement of corneal curvature is important to estimate refractive astigmatism, to obtain an impression of axial versus refractive ametropia, and to estimate the base curve needed in fitting rigid contact lenses. Irregular astigmatism found with refractive surgery, trauma, keratoconus, keratoglobus, or pellucid marginal degeneration or from contact lens wear can be assessed qualitatively with the keratometer* (Fig. 7-2).

*Although the term keratometer originally referred to a specific ophthalmometer made by Bausch & Lomb, keratometer has become the common jargon of practitioners. The word is used here in place of ophthalmometer for that reason.

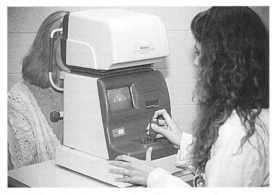

**FIGURE  7–2**  Automated  refractometer-keratometer measures central corneal curvature, estimates peripheral corneal curvature, and simultaneously provides ocular refraction.

The principle of keratometry relies on the reflective optical properties of the cornea. An object placed in front of the cornea produces a virtual image due to the diverging reflective properties of the cornea, which are a function of the corneal radius of curvature. For a given object distance, the location and hence the size of this image depends on the reflecting power of the cornea. One approach is to measure the height of the image using a reticule within a magnifying optical system. Such an approach is difficult, in part because of the continual, small, involuntary eye movements made by the patient. These eye movements may be negated by using the *doubling principle*. The reflected image is split into two images using a semisilvered mirror and a series of prisms. The relative displacement of the two images is adjusted until the top of one image is coincident with the bottom of the second, as described below.

Figure 7-3A shows the mires as viewed from the practitioner's side of a conventional keratometer. The task is to align the mires at the 9 o'clock position of the lower right hand circle to measure the horizontal meridian and at the 12 o'clock position of the lower right hand circle to measure the vertical meridian (Fig. 7-3B).

The specific procedure is as follows:

- □ Ask the patient to place his or her chin in the chin rest and forehead against the headrest.
- □ Have the patient fixate on the reflected image of his or her eye or the target in the instrument.
- □ With the keratometer in the straight-ahead position, sight down the outside of the instrument and adjust the instrument vertically until the leveling sight is aligned with the patient's temporal canthus.
- □ Occlude the eye not being tested. Release the knob for locking the instrument and rotate the instrument until it points directly at the eye to be tested. Instruct the patient to look into the instrument where he or she sees a reflection of his or her own eye.
- □ Adjust the focus of the instrument until the image of the mires is clear.
- □ Make fine vertical and horizontal adjustments necessary to place the reticule cross near the center of the lower right mire image.
- □ Lock the instrument in place.
- □ Rotate the instrument (to locate the horizontal or near horizontal principal meridian) until the horizontal bars of the two crosses to the left of the focusing mire are aligned. Maintain clarity of the image during this step by continual refinement of the focus.
- □ Turn the horizontal measuring knob (on the left of the instrument) until these two crosses are superimposed.
- □ Direct attention to the two horizontal lines above the focusing mire, and turn the vertical measuring knob (on the right of the instrument) until these lines are superimposed.
- □ Record the median readings as:
- □ 43.00/44.75 @ 090, mires regular or distorted, or
- □ 43.00 @ 180 44.75 @ 090, mires regular or distorted.

The keratometer measures an area of the central cornea with a diameter of approximately 3.50 to 3.75 mm. Using a fixation system or having the patient fixate on the "pluses" or "minuses" on the keratometer may assist the practitioner in estimating peripheral corneal curvature. Curvatures approaching 50.00 D should raise the suspicion of keratoconus, and inferior steepening and/or excess superior flattening may indicate a keratoconus suspect. Automated ophthalmometers may add an assessment of corneal asphericity as well as an apical radius of curvature estimate. If the corneal curvature is too

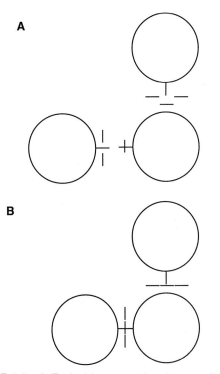

A

B

**FIGURE 7-3** *A,* Typical keratometric mires as viewed through the eyepiece. *B,* Keratometric mires aligned to measure the horizontal and vertical meridians.

steep, a plus lens can be placed over the opening on the mire face of the standard keratometer and secured with tape or special lens holders. A minus lens can be placed for curvature flatter than the standard range. Table 7–1 provides the values for extending the range of the keratometer with a +1.25 ophthalmic trial lens.[1] A hand-held keratometer (Alcon Laboratories, Ft. Worth, TX) is available for general patient use, which provides access to bedridden, obese, aged, or young patients who may otherwise be difficult to position in a typical instrument stand or table-mounted keratometer.

# Corneal Topography and Videokeratography

. . . . . . . . . . . . . . . . . . . . . . . . .
## QUALITATIVE ASSESSMENT OF CORNEAL SHAPE

The assessment of corneal shape can be as qualitative as using the reflection of the curved end of a paper clip off the cornea to the observation of a Placido's disc (Keeler Instruments, Inc.) image. One should recall that the normal corneal surface is steepest centrally and flattens asymmetrically in the periphery, simulating an irregular ellipse with an eccentricity value of 0.5. Superimposed on this asymmetrical aspherical geometry may be regular surface toricity or irregular surface toricity. In abnormal corneal shape, certain patterns may be pathognomonic for certain conditions.*

## PLACIDO'S DISC AND OTHER HAND-HELD CONCENTRIC RING OPTIONS

The examiner holds Placido's disc in the hand like a direct ophthalmoscope and views the rings reflected off the cornea through the lens in the center of Placido's disc. One should note the circularity and concentricity of the reflected rings in all meridians from central to peripheral rings. Circular rings indicate a regular spherical central cornea with regular peripheral corneal flattening. Oval-shaped rings indicate regular corneal toricity, with the steep meridian showing

---

*For example, in keratoconus patients and patients wearing flat-fitted, high-riding rigid contact lenses, the cornea may be steepest below the geometrical center of the cornea. In patients with pellucid marginal degeneration, the cornea shows marked against-the-rule astigmatism, with the horizontal meridian steeper in curvature.

**TABLE 7–1** Curves for Extending the Keratometer's Range With a +1.25 D Lens Over the Objective*

| Drum Reading With +1.25 D Lens Over Objective (D) | Corneal Power (D) |
|---|---|
| 43.00 | 50.12 |
| 43.25 | 50.37 |
| 43.50 | 50.75 |
| 43.75 | 51.00 |
| 44.00 | 51.25 |
| 44.25 | 51.62 |
| 44.50 | 51.87 |
| 44.75 | 52.12 |
| 45.00 | 52.50 |
| 45.25 | 52.75 |
| 45.50 | 53.00 |
| 45.75 | 53.37 |
| 46.00 | 53.62 |
| 46.25 | 53.87 |
| 46.50 | 54.25 |
| 47.00 | 54.75 |
| 47.25 | 55.12 |
| 47.50 | 55.37 |
| 47.75 | 55.62 |
| 48.00 | 56.00 |
| 48.25 | 56.25 |
| 48.50 | 56.50 |
| 48.75 | 56.87 |
| 49.00 | 57.12 |
| 49.25 | 57.50 |
| 49.50 | 57.75 |
| 49.75 | 58.00 |
| 50.00 | 58.25 |
| 50.25 | 58.50 |
| 50.50 | 58.87 |
| 50.75 | 59.12 |
| 51.00 | 59.50 |
| 51.25 | 59.75 |
| 51.50 | 60.00 |
| 51.75 | 60.37 |
| 52.00 | 60.62 |

*Rounded to the nearest 0.12 D.
From Mandell RB: Contact Lens Practice. Springfield, IL: Charles C Thomas, 1988.

"bunching" (less separation) of the rings. Rings that are more separated indicate the flatter meridian or axis of the steep meridian. The hand-held keratoscope designed for operating room use (Fig. 7–4) is held close to the patient's eyelids while the practitioner views through the center of the cone with the slit-lamp. The slit beam should be wide open, illuminating the rings from the side. The ring reflections from the cornea are observed to assess regularity, toricity, and displacement of the corneal apex where the steepened areas appear as bunched ring segments.

## CORNEASCOPE

The corneascope provides a Polaroid photograph keratoscopic image and photodocuments the

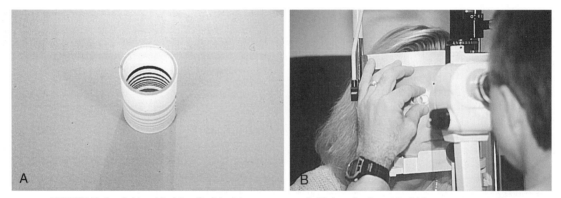

**FIGURE 7–4**   *A*, Hand-held cylindrical keratoscope. *B*, Using the hand-held keratoscope at the slit lamp.

patient's corneal diameter, iris color, and degree of bulbar conjunctival injection.

Corneascope photographs (Fig. 7–5) show corneal toricity and irregularity qualitatively and can be analyzed with a proprietary device (KeraScan) that measures the distance to the peripheral rings to estimate peripheral corneal curvature. However, this method has largely been replaced by modern computerized videokeratography.

## VIDEOKERATOGRAPHY

Computerized videokeratography is made possible by use of a curved Placido's disc or cone-shaped ring object to reflect rings off the cornea which are captured by a video system. Then, through the use of a "frame grabber" and a computer, the distances to many peripheral corneal points on the rings are determined to calculate peripheral corneal curvature and estimate peripheral corneal "power." When performing videokeratography, the clinician provides the necessary commands to the computer to prepare for image capture and carefully positions the patient

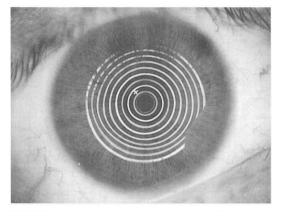

**FIGURE 7–5**   Representative corneascope Polaroid image.

behind the videokeratoscope. The patient is asked to fixate on a light within the system and to open his or her eye wide to prevent the upper eyelid from obscuring the superior corneal image. Multiple images are obtained and observed on the computer monitor until a clinically acceptable or optimal image is obtained. This image may then be stored for future reference and/or the results plotted to produce a color map or other output to be placed in the patient record or sent to another practitioner. Numerous outputs are available, including plots using normalized scales (curvatures are colored according to the average central curvature for that eye such that for most systems the central colors are similar regardless of how flat or how steep) and absolute (curvatures are always color-coded the same color) maps. Most clinicians prefer the absolute map (Fig. 7–6).

Although the peripheral curvature and power values are valuable for qualitative evaluation of the corneal shape, they should not be perceived as a precise map of corneal shape. For example, the radii may be only sagittal or axial radii, and powers calculated from these values may be of limited value for only one peripheral corneal radius.[7] Maps obtained from these systems (Fig. 7–7) may have blank areas where the cornea is too wrinkled for the frame grabber to find a reflected image for analysis. They also average from one zone to the next on the cornea, which results in some curve "smoothing" and stair steepening of the image. In some cases the system assumes that the cornea is a modified elliptical surface, whereas other systems assume that the cornea can flatten and then steepen again in a relatively short distance.

Benefits of videokeratography include the rapid evaluation of corneal shape for qualitative evaluation, especially the location and curvature of the apex in keratoconus. Some systems provide artificial intelligence programs for rigid con-

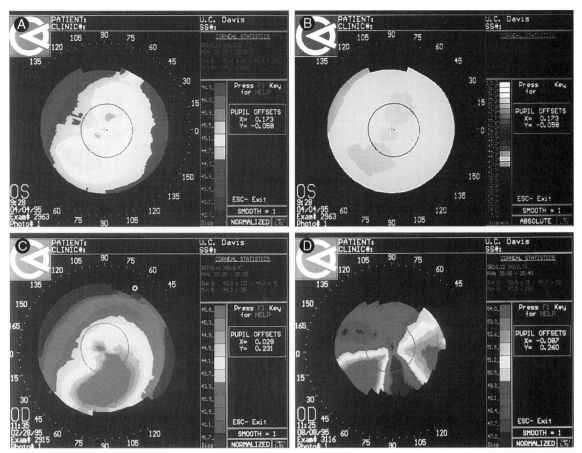

**FIGURE 7-6**   Corneal topography maps. *A*, Normal cornea (normalized scale). *B*, Normal cornea (absolute scale). *C*, Keratoconus (normalized scale). *D*, Distorted cornea (normalized scale).

tact lens fitting assistance and to "diagnose" keratoconus and other forms of corneal irregularity.

## SLIT-LAMP BIOMICROSCOPY

The most robust method to examine the cornea is with slit-lamp biomicroscopy. The slit-lamp may be mounted most conveniently on an ophthalmic instrument stand or at a table, separate from the stand, for slit-lamp photodocumentation. A hand-held slit-lamp may be used for children and those who cannot be positioned in a typical slit-lamp, such as the bedridden patient. Before using the slit-lamp, the practitioner should become familiar with the location of the on/

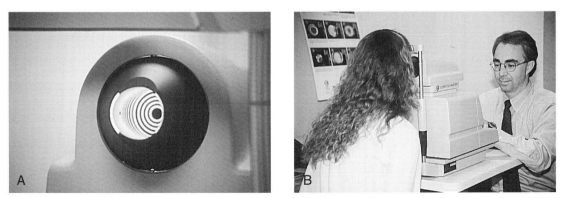

**FIGURE 7-7**   *A*, Conic (cylindrical) object, which is reflected off the cornea for videokeratoscope analysis. *B*, Computerized videokeratoscope during corneal modeling.

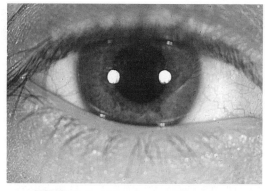

**FIGURE 7–8** Normal cornea and adnexa.

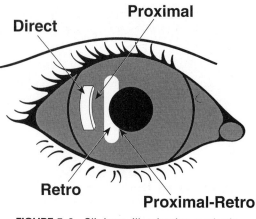

**FIGURE 7–9** Slit-lamp illumination methods.

off switch, the light intensity control, the filter controls (red free, cobalt, diffuser, and neutral density), the beam width and height controls, the magnification controls, and the joy stick and height adjustment control. The eyepieces should be focused. The optical cloth approved by the manufacturer should be used to clean the eyepieces as needed. The patient is positioned comfortably in the clean slit-lamp and the chin rest adjusted until the outer canthus is at the same level as the mark on the chin rest's vertical bars. This provides maximum vertical and horizontal range as the patient is examined. The slit-lamp should be turned off after each use, one should be familiar with how to change the light bulb

(for all instruments!), and it should be covered when not in use.

A consistent procedure is important to maximizing one's detection capabilities with the slit-lamp (Fig. 7–8):

☐ Start the examination with moderate illumination, enough to see ocular structures easily but just below the intensity that causes photophobia, at low magnification, and with a wide-open, maximum width beam.
☐ Beginning at the outer canthus and proceeding toward the nasal canthus, examine the

**TABLE 7–2** Types of Slit-Lamp Illumination

| Type of Illumination* | Structure to View | Viewing Method |
|---|---|---|
| Sclerotic scatter | Cornea for foreign body or opacity, edema, or haze | 2-mm slit straddles limbus; observe outside eyepieces; dark pupil as background |
| Diffuse | Lids, lashes, conjunctiva | Widest beam, low magnification |
| Direct | Cornea, conjunctiva | Moderate to high magnification; height of beam is maximum; observe directly where light strikes the object of regard |
| Slit/parallelepiped | Cornea at a specific surface or depth | 1- to 2-mm-wide slit; moderate illumination |
| Optic section | Cornea to judge depth | As narrow as possible with maximum illumination |
| Conic section | Anterior chamber for flare, cells | 1 mm wide and 1 mm high focused in anterior chamber |
| Specular reflection | Endothelium | Golden or dull reflection of hexagonal cells just next to the bright tear reflection |
| Indirect | | |
| Proximal | Cornea, any layer | 1- to 2-mm-wide beam; observe next to where the beam strikes the cornea using light scattered from a directly illuminated area |
| Retro | Cornea, any layer | Observe cornea backlighted by light reflected from iris |
| Proximal; retro | Cornea, any layer | Most sensitive; observe (with the pupil in the background) just adjacent to where the cornea is backlit by the iris |

*See Figures 7–9 and 7–10.[14, 15]

entire upper and lower eyelid margins, the
caruncle, and plica semilunaris.

☐ Evert the lower lid and examine the lower
cul-de-sac and the lower palpebral and bulbar conjunctiva.

☐ Observe the nasal and temporal bulbar
conjunctiva and then the superior bulbar
conjunctiva and limbus.

☐ Evert the upper eyelid, and observe the upper tarsal plate conjunctiva.

☐ With moderate magnification, examine the
temporal, inferior, and nasal limbus. Examination of the limbus and cornea may be
best done with a 1-mm slit-beam width.

☐ Examine the cornea from nasal to temporal
under moderate magnification. Examine the
entire corneal surface and, proceeding
across the cornea, observe all layers of the
cornea with direct illumination, proximal
illumination, retro- and proximal retro-illumination (Fig. 7–9). While examining the
cornea, higher magnification may be used
for viewing subtle, small objects of regard.
The endothelium is best viewed by specular
reflection adjacent to the bright tear reflection (Table 7–2).

Some clinicians begin the examination of the
cornea using sclerotic scatter illumination by
placing a 2-mm-wide slit beam at the limbus
(straddling the limbus) and observing outside the
slit-lamp eyepieces, that is, directly observing the
cornea grossly. Without magnification, look for
opacities or foreign bodies, which are highlighted as the cornea is internally illuminated like
a fiber optic (Fig. 7–10). Fluorescein may be
instilled prior to the slit-lamp examination or
after observing without fluorescein. Fluorescein
fills in the valleys between conjunctival folds,
papillae, and follicles and stains mucus. It also
highlights the dead, damaged, and missing epithelial cells of the cornea and conjunctiva. Fluo-

## TABLE 7–3  Grading of Clinical Slit-Lamp Observations*

| Grade | Observation |
| --- | --- |
| 0 | Not observed |
| 1.0 | Just noticeable, does not require treatment |
| 2.0 | Easily noticeable, requires monitoring |
| 3.0 | Advanced and requires immediate treatment (such as coalesced corneal epithelial staining) |
| 4.0 | Severe, (nearly) maximum, requires rigorous management |

*Modified from Mandell RB: Contact Lens Practice. Springfield, IL: Charles C Thomas, 1988.

rescein is especially effective if instilled repeatedly in the sequential staining technique.[8]

When corneal abnormalities are found, they
should be documented and drawn in the
patient's record.[9] Normal findings that are not
treatable should be noted but may not be graded.
Findings that can be treated should be graded on
a 0 to 4 scale. For example, normal findings such
as a Hudson-Stahli line, corneal striae in an aged
patient, an old childhood scar, and even arcus
senilis may not need to be graded. However,
abnormal findings from an active disease should
be graded (Tables 7–3 and 7–4).

Figure 7–11 provides the recently developed

## TABLE 7–4  Anterior Segment Observations to be Graded

Corneal staining (note type)
Conjunctival staining
Neovascularization
Infiltrates
Microcysts
Epithelial edema
Stromal edema
Limbal injection
Bulbar injection
Palpebral injection
Bulbar edema
Tarsal papillae
Lid margin/blepharitis
Endothelial polymegethism
Endothelial guttata
Corneal scar
Corneal haze
Flare/cells in anterior chamber
Other/specify

Edema and haze may be graded as:

| | |
| --- | --- |
| Grade 0 | None |
| Grade 1.0 | Just noticeable |
| Grade 2.0 | Easily noticeable |
| Grade 3.0 | Dense but iris detail is visible |
| Grade 4.0 | Obscures iris detail |

For all, note the location (drawing the finding in the appropriate zone)

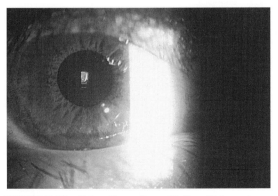

**FIGURE 7–10** Sclerotic scatter with the slit-lamp beam
straddling the limbus.

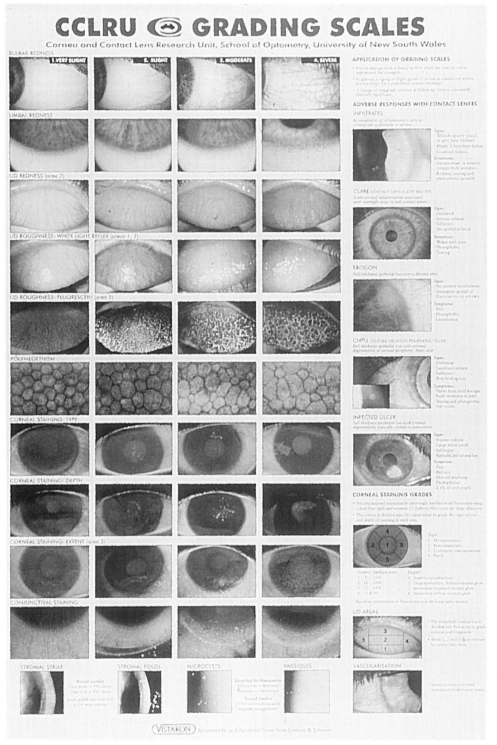

**FIGURE 7–11**   Slit-lamp grading scales. (From the Cornea and Contact Lens Research Unit, University of New South Wales.)

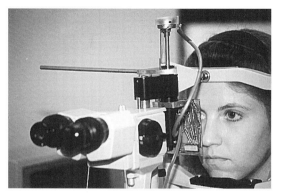

**FIGURE 7–12** Optical (non-contact) pachometry with a potentiometer provides computerized data analysis.

grading scale from the Cornea and Contact Lens Research Unit, University of New South Wales, for observation of corneal and conjunctival findings during slit-lamp biomicroscopy.

## CORNEAL THICKNESS

Corneal thickness is most typically measured for research or preoperatively in radial keratotomy patients. Optical pachometers (Fig. 7–12) require more operator training to reliably align the split image of the cornea where the anterior surface is aligned with the posterior surface. This physical distance is measured with the optical pachometer, which is then attached to a potentiometer. Multiple measurements of the central and peripheral cornea are averaged. In recent years the ultrasonic pachometer has been more accepted clinically because it is less user dependent. Unlike optical pachometry, it requires corneal anes-

thesia. Nevertheless, ultrasonic pachometry (Fig. 7–13) is probably no more invasive than applanation tonometry.

## CORNEAL SENSITIVITY

Corneal sensitivity is assessed clinically by making a cotton wisp from the sterile cotton on the end of a cotton-tipped applicator and touching the patient's cornea gently while keeping the examiner's hands away from the patient's line of sight (Fig. 7–14). Test the eye that has normal sensitivity first (if there is one), and then test the eye believed to be hypoesthetic. Patients with neuroparalytic keratitis or herpetic keratitis or contact lens wearers with hypoxia may have reduced sensitivity. A Cochet-Bonnet anesthesiometer may also be used (Fig. 7–15).

# Anterior Segment Photography

Photography of the eyelids, conjunctiva, or cornea for gross abnormalities such as lid bumps, ptosis, grossly observable conjunctival anomalies, large corneal scars, or grossly observable degenerative or dystrophic changes is possible with a Polaroid camera or—for better quality—a 35-mm camera with a close-up, macro lens. A 35-mm camera with close-up lens and ring flash, although expensive, is an excellent device. Photography stores and ophthalmic equipment suppliers stock these items. Polaroid film provides immediate feedback, and 35-mm photography

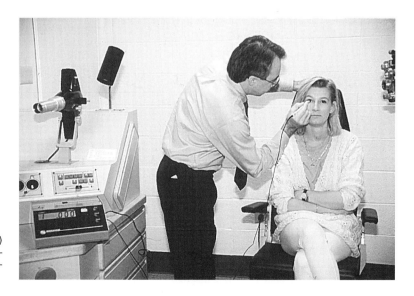

**FIGURE 7–13** Ultrasonic (contact) pachometer for central and peripheral corneal thickness measurement.

provides the highest contrast available for record-keeping purposes. ASA 100 or 200 is best for 35-mm photography for rapid (1 to 2 day) development, whereas ASA 25 or 64 provides the finest contrast but can take days to be returned.

Slit-lamp photodocumentation can be performed with Polaroid, 35-mm, videotape, or digital imaging, in which the image is immediately stored on a computer hard drive (Fig. 7-16). Table 7-5 lists the advantages and challenges of each system. Here are some tips to avoid poor photographs and obtain optimal photographs or video:

- Remember, most systems provide the magnification of the objective lens of the slit lamp and not the added magnification of the eyepiece(s). Therefore, take photographs at the maximum magnification at which good depth of focus can be maintained.
- Take three or four photographs of each image, so that at least one good image is assured.
- Use the lowest light to focus the object of regard to minimize the patient's photophobia.
- Use a yellow filter over the objective lenses when using a cobalt filter for best fluorescein exposure.
- The specular reflection from the first Purkinje image/tear film is very intense and can wash out an adjacent object, especially near the limbus or on the bulbar conjunctiva. The photographer's retina can adapt locally, but the photographic film cannot. The bright tear reflex may cause the light sensor in the video camera to turn down the sensitivity of the systems, which may reduce the contrast on the object of regard. In these situations, use a narrow slit or more oblique incident light to avoid this problem. Remember indirect and proximal

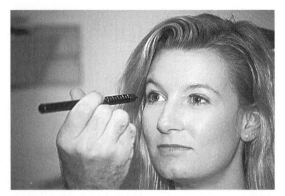

**FIGURE 7–15** Assessing corneal sensitivity with a Cochet-Bonnet anesthesiometer.

retro-illumination may pick up the most subtle observations.
- Bracket the exposure by using various flash intensities for each object.

Table 7-6 lists examples of how to obtain photodocumentation of various ocular structures. Slide sorting can be quite a chore. Keep a log of film type, date loaded, patient name, date and structure photographed, magnification, and flash intensity for each photograph. Select a fastidious person to sort and label the slides as soon as they are received. Plastic slide sleeves that store 20 slides are best for storage in three-ring binders or patient files.[10]

# Corneal Findings

· · · · · · · · · · · · · · · · · · · · · · · · · ·

Corneal findings can be due to infection, trauma, inflammation, or intrinsic disease (Table 7-7). The discussion that follows uses the corneal dystrophies and degenerations as examples of corneal conditions that can be evaluated using these techniques.

## CORNEAL DYSTROPHIES AND DEGENERATIONS

It is important to know the difference between a dystrophy and a degeneration (Table 7-8). This section reviews corneal dystrophies and degenerations[11] according to a **S**ubjective, **O**bjective, **A**ssessment **P**lan (SOAP) format, as would be recorded in a patient's chart (see Chapter 1).

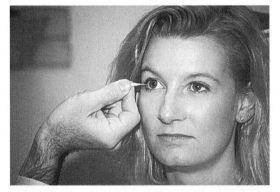

**FIGURE 7–14** Assessing corneal sensitivity with a cotton wisp.

**TABLE 7–5** Benefits and Challenges of Various Slit-Lamp Photodocumentation Systems (Excluding Expense)[20]

| System | Benefits | Challenges |
|---|---|---|
| Polaroid | Rapid evaluation | Poor contrast |
| 35 mm | Best contrast | Slowest evaluation |
| Videotape | Motion | Cumbersome to use |
| Digital imaging (Fig. 7–16) | Easy evaluation/access to many images | Some reduction of contrast |

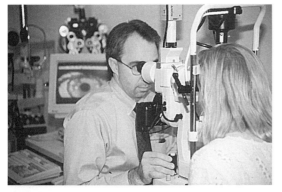

**FIGURE 7–16** Computerized digital imaging system allows rapid acquisition of multiple images and storage of images on computer media.

## Anterior Corneal Dystrophies

### Hereditary Epithelial Dystrophy (Meesmann's)

**S:** Asymptomatic in early stages; pain and photophobia in moderate to late stages when recurrent corneal erosions begin. Usually no loss in acuity unless the recurrent corneal erosions lead to subepithelial scarring and irregular astigmatism.

**O:** Upon slit-lamp examination, one sees multiple, fine round cysts in the epithelium, most prominently in the interpalpebral zone.

**A:** Rare, bilateral, symmetrical disorder of the corneal epithelium with autosomal dominant inheritance. It may be present within the first year of life but remains asymptomatic until early adult life or middle age, when the cysts begin to rupture and cause recurrent corneal erosions.

**P:** Loss of vision is rare, so treatment is not often required. However, lamellar or penetrating keratoplasty may be necessary in cases with severe scarring (see Fig. 7–31).

### Epithelial Basement Membrane Dystrophy (EBMD)

**S:** The patient may present in the third decade asymptomatically or with recurrent corneal erosions.

**O:** Upon slit-lamp examination, one sees maps, dots, and/or fingerprints in the corneal epithelium (see Fig. 7-28). *Maps* are curved or serpiginous lines with fairly sharp margins; *dots* are fine grey-white opacities that are oblong, round, or comma-shaped. *Fingerprints* appear as multiple maps that are somewhat parallel. Maps are the most common, dots are the next most common, and fingerprints are seen the least.

**A:** This is the most common of the anterior corneal dystrophies. It has no known pattern of inheritance, but it has been suggested that the inheritance pattern may be autosomal dominant. The etiology of this condition lies in an abnormal, redundant basement membrane with intraepithelial extensions. Normal maturation and desquamation of the underlying epithelial cells are blocked by these extensions, and focal degeneration and collection of cellular debris lead to the recurrent corneal erosions (Figs. 7-8 and 7-29).

**P:** Patients can remain asymptomatic. If recurrent corneal erosion occurs, typical treatment is with sodium chloride drops during the daytime and sodium chloride ointment at night. This helps to reduce epithelial edema and the recurrent corneal erosions. Ultimately, epithelial debridement or stromal puncture may be needed. Anterior corneal dystrophies may be successfully treated with excimer laser phototherapeutic keratectomy.[12]

### Reis-Bücklers' Dystrophy

**S:** Presenting early in childhood, the patient usually complains of ocular irritation and photophobia (caused by recurrent corneal erosions).

**O:** Early, the condition presents as a fine, reticular opacification at the level of Bowman's layer. Advanced cases show an irregular corneal surface and discrete bluish white subepithelial opacities on direct illumination.

**A:** This bilateral condition affects the central cornea and has an autosomal dominant inheritance pattern. A transient decrease in vision occurs at first, but later progressive visual loss ensues owing to anterior corneal opacification and

**TABLE 7-6** Examples and Illumination Set-Up for Various Structures

| Structure | Magnification | Illumination |
|---|---|---|
| Whole eye | Moderate | Moderate |
| Lids | Moderate | Moderate |
| Conjunctiva | Moderate | Low to moderate |
| Limbus | Moderate/high | Low |
| Whole cornea | Moderate/high | Moderate |
| Cornea | | |
|   Parallelepiped | High | Moderate/high; consider indirect illumination |
|   Sclerotic scatter | High | High |
|   Staining | High | High |
|   Endothelium (Figs. 7–17 and 7–18) | High | High (endothelial photography may require special endothelial photographic systems and requires specular reflection from the endothelium) |

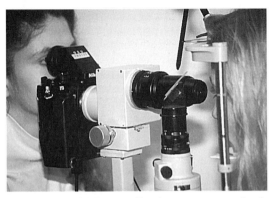

**FIGURE 7–17** High magnification non-contact (endothelial) camera.

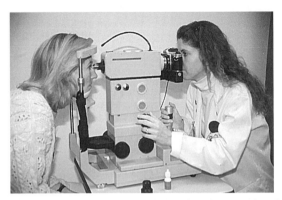

**FIGURE 7–18** Specular microscope for photography of the corneal endothelium and epithelium.

irregular astigmatism. Bowman's layer is gradually replaced by scar tissue. The recurrent corneal erosion attacks become less frequent, and the pain associated with the recurrent corneal erosions lessens, owing to decreased corneal sensitivity.

**P:** Advanced cases are treated with lamellar or penetrating keratoplasty. The excimer laser has shown some promise in treating some cases.

### Anterior Membrane Dystrophy (Grayson-Wilbrant)

**S:** Patients may present with recurrent corneal erosions, pain, and photophobia.

**O:** On slit-lamp examination, one finds grey-white, amorphous opacities of varying size in the central cornea at the level of Bowman's layer.

**A:** This disorder is autosomal dominant in inheritance, relatively rare, and very similar to Reis-Bücklers' dystrophy; but it differs in the following ways:

☐ Recurrent corneal erosions are less frequent.

☐ Visual acuity is less severely affected.
☐ Corneal sensation is normal.
☐ The disease is mostly in the central cornea, and the cornea between lesions remains clear.

**P:** Possibly lubricants at night.

## Stromal Dystrophies

### Lattice Dystrophy

**S:** Patients can present in the first to fourth decade with recurrent corneal erosions or visual disturbances.

**O:** Early findings include anterior refractive stromal dots, fine lines, and white spots. The stroma between the opacities is clear at first but gets progressively more hazy. This progression and the scarring lead to the erosions. Recurrent corneal erosions and scarring lead to decreased vision and decreased corneal sensitivity.

**A:** This autosomal dominant disorder has two categories, type I and type II.

**TABLE 7-7** Typical Cornea and Contact Lens Observations and Management Guidelines[16-19]

| Observation | Most Likely Etiology | Management Guidelines |
|---|---|---|
| Staining in aperture (Figs. 7–19 and 7–20) | Desiccation | Lubricants, blinking, lid therapy, punctal plugs, systemic hydration; low water content or thick soft lens |
| Staining along lid margin | Blepharitis | Lid therapy, hot compresses, lid scrubs, possible appropriate antibiotic |
| Staining at 3–4 and 8–9 o'clock near the limbus (Fig. 7–21) | Rigid lens wear | Thinner lens edge, more edge lift, blinking; lens cannot ride low; lubricants |
| Vascularized limbal keratitis | Mechanical | Same as above |
| Superior epithelial arcuate lesion ("epithelial split") (Fig. 7–22) | Contact lens–related (etiology unknown) | Remove contact lens until totally healed; use new lens with rigorous cleaning and disinfection |
| Focal staining (Fig. 7–23) | Crack in contact lens | Replace lens |
| Epithelial wrinkling (Fig. 7–24) | Contact lens | Change fit to prevent wrinkle |
| Limbal/corneal infiltrate (not ulcer) (Fig. 7–25) | Contact lens or staphylococcal exotoxin | Lid therapy, remove contact lens; possible antibiotic or possible appropriate antibiotic/steroid combination |
| Entire corneal surface (Fig. 7–26) | Toxic keratitis | Remove toxic agent; employ nonpreserved lubricant or irrigation |
| Superior limbic keratitis | Contact lens–related or thyroid disease | Remove contact lens if contact lens–related; if suspect thyroid disease, refer to appropriate primary care medical practitioner |
| Abrasion | Foreign body | Don't pressure patch if contact lens–related or if contact with vegetation was the cause; polish lens back surface on otherwise successful rigid contact lens wearer |
| Microcysts (Fig. 7–27) | Contact lens–related | Improve corneal oxygen supply |
| Dimple veiling | Bubbles under rigid contact lens | Change fit to avoid bubbles |
| Epidemic keratoconjunctivitis | Virus | Lubricants |
| Thygeson's disease | Virus? | Topical, low-dose corticosteroids; bandage contact lens |
| Recurrent corneal erosion (Figs. 7–28 and 7–29) | May be dystrophic | Lubricants; soft contact lens for pain; debridement; possibly excimer laser |
| Corneal scarring | Many causes | May be treated with excimer laser; consult refractive surgeon |
| Dendrite | Herpes simplex | No steroids if epithelial; antiviral medications as indicated |
| Infectious keratitis | Contact lens | Remove contact lens; culture; aggressive antibiotic therapy as indicated; consider corneal specialist consultation |

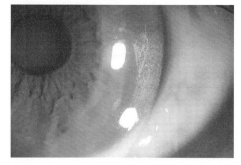

**FIGURE 7–19** Swirl staining of superficial epithelium. (Photograph by Lisa Badowski, OD, MS.)

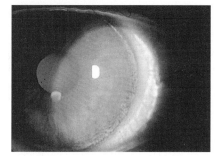

**FIGURE 7–20** Mild superficial staining and tear break-up.

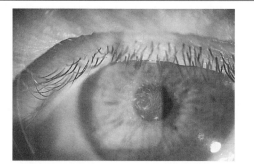

**FIGURE 7–21** Peripheral corneal desiccation (3 and 9 o'clock) staining and imprint in the corneal epithelium from a rigid contact lens.

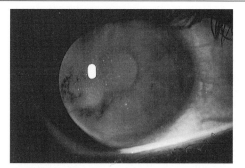

**FIGURE 7–22** Limbal epithelial (hypertrophy) hyperfluorescence from high minus soft contact lens wear.

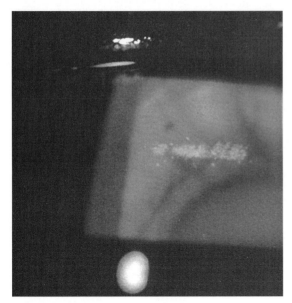

**FIGURE 7–23** Superficial epithelial erosion from a crack in a soft contact lens.

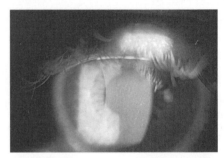

**FIGURE 7–24** Central corneal distortion from extended wear of RGP contact lens.

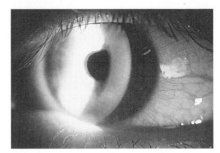

**FIGURE 7–25** Anterior stromal infiltrates from contact lens solution hypersensitivity.

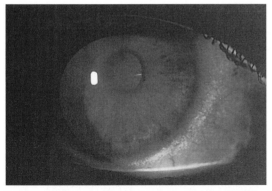

**FIGURE 7–26** Moderate corneal and conjunctival staining.

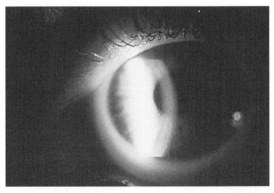

**FIGURE 7–27** Epithelial microcysts between slit-lamp beam and margin of iris viewed by proximal retroillumination.

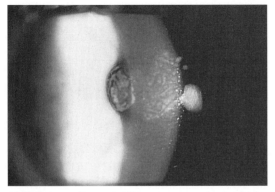

**FIGURE 7–28** Epithelial basement membrane dystrophy.

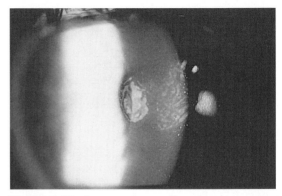

**FIGURE 7–29** Recurrent corneal erosion in a patient with epithelial basement membrane dystrophy.

**TABLE 7–8** The Defining Characteristics of Corneal Dystrophies and Degenerations

| Dystrophies | Degenerations |
| --- | --- |
| Bilateral | Unilateral |
| Symmetrical | Asymmetrical |
| Axial | Peripheral |
| Heritable | No inheritance |
| Early onset | Late onset |
| Primary corneal disease | Secondary disease |
| Noninflammatory | Inflammatory |

☐ Type I: Onset is usually in the first decade; it presents with recurrent corneal erosions and visual disturbance and has no systemic involvement.

☐ Type II: Less common, onset occurs in the fourth decade with similar presentation but with fewer lattice lines and systematically can involve various organs, the eyelids, and the lacrimal glands.

**P:** Penetrating keratoplasty, but recurrence after penetrating keratoplasty is more common than with other stromal dystrophies.

## Granular Dystrophy (Groenouw II)

**S:** Mild photophobia or asymptomatic. Recurrent corneal erosions are infrequent, and vision is usually not affected.

**O:** Fine, grey whole opacities in the anterior stroma, while the intervening stroma remains clear. As this dystrophy progresses, the opacities enlarge, coalesce, and increase in number. They also begin to resemble bread crumbs or snowflakes. The peripheral 2 to 3 mm of stroma are not involved.*

**A:** This is an autosomal dominant disorder with onset in the first or second decade of life. The deposits in the stroma are *hyaline* and are produced by abnormal keratocytes in the anterior stroma.

**P:** Treatment is not required in most cases, although penetrating keratoplasty may be necessary in a few advanced cases.

## Macular Dystrophy (Groenouw Type II)

**S:** Photophobia (early, first decade) and visual impairment (later, approximately fourth decade). Recurrent corneal erosions can occur but are much less frequent than with lattice.

**O:** The disorder initially presents as bilateral,

---

*This is important in the differential diagnosis of this disorder from macular dystrophy.

fine, superficial, central corneal haze. This eventually leads to the *entire stroma* being covered with multiple, irregular, grey-white nodules.

**A:** This is the least common of all the classic stromal dystrophies. The disorder is autosomal recessive and often occurs in consanguineous marriages. As the condition progresses, surface irregularity occurs and the cornea begins to lose sensation.

Macular dystrophy is differentiated from granular dystrophy (Groenouw I) by being recessive and by having haze between the opacities and early peripheral corneal involvement. This genetic disorder causes the keratocytes to deposit mucopolysaccharides.

**P:** Penetrating keratoplasty may be required by the fourth decade, but the disease can recur in the graft postoperatively.

## Central Cloudy Dystrophy (Francois')

**S:** No symptoms.

**O:** Deep, multiple grey stromal opacities separated by clear lines of stroma. These are best seen with oblique illumination or sclerotic scatter.

**A:** Central cloudy dystrophy is a bilateral, symmetrical, and nonprogressive disorder with autosomal dominant inheritance. It can occur as early as the first decade of life, but vision, corneal thickness, and sensation are not affected.

**P:** No treatment is necessary.

## Pre-Descemet's Dystrophy

**S:** No symptoms.

**O:** See Assessment just below.

**A:** There are four different types to this dystrophy.

1. Typical pre-Descemet's: This dystrophy usually occurs in the fourth to the seventh decades and appears as central diffuse opacities in the posterior stroma (pre-Descemet's area). The inheritance pattern of this dystrophy is autosomal dominant, and it is bilateral and symmetrical.

2. Pre-Descemet's associated with skin conditions: The cornea has grey, snowflake-like opacities deep in the stroma. The skin conditions with which it is associated are ichthyosis and pseudoxanthoma elasticum.

3. Polymorphic: This involves both the deep and the mid-stroma and appears as punctate and filament-like focal grey opacities.

4. Cornea farinata: An age-related degeneration in which the opacities are grey, yet smaller than the previous dystrophies.

It has been shown histologically by Curran et al[13] that pre-Descemet's dystrophies are an accumulation of lipofuscin-like material in posterior keratocytes. This supports the theory that these conditions may be degenerations, as opposed to true dystrophies.

**P:** All four examples are asymptomatic and require no treatment.

## Endothelial Dystrophies

### Fuchs' Dystrophy

Krukenberg's spindle is an hourglass-shaped pigmentation of the endothelium. Keratic precipitates are accumulations of inflammatory cells on the endothelium. Endothelial bedewing represents deposition of individual inflammatory cells on the endothelium.

**S:** Pain with progression to decreased vision.

**O:** Cornea guttata and pigment dusting of the endothelium. Later, bullae and edema.

**A:** There are three *clinical stages* to this dystrophy which need to be recognized: (1) cornea guttata, (2) stromal and epithelial edema, and (3) corneal scarring.

Fuchs' dystrophy is the most common endothelial dystrophy seen in practice. Fuchs' dystropy is an asymmetrical, bilateral condition that often presents in the sixth decade but can be seen clinically much earlier. It affects women three times more than men, and it is also more severe in women.

**P:** In the early stages, symptomatic relief from the edema may be observed with hypertonic saline drops in the daytime, and hypertonic ointment at bedtime. When the bullae begin to rupture and the patient experiences pain, it can be reduced by using a bandage soft contact lens (high water). Once the condition has progressed and vision is greatly affected, a penetrating keratoplasty is necessary.

### Posterior Polymorphous Dystrophy

**S:** Typically no symptoms occur prior to visual loss.

**O:** Slit-lamp examination may show a variety of findings, including vesicles, patches of abnormal endothelium, or a thickened Descemet's membrane. In severe cases there may be some corneal edema, and in a minority of patients changes may occur at the anterior chamber angle and the iris. These changes include growth of abnormal endothelium across the trabecular meshwork and onto the iris.

**A:** This bilateral condition is thought to be mainly autosomal dominant in inheritance but can be recessive in some cases. Onset is difficult to determine, but some cases have been seen at birth, suggesting that it may be congenital. Cases with growth into the trabecular meshwork need to be differentiated from iridocorneal endothelial syndrome.

**P:** Severe cases may require penetrating keratoplasty, although typically no treatment is needed. If accompanied by increased intraocular pressure due to chamber outflow problems, the glaucoma must be managed.

### Congenital Hereditary Endothelial Dystrophy (CHED)

**S:** There are two typical presentations: (1) at birth, corneal clouding and possibly nystagmus, and (2) later, the patient may present with photophobia and irritation.

**O:** Upon slit-lamp examination, the corneal epithelium and stroma exhibit marked edema, giving the cornea a ground glass appearance. Also, one can see dense white stromal opacities and a thickening of Descemet's membrane. Intraocular pressure and corneal sensation remain normal.

**A:** There are two distinct presentations. The first is at birth; it is autosomal recessive and presents with corneal clouding and possibly nystagmus. The second is seen later; it is autosomal dominant and is often preceded by irritation and photophobia. The opacification proceeds more slowly in this presentation, and nystagmus is seen less often. The underlying problem is deformation of the endothelium during fetal development.

**P:** Treatment is by penetrating keratoplasty, but its success is often limited by the presence of amblyopia. However, better results have been reported if treatment is initiated within the first few months of life.

### Keratoconus

**S:** The patient can present with spectacle blur, increased myopic or mixed astigmatism, or blurred vision.

**O:** Slit-lamp examination findings can include the following: Vogt's striae (vertical lines that represent folds in the deep stroma and Descemet's membrane) and/or Fleischer's ring (hemosiderin deposits in the deep epithelium which can completely surround the cone). Advanced cases can present with corneal scars and ultimately corneal hydrops (ruptures in Descemet's membrane which result in stromal edema [Fig. 7–30]). This edema usually resolves, leaving a residual scar.

**A:** Keratoconus is a progressive, non-inflammatory thinning of the cornea which leads to a conical protrusion of the cornea (the cone). The cone is usually located inferiorly. The condition may begin between the ages of 10 and 20 years, most typically between the ages of 20 and 30 years, and less often after age 30. The estimated incidence is 1 in 50,000 per year, and 90% of the cases are bilateral.

The diagnosis is made with the above subjective findings (see **S**), slit-lamp examination findings (see **O**), corneal topography (inferior cornea much steeper than superior), and/or the typical three-point-touch fluorescein pattern upon insertion of a lens parallel to the flat keratometric reading. The keratometric mires, retinoscopic reflex, or ophthalmoscopy reflex is distorted. The pathogenesis of keratoconus is not known. It is probably genetic, yet no family history is reported in 90% of the cases. Some of the ocular and systemic conditions associated with keratoconus are Down syndrome, atopy, and significant eye rubbing.

**P:** Management is with rigid lenses when spectacles and soft lenses are not adequate, and penetrating keratoplasty (Fig. 7–31) is necessary when rigid contact lenses can no longer provide good vision, can no longer be tolerated, or if thinning is too severe near the limbus.

## Age-Related Corneal Degeneration

### Vogt's Limbal Girdle

**S:** No symptoms.

**O:** Crescent-shaped, chalky white subepithelial deposits at the nasal and/or the temporal limbus within the palpebral fissure, with no clear zone between the deposits and the limbus.

**A:** These deposits represent a degeneration

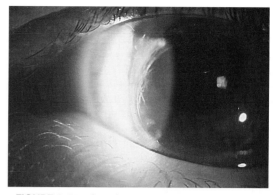

**FIGURE 7–31** Scar from penetrating keratoplasty.

of the subepithelial collagen, which is probably related to sun exposure. It is present in 55% of the population aged 40 to 60 years and 90% of the population over 70 years.

**P:** No treatment is necessary.

### Corneal Arcus (Arcus Senilis)

**S:** No symptoms.

**O:** A band of yellowish white deposits that can be seen inferiorly or around the corneal circumference, with a clear zone between the deposits and the limbus.

**A:** The most common age-related degeneration, it occurs in 60% of the normal population from 40 to 60 years and almost all people over the age of 80 years. The condition occurs earlier in blacks and 10 years earlier in men.

Arcus is related to the increased permeability of the limbal vessels with age and the deposition of low-density lipoproteins in the cornea.

**P:** The presence of arcus in a patient less than 40 years of age is an indication for a blood cholesterol evaluation.

### Cornea Farinata

**S:** No symptoms.

**O:** Upon slit-lamp examination there are fine dustlike opacities in the posterior stroma, usually in both eyes.

**A:** An age-related degeneration of the posterior stroma occurs where vesicles in posterior keratocytes contain lipofuscin (a degenerative pigment that accumulates in older cells).

**P:** No treatment.

### Cornea Guttata

**S:** No symptoms.

**O:** Small *peripheral* posterior guttate areas

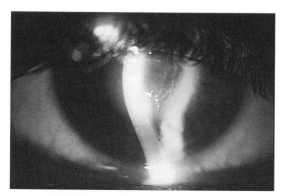

**FIGURE 7–30** Acute corneal hydrops.

appear dark upon retroillumination and first appear between 20 and 30 years of age.

**A:**   Greater than 70% of the population over age 40 years have one or more guttata. These guttata, or Hassall-Henle bodies, are differentiated from the guttata in Fuchs' dystrophy by their peripheral location. Guttata represent products of abnormal endothelial cells where localized thickenings in Descemet's membrane arise and disturb the endothelial mosaic. Familial cornea guttata can be present in younger patients.

**P:**   Monitor, no treatment is usually required.

### Crocodile Shagreen of Vogt

**S:**   Patients are usually asymptomatic, and their vision is not affected.

**O:**   Polygonal, greyish white opacities located in the anterior or posterior stroma separated by relatively clear spaces.

**A:**   This bilateral condition is usually located in the anterior stroma (anterior crocodile shagreen) but can be seen in the posterior stroma (posterior crocodile shagreen) at times.

**P:**   No treatment is needed.

### Band Keratopathy

**S:**   White area on the cornea, sometimes causing foreign body sensation, sometimes with decreased vision.

**O:**   Roughened, whitish yellow, dense deposits in the corneal epithelium.

**A:**   The calcium deposits associated with band keratopathy are extracellular and occur in the basement membrane of the epithelium, *in Bowman's membrane and in the superficial stroma*. It can occur as a degenerative change following a number of conditions, including chronic ocular disease, repeated ocular trauma, or systemic disorders with elevated levels of calcium or phosphate. In children, it is typically associated with the chronic uveitis involved with juvenile rheumatoid arthritis. In addition, band keratopathy is also seen with pilocarpine use or following use of solutions with phenylmercuric nitrate.

Band keratopathy begins in the periphery of the palpebral aperture and moves toward the central cornea; however, the band does not extend to the limbus i.e., a clear zone exists).

**P:**   Treatment of the underlying cause, with chelating agents and surgery, is required.

### Iron Pigmentation

**S:**   No symptoms unless caused by accompanying conditions.

**O:**   Deposition of brown pigment in the corneal epithelium.

**A:**   This degeneration is typically associated with conditions that alter the shape of the cornea, such as Fleischer's ring in keratoconus, the Stocker line at the head of a pterygium, the Ferry line around a filtering bleb, or with superficial, iatrogenic scars (e.g., penetrating keratoplasty or radial keratotomy). The alteration of the corneal surface allows the tear film to pool, and iron is deposited in the basal layer of the epithelium.

The most common iron deposition is a Hudson-Stahli line located at the junction where the lids meet. This is thought to be a degenerative age-related change.

**P:**   No treatment is required.

### Blood Staining of the Cornea

**S:**   Corneal discoloration, decreased vision.

**O:**   Rust-colored opacity in the cornea, either centrally or across the cornea.

**A:**   This serious degenerative change usually occurs with hemorrhages in the anterior chamber and prolonged elevated intraocular pressure. If extensive endothelial injury is present, blood staining can occur in the absence of high intraocular pressure.

**P:**   No treatment is required.

In the beginning, it is seen as a rust-colored opacity on the entire surface of the cornea or on just a small central portion. Later the opacity changes to greenish black to grey, and the clearing starts in the periphery and proceeds centrally.

Histologically, the blood causes extensive abnormalities in the endothelium, yet Descemet's membrane remains normal. Breakdown products are found in the intracellular and extracellular locations in the stroma, and degenerative changes occur in some keratocytes. Corneal hemorrhage can occur with neovascularization in contact lens wear. The staining takes two to three years to clear, and in some cases necrosis of keratocytes occurs, the staining does not clear, and a penetrating keratoplasty is necessary.

### Vortex Degeneration (Corneal Verticillata)

**S:**   No symptoms to decreased vision.

**O:**   Whorl-like powdery white or yellowish brown lines are seen in the central-inferior portion of the corneal epithelium.

**A:**   This is a degenerative change associated with toxic keratopathy from amiodarone, chloroquine, indomethacin, and chlorpromazine therapy.

**P:** Typically, no treatment is required. The patient's internist should be informed of this finding.

## Pterygium

**S:** White growth on the eye, extending across the cornea. Sometimes astigmatism, decreased vision.

**O:** A fibrovascular connective tissue overgrowth of conjunctival tissue onto the cornea.

**A:** This is typically triangle shaped and has the following three components:

1. The body: a flat pink sheet of connective tissue that is highly vascularized.
2. The head: white and slightly elevated and eventually firmly adherent to the superficial stroma.
3. The cap: a grey avascular zone that precedes the head and surrounds it like a halo.

A growing pterygium is red and inflamed, but an inactive one is less red and the inflammation decreases.

The cause of pterygium is not known exactly, but the prevalence is higher among people living close to the equator (i.e., the closer to the equator, the higher the prevalence). In addition to geographic location of those afflicted, another factor that implicates an environmental cause is the interpalpebral location of pterygia. Also, histologically pterygia are similar to solar radiation changes of collagen.

One should be able to differentiate malignancies of the conjunctiva, such as squamous cell carcinoma and pseudopterygium. Pseudopterygia can arise from peripheral inflammation (e.g., marginal keratitis), chemical burns, and cicatricial conjunctivitis. However, these can be differentiated by their lack of the classic pterygial components described above (cap, head, and body), atypical location, and lack of firm adhesion at the limbus.

**P:** Treatment is by surgical removal, and recurrence depends somewhat on the surgical method. Some advise sun and wind protection to avoid or slow the growth.

## Salzmann's Nodular Degeneration

**S:** Most cases are asymptomatic, yet some patients complain of irritation due to erosions.

**O:** Slit-lamp examination shows bluish-grey, elevated, fibrous, nodular lesions in the superficial stroma.

**A:** A gradually developing degeneration follows a history of prior ocular inflammation (phlyctenular keratitis, trachoma, vernal keratitis,

keratitis sicca, and exposure keratopathy). A few cases have presented without the patient having any prior knowledge of ocular inflammation.

This degeneration can occur at any age but occurs most frequently after the age of 50 years. It also occurs in females more frequently than males, and it is bilateral in 80% of all cases. The irritation comes from erosions of the epithelium over the nodules.

**P:** Penetrating or lamellar keratoplasty if the nodules are central and impair vision.

## Spheroidal Degeneration (Climatic Droplet Keratopathy)

**S:** Decreasing vision.

**O:** Subepithelial accumulations of clusters of yellow or grey droplets that form a band across the exposed area of the cornea.

**A:** This is another condition in which the environment is implicated as the causative factor. The most prominent factor is exposure to actinic radiation. Others factors include low humidity and exposure to wind, sand, or ice. Aging and corneal drying are additional factors.

There are three types of spheroidal degeneration:

1. Type I: This is the primary form. It is bilateral, age-related, and not associated with any other corneal diseases and affects only the periphery of the interpalpebral zone.
2. Type II: This type occurs secondary to previous corneal conditions and/or climactic exposure. The opacity spreads to the pupillary zone and decreases vision to the 20/100 to 20/200 range.
3. Type III: This is conjunctival spheroidal degeneration and occurs with pinguecula in 86% of cases. The opacities are large yellowish nodules that elevate the epithelium and decrease vision to worse than 20/200.

In all three types, men are affected in a ratio of 4:3 compared with women.

**P:** Penetrating and lamellar keratoplasty traditionally, but excimer laser has shown good results recently.

## Terrien's Marginal Degeneration

**S:** Decreasing vision in most and pain in younger patients.

**O:** Slit-lamp examination findings occur in the following order:

1. Fine punctate stromal opacities separated from the limbus by a clear zone.

2. Superficial vascularization of the involved area.

3. Slow, progressive stromal thinning forming a gutter at the peripheral edge of the cornea with a sharp central edge.

No staining is seen on the corneal epithelium.

**A:** This degeneration is bilateral in 86% of cases, and men are affected more than women. The epithelium over the gutter is normal and does not stain.

**P:** When corneal perforation is impending or has occurred, a lamellar or penetrating keratoplasty is necessary.

### Pellucid Marginal Degeneration

**S:** Decreasing vision due to against-the-rule astigmatism.

**O:** An inferior corneal protrusion above a band of stromal thinning is seen.

**A:** This uncommon corneal degeneration occurs between the second and fifth decades. It affects males and females equally and can generate as much as 20.00 D of against-the-rule astigmatism and/or irregular astigmatism. It can occur in conjunction with keratoconus, but some think it may be a variant or part of the continuum of keratoconus.

**P:** Rigid contact lenses when spectacles are not adequate and penetrating or lamellar keratoplasty when the patient cannot tolerate or be adequately corrected with contact lenses.

# Summary

. . . . . . . . . . . . . . . . . . . . . . . . .

Although it is only a very small area of tissue, the cornea represents the eye's "window to the world." By its very nature it needs to be clear, wet, and free of disease. These techniques allow the practitioner to evaluate the cornea, to categorize its abnormalities, and to apply treatment to restore it to provide functional vision.

#### ACKNOWLEDGMENTS

The author of this chapter acknowledges the significant contribution of Robert Steffen, OD, MS, to outline and simplify the reference material on corneal degenerations and dystrophies by Casey and Sharif[11] and of Karla Zadnik, OD, PhD, for the list of factors that discriminate degenerations and dystrophies.

# References

. . . . . . . . . . . . . . . . . . . . . . . . .

1. Mandell RB: Contact Lens Practice. Springfield, IL: Charles C Thomas, 1988.

2. Marquardt R, Stodtmeister R, Christ T: Modification of tear film break-up time test for increased reliability. *In* Holly FJ: The Preocular Tear Film in Health, Disease, and Contact Lens Wear. Lubbock, TX: The Dry Eye Institute, 1986.

3. Guillon JP, Guillon M: The role of tears in contact lens performance and its measurement. *In* Ruben M, Guillon M: Contact Lens Practice. London: Chapman & Hall, 1994.

4. Lemp MA, Mahmood MA, Weiler HH: Association of rosacea and keratoconjunctivitis sicca. Arch Ophthalmol 1984; 102:556-557.

5. Sakamoto R, Bennett ES, Henry VA, et al: The phenol red thread tear test: A cross-cultural study. Invest Ophthalmol Vis Sci 1993; 34:3510-3514.

6. Holly FJ: Diagnosis and treatment of dry eye syndrome. Cont Lens Spectrum 1989; 4:37-39.

7. Roberts C: Characterization of the inherent error in a spherically-biased corneal topography system in mapping a radially aspheric surface. J Refr Corn Surg 1994; 10:103-116.

8. Korb DR, Herman JP: Corneal staining, subsequent to sequential fluorescein instillation. J Am Optom Assoc 1979; 50:361-367.

9. Waring GO, Laibson PR: A systematic method of drawing corneal pathologic conditions. Arch Ophthalmol 1977; 95:1540-1542.

10. Martonyi C: Clinical Slit Lamp Biomicroscopy and Photo Slit Lamp Biomicroscopy. Ann Arbor, MI: Time One Ink, Ltd., 1985.

11. Casey TA, Sharif KW: A Colour Atlas of Corneal Dystrophies and Degenerations. London: Wolfe Publishing Limited, 1991.

12. Binder PS: Histological excimer laser keratectomy: Clinical and histopathological correlations. Ophthalmology 1985; 101:979-989.

13. Curran RE, Kenyon KR, Green WR: Pre-Descemet's membrane corneal dystrophy. Am J Ophthalmol 1974; 77:711-716.

14. Eskridge JB, Schoessler JP, Lowther GE: A specific biomicroscopy procedure. J Am Optom Assoc 1973; 45:400-409.

15. Brandreth RH: Clinical Slit Lamp Biomicroscopy. Berkeley: Multimedia Communications Center, School of Optometry, University of California, 1978.

16. Cullom RD, Chang B, Friedberg MA, Rapuano CJ: Wills Eye Hospital Office and Emergency Room Diagnosis and Treatment of Eye Disease. Philadelphia: JB Lippincott, 1994.

17. Dunn JP, Mondino BJ, Weissman BA: Immunologic complications of contact lens wear. *In* Bennett ES, Weissman BA: Clinical Contact Lens Practice. Philadelphia, JB Lippincott, 1991.

18. Dougal J: Abrasions secondary to contact lens wear. *In* Tomlinson A: Complications of Contact Lens Wear. St. Louis: CV Mosby, 1992.

19. Poggio EC, Abelson M: Complications and symptoms in disposable extended wear lenses compared with conventional soft daily wear and soft extended wear lenses. Contact Lens Assoc Ophthalmol J 1993; 19:31-39.

20. Barr JT, Gordon MO, Zadnik K, et al: A corneal scarring photodocumentation and reading method. J Refr Surg 1996; 12:492-500.

*Nina E. Friedman, OD, MS, and*
*Mark A. Bullimore, MCOptom, PhD*

8

# The Anterior Segment

The anterior chamber of the eye is the space defined by the cornea, sclera, ciliary body, iris, and lens. The angle where the anterior and posterior structures within the anterior chamber meet is occupied by the aqueous outflow apparatus: the trabecular meshwork and the canal of Schlemm. The anterior chamber structures have two basic functions: to act as optical elements in the formation of the visual image and to provide an appropriate level of aqueous drainage—thereby regulating intraocular pressure (IOP)—necessary for the maintenance of ocular structural integrity and health.

In the anatomically and physiologically normal eye, the refracting elements—the cornea, aqueous humor, and lens—are optically clear, the iris is opaque, and the aqueous humor produced in the posterior chamber by the ciliary body has ready access to well-functioning drainage channels in the anterior chamber angle. Abnormal anatomical configuration, changes associated with inflammatory or ischemic disease and aging, and both accidental and iatrogenic trauma can all compromise these tissues, adversely affecting the visual image, IOP, or both. The basic optometric tools for examination of the anterior chamber are slit-lamp biomicroscopic evaluation and tonometry. However, when these techniques reveal a patient with, or at risk for, glaucoma, gonioscopy is needed to assess the cause and extent of the risk.

In this chapter we present a brief, functional description of the anatomy of the anterior chamber in terms of the most common pathologies affecting the associated structures and the examination techniques required for the detection and differential diagnosis of these pathologies. Although corneal signs of the above-mentioned diseases are discussed, primary disorders of the cornea and their diagnosis, which are discussed in Chapter 6, are not included.

# Anatomy of the Anterior Chamber Angle and the Etiology of Glaucoma

The anterior chamber angle lies at the junction of the iris, ciliary body, sclera, and cornea; it contains the aqueous outflow apparatus, which is derived from these tissues. The crystalline lens, although not a component of the angle itself, plays a major role in the angle's anatomical configuration, because lens shape and position influence the contour of the iris and thus the relationship of the iris to other angle structures. The

state of the angle—the degree to which the iris allows access to the outflow apparatus and the patency of the outflow apparatus itself—determines the ease with which aqueous humor leaves the eye. The aqueous outflow rate is, in turn, the primary factor influencing IOP. Anything that interferes with aqueous outflow causes an increase in pressure and thus increases the risk of glaucomatous damage, with concomitant loss of visual field. Thus, examination of the angle is an important tool in investigating the cause of increased IOP, in identifying patients who are at risk for secondary open-angle glaucoma, and in assessing the chances of acute open- or closed-angle attacks—whether spontaneous, from ocular disease or trauma, or from pharmacological agents such as mydriatics and miotics.

Aqueous humor is produced by the ciliary processes in the posterior chamber of the eye, which is the space bounded by the anterior hyaloid face of the vitreous, the crystalline lens, the ciliary body, and the iris. From the posterior chamber the aqueous passes through the area of contact between the anterior surface of the lens and posterior surface of the iris and enters the anterior chamber through the pupil. The fluid pressure of the aqueous in the anterior chamber is the IOP. Because the aqueous humor is continuously being produced, it must drain from the eye at a rate sufficient to maintain the IOP. High IOP is nearly always due to abnormally high resistance to aqueous outflow, as opposed to abnormally high aqueous production. When elevated IOP is due to the anatomical obstruction of aqueous access to the trabecular meshwork by the iris, we speak of "angle-closure glaucoma." When the resistance to aqueous outflow is not due to limited access to, but rather to increased resistance within, the outflow apparatus, we speak of "open-angle glaucoma." That is, angle-closure glaucoma is caused by a macroscopic abnormality of the angle, whereas open-angle glaucoma is caused either by microscopic abnormalities of the drainage channels or, rarely, by an elevation in venous pressure. Obviously, how to care for a patient suffering from, or at risk for, glaucoma depends on the underlying cause; differential diagnosis requires an understanding of the basic anatomy—both gross and microscopic—of the anterior chamber angle.

# Gross Anatomy and Angle-Closure Glaucoma

The anterior surface of the peripheral iris forms the "floor" of the chamber angle. The iris root joins the ciliary body in front of the pars plicata, in the region where the longitudinal portion of the ciliary muscle inserts into the scleral spur (Fig. 8–1). The relative position of the iris insertion is an important factor in accessibility to drainage channels; the more anterior the iris insertion, the more likely that the peripheral iris will roll up into the angle and block the trabeculum when the pupil dilates. This situation is known as "plateau iris syndrome." In this condition, the depth of the anterior chamber may appear normal—that is, the plane of the iris is relatively flat centrally—but gonioscopically the angle is seen to be narrow. Patients with plateau iris syndrome are most likely to suffer the symptoms of angle closure (blurred vision, halos around lights, pain) in the dark or after the use of mydriatics.

One study has shown that the anteroposterior position of the iris root insertion varies significantly with ethnicity. On average, Asians have the most anterior iris insertion, Caucasians have the most posterior iris insertion, and African-Americans fall between the two. In addition, these investigators found a significant relationship between refractive error and iris insertion, with hyperopic eyes having more anterior insertions.[1]

Another important anatomical consideration in aqueous outflow is the position of the crystalline lens. The further forward the lens sits or the thicker the lens, the broader and tighter the zone of contact between the anterior surface of the lens and the posterior surface of the iris and the greater the resistance faced by the aqueous humor in moving from the posterior chamber to the anterior chamber. When the increased resistance causes an increase in posterior chamber pressure sufficient to push the peripheral iris forward into the trabecular meshwork (iris bombé), the situation is termed "pupil block." The difference between iris bombé and plateau iris is illustrated in Figure 8–2. In long, myopic eyes, the lens sits well back, and there is relatively little contact between iris and lens; narrow angles are extremely rare in myopic eyes. The prevalence of narrow angles due to pupil block increases in hyperopic eyes, which tend to have more crowded anterior chambers,[2] and with age, as the lens increases in size.[1, 2] Nevertheless, a narrow anterior chamber angle is a relatively rare finding, even in patients over the age of 60. Van Herick et al.[2] found that of 403 hyperopes (defined as refractive error > +1.00 D) aged 60 and older, only 14 (3.5%) had narrow (grade 2 or less) angles, and only 6 (2%) of 356 emmetropes (−1.00 D to +1.00 D) 60 years and older had narrow angles. Of 1350 myopes (< −1.00 D) of all ages, only 2 (0.15%) were found to have narrow angles.

Note that we have been talking about eyes in their "natural" state, that is, free of disease or trauma. There are pathological changes which, independent of eye shape or age, may cause secondary angle-closure glaucoma. Pupil block and resulting iris bombé may occur as a result of posterior synechiae, which are adhesions of the posterior iris epithelium (usually near the pupil margin, but more extensively in some cases) to the anterior lens surface as a result of trauma, iritis, exfoliation syndrome, previous angle closure, or prolonged use of miotics. Posterior synechiae can also form between the posterior iris and the anterior hyaloid face or lens capsule in aphakia. An anterior chamber intraocular lens, a displaced posterior chamber intraocular lens, vitreous prolapse through the pupil, or anything else capable of sealing off the route for the passage of aqueous humor between posterior and anterior chambers can cause iris bombé and increase the risk of angle closure. In such cases an opening must be made in the peripheral iris (iridectomy), either by Nd:YAG laser or surgery, to allow aqueous to leave the posterior chamber. Once the pressure difference between the anterior and posterior chambers is reduced, the peripheral iris falls away from the meshwork unless permanent peripheral anterior synechiae have already formed.

Peripheral anterior synechiae (PAS)—adhesions of the anterior iris base to the trabecular meshwork or posterior cornea—obstruct aqueous outflow by permanently sealing off access to the trabecular meshwork. PAS often form as a result of angle closure, trauma, inflammation, or retinal ischemia. The elevation in IOP varies directly with the extent of the PAS, which may range from small isolated sections to complete 360° obstruction.

A narrow angle by itself does not cause elevated IOP because even a slit-like angle allows aqueous enough access to the trabecular meshwork.[3] When the angle is narrow due to either pupil block or a plateau iris configuration, certain conditions may precipitate an acute or subacute elevation in IOP. That is, the only danger of the narrow angle is that it puts the patient at risk for angle closure, and it is only during angle closure that high IOP and the resulting glaucomatous damage to the optic nerve take place. If the attack is broken before anterior synechiae have a chance to form, then no significant damage is done to the outflow channels. On the other hand, once peripheral anterior synechiae have formed, the affected portion of the trabeculum is functionally lost and outflow resistance is per-

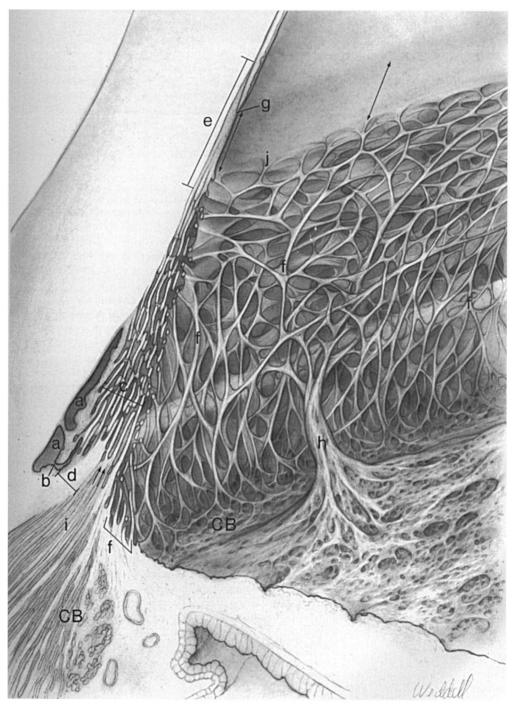

**FIGURE 8–1** Drawing of the aqueous outflow apparatus and adjacent tissues. Schlemm's canal (a) is divided into two portions. An internal collector channel (Sondermann) (b) opens into the posterior part of the canal. The sheets of the corneoscleral meshwork (c) extend from the corneolimbus (e) to the scleral spur (d). The rope-like components of the uveal meshwork (f) occupy the inner portion of the trabecular meshwork; they arise in the ciliary body (CB) near the angle recess and end just posterior to the termination of Descemet's membrane (g). An iris process (h) extends from the root of the iris to merge with the uveal meshwork at about the level of the anterior part of the scleral spur. The longitudinal ciliary muscle (i) is attached to the scleral spur but has a portion that joins the corneoscleral meshwork *(arrows)*. Descemet's membrane terminates within the deep corneolimbus. The corneal endothelium becomes continuous with the trabecular endothelium at (j). A broad transition zone (double-headed arrows) begins near the termination of Descemet's membrane and ends where the uveal meshwork joins the deep corneolimbus. (From Hogan MJ, Alvarado JA, Weddell JE: Histology of the Human Eye: An Atlas and Textbook. Philadelphia: WB Saunders, 1971.)

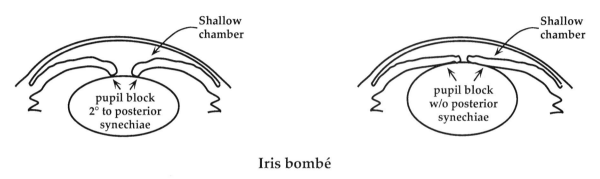

Iris bombé

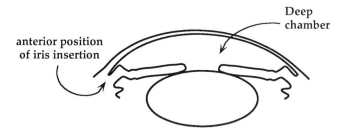

Plateau iris

**FIGURE 8–2** Iris bombé, showing pupil block with and without posterior synechiae, and plateau iris.

manently increased, creating a *chronic* state of elevated IOP. There is an important exception to the above comparison, however. In chronic primary angle-closure glaucoma with pupil block, the angle closes off progressively (usually beginning superiorly and making its way inferiorly), creating a situation of chronic, moderately elevated IOP which is proportional to the extent of the area of iris apposition to the meshwork.[3]

## Causes of Peripheral Anterior Synechiae

During acute angle-closure attacks or during anterior chamber collapse from penetrating trauma or surgery, the iris is pushed up tightly against the trabecular meshwork. If this contact continues for a prolonged period, that is, more than a few hours, exudates cause the iris to adhere permanently to the meshwork, almost ensuring a subsequent chronic elevation in pressure. For this reason, it is imperative that the angle be opened promptly. The presence of PAS in an asymptomatic patient with narrow angles is highly suspicious of previous, possibly unnoticed, angle-closure episodes.

In inflammatory processes such as those due to trauma or anterior uveitis, inflammatory exudates from leaky, congested iris vessels may end up in the angle where, as they organize and shrink, they pull up sections of the peripheral iris into the trabeculum, forming synechiae. Unlike PAS due to angle closure, the synechiae in iritis tend to be localized rather than extensive; furthermore, they occur in a minority of iritis patients.[4]

A particularly malignant form of glaucoma arises when iris neovascularization (rubeosis iridis) extends peripherally up over the meshwork. In the first phase, the fibrovascular membrane obscures the trabeculum and causes an increase in outflow resistance. Subsequently, fibrosis and shrinkage of the membrane draw the iris up into the angle, eventually causing complete and permanent angle closure and severe, intractable glaucoma. The most common cause of neovascular glaucoma is diabetes mellitus, followed by ischemic central retinal vein occlusion and then by carotid artery disease.[3] The common denominator is thought to be the angiogenic stimulus of retinal ischemia, and panretinal photocoagulation is often used prophylactically to slow or reverse the neovascular growth and lower the risk of progression to glaucoma. Not all untreated cases of rubeosis iridis become neovascular glaucoma.

Another potential cause of secondary angle-closure glaucoma is a group of disorders known as the iridocorneal endothelial (ICE) syndromes, the best known of which is essential iris atrophy, Chandler's syndrome, and Cogan-Reese syndrome. In the majority of patients, ICE dystrophies are unilateral or markedly asymmetrical disorders, with onset in early to middle adulthood. All are characterized by an abnormal corneal endothelium that appears on biomicroscopic examination to have a "hammered metal appearance;" the endothelial cell pattern is disorganized, and the cells lose their characteristic, normal polygonal shape. There may be fine guttata, especially in Chandler's syndrome, and corneal edema may occur even in the absence of elevated IOP from angle pathology. Abnormal endothelium grows posteriorly over the angle and onto the anterior iris surface. This membrane may cause moderately elevated IOP early by covering the angle and then cause severe angle-closure glaucoma as it shrinks, creating peripheral anterior synechiae. In essential iris atrophy, the formation of extensive PAS is associated with a tugging on the iris and results in displacement of the pupil (corectopia) toward the synechiae; thinning of the iris may in some cases become so severe that full-thickness holes appear (polycoria).

Posterior polymorphous dystrophy is a rare endothelial dystrophy that may be confused with ICE syndrome and may also cause glaucoma via membranous growth into the anterior chamber angle and the formation of anterior synechiae. This bilateral, inherited disorder is characterized by the presence of groups of endothelial vesicles which may be surrounded by areas of opacification.[5]

In addition to the above mechanisms of secondary angle closure, numerous congenital or developmental anomalies cause glaucoma, and many types of trauma, both accidental and iatrogenic, result in malformation of or damage to the angle. Intraocular tumors may also cause angle closure. Because these patients most likely have been previously diagnosed, or the cause of their glaucoma is obvious, we do not discuss them in detail here.

A closed angle or an angle at risk for closure can usually be diagnosed using gonioscopy; in most cases, the ease with which the examiner can see the trabecular meshwork reflects the ease with which aqueous can get to it. When a gross obstruction of the angle by the iris has been ruled out by gonioscopy in an eye with elevated IOP or glaucomatous optic nerve head damage, one must assume that the cause of the elevated pressure is either within the outflow apparatus itself or due to elevated episcleral venous pressure.

# Microscopic Angle Anatomy and Open-Angle Glaucoma

The angle recess is the name given the depression that forms in the first few months after birth at the anterior aspect of the junction between the iris and ciliary body. Uveal tissue originating from the iris root and ciliary body lines the recess and continues anteriorly to Schwalbe's line in two to three layers of cords known as the uveal meshwork. External to the uveal cords, that is, away from the chamber and toward the sclera, is the corneoscleral meshwork, which makes up the rest of the trabeculum. Extending anteriorly from the scleral spur to Schwalbe's line, it consists of five to nine fenestrated collagen sheets covered by endothelial cells. The outer two-thirds of the corneoscleral meshwork joins the scleral spur itself, with the remaining inner third joining the tendinous termination of those longitudinal ciliary muscle fibers which bypass the scleral spur. Although the effect ciliary contraction has on the meshwork is not precisely known, evidence suggests that facility of outflow is increased during accommodation in humans and by stimulation of the ciliary ganglion in cats. This would explain the observation that cholinergic agents such as pilocarpine increase outflow facility in both normal eyes and eyes with open-angle glaucoma, independent of any miotic effect.[4]

Just beyond the corneoscleral meshwork in the scleral sulcus lies the canal of Schlemm, a venous channel that runs circumferentially around the limbus and is responsible for collecting aqueous humor and draining it to the episcleral venous network. A thin layer of tissue separates the lumen of the canal from the outermost corneoscleral sheet; this "juxtacanalicular tissue" is composed of an amorphous ground substance with occasional collagen bundles, lined on both sides (one facing the last corneoscleral sheet, the other the lumen of Schlemm's canal) with endothelial cells. Aqueous makes its way across the meshwork—through the fenestrations and between the lamellae—in winding paths that can be conceptualized as "aqueous channels." These spaces terminate at the juxtacanalicular tissue in cul-de-sacs,[6] from which aqueous passes into the canal. There are many different theories concerning the mechanism of aqueous flow, such as through intercellular gaps in the endothelial lining of Schlemm's canal versus transcellular channels, and the site of outflow resistance in both normal and hypertensive eyes, such as trabeculum, canal, and collector channels. The fact is that how aqueous gets into Schlemm's canal and why it has trouble doing so in certain eyes are still basically unknown.

When reduced outflow facility in an unobstructed angle results in increased IOP, which in turn leads to progressive cupping and atrophy of the optic nerve head and visual field loss, we speak of "open-angle glaucoma."[3] When the elevation in IOP occurs in the absence of any related ocular or systemic disease, it is assumed due to an idiopathic decrease in outflow facility and is called "primary open-angle glaucoma." This is a diagnosis of exclusion. When there is an known ocular or systemic condition presumed responsible for the increased outflow resistance, we speak of "secondary open-angle glaucoma."

Perhaps the most common ocular condition associated with secondary open-angle glaucoma is exfoliation syndrome. This disease is found predominantly in older patients, is found roughly equally in men and women, and—although found to some degree in most countries—is a common cause of glaucoma in Scandinavian populations.[7] It manifests itself as the elaboration and deposition of a greyish-white fibrillar material involving many ocular tissues, including the ciliary body, zonules, lens capsule, iris, cornea, and trabecular meshwork. The associated glaucoma is characterized by higher IOPs, greater resistance to treatment, and a worse prognosis than the primary open-angle form.[7, 8] The classic presentation of exfoliation syndrome is the well-known three-zone pattern on the anterior surface of the lens capsule (seen during pupil dilation) or as dandruff-like flakes on the pupil margin. The gonioscopic appearance of the angle in exfoliation syndrome is characterized by an abnormal amount of pigment, both bound to clumps of exfoliative material (deposited by the exiting aqueous) in the superficial meshwork and within the cells of the posterior corneal endothelium ("Sampaolesi lines").[9] A recent study suggests that an additional cause of the elevated IOP in exfoliation syndrome is the elaboration of exfoliative material deeper within the angle by trabecular cells themselves, with subsequent clogging of and damage to the corneoscleral meshwork and juxtacanalicular tissue.[8]

The most likely source of the liberated pigment in exfoliation syndrome is the pupillary portion of the iris pigment epithelium, which rubs against the rough surface of the coated lens capsule during pupil movement and is the site of the transillumination defects characteristic of this disease. An increase in anterior chamber pigment is often in seen exfoliation patients after pharmacological dilation. Some studies have shown an association between the quantity of pigment in the angle and the severity of glaucoma in exfoliation patients.[9, 10] Interestingly, a higher than normal prevalence of occludable angles is found among patients with exfoliation syndrome, even in the absence of miotic therapy (used for treating their glaucoma) and posterior synechiae (which are a common associated finding).[11, 12]

Another cause of secondary open-angle glaucoma associated with abnormal angle pigmentation is pigmentary dispersion syndrome, which is characterized by loss of pigment from the posterior peripheral iris and deposition of this pigment on the anterior iris, on the corneal endothelium and in the trabecular meshwork. The mechanism of this pigment liberation is most likely the rubbing action of the lens zonules against the peripheral iris, which is typically observed to be concave in these patients. Seen most commonly in young, myopic, Caucasian males, the condition tends to decrease in severity with age, presumably when changes in the lens/iris relationship lead to increased pupil block and a lifting of the peripheral iris away from the zonules.

Chronic inflammatory disease, such as anterior uveitis, can also lead to open-angle glaucoma via microscopic damage to the trabecular meshwork by inflammatory by-products. This is in addition to the role of inflammatory disease in closed-angle glaucoma through the formation of both posterior and anterior synechiae.

A rather mysterious cause of secondary open-angle glaucoma is angle recession caused by blunt trauma. The injury causes a tear in the ciliary muscle, which can be seen gonioscopically as an area where the angle is excessively deep, exposing a wide band of ciliary body. A secondary open-angle glaucoma may develop months to years after the original injury; the mechanism is not known.

## MECHANISM OF SECONDARY OPEN-ANGLE GLAUCOMAS

Although it was long assumed that increased outflow resistance in eyes with pigmentary dispersion syndrome and exfoliation syndrome was due to a mechanical "clogging" of the trabecular meshwork, recent electron micrographic studies have suggested that exfoliative material and pigment granules within the trabecular meshwork and juxtacanalicular tissue may be responsible for damage at the cellular level.[6, 8, 9, 13] An obliteration of the aqueous channels and a reduction in the cul-de-sac area has been found in both primary open-angle glaucoma and pigmentary glaucoma,[6] with the implication that the corneoscleral meshwork and juxtacanalicular tissue are the sites of increased outflow resistance in these glaucomas. Alvarado and Murphy[6] propose that melanin is toxic to the trabecular cells and that their injury and death lead to the adhesion of the trabecular sheets to each other, with the resulting loss of intralamellar spaces and disappearance of the aqueous channels and cul-de-sacs.[6] Interestingly, they note that a similar loss of cellularity and trabecular collapse is found in primary open-angle glaucoma, even in the absence of pigment. Schlotzer-Schrehardt and Naumann[8] found endothelial cell damage and disorganization of the meshwork and juxtacanalicular tissue in eyes with exfoliation syndrome, as well.

## THE ROLE OF EPISCLERAL VENOUS PRESSURE IN OPEN-ANGLE GLAUCOMA

Whatever the physiological mechanism of outflow resistance, the driving mechanism for aqueous movement out of the eye is the hydrostatic pressure gradient from anterior chamber to the anterior ciliary veins.* The aqueous leaves Schlemm's canal via 20 to 30 collector channels, which carry it to the intrascleral venous plexus, then to the episcleral venous plexus, and out through the anterior ciliary veins. Aqueous veins also provide a direct route between Schlemm's canal and the episcleral venous plexus.

A typical episcleral venous pressure is 9 to 10 mm Hg; as IOP increases above this level, aqueous is driven out of the anterior chamber at a rate proportional to the pressure difference until a steady state is reached. It should be noted that the steady state is not the point at which the two pressures are equal, when flow would stop, but rather the point at which the pressure difference is just enough to maintain outflow at a rate equal to that of aqueous humor production. The

trabecular meshwork is believed to act as a valve that collapses when the IOP drops below the episcleral venous pressure, thereby increasing outflow resistance and IOP and preventing red blood cells and other inappropriate blood components from entering the anterior chamber. (In this way the outflow apparatus functions as part of the blood-aqueous barrier.)[3] Once the IOP rises above the episcleral venous pressure, the trabeculum "opens up" and aqueous flows out. Unfortunately, this negative feedback loop breaks down at very high IOP, when the trabeculum is pushed outward, collapsing the lumen of Schlemm's canal and increasing outflow resistance and increasing the pressure still further.

When the episcleral venous pressure rises above normal levels, the IOP also increases via the mechanism described above. The increase in IOP is similar in magnitude to the increase in the episcleral venous pressure.[3] Downstream obstruction of venous drainage by aneurysm or neoplasm, jugular vein obstruction, thyroid eye disease, trauma, arteriovenous fistulas, or Sturge-Weber syndrome may cause elevated episcleral venous pressure and IOP. The associated eye findings and laterality vary, depending on the cause. For a more complete discussion of the common causes, the reader is referred to *Becker-Shaffer's Diagnosis and Therapy of the Glaucomas*, 6th ed.[3]

# Normal-Tension Glaucoma and Ocular Hypertension

. . . . . . . . . . . . . . . . . . . . . . . .

Glaucoma is a disease in which the IOP is sufficiently high to cause damage to the optic nerve. Because the nerve's vulnerability to pressure (most likely a function of both mechanical and vascular factors) varies enormously between individuals, there is no absolute definition of "high" IOP. It stands to reason that eyes with good vascular perfusion of the nerve head and a strong lamina cribrosa may not be damaged at all by slightly elevated IOP and may suffer nerve damage only when subjected to chronic moderately elevated pressures or the extremely high pressures typical of acute angle closure. When the IOP is elevated (i.e., above an arbitrary 21 mm Hg) in a patient with no detectable ocular or systemic cause and no glaucomatous damage to the optic nerve, it is defined as "ocular hypertension."

When there is pre-existing vascular disease or a structural weakness (due to heredity, collagen disorder, or high myopia, for example), the nerve

---

*In addition to the conventional outflow route discussed here, a smaller proportion of aqueous leaves the eye via the "uveoscleral route" by passing through the anterior ciliary body. According to Moses, this unconventional route is responsible for only 0.2 to 0.5 μL/min of outflow, compared with 1.8 to 2.5 μL/min through the trabeculum. Furthermore, a very small amount of aqueous also makes its way from the anterior chamber to the tear film through the cornea, and from the posterior chamber back into the vitreous. (Moses RA: Intraocular pressure. *In* Adler's Physiology of the Eye, 7th ed. St. Louis: CV Mosby Co, 1985.)

head may be vulnerable to damage even at "normal" IOP. If glaucomatous damage—seen at the nerve head or as visual field loss—is occurring, the pressure is too high for that nerve. When damage occurs with IOP below 21 mm Hg, it is defined by the term "normal tension glaucoma."

# Slit-Lamp Examination of the Anterior Chamber

A basic slit-lamp examination contains the following elements, which are directly relevant to the identification of risk factors in both open-angle and angle-closure glaucoma.

## GRADING THE PERIPHERAL ANTERIOR CHAMBER DEPTH

The peripheral anterior chamber depth is used as an indicator of the risk of angle closure. This technique was shown by van Herick et al.[2] to have very good correlation with gonioscopic grading of angle width. The grading scheme compares the anterior chamber depth at the limbus with the corneal thickness. The vast majority of patients in a primary care practice have grade 3 and grade 4 peripheral anterior chamber depths.

Grade 4: The anterior chamber depth is at least as wide as corneal thickness; the angle is wide open, with essentially no risk of angle closure (with the possible exception of plateau iris, as described above).

Grade 3: The anterior chamber depth is between one-quarter and one-half the width of the corneal thickness; the angle is open with essentially no risk of angle closure.

Grade 2: The anterior chamber depth is one-quarter of the corneal thickness; the angle is moderately narrow, and closure is possible.

Grade 1: The anterior chamber depth is less than one-quarter of the corneal thickness; the angle is extremely narrow, and closure at some point is probable.

Grade 0: The clear space between the iris and the cornea is slitlike or absent; the chamber is extremely shallow or closed, and angle closure is imminent or present.

Start temporally using the narrowest possible optic section under moderate ($16\times$) magnification. The slit-lamp beam should be oriented so that the optic section is incident perpendicular to the limbus, and the microscope should be oriented 60° from the lamp. Move the slit beam laterally from the limbus until it just becomes visible on the iris. Grade the angle by comparing the width of the peripheral anterior chamber (the clear space between the back of the cornea and the illuminated surface of the iris) with the corneal thickness. Repeat for the nasal angle. It should be kept in mind that the angle is often narrower superiorly than laterally. Any eye having a grade 2 or smaller temporal or nasal peripheral anterior chamber depth should be evaluated gonioscopically to determine the risk of angle closure.

## EXAMINATION OF THE CORNEAL ENDOTHELIUM

Examine the back surface of the cornea in direct, indirect, and retro-illumination to look for pigment deposition. Pigmentation may be scattered or may form a vertical line (Krukenberg spindle) in the central cornea. Corneal endothelial pigmentation signals the possible presence of pigment in the angle from pigmentary dispersion syndrome, exfoliation syndrome, uveitis, or other pathology. Also look for keratic precipitates, which are clumps of inflammatory proteins and cells that have settled out onto the corneal endothelium and indicate either active or past inflammation. A "hammered silver" appearance of the endothelium or very fine guttata are typical of ICE syndromes and corneal dystrophies. Groups of small endothelial vesicles are typical of posterior polymorphous dystrophy.

Use specular reflection to examine the endothelial cells for irregularities characteristic of ICE syndromes: a loss of polygonal pattern with change in the size, shape, and density of the endothelial cells.

# Examination of the Iris

Begin by using diffuse illumination at low magnification. Note the contour of the iris. Is it relatively flat, with a deep central chamber, or is it pushed forward? Look for gross abnormalities in the anterior iris surface, such as a post-surgical peripheral iridectomy, iris atrophy, tumors, or nevi. Make sure to lift the upper lid so that the entire iris is examined. Narrow the slit beam to 1 to 2 mm and increase the magnification to inspect the anterior stroma, noting the presence and distribution of pigment granules; large particles over the iris sphincter region are characteristic of exfoliation syndrome, whereas finer, more

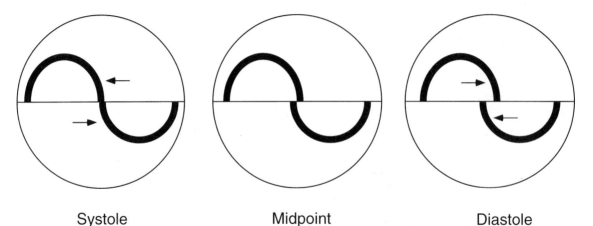

Systole                    Midpoint                    Diastole

**FIGURE 8–3**  Fluctuation in intraocular pressure with the cardiac cycle. Average intraocular pressure is measured when the amplitude of the movement is symmetrical around the tonometry end point.

peripheral deposits arranged along the contraction furrows are seen in pigmentary dispersion syndrome.[7] Carefully inspect the pupil margin for signs of exfoliation such as flakes and loss of the pigment ruff. Look for neovascular tufts signalling rubeosis iridis. Turn off the room lights, reduce the magnification, and, while dark adapting, use the slit beam to constrict the pupil, noting any asymmetries or irregularities that might indicate posterior synechiae.

When your eyes have dark adapted, move the lamp to the straight-ahead position and decrease the height of the slit, placing it just inside the pupil margin. Using retro-illumination off the fundus, look for iris transillumination defects, which appear as radially oriented slits in the ciliary portion of the iris. They are pathognomonic for pigmentary dispersion syndrome; a moth-eaten pattern of transillumination defects in the sphincter region is characteristic of exfoliation syndrome.

## Examination of the Aqueous

While the eyes are still dark adapted, reduce the slit beam to a conical section and angle the light source obliquely (45° to 60°). Using moderate to high magnification, bounce the focus back and forth between the posterior cornea and the anterior lens and iris, looking for cells in the anterior chamber and aqueous flare. Cells and flare in the aqueous indicate active inflammation. Inflammatory cells appear round and distinct, whereas flare—free-floating proteins—clouds the aqueous and scatters light, allowing the slit-lamp beam,

which is ordinarily invisible in optically empty space, to be seen. Pigment granules may also be found floating in the anterior chamber and may come from a number of sources, including pigmentary dispersion syndrome, exfoliation syndrome, and trauma.

At the conclusion of the slit-lamp examination, you should have a reasonably good idea of whether the patient is at risk for either angle-closure or secondary open-angle glaucoma. The next step, for all patients, is measurement of intraocular pressure.

## Tonometry

Tonometry should be performed routinely on all patients as part of a complete eye examination, and it is particularly important whenever other findings indicate the possibility of glaucoma. IOP should be measured before gonioscopy and dilation, because both may significantly affect it. On the other hand, because applanation tonometry may have both mechanical and pharmacological effects on the eye, it should always be performed *after* examination of the cornea and anterior chamber.

### PRINCIPLES OF GOLDMANN APPLANATION TONOMETRY

The clinical standard for measurement of IOP is the Goldmann tonometer. An understanding of the basic principles behind applanation tonometry should motivate the clinician to strive for the proper technique, which is necessary for accurate results.

This slit lamp–mounted applanation device measures the amount of force needed to counteract the IOP in flattening a circular corneal area 3.06 mm in diameter. When the face of the tonometer head is in contact with the cornea, four forces are operating: The fluid pressure behind the cornea (IOP) and the corneal resistance to deformation work *against* applanation, pushing the tonometer head away from the cornea, while the force of the tonometer head and the capillary attraction of the tear film for the tonometer head work *for* applanation, pushing or pulling the tonometer head toward the cornea. For a circular applanation area of diameter 3.06 mm, the force required to deform the cornea is counterbalanced by the capillary attraction of the tear film for the tonometer head, leaving the force of the tonometer and the IOP to counterbalance each other.[3]

The applanated area is visualized by the clinician as a ring of tear fluid surrounding the flattened area (made visible by the use of fluorescein and a cobalt filter). The inner diameter of this annulus is equal to the area of applanation. Just behind the face of the tonometer tip are two prisms, oriented so that the top half of a 3.06-mm tear ring is displaced one-half its diameter to the left, and the bottom half is displaced the same amount to the right (Fig. 8–4). Because the relative balance of the forces involved determines the size of the ring, only when the diameter of the applanation area is exactly 3.06 mm do the inner edges of the two half rings touch, and the dial reading is an accurate indicator of IOP.

Because only 0.5 μL of aqueous humor is dis-

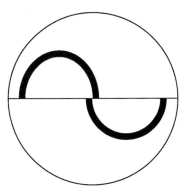

**FIGURE 8–4** In Goldmann tonometry, the applanated area is visualized by the clinician as a ring of tear fluid surrounding the flattened area. The inner diameter of this annulus is equal to the area of applanation. Just behind the face of the tonometer tip there are two prisms, oriented so that the top half of a 3.06-mm tear ring is displaced one-half of its diameter to the left, and the bottom half is displaced the same amount to the right.

placed by this deformation, the measurement is not very sensitive to differences in ocular rigidity; however, the measured IOP is slightly higher (about 3%) than the actual IOP.[3] Hand-held versions of this type of instrument, such as the Perkins tonometer, work on the same principle, with the advantage that they can be used on patients who cannot sit at a slit lamp.

## GOLDMANN TONOMETRY: TECHNIQUE

1. Place a clean, dry tonometer prism in the holder on the slit lamp, aligning the 180° mark on the prism with the white mark on the holder for patients with 3.00 D or less corneal toricity. For patients with higher corneal toricity, align the mark corresponding to the flat meridian of the cornea on the prism with the red mark on the prism holder. This is to provide a sufficient area of contact along the tonometer midline for highly toric corneas. Set the tonometer dial to 1 gram.

2. Swing the tonometer arm into place, making sure it is in the click stop position. Angle the lamp so that the tip of the tonometer head is well-illuminated, using a bright, wide-open beam and cobalt filter. Set the magnification to medium (10×), and turn down the room lights.

3. Anesthetize the cornea and instill fluorescein in one of the following ways:

☐ Instill one drop of topical anesthetic in each eye, wait a minute, then carefully apply fluorescein from a wetted strip into the lower fornices.

☐ Instill one drop of Fluress or other anesthetic/fluorescein combination to each eye.

4. Position the patient comfortably at the slit lamp, with chin and forehead firmly against the rests. Instruct the patient to blink to distribute the fluorescein, open his or her eyes widely, and look straight ahead. While looking from outside the slit lamp, bring the tonometer carefully toward the cornea by sliding the entire slit lamp forward, holding the joystick back to ensure enough forward play for applanation, until a blue limbal "glow" is seen and the tonometer just barely makes contact with the tear film. Approach the cornea slightly low, to avoid touching the upper lashes, then raise the tip to the level of the corneal apex.

5. Seat yourself behind the oculars and move the joystick gently forward until contact is

made. If the prism is far off-center, an intact circle is seen either above or below the center line. In this case, back off the cornea and use the joystick to move the slit lamp in the direction of the circle. Re-applanate, performing minor adjustments with the joystick so that the top and bottom semicircles are the same size and the entire pattern is centered. To center, always move the prism toward the larger segment of the tear circle (e.g., move prism up if top half is bigger).

As the tonometer head makes increasing contact with the cornea, the ring diameter increases. The size of the semicircles reflects whether the amount of contact is grossly appropriate, that is, whether you are within the "fine tuning" range provided by the force dial (Fig. 8-5). When there is far too little contact because the tonometer head is too far away from the cornea, the semicircles appear too small and too far apart, and the joystick should be used to move in closer. If the tonometer prism is pushed too far in, the circle appears to be too large; use the joystick to back off. Once the correct applanation area is approximately achieved (test for this by moving the dial in either direction to make sure you can both overlap and separate the rings), adjust the force dial until the *inner* edges of the two semicircles line up, forming a continuous curve.

6. Multiply the reading on the tonometer dial by 10 to get the intraocular pressure in millimeters of mercury (mm Hg).
7. Repeat the measurement; if not within 1 mm Hg, repeat again.

## RECORDING INTRAOCULAR PRESSURE

When recording IOP, always specify the time at which the measurement was taken. For glaucoma patients, also record the time(s) when glaucoma medication(s) were last instilled (for topical medications) or ingested (for oral medications).

## CAUSES OF INACCURATE MEASUREMENT OF INTRAOCULAR PRESSURE

☐ Pressure on the globe: Obviously, if it is necessary to hold the lids while performing tonometry, the examiner must be sure to avoid putting any pressure on the globe, as this significantly elevates the IOP.
☐ Systole/diastole pulsations: In some patients, the intraocular pressure fluctuates significantly with arterial pressure. This is seen as a pulsatile movement of the rings such that they are farther apart during systole, when the IOP is higher, and closer together during diastole, when the IOP is lower (see Fig. 8-4). To avoid overestimating or underestimating IOP in these patients, adjust the tonometer dial so that this movement "straddles" the usual end point; this reflects the average IOP.
☐ Uncalibrated tonometer: The tonometer should be periodically checked for calibration.
☐ Corneal pathology: Any condition that affects corneal thickness or corneal regularity (e.g., edema, scarring, thinning, surgery) affects the accuracy of the Goldmann tonometer. Other devices—such as the Mackay-Marg tonometer, the Tono-Pen, or the Pneuma-tonometer—may be more appropriate in such cases.
☐ Amount of fluorescein: The thickness of the tear meniscus can affect the measurement of IOP. The ring width should be approximately one-tenth the ring diameter (0.3 mm). If there is too little fluorescein in the eye, the rings are too narrow and pressure is slightly underestimated. Too much fluorescein results in rings that are too wide, and the IOP is slightly overestimated.

## ROUTINE ACTIVITIES THAT AFFECT INTRAOCULAR PRESSURE

☐ Alcohol and marijuana temporarily lower IOP.
☐ Excessive water consumption can raise IOP.
☐ While strenuous exercise generally tends to reduce IOP,[3] it can cause a sharp increase in pressure in patients with pigmentary dispersion syndrome.

## DISINFECTION OF THE TONOMETER TIP

The Goldmann tonometer tip must be disinfected after each use. It should be immersed in 3% hydrogen peroxide for 10 minutes.

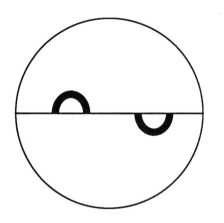

Applanation area far too small; gently increase pressure on cornea using joystick

Applanation area roughly correct; use force dial to align inner edges

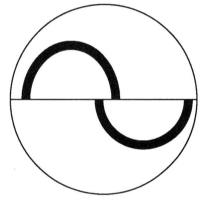

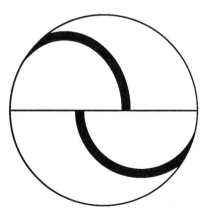

Applanation area far too large; reduce pressure on cornea using joystick

**FIGURE 8–5** In Goldmann tonometry, when there is far too little contact because the tonometer head is too far away from the cornea, the semicircles appear too small and too far apart, and the joystick should be used to move in closer. If the tonometer prism is pushed too far in, the circle appears to be too large; use the joystick to back off. Once the correct applanation area is approximately achieved, adjust the force dial until the *inner* edges of the two semicircles line up, forming a continuous curve.

## INTERPRETATION OF TONOMETRY RESULTS

IOP is only one—albeit significant—piece of information in assessing a patient's risk of having or developing glaucoma. Although elevated IOP is no doubt associated with visual loss due to damage to the optic nerve head, most ocular hypertensives do not develop visual loss. The decision to initiate treatment to lower IOP depends on the larger picture, which includes age, race, family history of glaucoma, refractive error, systemic health, ocular health, your ability to visualize the optic nerve head, and the patient's ability to perform reliable visual fields.

An IOP of 22 mm Hg or greater should certainly make you take notice. Having done a slit-lamp examination, you will already know whether the patient has pigmentary dispersion syndrome, exfoliation syndrome, uveitis, a corneal endothelial dystrophy, or a shallow peripheral anterior chamber. The first step, then, is to perform gonioscopy to gauge the effect these have had on the angle, and to look for other—possibly hidden—causes of aqueous obstruction such as plateau iris, peripheral anterior synechiae, neovascularization, or neoplasm. A normal, open angle leaves you with a high index of suspicion for primary open-angle glaucoma. The next step is a careful stereoscopic assessment of the optic nerve heads (noting cup to disc ratio, color, and health of the neuroretinal rim), and visual fields.

Once all the above information has been gathered, you need to make a decision regarding the disposition of the patient. The following guidelines are adapted from *Becker-Shaffer's Diagnosis and Therapy of the Glaucomas* (6th ed.). IOP between 22 and 30 mm Hg which is unaccompanied by gonioscopic abnormalities, suspicious cupping, visual field loss, or a positive family history of open-angle glaucoma puts the patient in the ocular hypertensive category. This patient should be followed every 1 to 2 years with tonometry, optic disc assessment, and visual fields. Baseline stereo optic disc photographs are helpful in judging whether change is taking place; increased disc cupping over time or the development of glaucomatous field loss warrants initiation of medical treatment to lower IOP. An ocular hypertensive with a family history of glaucoma may also be considered for treatment because he or she is at a much greater risk for the development of visual loss than an ocular hypertensive with no family history.

When IOP is over 30 mm Hg, treatment should be seriously considered even in the absence of other risk factors, based on studies that show that above this pressure a significant percentage of eyes (varying from 11% to 29%) have either optic nerve damage or visual field loss.[3] If you do not treat glaucoma yourself, patients with IOP over 30 mm Hg should be referred.

# Gonioscopy

By doing gonioscopy one is generally trying to answer one or both of the following questions: (1) Is this narrow angle in danger of closing? or (2) Is there some secondary process going on in this angle which is causing or which will someday cause glaucoma?

To develop the manual dexterity and the familiarity with angle structures necessary to be an effective gonioscopist, the clinician should make a point of performing this technique as often as possible. Although gonioscopy is optional for the majority of patients, examination of the anterior chamber angle is required under the following circumstances:

1. The suspicion that a patient is at risk for spontaneous angle closure may be based on slit-lamp grading of the peripheral anterior chamber depth (van Herick grade 2 or lower), the appearance of iris bombé, or a patient's report of symptoms suggesting transient episodes of angle closure.

   In the foregoing circumstances gonioscopy should be performed whether pupil dilation is anticipated or not. Once the angle has been examined, the decision of whether or not to dilate can be made based on the relative risks and benefits.
2. Previously undiagnosed elevated IOP, especially if it is unilateral.
3. Previously undiagnosed glaucomatous damage to the optic nerve head, even in the absence of elevated IOP.
4. When neovascularization of the iris is found.

Gonioscopy should also be used to document the state of the angle when the history, slit-lamp examination, or ophthalmoscopy indicates a risk of future secondary glaucoma. This would be the case with chronic inflammation (e.g., iritis), pigmentary dispersion syndrome, exfoliation syndrome, ischemic disease, ICE syndrome, and after blunt trauma (especially with hyphema). In other words, gonioscopy is performed whenever it is necessary to diagnose the cause of elevated IOP or to characterize the risk of developing acute or chronic glaucoma.

Gonioscopy should always be performed after

tonometry because the pressure of the gonioscopy lens on the anterior chamber may significantly alter (usually lower) the IOP. Unless the purpose is to observe the angle during dilation or to view the anterior ciliary body, gonioscopy should be done prior to dilation.

## GONIOSCOPIC LENSES

The anterior chamber angle cannot be viewed directly because in nearly all eyes light emerging from the angle undergoes total internal reflection at the interface between the pre-corneal tear film and the air. Two basic techniques are used to circumvent this problem. In direct gonioscopy, a lens is placed on the eye which replaces the tear film–air interface with a more steeply curved lens-air interface at which light is refracted rather than reflected. This type of lens (Koeppe lens) has the advantage of providing a 360° view of the angle. Unfortunately, the patient needs to be examined in the supine position, and the light source/magnification system must be either hand-held or suspended from the ceiling. For these reasons, direct gonioscopy has lost popularity over the years in clinical practice and has been replaced by indirect gonioscopy.

Indirect gonioscopy also uses a contact lens to neutralize the tear film–air interface, but illumination and visualization of the angle are accomplished using the slit lamp via angled mirrors within the lens, oriented opposite the portion of the angle being observed. The advantages of this technique are that the patient sits upright and that the slit lamp allows variable magnification and—perhaps most importantly—the use of a narrow beam of light to reveal the contour and position of angle structures. Indirect gonioscopy lenses come in two basic designs. The first is the Goldmann-type lens, which has either one or two mirrors specifically angled for gonioscopy (and thus needs to be rotated 270° or 90°, respectively, in order to view all four quadrants) and requires a viscous fluid such as methylcellulose (gonioscopy fluid) to fill the cornea-lens interface. The second is the Zeiss-type four-mirror lens, which allows viewing of all four quadrants without rotation and, because of its flat base curve, does not require gonioscopy fluid. Each type has its advantages and disadvantages. The use of gonioscopy fluid is fairly noxious to the patient, needs to be flushed from the eye to avoid both irritation and a compromised view in ophthalmoscopy, and is liable to problems with air bubbles. On the other hand, the suction achieved with a Goldmann lens makes it stable on the eye and thus easy to handle; it is a good

lens for beginning or occasional gonioscopists. It is hard for the patient to blink out these lenses. In addition, the center of all Goldmann lenses is an excellent fundus contact lens; the Goldmann three-mirror lens also has mirrors angled for the mid- and far periphery of the retina.

The Zeiss-type lens fits much more easily into the flow of the examination because the examiner can pick it up after tonometry and place it on the still-anesthetized eye to get an immediate look at the angle, then proceed with dilation without having to flush gonioscopic fluid from the eye. Its greatest advantage, however, is its small diameter, which allows indentation gonioscopy for distinguishing appositional angle closure from synechial angle closure, and makes it less intimidating to the patient. Because it is held against the eye only by pressure, the Zeiss lens requires a steady hand, good coordination, and considerable practice in order to maintain the proper amount of contact.

## INDIRECT GONIOSCOPY: TECHNIQUE

### Choice of Lens

The choice of lens depends on several factors, some of which are discussed above. Individual preference is undoubtedly the primary determinant. Another consideration is the size of the palpebral aperture; a patient with a small aperture and tight lids may do better with a smaller lens. One should be aware that different lenses give different vantage points of the angle: The smaller Goldmann-type lenses (the one- and two-mirror lenses) place the mirror higher relative to the angle—which allows a steeper view into a narrow angle—than does the larger three-mirror lens. Although this is an advantage when trying to see over an iris bombé or plateau iris, it foreshortens the view of the angle structures compared with the view given by the larger lens, which—because the lens is farther from the angle—is more nearly parallel to the (normal) iris plane. Therefore, the smaller lenses are better for narrow angles, whereas the larger lens is better when a detailed view of angle structure is required, that is, in the open-angle situation. In most situations this is not a critical decision, however, because the view into the angle can be varied by changing the position of the lens relative to the angle (Fig. 8-6).

### Application of the Gonioscopy Lens

The patient should be seated comfortably at the slit lamp with the chin rest adjusted so that the

Iris blocking view of angle structures                    Angle structures visible

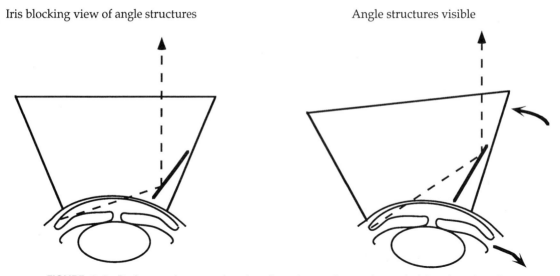

FIGURE 8–6  During gonioscopy, the view into the angle can be varied by changing the position of the lens relative to the angle. Sliding the lens toward the angle and/or having the patient look toward the mirror allows a steeper view into the angle.

outer canthus more or less lines up with the mark on the slit lamp. Set the magnification to $20\times$ with the lamp straight ahead and a 2- to 3-mm high narrow slit beam (optic section). If needed, place an elbow rest on the slit-lamp table to stabilize the arm that will hold the lens.

If using a Goldmann lens, turn the lens concave side up and fill the concavity with gonioscopy fluid, being extremely careful not to get air bubbles into the lens. Many clinicians store gonioscopy fluid bottles upside down to keep air out of the tip; some remove the tip and pour the fluid. Alternatively, start the stream going over a tissue, then move it over the lens when all the air has been forced out.

If the eyes are not still anesthetized from tonometry, instill anesthetic to both eyes. Seat yourself, have the patient look up, and reach around the slit lamp to pin the upper lid to the superior orbital rim. For the right eye, hold the lens in the left hand, with the gonioscopy mirror in the superior position, and use the right hand to hold the lid. Apply the edge of the lens opposite the gonioscopy mirror to the inferior bulbar conjunctiva, just below the limbus. As you do this, instruct the patient to look straight ahead, and as he or she does so gently rock the lens up against the cornea. Do not release the upper lid until the lens is in contact with the cornea superiorly. If using a Goldmann-type lens, hold the lens lightly with thumb, forefinger, and middle finger, and use the remaining two fingers to brace your hand on the patient's cheek. If a bubble under the lens interferes with the view, remove the lens and start over.

If using a Zeiss lens, hold the lens lightly but steadily against the eye, with thumb and forefinger holding the handle and the other three fingers braced against the cheek. Folds in Descemet's membrane mean that too much pressure is being used. Air under the lens means that the contact between lens and cornea is insufficient.

No matter which lens is used, be methodical in your examination. Begin with the inferior angle, and work your way around all four quadrants.

## The Gonioscopist's View: a "Tour" of the Anterior Chamber Angle

The gonioscopic "view" places you, the gonioscopist, in the anterior chamber of the eye, looking into the angle. Think of the view in the superior mirror, where it is as if you are standing on the anterior surface of the iris, just on the opposite side of the pupil from the (inferior) angle. Looking down, you see the pupil at your feet, the anterior lens capsule lying just below. Inspect the pupil margin for exfoliative material or neovascularization. As your gaze moves away toward the angle, you should note the pupillary ruff, the collarette, and the crypts and folds of the iris stroma beyond. Note any abnormalities in shape or color, any abnormal blood vessels, or any pigment deposition. Beyond the contraction furrows you encounter the last roll of the iris, behind which looms the dome of the cornea. At the place where the iris meets the corneoscleral junction lies the angle. In a wide-open angle the baseboard, so to speak, is a pigmented band—ranging in color from light grey to dark brown—which is the anterior face of the ciliary body. Just above it is the line of scleral spur, which may be evident only by its contrast with the ciliary body below and which may be pale grey, white, or yellowish. There may be an occasional iris process, or many, which follow the contour of the recess between floor and wall, or bridge the gap to insert near the spur. Above the spur lies the trabecular meshwork, which may be relatively featureless, or pigmented—most heavily in its bottom third—behind which lies the canal of Schlemm. (If the lens is compressing the episcleral veins, or the IOP is quite low, or there is elevated episcleral venous pressure, and if the meshwork is not too darkly pigmented, you might see Schlemm's canal, made visible by the red blood cells within.) The meshwork continues upward until it reaches the upper limit of the angle, Schwalbe's line. If Schwalbe's line is hard to locate, follow the optic section up to where it splits in two. When you have found the place where the fuzzy sweep of the anterior corneal reflex curves around to join the more distinct sweep of the posterior corneal reflex, you have found it. Follow the optic section back down the wall of the angle, and note the contour of the peripheral iris. Does the optic section disappear before it shows up again on the iris floor or is it visible as it makes the turn? If it is visible, does it seem to dip as it runs along the anterior iris surface? Now look at the angle formed by the optic section between the iris surface and the trabecular meshwork; this should give you a good idea of the angle width.

## Indentation Gonioscopy

One of the main advantages of the Zeiss four-mirror lens over the Goldmann design is that its smaller area of contact and flatter base curve allow the examiner to distinguish appositional narrowing or closure (due to iris bombé or plateau iris) from anterior synechiae by exerting pressure on the central cornea. The peripheral displacement of aqueous forces the peripheral iris away from the angle structures unless synechiae prevent it. This is known as indentation gonioscopy and should be performed by briefly exerting *gentle* pressure to avoid compromising vascular perfusion to an already at-risk nerve head.

## Grading the Angle

Along with viewing the angle, you need to be able to characterize it for the patient's record and/or for referral. Several grading schemes are used by gonioscopists. The Shaffer system grades the angle between the peripheral iris and the trabecular meshwork as follows:

| | |
|---|---|
| Grade 4 | 35°-45° |
| Grade 3 | 20°-35° |
| Grade 2 | 20° |
| Grade 1 | ≤10° |
| Slit | slit |
| Grade 0 | 0° |

Closure is considered possible for grade 2 angles and probable for grade 1 or slit angles; Grade 0 angles are already closed.

A more rigorous grading system was devised by Spaeth,[15] in which the angle is characterized in terms of the position of the iris attachment, the geometric relationship between the iris and trabecular meshwork, and the shape of the peripheral iris, as follows:

### The Spaeth Grading Scheme

1. Angle width is graded by estimating the angle between two imaginary lines, one tangential to the trabecular meshwork and the other tangential to the anterior iris surface about one-third of the way between the iris root and the pupil margin. Spaeth recommends 10° increments from 0° (iris up against cornea) to 40° (iris flat) (Fig. 8-7).
2. Peripheral iris contour is described by one of three letters (Fig. 8-8):
   r Iris has a mildly convex shape or flat shape (r stands for "regular"); this is the normal, common form.
   s Iris rises steeply from its root, as with iris bombé or plateau iris, obscuring the view of the angle structures (s stands for "steep" or "sharp").
   q Iris has a concave shape peripherally, which results in a wide angle recess (q stands for "queer"); this is seen in some myopic eyes and in pigmentary dispersion syndrome.
3. The position of the iris attachment is characterized using one of five capital letters (Fig. 8-9):
   A Iris attaches at or anterior to Schwalbe's line (i.e., to the peripheral cornea), thus obscuring the trabecular meshwork. This is pathological.
   B Iris attaches to trabecular meshwork (i.e., posterior to Schwalbe's line but anterior to scleral spur); this is also pathological.

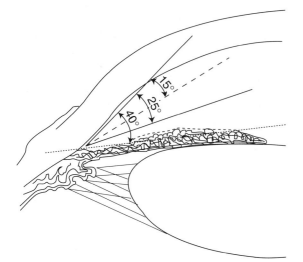

**FIGURE 8–7** Angle width is graded by estimating the angle between two imaginary lines, one tangential to the trabecular meshwork and the other tangential to the anterior iris surface about one-third of the way between the iris root and the pupil margin. Spaeth recommends 10° increments from 0° (iris up against cornea) to 40° (iris flat). (From Spaeth GL: The normal development of the human anterior chamber angle: A new system of descriptive grading. Trans Ophthal Soc UK 1971; 91:709–739.)

C Iris attaches at or just posterior to the scleral spur; this means that although there is essentially no angle recess and none of the anterior ciliary body is visible, the trabecular meshwork is not being obstructed. This is an anatomical variant seen mainly in young children.

D Iris attaches to the ciliary body such that a moderate band of ciliary body is visible; the angle is wide open. This is the most common finding in a normal population.

E Iris attaches to the ciliary body such that a wide band of ciliary body is visible; the angle is extremely deep. This is also a normal variant, seen mainly in myopes.

Note: If indentation gonioscopy shows the actual attachment to be further posterior than the apparent attachment, indicate the latter in parentheses, for example, (C)D.

As an example, consider an eye in which the peripheral iris obscures the view of the ciliary body, the scleral spur, and part of the trabecular meshwork. Indentation gonioscopy shows that the actual insertion of the iris is at the scleral spur. This angle is a (B)C. The optic section dives down behind the iris before re-emerging on the iris surface; that is, it has a steep, or "s," peripheral iris contour. At this point, we know that this is a narrow angle, but we do not know whether

it is due to iris bombé or plateau iris. This information is contained in the angle width. Whereas a bombé iris is something like "(B)C10s," a plateau iris—with its characteristically deeper central chamber—is more likely a "(B)C30s."

What do the above grades mean in terms of risk of angle closure? This depends on the combination of features seen. Any angle that is characterized primarily as an "A" or "B" is either at risk for closure or is already closed. A "C" is unlikely to close, and "D" and "E" angles will not close. An "s" iris is more problematic than an "r" or a "q," but whether or not closure is likely depends on the position of the iris attachment. Similarly, although a 40° angle width by itself seems to indicate a wide-open angle, "A40r" describes an angle completely closed by anterior synechiae.

The above scheme characterizes the angle as a whole with respect to its shape—that is, whether the angle is open, narrow, or closed. Pigmentation of the angle should also be graded, as this relates to the risk of secondary open-angle glaucoma. Spaeth[15] recommends grading the pigmentation of the posterior trabecular meshwork, as this is where the bulk of filtering takes place as aqueous passes to Schlemm's canal. In his system, a grade of 0 indicates no pigment, grade

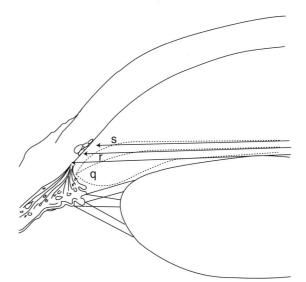

**FIGURE 8–8** Peripheral iris contour is described by one of three letters: r, The iris has a mildly convex shape or flat shape (r stands for "regular"); this is the normal, common form. s, The iris rises steeply from its root, as with iris bombé or plateau iris, obscuring the view of the angle structures (s stands for "steep" or "sharp"). q, The iris has a concave shape peripherally which results in a wide angle recess; this is seen in some myopic eyes and in pigmentary dispersion syndrome. (From Spaeth GL: The normal development of the human anterior chamber angle: A new system of descriptive grading. Trans Ophthal Soc UK 1971; 91:709–739.)

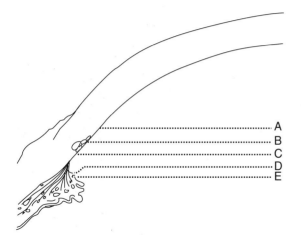

**FIGURE 8–9** The position of the iris attachment is characterized using one of five capital letters: A, The iris attaches at or anterior to Schwalbe's line (i.e., to the peripheral cornea), thus obscuring the trabecular meshwork; this is pathological. B, The iris attaches to trabecular meshwork, i.e., posterior to Schwalbe's line but anterior to scleral spur; this is also pathological. C, The iris attaches at or just posterior to the scleral spur; this means that although there is essentially no angle recess and none of the anterior ciliary body is visible, the trabecular meshwork is not being obstructed, an anatomical variant seen mainly in young children. D, The iris attaches to the ciliary body such that a moderate band of ciliary body is visible; the angle is wide open. This is the most common finding in a normal population. E, The iris attaches to the ciliary body such that a wide band of ciliary body is visible; the angle is extremely deep. This is also a normal variant, seen mainly in myopes. (From Spaeth GL: The normal development of the human anterior chamber angle: A new system of descriptive grading. Trans Ophthal Soc UK 1971; 91:709–739.)

1+ barely perceptible pigment, grade 2+ definite but mild pigment, grade 3+ moderately dense pigment, and grade 4+ "dense blackening of the posterior trabecular meshwork." Spaeth also recommends making this grading judgment in the superior angle because gravity makes the inferior angle a sort of "dumping ground" for pigment from many sources not necessarily important for the risk of open-angle glaucoma. Note also that while pigmentary dispersion syndrome and exfoliation syndrome both cause pigmentation of the trabecular meshwork, the appearance is usually somewhat different. In exfoliation syndrome, the pigment is bound to clumps of exfoliative material in large complexes that get stuck on the surface of the uveal meshwork, giving it a patchy, uneven coloration. In pigmentary dispersion syndrome, the fine pigment granules are phagocytized by, and therefore located within, the endothelial cells of the meshwork, resulting in a more uniform pigmentation. Keep in mind that usually other clues help in the differ-

ential diagnosis. For example, in pigmentary dispersion syndrome, the peripheral iris appears concave ("q"), and there is often deposition of fine pigment granules arranged circumferentially in the contraction furrows of the anterior iris. In exfoliation syndrome, the pupil margin may show flakes of exfoliative material, and there are often wavy lines of pigment anterior to Schwalbe's line ("Sampaolesi lines"), although this is not pathognomonic for the condition.

In addition to angle configuration and pigmentation, the location and extent of anterior synechiae, neovascularization, angle recession, tumors, or any other abnormality should all be documented.

## Narrow or Closed Angle

When gonioscopy reveals or confirms an angle at risk for spontaneous closure, the patient should be referred for appropriate treatment. Extremely narrow or closed angles due to either pupil block or plateau iris may be treated with mild miotics (pilocarpine 1% to 2%) to keep IOP down and pull the peripheral iris out of the angle until a peripheral iridectomy can be performed. Stronger miotics, such as the cholinesterase inhibitors, should be avoided, as they can exacerbate pupil block. If it is necessary to dilate these patients, sympathomimetics, such as phenylephrine, should not be used unless an α-blocking agent is available to reverse their effect in the event of acute angle closure. Furthermore, patients should be kept in the office until the mydriatic effect is completely gone, because the possibility of acute closure is highest in the mid-dilated state. Reversal of the mydriasis with pilocarpine is not a safe alternative to keeping the patient nearby, because the miotic agent may wear off before the mydriatic agent does, leaving the patient at risk. Patients with narrow angles should be educated with respect to the symptoms of acute and subacute angle closure and advised to seek immediate treatment if they occur.

## The Crystalline Lens

The crystalline lens lies posterior to the iris and anterior to the vitreous (see Fig. 8-1). With an equatorial diameter of 9 to 10 mm and a sagittal thickness of 3 to 4 mm, the biconvex lens is suspended from the ciliary muscle by zonular fibers. The lens is avascular, deriving its nutrition from the aqueous humor.

The primary function of the lens is refractive, accounting for one-third of the eye's optical power. The lens has the unique ability to increase its power. Contraction of the ciliary muscle causes relaxation of the zonules and results in an increase in both lens surface curvature and thickness. This change in power—accommodation—allows the younger eye to focus on near objects and/or to overcome hyperopia.

Aging brings with it a loss of accommodation, widely although not unanimously believed to be attributable to a loss of lens elasticity.[14] The aging process also results in a reduction in transparency. It is this opacification that leads to the pathology most commonly observed by the eye care practitioner—cataract.

## CRYSTALLINE LENS ANATOMY

The crystalline lens has a layered or *lamellar* structure, like an onion (see Fig. 8–1). New layers are laid down over a patient's life span, producing an age-related increase in sagittal thickness that, in some cases, can contribute to angle closure.

The external surface of the lens is a *capsule* that is highly elastic and non-cellular. Under the capsule is a layer of epithelial cells. The bulk of the lens is composed of *lens fibers*, long, prismatic, ribbon-like cells. The more superficial the fibers, the more recently they have been laid down. The deeper the cells, the older they are. Microscopically, the deeper cells exhibit an absence of nuclei.

The center of the lens is the *embryonic* nucleus. Successive layers comprise the *fetal, infantile*, and *adult* nuclei. The outermost layer is termed the *cortex*, which is formed after the adult nucleus is complete. The cortex and adult nucleus are very thin in childhood and adolescence. By observing the location of any opacities, the astute clinician can identify the developmental stage at which the insult occurred, much the same way as a botanist can derive information about the weather by looking at the rings in the trunk of a tree.

The lens fibers do not terminate at the poles of the lens but along the lens's suture lines. The paired suture lines in the center of the fetal nucleus are Y-shaped. The anterior suture is an erect Y, whereas the posterior is inverted. Both are readily visible using the slit lamp. As the lens and patient age, these *Y-sutures* become more visible.

The boundaries between the different layers or nuclei are also visible owing to variations in their refractive index. These boundaries are referred to as the *zones of discontinuity*.

## AGE-RELATED LENS OPACITIES

The most commonly observed abnormality of the lens is opacification, and the most common cause of the opacification is age. The quoted prevalence of lens opacities depends strongly on the criteria adopted to describe an opacity. Nonetheless, conventional wisdom suggests that 90% of patients over the age of 70 years have some sort of lens opacities. Age-related opacities may be divided into three categories: nuclear, cortical, and posterior subcapsular (Fig. 8–10).

Nuclear opacities are the most common and are often referred to as nuclear sclerosis. Nuclear opacification is an extension of the aging of the lens nucleus. The patient experiences a slow, gradual, progressive loss in vision. The nucleus begins to take on a milky appearance, owing to increased light scatter, and yellows as a result of absorption of blue light. The change in lens color is also referred to as brunescence. There may also be a concurrent increase in the refractive index of the nucleus, which can result in a myopic shift in refractive error. Finally, localized changes in refractive index may manifest as monocular diplopia.

Cortical opacities occur in the cortex of the lens and usually begin outside of the pupil area and in the inferior nasal quadrant. For this reason, the clinician is likely to observe them before the patient is aware they exist. Cortical opacities may begin as vacuoles, containing fluid, near the anterior adult nucleus. Another early change is the development of water clefts, which appear as radial spokes, or cuneiform opacities, pointing toward the center of the lens. During this process the lens is taking in water and swelling, causing a narrowing of the anterior chamber. At advanced stages when the cortex is completely opaque, the lens returns to its habitual size.

Posterior subcapsular, or cupuliform, opacities can be considered a subtype of cortical opacities. They are, however, categorized separately owing to their unique location and their greater effect on vision. Posterior subcapsular opacities develop near the posterior pole of the lens and can appear as a thin layer of vacuoles or crystals. They are best observed by retro-illumination, appearing as a dark shadow against the bright fundus reflex. Unlike the other age-related opacities, posterior subcapsular opacities can occur in younger patients and frequently have a dramatic effect on vision owing to their proximity to the visual axis and nodal point of the eye. Intuitively, vision should be more affected when pupil size is reduced, such as in bright illumination and during near vision. Posterior subcapsular opaci-

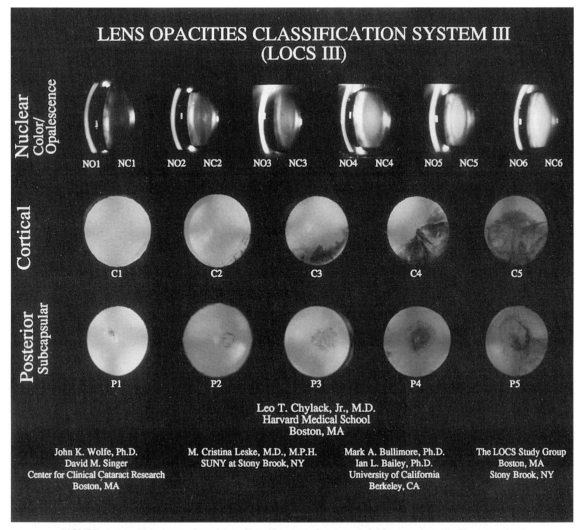

**FIGURE 8–10** The Lens Opacities Classification System (LOCS), version III. The standard photographs illustrate varying severity of nuclear, cortical, and posterior subcapsular opacities. Nuclear opacities are shown by direct focal illumination. Cortical and posterior subcapsular opacities are shown by retroillumination such that a bright red fundus reflex is observed. Any opacities appear as dark or translucent shadows against the bright background.

ties may also develop secondary to trauma or corticosteroid use.

## OTHER OPACITIES AND ABNORMALITIES

Like the cornea, the lens can be misshapen, although this occurs much less frequently. The lens can be abnormally small (microphakia) or have conical surfaces (lenticonus). The lens may be partially (Fig. 8–11) or completely displaced (ectopia lentis). This may be associated with trauma or a congenital syndrome such as Marfan syndrome.

Opacities may also be hereditary, develop-

mental, secondary to systemic disease or medication, or traumatic. A variety of other lens opacities have been documented, but this discussion is restricted to the most common types.

Congenital and developmental opacities are commonly observed and usually stable; for example, the Y-sutures may be more pronounced. Epicapsular stars (Fig. 8–12) appear as small specks of pigment on the anterior lens capsule.

On the posterior surface, remnants of the hyaloid artery may be visible, either as a white dot (Mittendorf's dot) or as a threadlike attachment on the nasal side of the posterior pole. Vision is rarely compromised.

More serious opacities include those secondary to systemic rubella infection occurring dur-

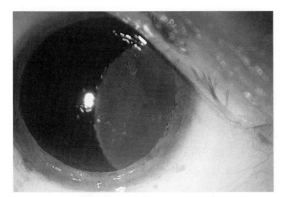

**FIGURE 8–11**   Ectopia lentis.

ing the first trimester of pregnancy. The opacities may be lamellar or nuclear in nature and can be extremely detrimental to vision and development. They require early extraction.

Opacification can occur secondary to ocular diseases. Retinitis pigmentosa and Fuchs' heterochromic iridocyclitis are both associated with posterior subcapsular opacities. Similarly, systemic disorders, particularly those that are metabolic in origin, can cause cataract. Juvenile onset diabetes that is poorly controlled or severe can lead to snowflake opacities in the anterior and posterior cortex which can progress to complete cortical opacification. Age-related opacities may also occur at a younger age in diabetes. Poorly controlled diabetes can also result in marked changes in refractive error. Hyperglycemia induces myopic shifts in refractive error, whereas hypoglycemia moves refraction in the hyperopic direction. Even when the patient's blood sugar is regulated appropriately, his or her refractive error may take weeks or months to stabilize.

Finally, drugs and toxins including phenothiazines and selenium can lead to lens opacities. The most common iatrogenic cataract is due to either topical or systemic corticosteroid use. Prolonged steroid use typically results in a posterior subcapsular opacity and thus affects vision at an early stage.

## WHEN IS A CATARACT NOT A CATARACT?

One of the issues in the ophthalmic examination is that of when a lens opacity should be considered a cataract. The AHCPR Clinical Practice Guidelines identify three criteria for cataract[16]:

1. Any opacification of the lens
2. An opacity that causes reduced visual acuity
3. An opacity that interferes with the patient's everyday activities

All of these definitions may be considered equally valid, depending on the circumstances to which they are applied. The clinician is probably best served by reserving the term *cataract* for patients who are experiencing some form of functional disability due to their lens opacities, such as difficulty with reading or driving. This is particularly germane when discussing findings with the patient. Telling a symptomless individual that he or she has a cataract may not represent the best option in patient management.

## PHOTOGRAPHIC SYSTEMS FOR GRADING LENS OPACITIES

Traditionally clinicians have used the ubiquitous 4-point scale to grade the severity of lens opacities. The grading has been referenced to line drawings or, more often, a clinician's own experience. Consequently, there was limited standardization between clinicians, particularly those trained at different institutions and with different levels of experience.

Clinical trials in ophthalmology and optometry expanded substantially during the 1980s, and a need for standardized classifications systems became obvious. Photographic reference systems were developed for the grading of cataract with three standard series of photographs to provide three reference levels of severity.

Several lens grading systems are currently available, including the Lens Opacities Classification System (LOCS),[17] the Wilmer System,[18] the Wisconsin System,[19] and the Oxford Clinical Cataract Classification and Grading System.[20] These systems typically include standards for nuclear, cortical, and posterior subcapsular opacities and can promote agreement between observers at different clinical sites. The clinician observes the patient's crystalline lens with a standardized ar-

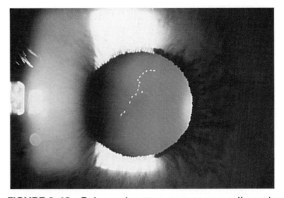

**FIGURE 8–12**   Epicapsular stars appear as small specks of pigment on the anterior lens capsule.

rangement of the slit-lamp biomicroscope and, by referring to the standard photographs, assigns a grade to any opacity. A grade of "2" is assigned to a nuclear opacity that appears to be equal to or greater than that shown in the "Grade 2" standard photograph but less than that shown in "Grade 3" standard photograph.

The numerical grading system and the use of standard reference photographs have undoubtedly enhanced the reproducibility of clinical estimates. Some authors have advocated interpolating between the numerical standards. Bailey et al.[21] suggested that clinicians use decimalization, dividing each integer scale unit into 10 equal parts, to interpolate between the benchmark grades shown in the reference photograph. Lenses with nuclear opacity greater than that shown in the standard photograph for grade 2 but less pronounced than the standard photograph for grade 3 could be assigned grades of 2.1 through 2.9. Bailey and co-workers demonstrated that this approach enabled clinicians to reliably detect smaller changes in the patient than the traditional integer grading approach.

The development of photographic standards for subjective grading has coincided with advancements in image processing which have facilitated the objective assessment of changes in the crystalline lens. Objective techniques are now available for the assessment of the color, density, and extent of lens opacities.[22, 23]

The LOCS III system (see Fig. 8–10) established an objective basis for the interval steps used in the grading of different features of cataract.[17] Scaling intervals for grading nuclear opalescence and color have been chosen to represent equal differences in optical density and color purity, and the standards for cortical and posterior subcapsular opacities are based on a monotonic function relating the grade to the area of opacification.

## SYMPTOMS

Depending on the type and location of the opacity, patients may report decreased vision, distortion, monocular diplopia, difficulties with color discrimination, glare disability, and/or problems with night driving. Conversely, the patient may have a marked opacity but be symptom-free, particularly with cortical opacities.

The challenge for the clinician is to determine whether the decreased vision is due to the lens or has some other cause. The first step should be to perform a careful refraction. The first opportunity to observe the clarity of the media is when observing the retinoscopic reflex. A crisp reflex implies clear media. Nuclear opacities dull the retinoscopic reflex, whereas cortical and posterior subcapsular opacities may appear as dark spokes or dots against an otherwise bright reflex. Subjective refraction can be more difficult in patients with lens opacities, requiring the clinician to abandon his or her usual ±0.25 D refinement approach in favor of larger changes in refracting lens power which are easier for the patient to discriminate from one another.

The direct ophthalmoscope is another useful tool for observing lens opacities. With a low plus lens (+6.00 to +8.00 D) dialed into the instrument, the clinician can observe the light reflex from 6 inches (15 cm). With a higher plus lens, say +20.00 D, opacities can be viewed by direct illumination. Finally, the fundus is viewed by direct ophthalmoscopy. The clinician should determine whether his or her view of the retina agrees with the patient's visual acuity. A "20/30 view" in a patient with 20/100 visual acuity should prompt the clinician to investigate explanations other than cataract for the vision loss.

## SLIT-LAMP EXAMINATION OF THE LENS

The primary tool for the examination of the crystalline lens is the slit-lamp biomicroscope. This is best done with the pupils dilated to ensure a wide view for the detection of off-axis opacities. A narrow slit beam should be used to minimize patient discomfort and to facilitate the localization by layer of any opacities as the clinician "slices" through the lens.

The examination should commence with an angle of 30° between the illumination tower and the microscope objective lenses. The clinician should sweep slowly across the lens. On the first pass, care should be taken to focus on the anterior surface of the lens. On the second pass, the slit beam should be focused on the posterior surface. Failure to do so causes the clinician to miss subtle posterior subcapsular opacities, Mittendorf's dots, hyaloid remnants, and posterior cortical irregularities.

Next, illuminate the nucleus, observing the degree of opacification and color. The Y-sutures should be visible, as should the zones of discontinuity. Finally, move the beam to concentrate on the cortex. Are there any vacuoles visible? They have the appearance of little air bubbles except that they are refractile, filled with fluid. The clinician can determine the refractive index of the vacuole relative to the surrounding tissue by observing the reflected light (Fig. 8–13). If the reflex from the vacuole is on the same side as the

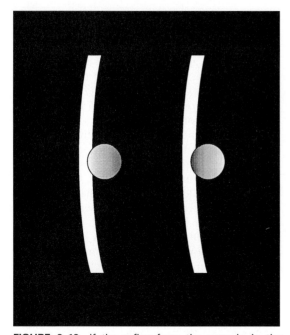

FIGURE 8–13 If the reflex from the vacuole in the crystalline lens is on the same side as the reflected beam, the vacuole has a lower refractive index. Conversely, a body with a higher refractive index gives a light reflex on the opposite side to the beam.

incident beam, the vacuole has a lower refractive index. Conversely, a body with a higher refractive index gives a light reflex on the side opposite to the beam.

The examination should conclude by viewing the lens using retro-illumination. The angle between the illumination tower and the microscope should be set at less than 5° such that a bright red fundus reflex is observed. Any opacities appear as dark or translucent shadows against the bright background (see Fig. 8-10). A useful approach is to focus the slit on the anterior surface of the lens, broaden it slightly, and then rotate it about the 0° position. It is unlikely that more than half of the pupil area can be retro-illuminated at any one time (the lower photographs in Figure 8-10 were taken with a special Neitz camera), so the lens must be viewed with illumination from both the nasal and temporal sides. Care must be taken to focus first on the anterior lens surface and then on the posterior surface. Maintaining focus on a virtually clear posterior surface can be difficult. A useful approach is to use direct focal illumination to locate the posterior lens surface and then switch to retro-illumination while locking the position of microscope or restricting yourself to small lateral movements.

Supplementary tests can also be used to deter-

mine the severity of the cataract. Disability glare testing can be done to elucidate symptoms such as difficulty with night driving (see Chapter 11). The introduction of a glare source into the field of vision can markedly reduce visual acuity, particularly with posterior subcapsular opacities.

When the lens opacity makes it difficult to view the fundus, a range of techniques can be used to assess the viability of the retina and optic nerve, including laser interferometry and the Potential Acuity Meter. These and other techniques are describe comprehensively in Chapter 11.

## CATARACT EXTRACTION

Cataract extraction is the most commonly performed surgical procedure in the United States. The cataractous lens is extracted and replaced with a synthetic intraocular lens, creating the condition of *pseudophakia*. The visual outcome is usually excellent, and serious complications are rare. Most extractions are extracapsular, wherein the lens capsule is left behind. One common complication to the procedure is opacification of the remaining posterior lens capsule. This is easily treated by non-invasive YAG laser capsulotomy. The YAG laser easily "punches" a hole in the capsule, producing an instantaneous improvement in visual acuity. The reader is referred to other texts for a more complete description of the postoperative management of the cataract patient and common complications.[24]

The high success rates of modern cataract surgery mean that clinicians should have no reservations about referring a patient for the procedure as soon as the patient is impaired by his or her cataracts. This can be when vision is still 20/40 or better. The patient's occupation, hobbies, visual demands, and physical health should all factor into the decision, which should be based on an intelligent dialogue between doctor, patient, and, if appropriate, the patient's family.

## References

1. Oh YG, Minelli S, Spaeth GL, Stein WC: The anterior chamber angle is different in different racial groups: A gonioscopic study. Eye 1994; 8:104-108.
2. van Herick W, Shaffer RN, Schwartz A: Estimation of width of angle of anterior chamber: Incidence and significance of the narrow angle. Am J Ophthalmol 1969; 68:626-629.
3. Becker BL: Becker-Shaffer's Diagnosis and Therapy of the Glaucomas. St. Louis: CV Mosby, 1989.
4. Becker B: Becker-Shaffer's Diagnosis and Therapy of the Glaucomas. St. Louis: CV Mosby, 1983.

5. Alward WLM: Color Atlas of Gonioscopy. London: Wolfe Publishing—An imprint of Mosby-Year Book Europe, Ltd., 1994.

6. Alvarado JA, Murphy CG: Outflow obstruction in pigmentary and primary open angle glaucoma. Arch Ophthalmol 1992; 110:1769-1778.

7. Ritch R: Exfoliation syndrome and occludable angles. Trans Am Ophthalmol Soc 1994; 92:845-944.

8. Schlötzer-Schrehardt U, Naumann GOH: Trabecular meshwork in pseudoexfoliation syndrome with and without open-angle glaucoma. Invest Ophthalmol Vis Sci 1995; 36:1750-1764.

9. Sampaolesi R, Zarate J, Croxato O: The chamber angle in exfoliation syndrome. Acta Ophthalmol (Suppl 184) 1988; 66:48-53.

10. Rouhiainen H, Teräsvirta M: Pigmentation of the anterior chamber angle in normal and pseudoexfoliative eyes. Acta Ophthalmol 1990; 68:700-702.

11. Wishart PK, Spaeth GL, Poryzees EM: Anterior chamber angle in the exfoliation syndrome. Br J Ophthalmol 1985; 69:103-107.

12. Gross FJ, Tingey D, Epstein DL: Increased prevalence of occludable angles and angle-closure glaucoma in patient with pseudoexfoliation. Am J Ophthalmol 1994; 117:333-336.

13. Murphy CG, Johnson M, Alvarado JA: Juxtacanalicular tissue in pigmentary and primary open angle glaucoma: The hydrodynamic role of pigment and other constituents. Arch Ophthalmol 1992; 110:1779-1785.

14. Gilmartin B: The aetiology of presbyopia — a summary of the role of lenticular and extralenticular structures. Ophthal Physiol Opt 1995; 15:431-437.

15. Spaeth GL: The normal development of the human anterior chamber angle: A new system of descriptive grading. Trans Ophthalmol Soc UK 1971; 91:709-739.

16. AHCPR Pub. No. 93-0542: Cataract Management Guideline Panel. Cataract in Adults: Management of Functional Impairment. Clinical Practice Guideline, Number 4. Rockville, MD: US Department of Health and Human Services, Public Health Service, Agency for Health Care Policy and Research, 1993.

17. Chylack LT Jr., Wolfe JK, Singer D, et al.: The Lens Opacities Classification System, version III (LOCS III). Arch Ophthalmol 1993; 111:831-836.

18. Taylor HR, West SK: A simple system for the clinical grading of lens opacities. Lens Res 1988; 5:175-181.

19. Klein BEK, Klein R, Linton KLP: Assessment of cataract from photographs in the Beaver Dam Eye Study. Ophthalmology 1990; 97:1428-1433.

20. Sparrow JM, Bron AJ, Brown NAP, et al.: The Oxford clinical cataract classification and grading system. Int Ophthalmol 1986; 9:207-225.

21. Bailey I, Bullimore M, Raasch T, Taylor H: Clinical grading and the effects of scaling. Invest Ophthalmol Vis Sci 1991; 32:422-432.

22. Hockwin O, Dragomirescu V, Laser H: Measurements of lens transparency or its disturbances by densitometric image analysis of Scheimpflug photographs. Graefes Arch Clin Exp Ophthalmol 1982; 219:225-262.

23. Sparrow JM, Brown NAP, Shun-Shin A, Bron AJ: The Oxford modular cataract image analysis system. Eye 1990; 4:638-648.

24. Murrill CA, Stanfield DL, Van Brocklin MD: Primary Care of the Cataract Patient. Norwalk, CT: Appleton & Lange, 1994.

9

*Robert B. DiMartino, OD, MS*

# The Posterior Segment

The abnormalities observed by the clinician with funduscopy fit into one or more general groups of findings: (1) blood vessel abnormalities, (2) opacities in the otherwise transparent retina (hemorrhages, exudates, edema, nerve fiber layer infarcts, and vascular and glial tissue proliferation), (3) disturbances in the position of the sensory retina (rhegmatogenous or non-rhegmatogenous detachments), (4) derangements in the retinal pigment epithelium, and (5) abnormalities in Bruch's membrane and choroid. Discussion of the diseases in the groups identified above is beyond the scope of this chapter. Instead, this chapter reviews the normal findings present in the funduscopic examination and details the techniques implemented in this evaluation, providing the reader with a foundation upon which to build examination of the human fundus.

The ophthalmic clinician has two goals in the funduscopic evaluation of a patient's fundus. The first is to critically evaluate the greatest expanse of tissue possible. The second, and nearly as important, goal is to execute this evaluation in an efficient, methodical manner and, in doing so, to limit patient discomfort. These goals are occasionally in opposition to each other. For example, the light used to evaluate the retina with the binocular indirect ophthalmoscope is bright and often uncomfortable for the patient. In comparison, most clinicians believe that evaluating the retina with scleral indentation is uncomfortable for the patient. In reality, even the novice clinician can use scleral indentation of the retinal periphery with minimal awareness by the patient. This expands and expedites the examination process. The first step in accomplishing both goals is to understand the functional anatomy of the fundus.

## Relevant Anatomy

. . . . . . . . . . . . . . . . . . . . . . . . .

The posterior segment is defined anteriorly by the patellar fossa, a circular depression in the vitreous face that accommodates the posterior lenticular surface.[1] At the perimeter of this depression lies the ligamentum hyaloideocapsulare (Wieger's circular attachment), an annular thickening 8 mm in width. In young eyes, the ligamentum hyaloideocapsulare creates a firm attachment with the posterior lenticular surface (Egger's line). This attachment forms a well-defined region, the retrolental space of Berger, between the posterior surface of the crystalline lens and the anterior vitreous face. With increasing age, the attachment of the ligamentum hya-

loideocapsulare loses its attachment to the crystalline lens, and the definition of the region becomes obscured. When intracapsular cataract extraction was the procedure of choice, a loose or absent vitreal attachment was an important prognostic finding in the success of the procedure.

Peripherally, the posterior segment is formed by the anterior vitreous, which is in contact with the zonules of the crystalline lens and the pars plicata or ciliary processes of the ciliary body. This surface creates the boundary between the posterior chamber and the posterior segment. This vitreal surface is known as the anterior hyaloid, which extends to the posterior aspect of the ora serrata. Posteriorly, the vitreous is closely adherent to the internal limiting membrane of the retina. The posterior segment thus includes all the ocular structures extending posteriorly to this anterior vitreal border, limited by the intraocular portion of the optic nerve.

The origin of the vitreous is unclear. The primary vitreous has formed by about the sixth week of embryonic development. The secondary vitreous begins to form in the ninth week of development. It originates as parallel rows on the inner retinal surface. As the secondary vitreous continues to develop, the primary vitreous is forced into the central aspect of the optic cup, forming what becomes Cloquet's canal. This canal originates at the optic disc in the area of Martegiani and terminates in the patellar fossa. The hyaloid artery and vein pass through this canal and serve as a developmental vascular structure, the tunica vasculosa lentis, which supplies the rapidly growing crystalline lens. By the eighth month of gestation, the hyaloid vascular system has completely atrophied, leaving the canal devoid of structures. Lenticular and posterior remnants of this vascular structure are present in some eyes. A Mittendorf's dot is the posterior capsular remnant of this vascular structure. Bergmeister's papilla can be seen in a small percentage of eyes as an opaque stalk extending from the optic disc into the vitreous.

The vitreous is attached to the retina in three locations.[2] The vitreous base extends about 2 mm anterior and 4 mm posterior to the ora serrata. It is a relatively firm attachment and contributes in part to the etiology of peripheral retinal breaks and rhegmatogenous detachments. The second important attachment lies between the vitreous and the internal limiting membrane at the edge of the optic nerve. This peripapillary attachment weakens and eventually disappears with advancing age. Posterior vitreous detachment (PVD) rarely occurs before 45 years of age.[3] It is more common in women than in men.[4, 5]

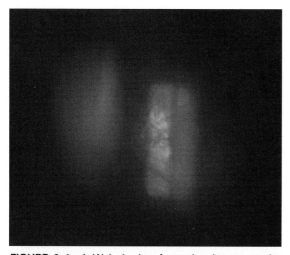

**FIGURE 9–1** A Weiss's ring formation in a posterior vitreous detachment.

No obvious predilection is associated with race. After the age of 50 years, the prevalence of PVD is approximately equal to the patient's age in years. During a PVD, the patient may experience photopsia. Following a PVD, patients may report a translucent obscuration of their vision. Funduscopically, the previous peripapillary attachment of the vitreous can be observed anterior and slightly inferior to the optic nerve head as a translucent and roughly oval structure. This is known as Weiss's ring[6] (Fig. 9–1).

The third attachment of the vitreous to the retina is at the macula. This attachment is irregular but roughly annular with a diameter of 3 to 4 mm. This attachment is the weakest of the three and is not visible on ophthalmoscopic or slit-lamp examination (Table 9–1). It does not play a significant clinical role, except in pathological conditions, which include macular holes and epiretinal membrane formation.

A fourth attachment of the vitreous to the retina is at the major retinal blood vessels. This attachment is usually unimportant except in conditions like persistent hyperplastic primary vitreous or the avulsion of retinal vessels. This latter condition demonstrates the dramatic strength of this adhesion because it is strong enough to tear vessels from the retina.

The vitreous undergoes a number of age-related, degenerative changes in addition to the loss of these anatomical attachments. One of these changes is liquefaction, the movement of fluid into pockets known as lacunae. This coalescence results in syneresis, a shrinkage of the vitreous. Finally, an increased density of the vitreous fibers occurs with age. All of these changes—loss of attachments, liquefaction, syneresis, and increased fibril density—contribute to making the vitreous more visible with age.

The sclera forms 80% of the wall of the eye. It varies in thickness from 0.3 mm posterior to the insertions of the rectus muscles to 0.4 to 0.6 mm at the equator, 0.8 mm at the limbus, and 1.0 mm at the optic nerve. The sclera is the white "backdrop" against which the fundus is viewed. Its contribution to the appearance of the fundus does not vary from individual to individual or across races. It is upon this scleral stage that the remainder of the fundus is set.

The choroid is adjacent to the sclera and provides the outer third of the retina with oxygen and nutrients, as well as removing carbon dioxide and waste products. Per unit volume, the choroid has the highest blood flow of any tissue in the body. Electromagnetic energy is focused by the optical elements of the eye on the photoreceptor layer of the retina, which results in the concentration of heat energy. If sufficient heat were to accumulate in this delicate tissue, it would become damaged. Therefore, in addition to its role in maintaining retinal nutritional homeostasis, the choroidal blood flow helps to prevent the retina from overheating. The blood in

| **TABLE 9–1** Vitreal Attachments | | |
| --- | --- | --- |
| **Attachment** | **Structure** | **Adhesion** |
| Ligamentum hyaloideocapsulare | Anterior face of vitreous with posterior capsule of the crystalline lens | Firm in the young, absent in the elderly |
| Vitreous base | Vitreous with the pars plana and peripheral anterior retina | Very firm attachment throughout life |
| Peripapillary | Vitreous and the edge of the optic nerve head | Relatively firm in the young, lost in a majority of adults over 50 years (PVD) |
| Macular | Annular vitreous attachment to the retina around the macula | Firm attachment that is lost with advancing age or secondary to trauma or inflammation in the young |
| Retinal vasculature | Major mid and peripheral retinal blood vessels | Firm attachment that can result in avulsed vessels under appropriate conditions |

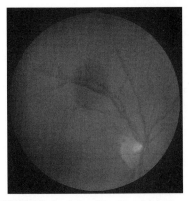

**FIGURE 9–2**    A benign choroidal nevus.

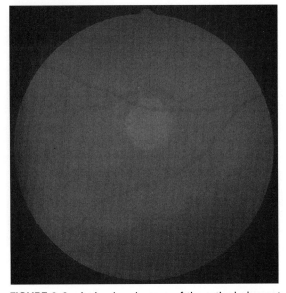

**FIGURE 9–3**    A circular absence of the retinal pigment epithelium, referred to as a window defect. Note the increased detail of the choroidal vasculature and the pale pink fundus appearance.

the choroid is supplied by the 20 short posterior ciliary arteries that pierce the sclera around the optic nerve in a ring formation, the circle of Haller-Zinn. Each quadrant of the choroid is drained by a vortex ampulla and vein.

The choroid varies in both the pattern and intensity of the vessel pattern as well as the amount of melanin between the vessels. Its contribution to the fundus presentation is the orange-red color in the texture of its vessel pattern. In addition to melanin, the choroid is also the site of pigment tumors or melanomas. As with tumors elsewhere in the body, melanomas can be either benign or malignant. Clinically, the term "melanoma" should be used with great caution, as it alarms patients and can be misinterpreted by other health care providers. A better term for a benign melanoma is a nevus or mole (Fig. 9-2).

The choroid's vascular bed, the choriocapillaris, has finer vessels that form a thin film of fluid against the next layer, Bruch's membrane. Overlying the vascular bed of the fundus is the pigment epithelium of the retina. This single layer of cells is responsible for the phagocytosis of the used outer segments of the rods and cones. As its name implies, this epithelial layer contains pigment, which varies from individual to individual. The pigment in this layer is rela-

tively uniform throughout the fundus. Notable exceptions to this uniformity are in the macula and the periphery. In the macula, the retinal pigment epithelium has increased melanin, which gives this region its characteristic granulated, dark appearance. In the periphery, there is less melanin in the retinal pigment epithelium.

The overlying, transparent to translucent retina is formed by 10 distinct layers. The term "retina" is synonymous with the neurosensory or sensory retina. A physiological and anatomical distinction can be made, however, by separating the retina into vascular and avascular regions (Table 9-2).

Under varying conditions one or more of the fundus layers may be absent. The absence or abundance of a particular tissue(s) can confuse a

| TABLE 9–2    Layers of the Retina | | |
| --- | --- | --- |
| Pigment epithelium | | |
| Photoreceptors | | |
| Outer limiting membrane | | |
| Outer nuclear layer | | |
| Outer plexiform layer | Avascular retina ↑ | |
| Inner nuclear layer | Vascular retina ↓ | |
| Inner plexiform layer | | |
| Ganglion cell layer | | |
| Nerve fiber layer | | |
| Inner limiting membrane | | |

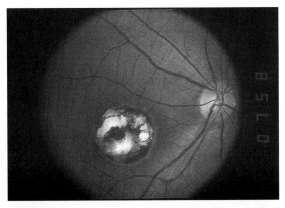

**FIGURE 9–4**    A macular lesion resulting from a retinal choroiditis, presumably *Toxoplasma gondii*.

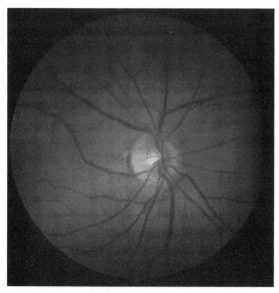

**FIGURE 9-5** Linear radial hyperplasia of the retinal pigment epithelium resulting from a connective tissue disorder referred to as angioid streaks.

clinician who does not have a solid understanding of fundus anatomy (Figs. 9-1 through 9-5).

# The Optic Nerve Head

. . . . . . . . . . . . . . . . . . . . . . . . . .

The optic nerve head (optic disc) is located 12° to 14° nasal and 1° superior to fixation. The optic disc is oval in shape and subtends roughly 5° horizontally and 7° vertically. The optic disc is used as a reference for both the location and the size of other fundus findings. Frequently lesions are described using the notation of disc diameters (DD). One disc diameter corresponds to approximately 1.5 mm. The central retinal artery and vein—or the branches of these vessels if they bifurcate prior to the disc surface—are in the optic nerve head. A sketch of the optic disc is sometimes included in the patient's medical record. Patient record forms have a diagram designed for this purpose. The perimeter of the optic disc is represented by a circle. A grid is superimposed on the area contained by this cir-

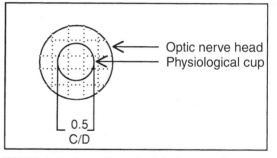

**FIGURE 9-7** Recording physiological cupping on a template.

cle such that each square represents 0.20 of the disc diameter (Fig. 9-6).

The optic disc is formed from the right-angle bending of the nerve fiber layer as it alters its course in preparation for exiting the eye. The optic nerve is composed of nerve fiber axons that range in number from 0.75 to 1.25 million, with a mean of slightly less than 1.0 million.[1, 7-9] Rarely do these axons fill the entire surface of the nerve head, resulting in a depression in the plane of the optic disc. This depression, which is formed by the void of nerve fibers, is referred to as the physiological cup. A portion of the clinical examination of the fundus is dedicated to estimating the dimensions of the physiological cup as a function of the optic disc. Classically, this estimation is performed by measuring the horizontal dimension of the cup as a function of the disc horizontal diameter. This value is expressed as a decimal and referred to as the cup-to-disc ratio (C/D) (Figs. 9-7 to 9-12).

The estimation process in determining the C/D ratio has at least two separate components. One component is the determination of the borders of the disc and the cup, which is greatly enhanced by using stereoscopic examination

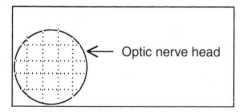

**FIGURE 9-6** Optic nerve recording template.

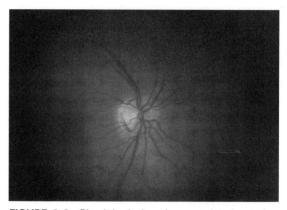

**FIGURE 9-8** Physiological optic nerve head cupping 0.0 C/D.

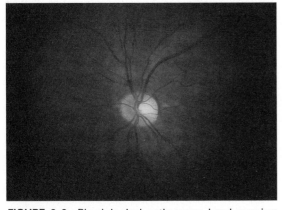

**FIGURE 9–9** Physiological optic nerve head cupping 0.2 C/D.

techniques. The second component is the mental formation of a fraction of these two distances. Good and Quinn and others have demonstrated that—even under ideal conditions—each component in the estimation process contributes an error to the final value.[10, 11]

Another criticism of the C/D ratio, as presented above, is that it records only one aspect of the relative cup size—its horizontal dimension. Twice as much information about the cup size can be obtained by recording a vertical C/D ratio (Fig. 9–13). This simple and efficient additional step is seldom followed in clinical practice. Another variant on the single, horizontal C/D ratio is to remove the constraint of recording dimensions in the cardinal geometric planes. In this approach, the largest and smallest C/D ratios are recorded with their associated clock hours (Fig. 9–14).

Some additional comments are important regarding C/D ratios. It is crucial that the clinician recall that a C/D ratio is an estimation of the void of nerve fiber axons. What is vital to vision is the

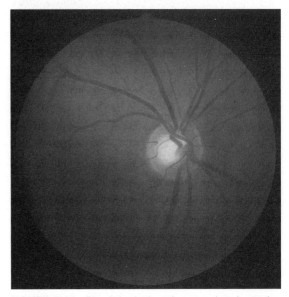

**FIGURE 9–11** Physiological optic nerve head cupping 0.6 C/D.

*presence* of neural tissue, or a "rim-to-disc" ratio. A shortsighted argument is that simple geometry implies that these two estimations are reciprocal. This author would argue that the philosophical approach is different, and the clinician should always be directed in assessing what tissue is present, as this is what provides the patient with vision.

A number of techniques are available for viewing the optic nerve head to determine the C/D ratio. Technology is advancing in this area at an impressive rate. New digitizing and laser scanning instruments continue to be developed and may become more cost effective. If this trend continues, these instruments will become invaluable in assessing the C/D ratio. However, until they are readily available, the best and current

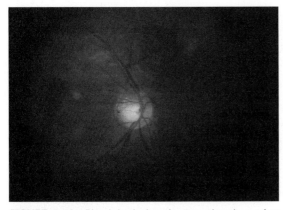

**FIGURE 9–10** Physiological optic nerve head cupping 0.4 C/D.

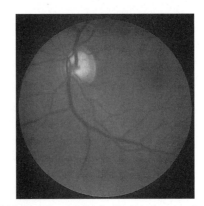

**FIGURE 9–12** Non-physiological optic nerve head cupping 0.8 C/D.

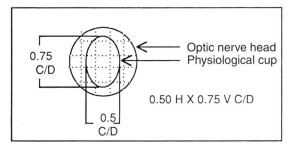

**FIGURE 9–13** Recording physiological cupping on a template.

standard is a stereoscopic view of the nerve head with image enlargement.

Under normal conditions, the insertion of the optic nerve into the eye is nearly orthogonal to the tangent of the globe in this location. This means the margins of the optic nerve head are flat with the plane of the retina. In some eyes, the insertion of the optic nerve is oblique temporally to the globe. In these eyes, the nasal margin of the nerve is more pronounced than the temporal edge. Occasionally, the optic nerve inserts from a superior position, which results in a more pronounced superior margin. In various disease states the margins of the optic nerve appear elevated or blurred in their presentation (Table 9-3 and Figs. 9-15 and 9-16).

# Peripapillary Retina

· · · · · · · · · · · · · · · · · · · · · · · · · · ·

The peripapillary region has important clinical and diagnostic features. One of the most com-

| TABLE 9–3 Sources of Blurred or Elevated Nerve Head Margins | |
|---|---|
| **Etiology** | **Significance** |
| Buried nerve head drusen | Little/no vision disturbance |
| Nerve head drusen | Little/no vision disturbance Occasionally choroidal (subretinal) neovascularization can occur |
| Pseudotumor cerebri (benign cranial hypertension) | Chronic elevation of cerebrospinal fluid leads to optic atrophy |
| Advanced systemic hypertension | Grave prognosis from the systemic complications unless systemic blood pressure is controlled quickly |
| Space-occupying cranial lesion | Grave prognosis requiring neuro-surgical evaluation |

mon anatomical variations is a crescent at the margin of the optic nerve head. Crescent formation can occur if various fundus tissues do not reach the optic nerve or have an incomplete extension to it. In some myopic individuals, the retinal pigment epithelial layer does not reach the optic disc. The remaining layers, the sclera and choroid, remain and form what is referred to as a choroidal crescent. The absence of the retinal pigment epithelium in this crescent exposes the coarse, patchy pigmentation characteris-

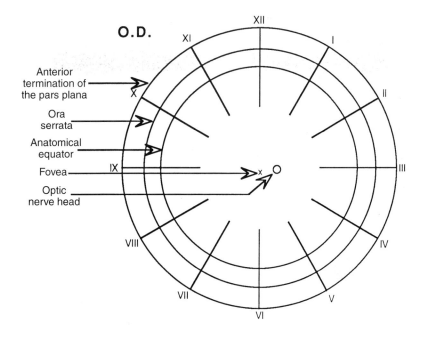

**FIGURE 9–14** The fundus mapping system.

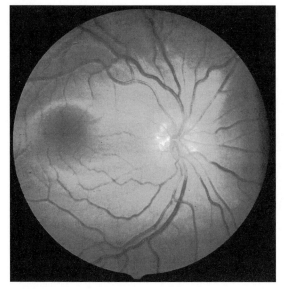

**FIGURE 9–15** Surface optic nerve head drusen. Note the blurred margins of the disc.

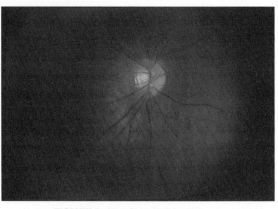

**FIGURE 9–17** Choroidal crescent.

tic of the choroid (Fig. 9–17). In some eyes the retinal pigment epithelium and vascular tunic do not reach the optic nerve, resulting in a white crescent, which is completely attributable to the sclera (Fig. 9–18). Occasionally, an abundance of melanin is associated with the retinal pigment epithelium at the optic nerve head margin. This excessive pigmentation obscures the underlying choroid and sclera. It is referred to as a pigment crescent or retinal pigment epithelial crescent (Fig. 9–19).

The peripapillary area can undergo age-related changes, including pigment migration, clumping, and atrophy. Additionally, the peripapillary area can undergo significant atrophy that radiates from the disc in tonguelike projections. The latter atrophy—geographic helicoid peripapillary choroidopathy—is not age-related and is subject to recurrence (Fig. 9–20). Atrophy of the peripapillary area has been associated specifically with low-tension glaucoma.[12]

A high concentration of nerve fibers is found in the inner retinal layer associated with the peripapillary area. As a result, the peripapillary region has the greatest nerve fiber layer thickness of the fundus. The nerve fibers at the disc are radial in their orientation. The fibers originating on the nasal retina continue to fan out in a radial pattern. The temporal retinal fibers have a less direct pattern. Macular fibers run a straight course from their origin to the nerve head. The

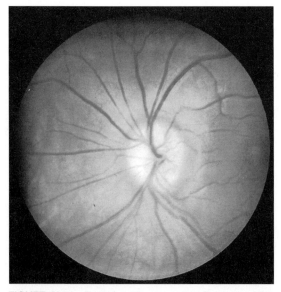

**FIGURE 9–16** Buried optic nerve head drusen. Note the blurred margins of the disc.

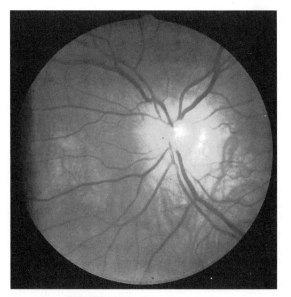

**FIGURE 9–18** Scleral crescent.

remaining temporal fibers follow an arcuate path from their synapse in the retina to their radial entry to the optic nerve. Temporal to the macula, the fibers from the superior and inferior retina form a natural line, the horizontal raphe. This correlates with visual field defects that respect this horizontal separation of retinal hemispheres.

## Nerve Fiber Layer

Defects in the arcuate fibers within 3 DD of the optic nerve head have been implicated in glaucoma.[13] The loss of nerve fibers is thought to occur before the visual field defects are detectable.[14] Nerve fiber layer defects can be difficult to see. A monochromatic (red-free) filter can improve the clinician's chances of detecting these defects by increasing contrast and decreasing the depth of field.[15]

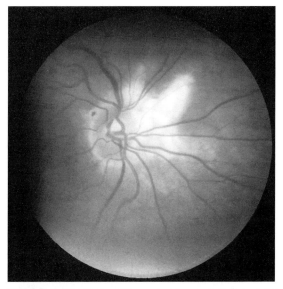

**FIGURE 9–20** Peripapillary atrophy, possibly a mild presentation of geographic helicoid peripapillary choroiditis.

## Retinal Vascular System

The central retinal artery, the corresponding vein, and their capillary communication have the task of supplying the nerve fiber layer and inner two-thirds of the retina with the necessary metabolites. The central retinal artery is the first branch of the ophthalmic artery. The internal carotid supplies the ophthalmic artery. About 10 mm posterior to the globe, the central retinal artery enters the optic nerve. Once inside the

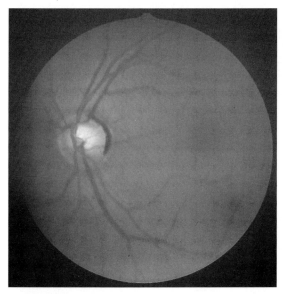

**FIGURE 9–19** Retinal pigment epithelial crescent.

nerve, it travels to its target tissue centrally. The intraneural artery has all of the components of other small arteries throughout the body. As the central retinal artery, or its branches if it bifurcates before the optic nerve head, reach the internal eye, the internal elastic lamina is replaced by an increased muscularis. This differentiates the central retinal artery from other arteries of similar size elsewhere in the body. The exchange of internal elastic lamina for muscularis gives the vessel the potential for greater response to pressure and chemical stimuli. The anatomical difference is significant in various disease processes. Unlike the intraneural portion of the vessel, the intraocular extension is not at risk for giant cell arteritis, which results from an inflammation of the internal elastic lamina. However, changes associated with atheromas and arteriosclerosis can be present in both the interneural and intraocular vessel. Before proceeding further in this discussion of retinal vasculature, the reader should recall that blood vessels in the retina and elsewhere in the body are transparent. Their observation is possible only because they contain blood. When blood vessels are examined, what is observed is the blood within the vessel, not the vessel wall.

The central retinal artery bifurcates at or before the optic disc into its superior and inferior branches. A second bifurcation occurs, splitting the superior and inferior branches each into a temporal and nasal subordinate extension. Thereafter bifurcations are random and continue throughout the extent of the vessel.

At a bifurcation site the artery undergoes a rapid decrease in caliber which requires careful scrutiny during funduscopy. Calcific plaques from the internal carotid or the heart have the greatest likelihood of lodging where the artery vessel undergoes a rapid decrease in caliber. These emboli are referred to as Hollenhorst's plaques (Fig. 9–21). Previously the standard of care for a Hollenhorst plaque was a carotid endarterectomy. More recent studies have indicated that more than one-third of patients with no symptoms have normal internal carotid arteries by duplex ultrasound evaluation.[16] However, all patients with a Hollenhorst's plaque require carotid auscultation and further medical work-up.

In the retina, branches of the central retinal artery and vein travel in pairs. Two veins are always separated by an artery and vice versa. Often branches from an artery and its corresponding vein cross. In the vast majority of these vessel crossings, the artery passes anterior to the corresponding vein. At the site of a vessel crossing, the artery and vein share a common adventitial sheath. Therefore distention of the higher pressure arterial vessel results in alteration in the appearance of the vein at crossings. Additionally, changes in arterial vessel wall rigidity and vessel pressure result in "pinching" or "crimping." These changes are most notable in systemic hypertension.

Many systems have been developed to grade hypertensive retinal vessel changes.[17, 18] Although vessel crossing changes are indicative of systemic hypertension, they are not found initially in every patient with the condition. Therefore, the ab-

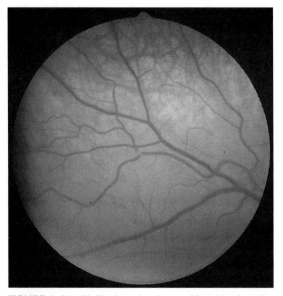

**FIGURE 9–21** Hollenhorst's plaque. Note the location and reflective nature of this calcific embolus.

sence of vessel crossing changes does not rule out the possibility of elevated blood pressure. The responsible ophthalmic practitioner measures arterial blood pressure on every patient.

The branches of the central retinal vein coalesce to form larger vessels as they approach the optic nerve head. On the optic nerve head, the central retinal vein or its major contributory branches can be observed to spontaneously pulsate in a rhythmic fashion. This pulsation can usually be observed at points where the vessel undergoes changes in direction. The most abrupt direction change occurs as the vessel descends into the physiological cup. The range or extent of this pulsation in the normal patient population is significant. This pulsation need not be present in the normal state. It may also include dramatic collapse and expansion of a central retinal vein segment.

During systole, blood under high pressure is pumped from the heart and enters the aortic arch. During diastole, the blood pressure in the aortic arch diminishes. The difference between these two pressures is referred to as the pulse pressure. As the arterial system divides into smaller and smaller arteries, the systole, diastole, and pulse pressure all diminish. In the venous portion of the vascular system, the pulse pressure is absent, and the blood pressure is further diminished. The central retinal vein has an approximate pressure of 18 mm Hg and notably absent pulse pressure. Recall that the choroid is a highly vascularized structure that is supplied by the internal carotid, a high-pressure branch in the arterial system. During systole, the choroid receives a rush of blood resulting from the pulse pressure of the arterial system. This vascular bed becomes "engorged" during systole. Because the eye has an essentially limited volume, this addition of fluid results in an increase in intraocular pressure. This shift is not sustained but remains rhythmically transient, corresponding with systole. During the increase in intraocular pressure, the central retinal venous pressure is exceeded and the wall yields, resulting in the observation of pulsation. During this rhythmic alteration of intraocular pressure with the cardiac cycle, the central retinal artery does not pulsate.

The presence of spontaneous venous pulsation is a normal finding and suggests that the resting intraocular pressure is slightly lower than the central retinal venous pressure. Of clinical significance is the absence of spontaneous venous pulsation in an individual who has a well-documented history of this observation. This "loss" of pulsation suggests the presence of increased back pressure in the local venous system. This change in pressure can be related to an intracranial mass and warrants further evaluation.

Spontaneous arterial pulsation is significant and always an indication of pathology. There are two etiological possibilities for this finding. One is substantially elevated intraocular pressure. The incremental addition in intraocular pressure from the cardiac cycle can then exceed the diastolic pressure of the central retinal vessel, resulting in pulsation. A second possibility is that of reduced perfusion pressure of the central retinal artery. In this case the arterial pressure is low enough that it yields to the diastolic intraocular pressure. If left untreated, both of these conditions have grave consequences and therefore require immediate evaluation and intervention.

# Topography of the Posterior Pole

The histological definition of the posterior pole, macula, and fovea differs from generally accepted clinical definitions[19] (Table 9-4). From the histologist's perspective, the anatomical region of the retina that has more than one layer of ganglion cells is the area centralis. This roughly circular region is approximately 6 mm in diameter. Its center is located at fixation. The clinician defines this same region as the posterior pole. Clinically this is the region of the fundus that spans from the optic disc to a point roughly 2.5 DD temporal of fixation. Funduscopically, the vertical boundaries of the posterior pole are formed by the superior and inferior temporal vascular arcades. The central 1500 μ of the area centralis is referred to as the fovea by the histologist. Clinically, this same area is defined as the macula. Regardless of the terminology, this region is characterized by the absence or termination of the major retinal vessels. In the center of the central 1500 μ is a region called the foveola by histologists. It represents slightly thickened retinal tissue surrounding a depression measuring 350 μ in diameter. This depression is essentially devoid of rod photoreceptors.

Funduscopically, the clinician-defined fovea is located in the center of the macula. As previously described, the retinal topography is characterized by a small concave depression in this location. This small, regular concavity combined with the internal limiting membrane resembles a concave mirror. Clinicians are observing the fovea when they see a small but bright reflection in the center of the macula. This pinpoint reflection is present in young normals but may diminish or disappear completely as a normal, age-related change.

# Diabetic Retinopathy

The majority of ocular complications from diabetes present as some variation of retinopathy. The traditional terms for diabetes—adult versus juvenile and Type I versus Type II—have been replaced by classifying diabetic patients according to their dependence upon insulin for survival. The current terms are insulin-dependent diabetes mellitus (IDDM) and non–insulin-dependent diabetes mellitus (NIDDM).

The classification of retinopathy has also evolved. Currently, diabetic retinopathy is classified into non-proliferative diabetic retinopathy (NPDR) and proliferative diabetic retinopathy (PDR) groupings, each of which has subcategories (Table 9-5). The correct staging of the retinopathy aids the practitioner in the appropriate management of this condition. Standard photographs have been adopted to aid the practitioner in staging the level of retinopathy. (Note: These stereo photographs are available through the Fundus Photograph Reading Center, Department of Ophthalmology, University of Wisconsin, Madison Medical School.)

Diabetic retinopathy is classified into three broad categories. The first group includes changes associated with branches of the central retinal artery and vein or with the capillary bed that provides the link between them. Included in this group are microaneurysms and dot-blot hemorrhages. Venous caliber changes such as venous beading, dilation, and loop formation are also included and represent retinal response to hypoxia. Intraretinal microvascular abnormalities (IRMA) represent neovascularization within the retina. Closure of retinal capillaries and arterioles, which has the poorest prognosis for vision, completes this category.

The second category of changes is a function of leakage from capillaries and can occur at any level of retinopathy. This causes a localized thickening or edema of the adjacent retina. Subsequently, a residual yellow lesion forms as a

**TABLE 9–4** Terminology Used in the Topology of the Central Retina

| Structure | Histologist | Clinician |
|---|---|---|
| Central 6000 μ | Area centralis | Posterior pole |
| Central 1500 μ | Fovea | Macula |
| Central 500 μ | Foveola | Fovea |

**TABLE 9–5** Levels of Diabetic Retinopathy

**Non-Proliferative Diabetic Retinopathy (NPDR)**

| | |
|---|---|
| Mild | At least one microaneurysm (but less than the requirements for moderate, severe, or very severe NPDR or early/high-risk PDR) |
| Moderate | Hemorrhage/microaneurysm greater than standard photograph 2A or cotton wool spots, venous beading, or IRMA definitely present (but less than the requirements for severe/very severe NPDR or early/high-risk PDR) |
| Severe | Hemorrhage/microaneurysm greater than standard photograph 2A in all four quadrants or venous beading equal to standard photograph 6B on two or more quadrants, or IRMA greater than standard photograph 8A in one quadrant (but less than the requirements for very severe NPDR or early/high-risk PDR) |
| Very severe | Any two of the requirements for severe NPDR (but less than the requirements for early/high-risk PDR) |

**Proliferative Diabetic Retinopathy (PDR)**

| | |
|---|---|
| Early | New vessels (but the definition not met for high-risk PDR) |
| High risk | NVD ≥ 1/3–1/4 disc area or NVD and vitreous or preretinal hemorrhage, or NVE ≥ 1/2 disc area and preretinal or vitreous hemorrhage |

marker of prior or concurrent leakage. This finding is called hard exudate because of its well-circumscribed borders. Macular edema is defined as leakage within 2 DD of the fovea. When the leakage is more proximal to the fovea, the complications for vision become more serious. Clinically significant macular edema (CSME) has a well-established definition. To be clinically significant, at least one of the following must exist: (1) retinal thickening at or within 500 μ of the center of the macula, (2) hard exudates at or within 500 μ of the center of the macula if associated with retinal thickening, and/or (3) a region of retinal thickening 1 DD or greater at or within 1 DD of the macular center. Retinopathy meeting any one these three requirements is defined as CSME. Patients with CSME are at risk of losing vision and must be evaluated for focal or grid laser treatment.

The third category of retinal changes associated with diabetes is neovascularization and the subsequent fibrovascular proliferation. As indicated by the prefix "neo," these new vessels are created in response to retinal hypoxia. The serious complications of proliferative retinopathy are not specifically the new vessels but are a result of the contraction of the fibrovascular tissue from these vessels.

Extensive studies have been conducted in the management of diabetes and its associated retinopathy. The reader is directed to the Diabetic Retinopathy Study (DRS),[20-30] the Early Treatment Diabetic Retinopathy Study (ETDRS),[31-42] the Diabetic Retinopathy Vitrectomy Study (DRVS),[43-47] and the Diabetic Control and Complications Trial (DCCT).[48, 49]

# The Retinal Periphery

The retinal periphery is divided into four quadrants for ease of examination recording and communication with other practitioners. This artificial compartmentalization of the retina has also evolved from epidemiological studies that have examined the prevalence of disease processes. Another useful descriptive tool is to refer to a funduscopic location by the clock hour which describes its orientation. The reference clock is oriented from the clinician's point of view, not the patient's. A final descriptive system uses both geographic terminology and anatomical structure to identify location (Fig. 9–14 and Table 9–6). The equator is the greatest sagittal circumference of the eye and is utilized in this system. The two anatomical structures in this system are the ora serrata and the anterior border of the pars plana. Both of these anatomical structures are anterior to the equator. Unlike the equator, which has only rough funduscopic landmarks, the ora serrata and pars plana can readily be determined.

**TABLE 9–6** Distance from the Optic Nerve Head to Peripheral Retinal Locations and Landmarks

| Direction | Anatomical Equator | Anterior Edge of the Ora Serrata |
|---|---|---|
| Superior | 9 DD (16 mm) | 11.7 DD (21 mm) |
| Inferior | 8.6 DD (15.5 mm) | 11.3 DD (20.3 mm) |
| Temporal | 10.7 DD (19.25 mm) | 14 DD (24.25 mm) |
| Nasal | 7.8 DD (14 mm) | 11 DD (19.9 mm) |

Perhaps the astute reader has already formulated a criticism of this common system: by definition, the equator represents the greatest circumference and yet is represented by the smallest circle on this diagram. Even given this well-founded criticism, this system enjoys wide utilization among ophthalmic practitioners.

Other useful anatomical landmarks of the periphery include the four vortex ampullae. These choroidal collection reservoirs usually number one to a quadrant. Occasionally, two small ampullae are in close proximity in one quadrant. These structures are quite variable in appearance. The notable exception to this is the "swirling" appearance (and hence the name vortex) of the large choroidal vessels that drain into these structures. The vortex ampullae are posterior to the equator and provide the clinician with a convenient reference location.

Additional anatomical references include the long and short posterior ciliary nerves. The two long posterior ciliary nerves enter the globe near the equator at the 3 and 9 o'clock positions. They continue anteriorly through the sclera and choroid en route to innervate anterior ocular structures. At their entrance to the inner choroid, they become visible funduscopically. This corresponds roughly to the region between the equator and ora serrata. Their appearance is characteristic as a linear cream-colored structure that is usually bounded by pigment (Fig. 9–22).

The short posterior ciliary nerves are more numerous, random in their orientation, and shorter than the long posterior ciliary nerves.

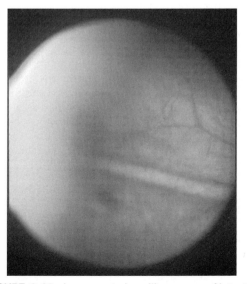

**FIGURE 9–22** Long posterior ciliary nerve. Note the appearance of a linear cream-colored structure bounded by a pigment band on either side.

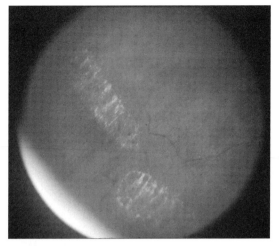

**FIGURE 9–23** Lattice degeneration of the retinal periphery.

Occasionally, they can be observed in the vicinity of the vortex ampullae.

The retinal periphery can undergo a large range of pathological changes. The vast majority of the changes are a function of the retinal traction at the vitreous base. As the vitreous undergoes age-related liquefaction, focal attachments remain with the peripheral retina. These attachments exert increased traction on the retina. When the retina yields to traction, a break is created in the tissue. Breaks in retinal tissue are described as "rhegmatogenous." Breaks in the sensory retina allow pigment granules from the epithelial layer to be dispersed into the vitreous. This is referred to as Shaffer's sign, or tobacco dust, and represents a clear message to the clinician that a rhegmatogenous retinal change has occurred. The retina can respond to this increased mechanical force in a number of ways.

The most common peripheral retinal change is the broad category of lattice degeneration. Classically, the lattice appears as band- or cigar-shaped, circumferential lesions. Often the fine vessels in these lesions undergo sclerosis, yielding a fine criss-cross pattern of white lines (Fig. 9–23), hence the term "lattice." Variations in lattice degeneration include pigmentation from hyperplasia of the retinal pigment epithelium. Atrophic holes, which are associated with lattice degeneration, are prognostic for more significant rhegmatogenous changes. Holes located *within* lattice lesions are of little significance. Atrophic holes on the border of or outside lattice lesions carry with them greater concern and greater risk of retinal detachment.

The release of focal traction can be observed in retinal hole formation. Focal traction can weaken a well-circumscribed region of retina, resulting in separation of the sensory retina. Often, the liberated tissue can be seen in the immediate vicinity of the overlying vitreous as a free-floating opacity referred to as an operculum.

Once the focal traction has been eliminated, the patient is usually free from additional complications. However, the retina that remains attached can undergo changes, including the influx of vitreal fluid. This results in a local delamination, elevation, and weakening of the retina. This fluid appears as a grey annulus that encircles the retinal hole formation. Scleral indentation is indicated to determine the extent to which this annular region is elevated.

Tears in the peripheral retina have a classic "horseshoe" appearance. This rhegmatogenous change represents a more serious presentation than lattice or peripheral hole formation. The torn flap remains attached to the vitreous and is subject to additional traction. This continued traction and insult increase the likelihood of true retinal detachment. Peripheral retinal tears are radial in their orientation. The arch of the tear points to the central retina. Tears are more common in the superior temporal quadrant. They are associated with patients' observations of photopsia, grey/black dots, and increased floaters. Therapy includes thermal laser and cryopexy surgery.

True retinal detachments represent the most serious complication of rhegmatogenous findings. In this condition, the retina has lifted free of its pigment epithelium. The symptoms of a retinal detachment include those for a retinal tear, with the notable addition of a "curtain" or "shadow" across the patient's vision. Funduscopically, retinal detachments appear as elevated and undulating retinal tissue that has lost its transparency.

If re-attachment is not successful in a short period of time—1 or 2 days—retinal function and the associated visual function are permanently lost. Therefore, a retinal detachment is an ocular emergency. It requires immediate evaluation and intervention. Patients presenting with the symptoms of a retinal detachment or tear more frequently have vitreous traction without a rhegmatogenous finding. However, these patients require a full mydriatic evaluation with thorough binocular indirect ophthalmoscopy and scleral indentation. Treatment includes scleral buckling surgery with cryopexy, a combination of cryopexy and intraocular gas bubble, or a combination of all three modalities.

# Ophthalmic Funduscopic Instruments

The instruments used in funduscopic evaluation have two essential properties. First, the patient's retina must be illuminated. Second, an image of the patient's retina must be formed on the observer's retina. Regardless of the level of sophistication, all of these instruments described below accomplish both these requirements.

## DIRECT OPHTHALMOSCOPE

The first instrument to gain widespread popularity was the direct ophthalmoscope. Although it continues to have a limited place in ophthalmic practice, the direct ophthalmoscope is the centerpiece for pediatricians' and primary care providers' funduscopic evaluation. In this sense, the direct ophthalmoscope has withstood the test of time.

In optical terms, the direct ophthalmoscope creates conjugacy between the patient's and the observer's retina. This is accomplished by altering light exiting from the patient's eye to focus it on the observer's retina. The alteration in vergence is possible by interposing lenses of varying dioptric power (Fig. 9–24). These lenses are located in a wheel that is manipulated by the observer. Illumination of the patient's fundus is provided by a light source within the neck of the instrument. Light is reflected into the observation path before the dioptric wheel by a half-silvered mirror or reflecting prism (Fig. 9–25). The intensity of the light is controlled by a rheostat on the top of the battery handle. The light and hence the viewing system are controlled by

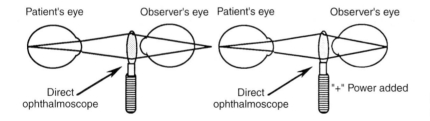

Patient's eye          Observer's eye  Patient's eye          Observer's eye

Direct ophthalmoscope          Direct ophthalmoscope          "+" Power added

**FIGURE 9–24** Schematic of direct ophthalmoscope.

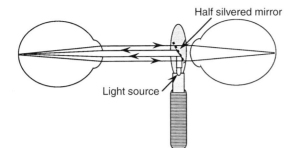

**FIGURE 9-25** Light source in the direct ophthalmoscope.

a range of adjustable apertures. Modern instruments have a standard set of small, medium, and large circular apertures. More sophisticated instruments have slits, grids, or half-moon apertures in addition to the standard circular set.

The procedure for direct ophthalmoscopy is described in a stepwise fashion in this text. One of the criticisms of the direct ophthalmoscope is its small field of view. Mydriatic evaluation with the large circular aperture is a step that the practitioner can take to address this concern. Regardless of the status of pupillary dilation, the practitioner can maximize the field of view by keeping the instrument close to his or her eye. Close proximity to the patient's eye further enlarges the field of view with the direct ophthalmoscope.

Direct ophthalmoscopy has additional limitations resulting from corneal aberrations and vignetting. It produces about a 15× enlargement of retinal detail and a field of view of about 10° (Table 9-7). Myopes have slightly larger-appearing retinal details than do hyperopes. The direct ophthalmoscope is useful for evaluating the posterior pole with high magnification. Approximately 60° of the fundus can be evaluated with this instrument.

Direct ophthalmoscopic fundus evaluation begins at the optic nerve head. Cupping, margins, color, and the blood vessels at the disc are evaluated. After evaluating the nerve head, the vascular branches out to at least the third bifurcation are followed and observed. The last region to be evaluated is the macula.

## Procedure for Direct Ophthalmoscopy

☐ Prepare the patient by seating him or her comfortably at the right height to ensure both patient and doctor comfort.
☐ Examine the patient's eye with the same eye you are using, that is, patient's right eye and practitioner's right eye.
☐ Cradle the instrument with the hand on the same side as the eye with which you are viewing.
☐ Place your index finger on the dioptric power wheel, your middle finger around the neck of the instrument, and your lower two fingers around the battery handle.
☐ Turn on the instrument and adjust the light intensity to the necessary level.
☐ For the emmetropic patient and practitioner, set the optical power wheel to +3.00 D.
☐ Holding the instrument close to your eye, sight through the ocular.
☐ Starting at about 30 cm from the patient, direct the light into the patient's eye.
☐ Note the patient's fundus reflex within the pupil while advancing slowly toward the patient and adjusting the power wheel to bring fundus details into view.
☐ Locate a fundus vessel and follow its path in the direction in which it increases in size using the patient's pupil as your center of rotation.
☐ Locate the optic nerve head.
☐ Continue with funduscopic screening.
☐ Record your findings.

## MONOCULAR INDIRECT OPHTHALMOSCOPY

This instrument, developed by American Optical, is used almost exclusively by optometrists. It has a number of distinct advantages over direct ophthalmoscopy. In addition, before diagnostic pharmaceutical agents were widely used in optometry, the monocular indirect ophthalmoscope

| TABLE 9-7 Comparison of Various Fundus Instruments | | | |
|---|---|---|---|
| Technique | Enlargement | Field of View | Viewing Limitations |
| Direct ophthalmoscopy | 15× | 8–10° | Central 60° |
| Indirect ophthalmoscopy | 7.5× | 20° | Anatomical equator |
| Binocular indirect ophthalmoscopy | 2–4× | 40–75° | None |
| Fundus contact lens | Variable | Variable | None |

permitted a non-mydriatic evaluation of the retinal periphery.

The monocular indirect ophthalmoscope overcomes the limitations of direct ophthalmoscopy by focusing its illumination system at the plane of the pupil. This illuminates a larger region of retina. Light exiting the patient's pupil is captured by the same convergent lens that focuses the illumination system. These image rays form an image on the practitioner's side of this optical element. This image of the retina is inverted and reversed. The image rays deviate from this initial focus and strike a second convergent lens. This latter optical element has sufficient vergence to focus the divergent image a second time. The second image is now upright and unreversed (Fig. 9–26). An ocular allows parallel rays to exit the instrument.

The initial goal of monocular indirect ophthalmoscopy is, like direct ophthalmoscopy, to locate the optic disc. Once the disc has been evaluated, excursions are made into the periphery as though outlining the petals on a flower. Again, the last region to be evaluated should be the macula.

As has been discussed, the monocular indirect ophthalmoscope represented significant improvements over its predecessor (Table 9-7). It has a larger field of view and brighter illumination and allows greater access to the periphery. With all these advantages, its major drawback remains a monocular image.

## Procedure for Monocular Indirect Ophthalmoscopy

☐ Prepare the patient by seating him or her comfortably at the right height to ensure both doctor and patient comfort.

☐ Examine the patient's eye with the same eye you are using, that is, patient's right eye with practitioner's right eye.

☐ Hold the instrument battery handle with the hand on the same side as the eye with which you are viewing.

☐ Place your index and middle fingers of the opposite hand on the head of the instrument.

☐ Turn on the instrument and adjust the light intensity to the necessary level.

☐ Place the edge of the hand that is holding the instrument head against the patient's forehead.

☐ Sight through the instrument, adjusting the focus with the thumb of the hand holding the battery handle.

☐ Locate a fundus vessel and follow its path in the direction in which it increases in size.

☐ Locate the optic nerve head.

☐ Continue with funduscopic screening.

☐ Record your findings.

## BINOCULAR INDIRECT OPHTHALMOSCOPE AND CONDENSING LENSES

This instrument is the premier choice for evaluating the fundus. Its wide and bright field of view permits a rapid assessment of the retinal periphery. The instrument is quite simple in design. What the binocular indirect ophthalmoscope lacks in complexity is compensated for by the skill and training of the practitioner. Most individuals can gain an adequate view of the fundus with the direct or indirect monocular ophthalmoscopes early in their training. The binocular indirect ophthalmoscope, however, requires much more than an initial effort to obtain a satisfactory view. This instrument requires years of daily use for its full potential to be realized. Novices should take some comfort in recalling that their more experienced colleagues would not set this instrument aside for another, suggesting that the results are more than worth the effort.

Optically, the binocular indirect ophthalmoscope is similar to the monocular instrument, with two notable exceptions. The image the practitioner sees is inverted and reversed with the binocular indirect ophthalmoscope. Second, the lens that is used in this procedure is hand-held and as such can be of various dioptric values and diameters. In fact, as the reader will discover, the condensing lens—not the binocular indirect ophthalmoscope—plays the major role in this form of funduscopy.

The condensing lenses used in binocular indirect ophthalmoscopy are biconvex in design, regardless of their manufacturer. To minimize aberration, the lenses have a designated patient surface. By convention, this is marked on the lens as a white ring. Although a view can be obtained with the lens inverted, the image is of

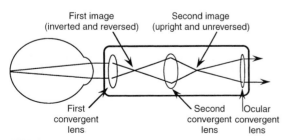

**FIGURE 9–26** The optics of the monocular indirect ophthalmoscope.

poorer quality. The lens should be held between the thumb and index finger of one hand. This allows the additional fingers of that hand to rest on the patient's face for stability. The other hand can be used to retract the patient's eyelids, apply a scleral indentor, and/or steady the lens.

The condensing lens used in binocular indirect ophthalmoscopy controls the image size and the field of view. The dioptric power of the condensing lens and image enlargement are inverse properties. A good approximation of the magnitude of image enlargement is the quotient resulting from the dioptric power of the eye divided by the dioptric power of the lens. Hence, a 28.00 D lens and a roughly 60.00 D eye result in approximately an image enlargement of two times. A 14.00 D lens and the same eye result in an enlargement of four times. A 20.00 D lens has three times enlargement. The diameter and power of the condensing lens control the field of view. As a rule, increasing the dioptric power results in a larger field of view. Conversely, increasing the diameter also increases the field of view. Hence, a very large diameter 28.00 D lens would yield a larger field of view than a small 14.00 D lens. Lenses can be clear or tinted yellow. Clinical studies have indicated a patient preference for yellow lenses.[50]

Light from the binocular indirect ophthalmoscope headset is projected through the condensing lens. This light is focused by the lens at the plane of the pupil. This allows a large column of light (the diameter of the condensing lens) to be directed through a small region (the pupil) (Fig. 9-27). After passing through this plane, the light reaches the fundus.

Light leaves the fundus and is acted upon by the optics of the eye. In the simple case of the emmetrope, this light leaves the patient's eye as parallel rays. This parallel light is captured by the condensing lens, and an image is formed at the posterior focal point. For a 20.00 D lens, the image of the fundus is formed 5 cm from the lens (Fig. 9-28).

The condensing lens plays other key roles that are less obvious. One of these is creating the optical situation in which the patient's pupil and

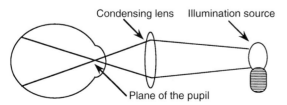

**FIGURE 9–27** The binocular indirect ophthalmoscope illumination system.

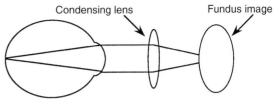

**FIGURE 9–28** The binocular indirect ophthalmoscope imaging system.

the observer's pupils are conjugate points. This negates the patient's pupil as a limiting aperture. In effect, it is as if the observer's pupils are in the same optical plane as the patient's pupil. The contribution of the headset, in addition to supplying the illumination source, is to optically reduce the pupillary separation of the observer from an average of 60 mm to about 15 mm. Because the lens is closer to the patient's pupil than the observer, there is a resultant relative magnification of its diameter. The optical enlargement of the patient's pupil in combination with the pupillary separation reduction of the headset has a critical role in the usefulness of this instrument. These two factors allow both of the observer's pupils to "fit" within the patient's pupil, facilitating the binocular view.

The high dioptric value and large diameter of these condensing lenses give them both beneficial and detractive properties. The lens need be tilted only slightly to minimize reflections from its surface. Moving the lens while an image is formed allows the observer to cover a greater fundus region in nearly the same time. Unfortunately for the novice, seemingly small lens movements result in the loss of the image. As the dioptric power of the lenses is increased, these advantages and disadvantages become more pronounced. Experience and practice minimize the disadvantages and enhance the advantages inherent in the use of condensing lenses.

The binocular indirect ophthalmoscope headset is essentially static during this entire procedure. Other than optically reducing the observer's interpupillary distance and providing an illumination source, the headset has a small role to play. However, it is essential that the headset have the proper alignment and ocular separation. If the illumination source is adjustable, it should be just lower than center to minimize reflections.

Binocular indirect ophthalmoscopy has a number of pitfalls. One of the earliest mistakes practitioners make is not "tromboning" the condensing lens. A second mistake is the failure to keep arm's length distance from the patient. Novice practitioners often think that they need to adjust their position inward from full arm extension to obtain a clear view. Another mistake is not attempting to use condensing lenses of higher or lower power than the ubiquitous 20.00 D lens. A final mistake is not using sufficient illumination to view the patient's fundus.

The view with the binocular indirect ophthalmoscope is reversed and inverted. This initially can be quite confusing and takes some adjustment. Because of the reversal, the practitioner needs to move in the same direction as the point of interest. It is important to note that only the view in the lens is reversed and not the region of the retina. If the patient is looking superiorly and you are looking at his or her eye from an inferior position, what you see in the lens is reversed and inverted, but the area of the fundus you are visualizing is in the superior hemisphere of the patient's eye.

Scleral indentation brings a dynamic characteristic to the binocular indirect ophthalmoscope examination. This technique is used for two reasons. It allows the practitioner to examine regions of the far periphery that otherwise may have been inaccessible. Second, it allows the practitioner to dynamically examine retinal pathology, specifically peripheral retinal degenerations and retinal breaks. Initially, the practitioner may have some reservations about scleral indentation (a preferable term to scleral depression) as it relates to patient comfort. Even for the novice practitioner, this procedure can be all but free of patient discomfort. Scleral indentors come in two varieties. The thimble style is useful for practitioners with small hands. The stylus type indentor is useful for practitioners with larger hands.

## Procedure for Binocular Indirect Ophthalmoscopy

☐ Prepare the patient by seating or reclining him or her comfortably to ensure both doctor and patient comfort.

☐ Adjust the headset on your head, ensuring that the correct ocular separation has been selected and you are fusing an object at 40 cm.

☐ Adjust the rheostat on the transformer to an appropriate setting.

☐ With your arms nearly fully extended near the patient's face, direct the light from the headset into the patient's eye.

☐ Note the fundus reflex.

☐ Bring the condensing lens with the white marking toward the patient into the illumination beam near the patient's eye. You should note that the image within the lens

includes both the fundus reflex and the patient's adnexa.

☐ Draw the lens away from the patient slowly. As you do so, the condensing lens "fills" with the patient's fundus image.

☐ As you continue to draw the lens away from the patient, a point is reached where the image again contains adnexa. When this occurs, reverse the direction of lens movement.

☐ Continue to move the lens between the points where the image contains adnexa to find the best image.

☐ Remember to keep the patient at about arm's length distance.

☐ Direct the patient's gaze in the same direction as the region of the retina you wish to evaluate; for example, for superior retina, have the patient look up.

☐ Tilt the lens slightly to minimize reflections and maximize the image quality.

☐ Begin a systematic funduscopic screening, superior, superior-nasal, nasal, inferior-nasal, inferior, inferior-temporal, temporal, superior-temporal, and then the posterior pole.

☐ Record your findings.

## Procedure for Binocular Indirect Ophthalmoscopy and Scleral Indentation

☐ Follow all the set-up directions described above for binocular indirect ophthalmoscopy.

☐ Direct the patient's gaze in the opposite direction from the region of the retina you wish to evaluate; for example, if the target tissue is the superior retina, ask the patient to look inferiorly.

☐ Place your scleral indentor on the lid at the inner border of the tarsal plate.

☐ Direct the patient to slowly resume a gaze in the direction of the tissue you wish to evaluate; for example, if the target tissue is the superior retina, ask the patient to look superiorly.

☐ As the patient alters his or her gaze, follow the eye movement with the indentor. The action of the indentor should be along the globe, not against it.

☐ For lateral views, drag the superior or inferior lid into the canthal areas.

## SLIT-LAMP FUNDUSCOPY

The slit-lamp biomicroscope is a useful addition for certain funduscopic examinations. In all cases, a lens must be used in conjunction with the slit-lamp to visualize the fundus. The lenses can be separated into two groups. Non–contact lenses constitute the first of these groups. These lenses are useful for a rapid binocular screening of the central retina. The main feature of these lenses is that they overcome the substantial refractive power of the cornea. The initial entry in this group was the Hruby lens. It is a −58.60 D lens that is attached to the slit-lamp biomicroscope. Its large divergent power allows the slit-lamp biomicroscope to be focused on the fundus. Its use is limited to the posterior pole, and it requires a mydriatic pupil for adequate evaluation. The Hruby lens has been replaced by the highly convergent lenses commercially available from Volk, Ocular Scientific, and Nikon. They are biconvex and range in power from +60.00 to +90.00 D. The optics of slit-lamp funduscopy are identical to those of the binocular indirect ophthalmoscope.

The primary use for these lenses is the magnified and binocular evaluation of the posterior pole and optic nerve. The stereoscopic effect is remarkable, and with practice, a rapid and exceptional screening examination of this portion of the retina can be performed. These condensing lenses have the same characteristics as those used with the binocular indirect ophthalmoscope. Increasing dioptric power decreases magnification but increases the field of view.

Contact lens evaluation with the slit-lamp has two distinct lens groups. Direct lenses, like the traditional Goldmann variety, have mirrors of various shapes that are inclined at specific angles (Table 9–8). These mirrors are enclosed within the body of the lens. The ocular surface of the lens is concave and has a radius of curvature which is slightly steeper than the corneal surface. The central "non-mirrored" region of this lens is used to evaluate the central 30° of the fundus. This lens requires both a corneal anesthetic and a viscous gel such as gonioscopic prism solution or Celluvisc to cushion the cornea. The cornea's refractive power is neutralized by the lens's concave-plano surfaces.

The novice practitioner may become confused regarding which mirror to use. A simple means of recalling the correct application for each lens is using the mnemonic "APE." Beginning with the parabolic mirror and continuing clockwise around the lens, their purposes are angle, periphery, and equator. Further confusion exists because the view, unlike that with the binocular indirect ophthalmoscope, is reversed anteroposteriorly but not laterally.

Indirect lenses are a newer entry into the slit-lamp funduscopy arena. They typically employ multiple refractive surfaces to create a highly magnified and stereoscopic view of the fundus. A topical anesthetic is required for the use of these lenses, and many practitioners use cushioning solution as well. These lenses are notable for their stable, stereoscopic, and magnified image of the fundus. Usually a series of lenses is available with varying uses. A series may have a central lens with high magnification and stereopsis and a wide field lens that yields a panoramic view with reduced magnification. Indirect lenses produce an inverted and reversed image of the fundus.

Using direct or indirect fundus contact lenses for routine screening is impractical, however, because of their physical requirements and limitations. In addition, the illumination used with these lenses is uncomfortable for the patient. Their application is almost exclusively for more detailed investigation once an abnormality is seen with the binocular indirect ophthalmoscope.

## Procedure for Slit-Lamp Funduscopy with Non-Contact High Plus Lenses

- ☐ Seat the dilated patient behind the slit-lamp in the middle of the vertical travel range of the instrument.
- ☐ Reduce the horizontal and vertical dimension of the slit beam.
- ☐ With the slit-lamp in a "full back" position, direct the light into the patient's pupil.
- ☐ Introduce the lens into the beam of light near the patient's eye.
- ☐ Manipulate the slit-lamp forward until retinal detail comes into focus.
- ☐ Tilt the lens slightly to minimize reflections and maximize the image quality.
- ☐ Manipulate the slit-lamp and the lens together to obtain the best view and to evaluate the fundus.

**TABLE 9–8** Geometry and Function of Mirrored Fundus Lenses

| Mirror | Mirror Inclination | Structures |
|--------|--------------------|-----------|
| Parabolic | 59° | Anterior chamber—pars plana |
| Rectangular | 67° | Anterior equator to posterior ora serrata |
| Trapezoidal | 73° | Equatorial fundus |

## Procedure for Slit-Lamp Funduscopy with a Direct Mirrored Lens

- ☐ Seat the dilated patient behind the slit-lamp in the middle of the vertical travel range of the instrument.
- ☐ Instill a corneal anesthetic drop.
- ☐ Add two or three drops of cushioning solution to the concave surface of the lens, ensuring that the solution is bubble-free.
- ☐ Reduce the horizontal and vertical dimensions of the slit-lamp beam.
- ☐ Direct the patient's gaze into the inferior field. Retract the patient's lid with the hand that will manipulate the slit-lamp once the lens is in place.
- ☐ Direct the patient's gaze into the superior field. Hold the lens between the index finger and thumb. With the other fingers of this hand, retract the patient's lower lid.
- ☐ Place the lower edge of the lens against the lower lid margin. In a smooth and directed movement, manipulate the lens from a vertical position onto the ocular surface as the patient is directed to return to primary gaze. Release the superior and inferior lids.
- ☐ Rotate the lens to position the mirror of choice in the opposite field; for example, to look at the superior field, place the mirror in an inferior position.
- ☐ With the slit-lamp in a "full back" position, direct the light into the mirror of choice.
- ☐ Advance the slit-lamp until the retinal detail is in focus.
- ☐ Manipulate the slit-lamp and the lens together to obtain the best view and to evaluate the fundus abnormality of interest.

## Procedure for Slit-Lamp Funduscopy with an Indirect Mirrored Lens

- ☐ Seat the dilated patient behind the slit-lamp in the middle of the vertical travel range of the instrument.
- ☐ Instill a corneal anesthetic drop.
- ☐ Add two or three drops of cushioning solution to the concave surface of the lens, ensuring that the solution is bubble-free.
- ☐ Reduce the horizontal and vertical dimensions of the slit-lamp beam.
- ☐ Direct the patient's gaze into the inferior field. Retract the patient's lid with the hand that will manipulate the slit-lamp once the lens is in place.

- ☐ Direct the patient's gaze into the superior field. Hold the lens between the index finger and thumb. With the other fingers of this hand, retract the patient's lower lid.
- ☐ Place the lower edge of the lens against the lower lid margin. In a smooth and directed movement, manipulate the lens from a vertical position onto the ocular surface as the patient is directed to return to a primary gaze. Release the superior and inferior lids.
- ☐ With the slit-lamp in a "full back" position, direct the light into the region of the lens opposite the area of the retina you wish to evaluate.
- ☐ Advance the slit-lamp until retinal detail is in focus.
- ☐ Manipulate the slit-lamp and the lens together to obtain the best view and to evaluate the fundus abnormality of interest.

# References

1. Hogan MJ, Alvarado JA, Waddell JE: Histology of the Human Eye: An Atlas and Textbook. Philadelphia: WB Saunders, 1971, pp 611–613.
2. Hogan MJ: The vitreous, its structure, and relation to the ciliary body and retina. Invest Ophthalmol Vis Sci 1963; 2:418–445.
3. Alexander IJ: Primary Care of the Posterior Segment. 2nd ed. Norwalk, CT: Appleton & Lange, 1994, p 349.
4. Foos RY, Wheeler NC: Vitreoretinal jucture; synchysis senilis and posterior vitreous detachment. Ophthalmology 1982; 89:1502–1512.
5. Marakami K: Vitreous floaters. Ophthalmology 1983; 90:1271–1276.
6. Cline D, Hofstetter HW, Griffin JR: Dictionary of Visual Science. 3rd ed. Radnor, PA: Chilton Book Co., 1980.
7. Balazsi AG, Rootman J, Drance SM, et al.: The effect of age on the nerve fiber population of the human optic nerve. Am J Ophthalmol 1984; 97:760–766.
8. Repka MX, Quigley HA: The effect of age on normal human optic nerve fiber and diameter. Ophthalmology 1989; 96:26–32.
9. Jonas JB, Muller-Bergh JA, Schlotzer-Schrenhardt UM, et al.: Histomorphometry of the human optic nerve. Invest Ophthalmol Vis Sci 1990; 31:736–744.
10. Good TW, Quinn TG: Component evaluation of cup/disc ratio estimation. J Am Optom Assoc 1984; 55:889–893.
11. Aldredge B, Lum R, DiMartino RB: Intraclinician variability in the estimation of the cup to disc ratio. Doctor of Optometry thesis, University of California, Berkeley, School of Optometry, 1989.
12. Fantes FE, Anderson DR: Clinical histologic correlation of human peripapillary anatomy. Ophthalmology 1989; 96:20–25.
13. Airaksinen PJ, Drance SM, Douglas GR, et al.: Diffuse and localized nerve fiber loss in glaucoma. Am J Ophthlamol 1984; 98:566–571.
14. Sommer A, Katz J, Quigley HA, et al.: Clinically detectable nerve fiber atrophy precedes the onset of glaucomatous field loss. Arch Ophthalmol 1991; 109:77–83.
15. Miller NR, George TW: Monochromatic (red free) photography and ophthalmoscopy of the peripapillary retinal

nerve fiber layer. Invest Ophthalmol Vis Sci 1978; 17:1121-1124.

16. Schwarcz TH, Eton D, Ellenby MI, et al.: Hollenhorst plaques: Retinal manifestations and the role of carotid endarterectomy. J Vasc Surg 1990; 11:635-641.

17. Keith NM, Wagener HP, Barker NW: Some different types of essential hypertension: Their course and prognosis. Am J Med Sci 1939; 197:332-343.

18. Scheie HG: Evaluation of ophthalmoscopic changes of hypertension and arteriolar sclerosis. Arch Ophthalmol 1953; 49:117-138.

19. Sigelman J, Ozanics V: Retina. Duane's Biomed Found Ophthalmol 1983; 19:2-3.

20. Diabetic Retinopathy Study Research Group: Preliminary report on effects of photocoagulation therapy. Am J Ophthalmol 1976; 81:383-396.

21. Diabetic Retinopathy Study Research Group: Photocoagulation treatment of proliferative diabetic retinopathy. The second report of Diabetic Retinopathy Study findings. Ophthalmology 1978; 85:82-106.

22. The Diabetic Retinopathy Study Research Group: Four risk factors for severe visual loss in diabetic retinopathy. The third report from the Diabetic Retinopathy Study. Arch Ophthalmol 1979; 97:654-655.

23. Diabetic Retinopathy Study Research Group: Photocoagulation treatment of proliferative diabetic retinopathy: Relationship of adverse treatment effects to retinopathy severity. Diabetic Retinopathy Study Report No. 5. Dev Ophthalmol 1981; 2:248-261.

24. Diabetic Retinopathy Study Research Group: Diabetic retinopathy study. Report No. 6. Design, methods, and baseline results. Report No. 7. A modification of the Airlie House classification of diabetic retinopathy. Invest Ophthalmol Vis Sci 1981; 21:1-226.

25. Diabetic Retinopathy Study Research Group: Photocoagulation treatment of proliferative diabetic retinopathy. Clinical application of Diabetic Retinopathy Study (DRS) findings. Diabetic Retinopathy Study Report No. 8. Ophthalmology 1981; 88:583-600.

26. Ederer F, Podgor MJ: Assessing possible late treatment effects in stopping a clinical trial early: A case study. Diabetic Retinopathy Study Report No. 9. Control Clin Trials 1984; 5:373-381.

27. Rand LI, Prud'homme GJ, Ederer F, Canner PL: Factors influencing the development of visual loss in advanced diabetic retinopathy. Diabetic Retinopathy Study (DRS) Report No. 10. Invest Ophthalmol Vis Sci 1985; 26:983-991.

28. Ferris FL, Podgor MJ, David MD: Macular edema in Diabetic Retinopathy Study patients. Diabetic Retinopathy Study Report No. 12. Ophthalmology 1987; 94:754-760.

29. Kaufman SC, Ferris FL, Siegel DG, et al.: Factors associated with visual outcome after photocoagulation for diabetic retinopathy. Diabetic Retinopathy Study Report No. 13. Ophthalmology 1989; 96:746-750.

30. Diabetic Retinopathy Study Research Group: Indications for photocoagulation treatment of diabetic retinopathy. Diabetic Retinopathy Study Report No. 14. Int Ophthalmol Clin 1987; 27:239-253.

31. Early Treatment Diabetic Retinopathy Study Research Group: Photocoagulation for diabetic macular edema. Early Treatment Diabetic Retinopathy Study Report No. 1. Arch Ophthalmol 1985; 103:1796-1806.

32. Early Treatment Diabetic Retinopathy Study Research Group: Treatment techniques and clinical guidelines for photocoagulation of diabetic macular edema. Early Treatment Diabetic Retinopathy Study Report No. 2. Ophthalmology 1987; 94:761-774.

33. Early Treatment Diabetic Retinopathy Study Research Group: Techniques for scatter and local photocoagulation treatment of diabetic retinopathy. Early Treatment

of Diabetic Retinopathy Study Report No. 3. Int Ophthalmol Clin 1987; 27:254-264.

34. Early Treatment Diabetic Retinopathy Study Research Group: Photocoagulation for diabetic macular edema. Early Treatment Diabetic Retinopathy Study Report No. 4. Int Ophthalmol Clin 1987; 27:265-272.

35. Kinyoun J, Barton F, Fisher M, et al.: Detection of diabetic macular edema. Ophthalmoscopy versus photography. Early Treatment Diabetic Retinopathy Study Report No. 5. Ophthalmology 1989; 96:746-750.

36. Early Treatment Diabetic Retinopathy Study Research Group: Early Treatment Diabetic Retinopathy Study design and baseline patient characteristics. Early Treatment Diabetic Retinopathy Study Report No. 7. Ophthalmology 1991; 98:741-756.

37. Early Treatment Diabetic Retinopathy Study Research Group: Effects of aspirin treatment on diabetic retinopathy. Early Treatment Diabetic Retinopathy Study Report No. 8. Ophthalmology 1991; 98:757-765.

38. Early Treatment Diabetic Retinopathy Study Research Group: Early photocoagulation for diabetic retinopathy. Early Treatment Diabetic Retinopathy Study Report No. 9. Ophthalmology 1991; 98:766-785.

39. Early Treatment Diabetic Retinopathy Study Research Group: Grading diabetic retinopathy from stereoscopic color fundus photographs—an extension of the modified Airlie House classification. Early Treatment Diabetic Retinopathy Study Report No. 10. Ophthalmology 1991; 98:786-806

40. Early Treatment Diabetic Retinopathy Study Research Group: Classification of diabetic retinopathy from fluorescein angiograms. Early Treatment Diabetic Retinopathy Study Report No. 11. Ophthalmology 1991; 98:807-822.

41. Early Treatment Diabetic Retinopathy Study Research Group: Fundus photographic risk factors for progression of diabetic retinopathy. Early Treatment Diabetic Retinopathy Study Report No. 12. Ophthalmology 1991; 98:823-833.

42. Early Treatment Diabetic Retinopathy Study Research Group: Fluorescein angiographic risk factors for progression of diabetic retinopathy. Early Treatment Diabetic Retinopathy Study Report No. 13. Ophthalmology 1991; 98:834-840.

43. The Diabetic Retinopathy Vitrectomy Study Research Group: Two-year course of visual acuity in severe proliferative diabetic retinopathy with conventional management. Diabetic Retinopathy Vitrectomy Study (DRVS) Report No. 1. Ophthalmology 1985; 92:492-502.

44. The Diabetic Retinopathy Vitrectomy Study Research Group: Early vitrectomy for severe vitreous hemorrhage in diabetic retinopathy. Two-year results of a randomized trial. Diabetic Retinopathy Vitrectomy Study Report No. 2. Arch Ophthalmol 1985; 103:1644-1652.

45. The Diabetic Retinopathy Vitrectomy Study Research Group: Early vitrectomy for severe proliferative diabetic retinopathy in eyes with useful vision. Results of a randomized trial. Diabetic Retinopathy Vitrectomy Study Report No. 3. Ophthalmology 1988; 95:1307-1320.

46. The Diabetic Retinopathy Vitrectomy Study Research Group: Early vitrectomy for severe proliferative diabetic retinopathy in eyes with useful vision. Clinical application of results of a randomized trial. Diabetic Retinopathy Vitrectomy Study Report No. 4. Ophthalmology 1988; 95:1321-1324.

47. The Diabetic Retinopathy Vitrectomy Study Research Group: Early vitrectomy for severe vitreous hemorrhage in diabetic retinopathy. Four-year results of a randomized trial. Diabetic Retinopathy Vitrectomy Study Report No. 5. Arch Ophthalmol 1990; 108:958-964.

48. The Diabetes Control and Complications Trial Research

Group: The effect of intensive treatment of diabetes on the development and progression of long-term complications in insulin-dependent diabetes mellitus. N Engl J Med 1993; 329:977–986.

49. Diabetes Control and Complications Trial Research Group: Progression of retinopathy with intensive versus conventional treatment in the Diabetes Control and Complications Trial. Ophthalmology 1995; 102:647–661.

50. Griffith T, Semes L, Cutter G: Patient preference between yellow and clear glass condensing lenses for binocular indirect ophthalmoscopy. Clin Eye Vis Care 1989; 1:163–165.

*Chris A. Johnson, PhD*

# 10

# Perimetry and Visual Field Testing

Assessment of the peripheral visual field by perimetry and visual field testing has been a part of clinical ophthalmic diagnosis for more than 100 years. Although instrumentation and testing strategies have changed dramatically, the basic premise remains the same: Threshold sensitivity to detection of a stimulus is measured at locations throughout the peripheral visual field. Losses of sensitivity, either for the entire visual field (diffuse loss or generalized depression) or in specific regions of the visual field (localized loss), thereby *noninvasively* evaluate pathology or dysfunction of the visual pathways. The ability of perimetry and visual field testing to provide this type of useful clinical information is responsible for their long-term survival as important ophthalmic diagnostic procedures.

Perimetry and visual field testing subserve a number of important diagnostic functions. Because many eye diseases, such as glaucoma, have their initial effects on peripheral vision, perimetry is important in the early detection of pathological ocular conditions. Perimetry is the only standard clinical diagnostic test that evaluates the status of visual function for locations outside the foveal and macular regions. The spatial pattern of visual field deficits and comparison of patterns of visual field loss between the two eyes also provide valuable differential diagnostic information. Not only can this information be helpful in defining the locus of involvement along the visual pathways from the retina to the primary visual cortex, but it can also assist in identifying the specific type of disease entity that is present. In addition, perimetry and visual field testing are important for monitoring the status of visual function over time. In glaucoma, monitoring a patient's visual field is one of the most important factors in determining the efficacy of therapeutic management. There are many other neuro-ophthalmologic and retinal diseases in which monitoring the visual field is critical for determining whether a condition is stable or progressive.

Perhaps the most important role subserved by perimetry and visual field testing is their ability to reveal visual loss that may not be consciously apparent to the patient. Changes in foveal visual function are usually quite noticeable, and patients typically have a specific set of complaints about their vision. Peripheral vision loss, on the other hand, can often go unnoticed. This is especially true if the peripheral visual field loss is gradual and is primarily affecting only one eye, which is common in the early stages of glaucoma and other ocular diseases. In a study involving visual field screening of 10,000 California drivers' license applicants, only a small proportion (approximately 2 to 3%) had visual field loss, but

nearly 60% of those individuals with peripheral visual field loss were not aware that they had any problem with their vision.[1] A variety of causes of visual field loss were found, but the majority of cases had glaucoma, with various types of retinal disorders as the next most common cause. Paradoxically, even though the patient may be unaware of peripheral visual field loss, it can significantly impair performance of daily activities such as driving[1-4] and orientation and mobility.[5] Perimetry and visual field testing are therefore important to identify visual abnormalities that might not otherwise be detected by other parts of a standard eye examination or a careful case history.

Practically, it is not feasible to perform a thorough quantitative visual field examination on all patients. A quick confrontation visual field evaluation can usually be performed as part of a standard eye examination. Depending on the particular procedure, this detects moderate to advanced visual field losses, but it does not identify early visual field deficits. Quantitative screening procedures using either a manual or an automated perimeter can produce excellent detection of early visual field deficits using a strategy requiring only a few minutes, *provided that the test procedure is one that has been clinically validated.* Do not rely on the device manufacturer's recommendations unless they are supported by published clinical results. Quantitative threshold perimetry is the most time-consuming test procedure, requiring 15 to 20 minutes per eye, but it yields the best results. Again, only those procedures and devices that have published clinical validation studies should be used.

It is especially important periodically to examine the visual field in those patients who are at greater risk of having or developing visual field loss with quantitative screening or threshold methods. This includes (1) patients over the age of 60 because visual disorders are approximately five times more prevalent in the population over 60 and become even more common with advancing age beyond 60; (2) African-Americans over the age of 40 because glaucoma is more prevalent in African-Americans and tends to occur at an earlier age in these individuals than for other ethnic groups; (3) patients with high myopia, elevated intraocular pressure, diabetes or other vascular disease, family history of glaucoma or other eye disease, or any other "risk factors" for the development of ocular or neurological disorders; (4) patients with symptoms, complaints, results from ophthalmoscopy or other portions of their ocular examination that would suggest the presence of visual field loss; and (5) patients with significant problems involving orientation and mobility, balance, driving, night vision, and related everyday activities.

Recently, the development of automated procedures for visual field testing has increased the interest in and use of visual field test procedures. As a consequence, automated perimetry is now considered to be the "gold standard" for visual field testing. This chapter therefore emphasizes automated techniques and their methods of data representation. Automated perimetry has unquestionably had a dramatic impact on improving the quality of care for patients with ocular disorders. Automatic calibration of instruments, standardized test procedures, high sensitivity and specificity, reliability checks ("catch trials"), and quantitative statistical analysis procedures are some of the advantages of automated perimetry. However, there are also disadvantages, such as prolonged test time, increased cognitive demands, fatigue, and lack of flexibility for evaluating challenging patient populations. It should be strongly emphasized that no single method of visual field testing is best for all clinical circumstances.

Although automated perimetry is currently the most popular form of visual field testing, it is but one of many tools that the clinician can use to evaluate peripheral visual function. Various forms of visual field testing should be regarded as complementary techniques whose utility and appropriateness are determined by the clinical circumstances, the patient's abilities and willingness to cooperate, and the question that is being addressed. No single method of data representation, analysis procedure, visual field index, or other method of evaluating visual field data provides all the essential clinical visual field information. It is important to consider all the information available, including reliability characteristics, and the most important factor of all—the appropriate subjective clinical interpretation of the visual field results.

Finally, although the test may be automated, the patient is not. It is unreasonable to begin a visual field test, leave patients alone in a dark room for 15 minutes or more, and expect them to remain alert, energetic, attentive, interested, and maintaining proper ocular alignment and fixation throughout the test procedure. Some patients require periodic rest breaks, encouragement, and personal contact in order for visual field examinations to be performed in a reliable manner. In addition, it is incumbent on the examiner to ensure that proper test conditions, refractive characteristics, and other factors have been properly established prior to initiating the examination. When these factors are accounted for, perimetry can be a powerful clinical diagnostic tool. In addition to the operations manuals provided by automated perimetry manufacturers, a variety of sources are available to assist in proper testing of the visual field.[6-16]

This chapter provides a brief overview of the psychophysical basis for perimetry and visual field testing, the different types of perimetry and how they are performed, the interpretation of visual field information, and new perimetric tests that have recently been developed. It is not intended to be a comprehensive treatment of any of these topics but rather an introduction to visual fields and a synopsis of some of the main issues regarding perimetric testing and interpretation of visual field information. For a more detailed discussion of these issues, the reader is directed to several excellent sources.[6-18]

# The Psychophysical Basis of Perimetry and Visual Field Testing

The predominant psychophysical basis for perimetry and visual field testing is the increment or differential light threshold, which refers to the minimum amount of light that must be added to a stimulus ($\Delta L$) to make it just detectable on a uniform background (L). In darkness or for low background luminances, the amount of light needed to detect a stimulus is not influenced by the background luminance level, that is, $\Delta L = C$ (a constant). At higher background luminances, the increment or differential light threshold ($\Delta L$) increases in direct proportion to the background luminance; that is, a doubling of the background luminance requires a doubling of the stimulus luminance in order for it to be detected. This relationship, $\Delta L/L = C$, is known as Weber's Law or the Weber fraction in honor of the German scientist who initially described it.[19] Weber's Law holds over a large range of background luminance levels.

The standard background luminance used by most perimetric devices is 31.5 apostilbs (asb), or 10 cd/m². This luminance level is within the range of background luminance levels for which Weber's Law is valid. There are several advantages to the use of this background luminance level. First, this background level is close to the ambient lighting conditions found in offices and waiting rooms, and therefore a minimal amount of adaptation time is necessary. Usually the 1 to 2 minutes required to align the eye for testing is sufficient adaptation time. Second, the background luminance is one that is comfortable (not too bright or too dim) for nearly all patients. Third, patients demonstrate the least variability in responses at this adaptation level. The final and most important advantage of this background luminance level is that factors that influence the amount of light reaching the retina (e.g., changes in pupil size and absorption of light by the ocular media) affect the background and stimulus luminance equally. Thus, for the range of background luminances over which Weber's Law pertains, these changes in retinal illumination do not affect the increment threshold measure.

For a normal visual field, the increment threshold varies as a function of visual field location. With the 31.5 asb background luminance, the fovea has the highest sensitivity, that is, it is able to detect the dimmest and/or smallest targets. Increment threshold sensitivity drops somewhat rapidly between the fovea and 3° eccentricity and then decreases gradually out to 30° eccentricity. Beyond 30° eccentricity, the decrease in sensitivity again drops off more rapidly, and beyond 50° the slope of visual field sensitivity is very steep. A three-dimensional representation of sensitivity for a normal visual field of a left eye is shown in Figure 10-1. The temporal visual field is therefore to the left of the foveal peak, and the nasal visual field is to the right of the foveal peak. It is important to keep in mind that visual field coordinates are the opposite of retinal coordinates: for example, stimuli in the superior visual field project to the inferior retina, and stimuli in the temporal visual field project to the nasal retina.

In addition to the eccentricity-dependent changes in the slope of the visual field profile, note that the temporal visual field extends farther than the nasal visual field. Similarly, the inferior visual field extends farther than the superior visual field. The location of the blind spot (corresponding to the optic nerve head where the nerve fibers exit the eye) is approximately 15° temporal to the foveal peak and is indicated by the darkened oval area. This characteristic shape of the visual field sensitivity profile has often been referred to as the "hill of vision" or the "island of vision in a sea of blindness."

A number of stimulus factors affect the differential sensitivity to light, such as background luminance,[11, 13, 15, 17, 18, 20, 21] stimulus size,[10, 11, 13, 15, 17, 18, 20-23] stimulus duration,[11, 13, 15, 17, 18, 24] chromaticity,[8, 11, 15, 17, 18, 25-29] and other test parameters.[11, 12, 17, 18] Of these test attributes, stimulus size is the most typically adjusted or varied during perimetric testing. Not only does a change in stimulus size affect the overall sensitivity to light, but the slope of the sensitivity profile is also changed. Small targets produce steeper sensitivity profiles, and larger targets result in a flatter sensitivity profile, especially for the central 30 to 40° eccentricity.

Certain patient characteristics also influence the increment or differential light threshold. Pupil size,[30-32] refractive error,[33, 34] media opacities (cataract, corneal anomalies),[35-40] droopy eyelids or heavy brows,[41, 42] trial lens rim artifacts,[43] and related factors[44] can affect visual field sensitivity characteristics. Examples of the type of visual field characteristics produced by some of these conditions are presented in the section entitled Pre-retinal Conditions.

In addition to the influences mentioned above, a variety of cognitive and higher order functions in patients undergoing visual field testing can influence sensitivity to light. Attention and learning effects can alter increment threshold sensitivity.[45-48] Several studies have also demonstrated that fatigue can reduce visual field sensitivity, particularly after the test procedure has gone beyond 5 to 7 minutes.[49-52] Patients with visual field loss typically demonstrate greater fatigue

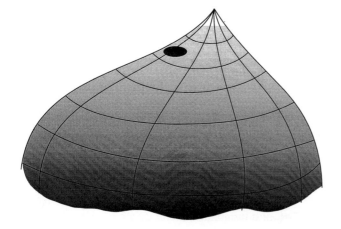

**FIGURE 10–1** Three-dimensional representation of visual sensitivity for a normal visual field, left eye.

effects than those with normal visual fields. The stability of prolonged steady fixation can also be a factor in the sensitivity and reliability of visual field threshold measurements.[53-55]

# Types of Perimetry and Visual Field Testing

Because perimetry and visual field testing have a history that dates back more than 100 years, a number of methods and test strategies have been developed over that time. The procedures in use today have been derived from a variety of development, validation, modification, and refinement efforts. This section presents a brief overview of the various types of perimetry and test strategies used to test the visual field, although the details of such procedures require more than just a portion of a chapter to appropriately cover the material. A more thorough discussion of perimetric methods is presented in other publications.[6-9, 17, 56]

Various forms of perimetry and visual field testing can be classified or differentiated in several ways. One means of distinguishing among visual field test procedures is the type of information provided. Screening procedures are primarily concerned with determining whether the visual field is normal or abnormal (or, for more elaborate procedures, whether abnormal visual fields are consistent with glaucoma or other ocular disorders). These techniques provide limited information about visual field status, but they can be performed very efficiently. Confrontation visual field examinations are examples of very rapid but limited visual field assessments. Quantitative visual field assessment procedures not only are concerned with whether the visual field is normal or abnormal but also are designed to provide information about sensitivity to light at numerous visual field locations. Thus, information from quantitative test procedures can provide detailed information concerning the pattern of loss for differential diagnosis, can characterize the amount of loss for evaluating severity, and can be monitored over time to look for changes. Several "hybrid" procedures have also been introduced that provide semiquantitative visual field information. The primary purpose of these procedures is to determine whether various portions of the visual field are normal or abnormal. However, in abnormal regions, additional testing is performed to ascertain whether the deficit is relative (mild to moderate loss) or absolute (severe loss), thereby providing semiquantitative visual field information.

Another means of classifying visual field tests is on the basis of their stimulus properties. Basically, there are three major forms of visual field testing: kinetic perimetry, static perimetry, and suprathreshold static perimetry. Kinetic visual field testing is most commonly performed by a highly trained and skilled perimetrist using a Goldmann perimeter, consisting of a white hemispherical bowl of uniform luminance (31.5 asb) onto which a small bright stimulus is projected. An eye patch is used to occlude the non-tested eye, while the eye to be tested is centered within the hemispherical bowl. The patient fixates a small target in the center of the bowl, and the perimetrist monitors eye position by means of a telescope. A stimulus of particular size and luminance is projected onto the bowl, and the target is moved from the far periphery toward fixation at a constant rate of speed, typically 4 to 5° per second.[57] Patients are instructed to press a response button when they first detect the stimulus. The location of target detection is noted on a chart, and the process is repeated for different meridians around the visual field, as shown in Figure 10-2. This yields an isopter (region of equal sensitivity).

Typically a number of isopters are produced by changing the size and intensity of the target to vary its detectability. In addition, scotomas, or areas of non-seeing, to particular stimuli are also plotted. This produces a two-dimensional representation of the hill of vision that is basically a topographical contour map of the eye's sensitivity to light. An example of this type of visual field representation is shown in the lower portion of Figure 10-3, in relation to the three-dimensional

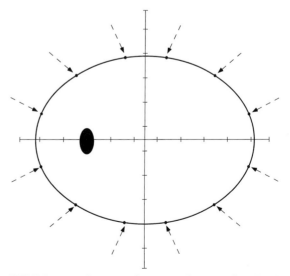

**FIGURE 10–2** Plotting of a single isopter of a visual field.

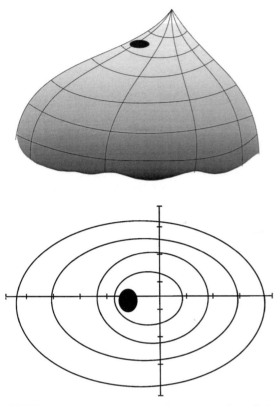

**FIGURE 10–3** Three-dimensional representation of visual sensitivity for a normal visual field, left eye *(top)* and two-dimensional representation of the "hill of vision" for the same eye *(bottom).*

visual field sensitivity surface plot shown in the top part of Figure 10-3. Kinetic perimetry is a highly acquired skill (and an art) that has many complexities in terms of mapping strategies, proper technique, and related factors. An outstanding, thorough description of the techniques used for kinetic perimetry may be found in Anderson's perimetry book.[6]

Static perimetry uses a stationary target, the luminance of which is adjusted to vary its visibility. Increment threshold measurements are obtained at a variety of visual field locations that are typically arranged in a grid pattern or along meridians. The representation of visual field sensitivity for grid patterns is typically a grey scale representation, as shown in the lower portion of Figure 10-4 in relation to the three-dimensional visual field sensitivity surface plot in the upper portion of Figure 10-4. Areas of high sensitivity near the peak of the hill of vision are denoted by lighter shading, and areas of low sensitivity are indicated by dark shading. Static perimetric determinations along meridians are usually represented by a sensitivity profile plot, as shown in the lower portion of Figure 10-5 in relation to

the three-dimensional visual field sensitivity surface plot in the upper part of Figure 10-5.

Both static and kinetic perimetry are quantitative procedures that require a considerable amount of testing time. Suprathreshold static perimetry is a procedure that is faster than quantitative techniques and is typically used for screening purposes. There are a large number of variations in test procedures, strategies, and theoretical foundations for suprathreshold static perimetry.[8, 56] However, the basic premise is that stimuli that can be readily detected by patients with normal peripheral vision are presented at selected locations throughout the visual field. Specific locations are usually selected to evaluate areas that are frequently affected by glaucoma and other ocular or neurological disorders that damage the visual pathways. Locations at which the target is seen are denoted by one symbol and locations where the target is not seen are denoted by another. In some instances, two target intensities are presented to each location. If neither target is seen, the deficit is recorded as absolute. If both targets are seen, the location is denoted as normal, and if the more intense target

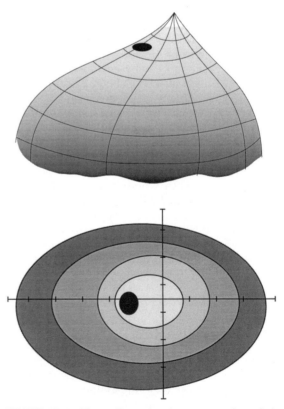

**FIGURE 10–4** Three-dimensional representation of visual sensitivity for a normal visual field, left eye *(top)* and two-dimensional representation of the "hill of vision" for the same eye as a grey scale *(bottom).*

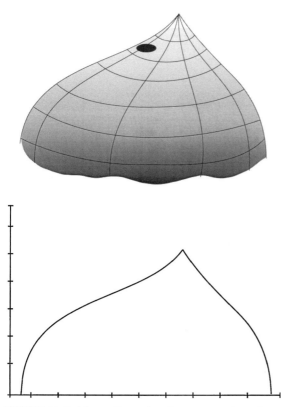

**FIGURE 10–5** Three-dimensional representation of visual sensitivity for a normal visual field, left eye *(top)* and two-dimensional sensitivity profile plot from static perimetry *(bottom)*.

ses, and makes it possible to have standardized protocols for multicenter clinical trials using perimetry. Secondly, the test procedures can be administered by personnel with more limited technical skills and training in perimetry and visual field testing. A third advantage is that statistical analyses and comparisons can be conducted automatically. Disadvantages of automated perimetry include its greater cognitive and attentional demands on the part of the patient and its diminished flexibility and interactive capabilities. The most common form of automated visual field testing is static perimetry, using a staircase threshold determination strategy. A number of suprathreshold static test procedures are also available with automated perimetry. Although several kinetic visual field test procedures have been developed for automated perimetry,[58-61] they have not been very successful. Manual visual field testing can be performed with kinetic, static, or suprathreshold static test strategies. Kinetic perimetry, using a Goldmann-type projection perimeter or a tangent screen, is the most common form of manual perimetry. Suprathreshold static procedures are also quite common. The widespread popularity and efficiency of automated static perimetry have now made the use of manual procedures for performing static threshold perimetry obsolete.

## Interpretation of Visual Field Information

A large amount of visual field information is derived from perimetric testing, especially for automated perimetry. Test conditions and stimulus parameters employed, indicators of patient reliability and cooperation, physiological factors (e.g., pupil size, refractive state, visual acuity), summary statistics and visual field indices, and other items are presented in conjunction with sensitivity values for various locations in the patient's visual field. Visual field sensitivity can also be represented in many different forms (e.g., numerical values, deviations from normal, grey scale representations, probability plots). The following discussion presents a brief overview of the various types of information provided on the final hard copy output of visual field results. Because of its current popularity, this discussion and the examples are directed toward automated static perimetry results.

It should be emphasized that no single type of data representation or item of visual field information provides a sufficient or complete description of visual field properties. All of the available information from the visual field output needs to

is seen but the lower intensity target is not, the deficit is denoted as relative loss.

A number of different methods of representing visual field data from suprathreshold static perimetry are available, although all of them generally adhere to the above-mentioned principles. An example of this type of data representation is presented in Figure 10–6. In this example, targets that were seen are denoted by open circles, whereas locations at which targets were not seen are represented by filled squares.

A third method of classifying visual field tests is manual procedures, usually conducted by a skilled perimetrist, versus automated perimetry. Today, the majority of visual field examinations use automated test procedures. Several distinct advantages are associated with the use of automated perimetry. First, automated perimetry provides a standardized diagnostic test procedure. This makes it possible to have the same procedures used worldwide, allows practitioners to compare their test results with those obtained at different sites, makes it possible to use the same normal population database for assessment of a patient's results and to perform statistical analy-

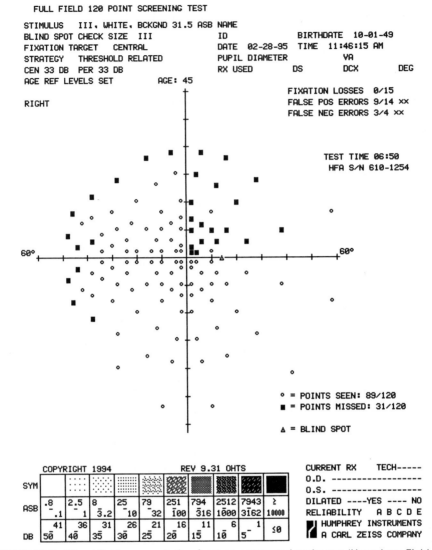

**FIGURE 10-6** Visual field representation from an automated perimeter (Humphrey Field Analyzer).

be evaluated in order to have a proper interpretation of the test results. Just as the findings from individual components of a standard eye examination need to be combined to render an appropriate clinical impression and diagnosis, all the individual components of perimetric results must be considered to properly interpret visual field findings. No single element of the visual field results provides all of the salient information in all cases. A thorough description of the information contained on the visual field printout for the Humphrey Field Analyzer is available from literature sources.[7, 62]

## ANCILLARY INFORMATION

Several important pieces of information that should be checked on each visual field examination are the patient's pupil size during testing, the refractive correction used for visual field testing (and whether the patient was cyclopleged and/or dilated for the test procedure), and the patient's visual acuity. Small pupils (less than 2 mm in diameter) can produce spurious test results, especially in older individuals who may have early crystalline lens changes. If pupil size is less than 2 mm, the patient's pupil should be dilated to minimize the possibility of a small pupil as a confounding variable for visual field interpretation. Proper near refractive corrections that are appropriate for the test distance of the perimeter bowl and the patient's age must be used to minimize the likelihood of refraction scotomas and sensitivity reductions due to blur. In addition, high refractive corrections (greater than ±6.00 D spherical equivalent) can sometimes produce trial lens rim artifacts. When a patient's spherical equivalent correction for perimetric testing exceeds $\pm 6.00$ D, it is advisable to use a soft contact lens correction that is appropriate for the test distance to avoid lens rim artifacts. The patient's visual acuity can also be useful information when assessing generalized visual field sensitivity loss and the potential causes of the loss.

## RELIABILITY INDICES

Visual field testing, as with all psychophysical test procedures, is based on subjective responses on the part of the patient. The quality of information obtained from perimetry and visual field testing thus depends on the patient's cooperation, willingness, and ability to respond in a reliable fashion and to maintain a consistent response criterion. Psychophysical test procedures that are criterion-free and minimize bias are generally too time-consuming to be used for clinical visual field testing. Thus, alternative methods must be used to assess the degree of reliability and consistency exhibited by the patient during perimetry and visual field testing. It is important to have some type of evaluation of patient reliability and consistency in order to be able to properly determine the significance of visual field information.

With manual perimetry, it is possible to directly monitor the patient's fixation behavior by means of a telescope viewer that can be used to observe the patient's eye during testing. The use of "catch" trials can be employed to determine the patient's reliability in properly responding to stimuli. False-positive errors (responses when no stimulus is presented) and false-negative errors (failure to respond to a stimulus presented in a region previously determined to be able to detect equal or less detectable targets) can be monitored throughout the test procedure.

Automated test procedures not only have the capability of monitoring false-positive errors, false-negative errors, and fixation behavior, but also can obtain an assessment of response fluctuation by testing a sample of visual field locations twice. Also, indirect indicators of fixation accuracy (e.g., whether or not a patient responds to a target presented to the physiological blind spot) can be monitored as well. An additional advantage of automated test procedures is that these reliability indices (false positives, false negatives, fixation losses and short-term fluctuation) can be immediately compared with the properties exhibited by age-matched normal control subjects and thereby provide an assessment as to whether the patient's reliability parameters are within normal population characteristics.[63]

It should be cautioned, however, that some of the reliability indices for automated perimetry are not always accurate indicators of a patient's performance characteristics. For example, false-negative rates are correlated with visual field deficits; that is, an increase of false-negative responses is seen as visual field losses become greater.[64] Thus, high false-negative rates may be more indicative of disease severity than unreliable patient response characteristics. Excessive fixation losses can be due to factors such as mislocalization of the blind spot during the initial phases of testing, misalignment of the patient midway through testing, or inattention on the part of the technician administering the visual field examination. In the Optic Neuritis Treatment Trial (ONTT), it was found that technician quality control score (based on adherence to the testing protocol and proper administration of the test) and the number of days since the last clinical center site visit were two of the strongest predictors of excessive fixation losses.[65] These two factors are related to the degree of care and attention demonstrated by the technician administering the test rather than any factors related to the patient. The ONTT results are encouraging because it was found that when a standardized protocol and rigorous quality control and training procedures were used, visual field reliability was excellent. Only 6 of 458 patients in the ONTT study were excluded on the basis of unreliable visual field results at the eligibility examination.[16]

## VISUAL FIELD INDICES

Another distinct advantage afforded by automated perimeters such as the Humphrey Field Analyzer and the Octopus is the ability to provide summary statistics pertaining to visual field information, known as visual field indices.[6, 7] Mean deviation (MD) on the Humphrey Field Analyzer and mean defect (MD) on the Octopus perimeters refer to the average deviation of sensitivity at each test location from age-adjusted normal population values. It is intended to provide an indication of the degree of generalized or widespread loss present in the visual field.

Pattern standard deviation (PSD) on the Humphrey Field Analyzer and loss variance (LV) on the Octopus perimeters present a summary measure of the average deviation of individual visual field sensitivity values from the normal slope of the visual field after correcting for any overall sensitivity differences, that is, MD. It is an index of the degree of irregularity of visual field sensitivity about the normal slope and is therefore intended to be an indication of the amount of localized visual field loss, because scotomas produce significant departures from the normal slope of the visual field with eccentricity. Corrected pattern standard deviation (CPSD) and corrected loss variance (CLV) take into account the patient's short-term fluctuation (STF), which is derived from testing a sample of 10 locations twice to determine the average deviation of repeated measures. This correction minimizes the influence of the patient's variability on the local deviation measures.

Another analysis procedure that is available for the Humphrey Field Analyzer is the glaucoma hemifield test (GHT).[66] This analysis procedure is specifically designed to detect glaucomatous visual field loss. The procedure evaluates the sensitivity characteristics of five clusters of points above and below the horizontal midline that resemble nerve fiber bundle patterns, because glaucomatous visual field deficits typically adhere to the nerve fiber bundle patterns. The sensitivity values for these clusters above and below the horizontal midline are compared with those of age-adjusted normal population values because the amount of glaucomatous visual field loss is usually asymmetrical about the horizontal midline. The analysis is identified as abnormal if one or more of the five regions demonstrate asymmetries across the horizontal midline that are beyond the 1% probability level for normal population values, and as borderline if asymmetries are within the 1% probability level for all five regions but are beyond the 3% probability level for one or more regions. Other types of analysis procedures using clusters of abnormal visual field locations and related criteria have been developed, but they are not automatically calculated by the Humphrey Field Analyzer or the Octopus perimeters.

## PROBABILITY PLOTS

One of the distinct advantages of automated static perimetry using projection devices such as the Humphrey Field Analyzer or the Octopus is that a patient's test results are compared with age-matched normal population values. Thus, it is possible to determine the amount of deviation from normal population sensitivity values on a point-by-point basis for all visual field locations tested. A useful means of expressing this information is probability plots. The Humphrey Field Analyzer has two very helpful methods of presenting this type of information. One of them is

the total deviation plot, and the other is the pattern deviation plot. For the total deviation plot, each visual field location has one of a group of different symbols indicating whether the sensitivity is within age-adjusted normal limits or is below the 5%, 2%, 1%, or 0.5% normal limits, respectively. This provides an immediate graphical representation of the locations that are abnormal and the degree to which they vary from normal levels.

The pattern deviation plot is similar, except that the determinations are performed after the average or overall sensitivity loss has been subtracted, thereby revealing the locations with localized deviations from normal sensitivity values. The value of these representations is twofold. First, they provide an immediate indication of the locations with sensitivity loss. Second, the comparison of the total and pattern deviation plots characterizes the degree to which the loss is diffuse/widespread or localized. If the deficit is predominantly localized, the total and pattern deviation plots look virtually identical, as illustrated in the top portion of Figure 10–7. If the loss is predominantly widespread, the abnormal locations appear on the total deviation plot, but all or most of these locations are within normal limits on the pattern deviation plot. An example of this is shown in the lower portion of Figure 10–7. The degree of similarity between the total and pattern deviation plots thus gives an indication of the proportions of widespread and localized loss.

## GRAPHICAL REPRESENTATION OF VISUAL FIELD DATA

In most instances, the numerical representation of visual field information, either by means of summary values such as visual field indices or by sensitivity values for individual visual field locations, is difficult to interpret. A graphical representation of visual field data makes it easier to evaluate, particularly for detecting specific patterns of visual field loss or for assessing progression or visual field changes over time. There are three primary methods of graphically representing visual field data: isopter/scotoma plots, profile plots, and grey scale plots, as illustrated in Figures 10–2 through 10–4. The graphical representation of visual field information is extremely important for the purposes of interpretation and diagnosis. The clinician's qualitative judgment of visual field patterns and changes is still the most critical aspect of visual field interpretation, in spite of the benefits afforded by quantitative statistical analyses and comparisons.

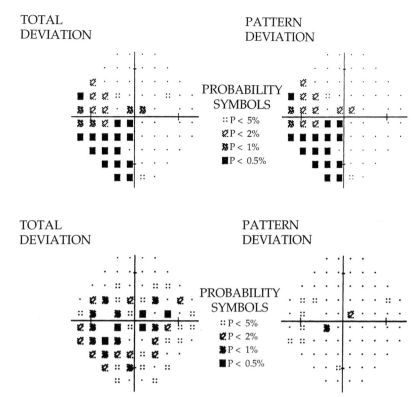

TOTAL
DEVIATION

PATTERN
DEVIATION

PROBABILITY
SYMBOLS

:: P < 5%
🌣 P < 2%
🌑 P < 1%
■ P < 0.5%

TOTAL
DEVIATION

PATTERN
DEVIATION

PROBABILITY
SYMBOLS

:: P < 5%
🌣 P < 2%
🌑 P < 1%
■ P < 0.5%

**FIGURE 10–7** The Humphrey Field Analyzer's total deviation and pattern deviation plots for localized loss of sensitivity *(top)* and diffuse loss of sensitivity *(bottom).*

## PRE-RETINAL CONDITIONS

Figure 10–8 presents examples of several pre-retinal factors that affect visual field sensitivity. The top set of figures *(A)* shows the effects of pupil size on visual field sensitivity. The left graph presents the results obtained for a patient with a 1-mm pupil, and the right graph presents the results for the same patient with a 3-mm pupil. Note the general improvement in sensitivity with the larger pupil size. The next set of visual fields *(B)* demonstrates the effects of superior visual field constriction produced by ptosis (left graph) and the subsequent improvement in the superior visual field after taping the upper lid (right graph). Droopy lids and prominent brows are common in elderly patients and can be problematic in evaluating visual fields for early glaucomatous losses. When in doubt, it is best to tape up the eyelid using easily removable surgical tape.

The third set of visual fields *(C)* shows the effects of 2.00 D of spherical refractive error due to the use of an improper lens correction (left) and the subsequent use of a proper refractive correction (right) on visual field sensitivity. The primary effects of refractive error on visual field sensitivity consist of a generalized reduction in sensitivity, as indicated by the slightly darker grey scale representation on the left compared with

the right graph. The bottom visual field examples *(D)* show a visual field depression produced by a cataract (left graph) and an example of a trial lens rim artifact produced by obstruction of a portion of the visual field by the lens holder (right graph). In general, pre-retinal factors that influence the visual field produce artifactual test results that complicate the proper diagnosis of visual field deficits produced by other ocular conditions. Other test procedures, such as visual acuity, contrast sensitivity, and glare disability, are more useful methods for monitoring cataract, corneal disorders, and other pre-retinal abnormalities.

## COMMON RETINAL DISORDERS

Figure 10–9 presents examples of visual field deficits produced by several common retinal disorders. The upper *(A)* left figure shows an example of visual fields in diabetic retinopathy. Typically, the initial visual field deficits in diabetic retinopathy occur in the midperiphery at about 25 to 30° eccentricity in a patchy fashion. The upper *(A)* right figure presents an example of age-related macular degeneration, which has a prominent area of central visual loss. The middle *(B)* graph on the left shows an example of visual field loss in retinitis pigmentosa, which depicts

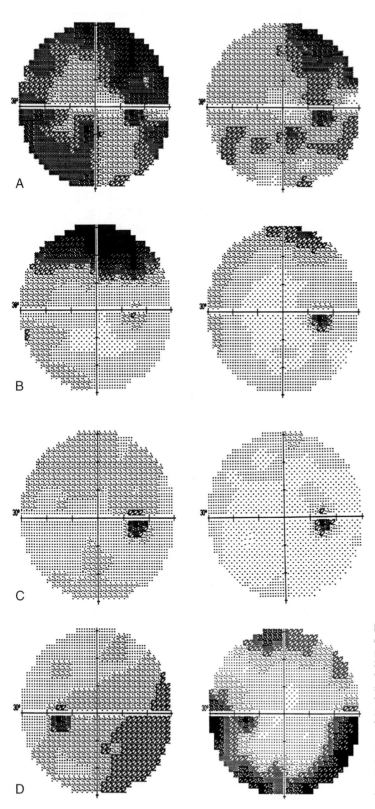

**FIGURE 10–8** Visual fields showing the effects of preretinal factors. *A,* Effects of pupil size with a 1-mm pupil *(left)* and a 3-mm pupil *(right). B,* Effects of superior visual field constriction produced by ptosis *(left)* and improvement produced by taping the upper lid *(right). C,* Effects of 2.00 D of spherical refractive error due to the use of an improper lens correction *(left)* and the proper refractive correction *(right). D,* Effects of a cataract producing a visual field depression *(left)* and an example of a trial lens rim artifact produced by obstruction of a portion of the visual field by the lens holder *(right).*

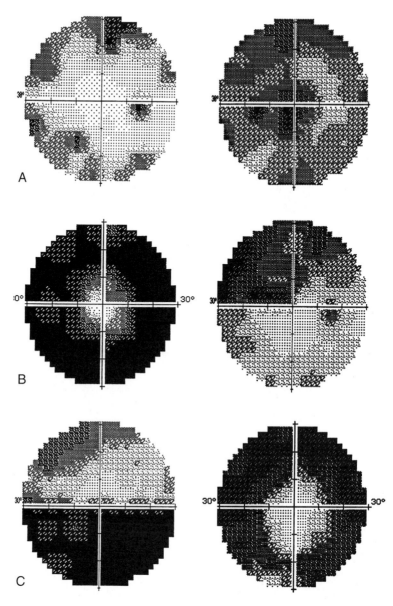

**FIGURE 10–9** Visual fields showing the effects of retinal disorders. *A,* Diabetic retinopathy *(left)* and macular degeneration *(right). B,* Retinitis pigmentosa *(left)* and branch retinal artery occlusion *(right). C,* Central retinal vein occlusion *(left)* and retinal cone dystrophy *(right).*

the classic "ring" scotoma. The middle right figure shows an example of a visual field deficit produced by a branch artery occlusion, which corresponds to the arcing pattern of the vascular arcade branching out from the optic disc. The lower *(C)* left graph shows an example of an inferior altitudinal visual field deficit produced by a central retinal vein occlusion, and the lower *(C)* right graph shows visual field loss produced by a retinal cone dystrophy.

In general, only a few retinal disorders produce characteristic patterns of visual field loss. The ring scotoma in retinitis pigmentosa and the deficit shown for a branch artery occlusion corresponding to the vascular arcade are examples of distinct patterns. Diseases that affect the macular region produce central scotomas, but their size and shape vary considerably from one patient to another. A common characteristic of visual field deficits produced by retinal disorders is that the loss is quite irregular and does not correspond to the distinct anatomically based patterns found for other portions of the visual pathway.

## GLAUCOMA

Examples of typical glaucomatous visual field deficits are presented in Figure 10-10. The top graphs *(A)* show examples of early glaucomatous visual field loss in the form of an inferior (left

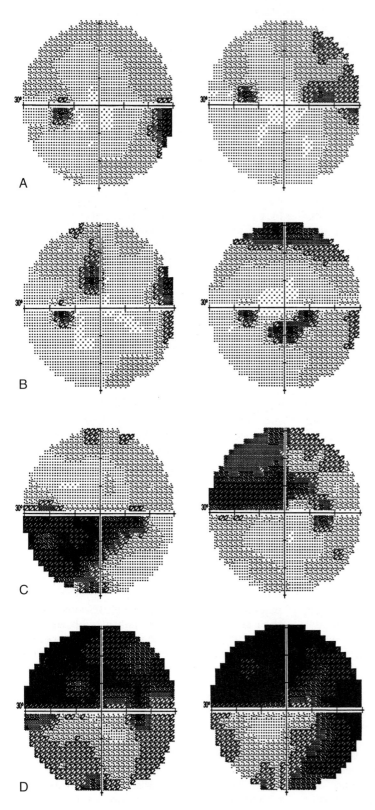

A

B

C

D

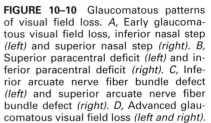

**FIGURE 10–10** Glaucomatous patterns of visual field loss. *A,* Early glaucomatous visual field loss, inferior nasal step *(left)* and superior nasal step *(right). B,* Superior paracentral deficit *(left)* and inferior paracentral deficit *(right). C,* Inferior arcuate nerve fiber bundle defect *(left)* and superior arcuate nerve fiber bundle defect *(right). D,* Advanced glaucomatous visual field loss *(left and right).*

graph) and a superior (right graph) nasal step. The next graphs (*B*) show an example of a superior (left graph) and an inferior (right graph) paracentral deficit, representing partial nerve fiber bundle losses. More extensive forms of glaucomatous visual field loss are shown in the next set of graphs (*C*). The left graph shows an inferior arcuate nerve fiber bundle defect, whereas the right graph depicts a superior arcuate nerve fiber bundle defect. The bottom graphs (*D*) depict more advanced forms of glaucomatous visual field loss, with extensive losses for both the superior and inferior arcuate nerve fiber bundle regions.

Several features present in the examples shown in Figure 10-10 are typical of glaucomatous patterns of visual field loss. First, note that in most instances, the visual field loss "respects" the horizontal meridian in the nasal visual field; that is, an abrupt transition in sensitivity occurs along the horizontal midline. For early deficits, the sensitivity loss is often clustered near the horizontal meridian and thus has the appearance of a stairstep. Because of this, the deficit is often referred to as a nasal step. In addition, glaucomatous visual field deficits are most commonly found in the region between 10 and 30° from fixation, particularly for early to moderate visual field loss. Another pattern of visual field loss that is characteristic of glaucoma is the arcuate nerve fiber bundle defect. This type of deficit "fans out" in an expanding arc from the blind spot toward the nasal horizontal midline in the region between 10 and 30° eccentricity. It basically reflects the pattern of the arcuate nerve fiber bundles as they enter the superior and inferior regions of the optic nerve head and indicates partial or complete damage to nerve fibers at the optic nerve head.

Note also that for both partial and complete arcuate nerve fiber bundle defects, the deficit is typically longer (along the arc) than it is wide and the deficit "points" to the blind spot. These patterns of visual field loss thus reflect the underlying glaucomatous pathophysiology occurring at the optic nerve head. Another characteristic of glaucomatous visual field defects is that they are usually asymmetrical both across the horizontal midline in the same eye and between the two eyes. Typically, glaucomatous visual field loss is more advanced in one eye than the other, or it is present in one eye and the visual field of the other is normal.

In the vast majority of cases, these patterns of visual field loss are indicative of glaucoma. Several other conditions (e.g., optic nerve drusen, optic neuritis, and ischemic optic neuropathy) can sometimes produce these types of deficits.

In most of these instances, the locus of involvement is still the optic nerve head.

## OTHER OPTIC NEUROPATHIES

Examples of the types of visual field deficits that are encountered with optic neuritis are presented in Figure 10-11. It can be readily observed that a wide variety of patterns of visual field loss can be present for optic neuritis. Some of this variation is related to exactly when during the acute phase of an optic neuritis attack the visual field examination is performed. Soon after the initial optic neuritis attack, severe visual field loss in the form of a dense central scotoma is frequently observed. This can produce an absolute sensitivity loss for the entire central 30° visual field. The upper (*A*) left and right graphs present examples of central scotomas of moderate severity associated with optic neuritis. The next set of visual fields (*B*) in optic neuritis depict a nasal step (left graph) and a centrocecal deficit (right graph). A centrocecal defect includes the blind spot, the macular region, and the area of visual field between the blind spot and fixation. It is often characterized by a candle-flame shaped pattern of visual field loss that encompasses the macular region, the blind spot, and the area between them. This pattern corresponds to the papillomacular bundle, a group of nerve fibers subserving the macular region and adjoining areas toward the optic nerve head.

The visual field deficit shown on the left portion of Figure 10-11*C* depicts visual field loss around the 30° peripheral rim of the central visual field. This pattern of loss is often encountered at various stages of recovery in optic neuritis. Another pattern of visual field loss that is frequently encountered in optic neuritis is an altitudinal loss of the superior or inferior hemifield, as shown in Figure 10-11*C* on the right. An altitudinal visual field deficit is differentiated from an arcuate defect in that it respects the horizontal meridian across the entire central visual field, cutting across the foveal region. Arcuate nerve fiber bundle defects resembling typical glaucomatous deficits can also sometimes be observed in optic neuritis. Examples of these deficits have been shown for glaucoma. The lower left graph of Figure 10-11*D* shows an example of a superior arcuate type deficit in optic neuritis, and the lower (*D*) right graph shows an example of a double arcuate type of defect.

Examples of visual field deficits for several other optic neuropathies are presented in Figure 10-12. The two top graphs (*A*) show an example of a superior (left) and an inferior (right) altitudi-

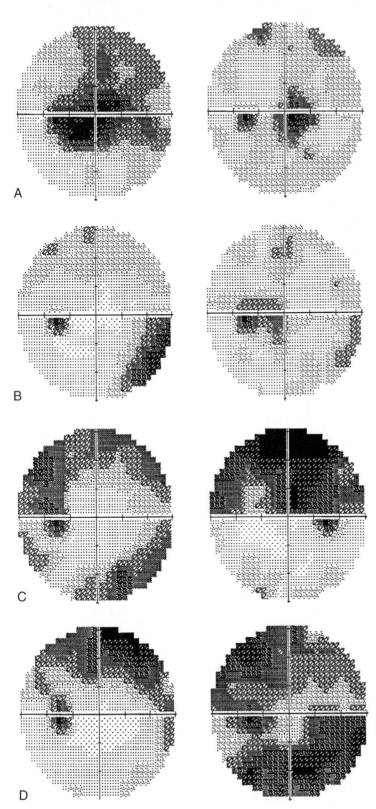

**FIGURE 10–11** Visual field deficits in optic neuritis. *A,* Central scotomas of moderate severity. *B,* Nasal step *(left)* and centrocecal deficit *(right). C,* Visual field loss around the 30-degree peripheral rim of the central visual field *(left)* and altitudinal loss of the superior hemifield *(right). D,* Superior arcuate-type defect *(left)* and double arcuate-type defect *(right).*

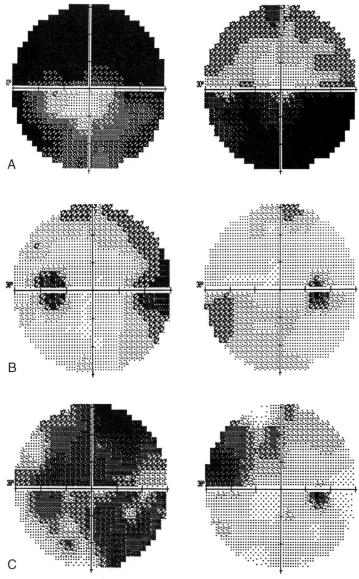

A

B

C

**FIGURE 10–12** Visual field deficits for other optic neuropathies. *A,* Superior altitudinal visual field deficit in anterior ischemic optic neuropathy *(left)* and inferior altitudinal visual field deficit in anterior ischemic optic neuropathy *(right)*. *B,* Enlarged blind spot and depressed sensitivity in the nasal visual field in papilledema *(left)* and nasal step in papilledema *(right)*. *C,* Glaucoma-like defects in optic nerve head drusen.

nal visual field deficit associated with anterior ischemic optic neuropathy. As mentioned earlier, note that the altitudinal deficit respects the horizontal midline across the entire central visual field. The middle two graphs *(B)* show visual field deficits that occur in papilledema. The left graph demonstrates an enlarged blind spot, which is a common visual field defect for papilledema, along with a region of depressed sensitivity in the nasal visual field. The right graph shows an example of papilledema in which the visual field deficit resembles a nasal step. In some instances, glaucoma-like deficits can also be obtained for patients with optic nerve head drusen, as shown in the lower graphs *(C)* in Figure 10–12. Many other optic neuropathies produce vi-

sual field loss, most of which resemble one of the examples shown for optic neuritis and other optic neuropathies in Figures 10–11 and 10-12.

## CHIASMAL LESIONS

At the optic chiasm, fibers from each nasal retina cross over to join the ipsilateral fibers from the temporal retina of the other eye. The separation of nerve fibers from the nasal and temporal retinas occurs along the vertical midline traveling through the fovea. Thus, one prominent feature of both chiasmal and post-chiasmal disorders is that the visual field loss "respects" the vertical meridian. In other words, an abrupt transition in sensitivity or "vertical step" is present for both eyes.

Disorders occurring at the optic chiasm typically affect the crossing fibers from the nasal retinas of each eye (representing the temporal visual fields). This results in a bitemporal visual field loss. The top graphs *(A)* in Figure 10-13 show the left and right eyes of a patient with a superior temporal visual field loss in both eyes due to a pituitary adenoma. Note the distinct vertical step in both eyes. Also, the defect in the left eye (left graph) resembles a wedge that "points" toward fixation. The deficit in the right eye includes the entire temporal hemifield. Pituitary adenomas are the most common type of disorder affecting the optic chiasm. Because they typically compress the inferior fibers (representing the superior visual field) crossing at the chiasm, subtle superior temporal deficits are often found on visual field testing. Thus, whenever superior temporal visual field loss occurs in both eyes, one should carefully look for evidence of a vertical step. The example shown in Figure 10-13 depicts a fairly marked amount of visual field loss, although chiasmal deficits can often manifest themselves as a subtle temporal visual field loss in both eyes which includes a small vertical step.

Although other types of visual field loss can occur for chiasmal lesions, they are very uncommon. Junction scotomas consist of a dense central visual field loss in one eye and a temporal visual field cut in the other eye. They are typically produced by a compressive lesion affecting the optic nerve of one eye and extending to the "junction" of the optic nerve and chiasm, where it affects the crossing fibers from the other eye. It is also possible to obtain binasal visual field deficits from bilateral compression of both outer sides of the chiasm, but this is extremely rare.

## POST-CHIASMAL LESIONS

Lesions of the visual pathways that occur after the optic chiasm produce homonymous defects, meaning that they occur on the same side (left or right) for both eyes. In this view, the deficit thus is present in the nasal visual field of one eye and the temporal visual field of the other eye. The second set of graphs *(B)* in Figure 10-13 shows a small, localized homonymous visual field defect in the left and right eyes resulting from an occipital lobe lesion. Note that the deficit in the right eye (right graph) extends over to the normal blind spot. The third set of graphs *(C)* in Figure 10-13 shows a homonymous superior quadrant deficit in both eyes. The

lower set of graphs *(D)* presents an example of a total homonymous hemianopsia in which the patient is no longer able to see anything to the left of fixation. As with chiasmal lesions, the vertical meridian is respected in each case.

Another factor that is important in the interpretation of post-chiasmal visual field loss is the degree of similarity or "congruity" between the visual field appearance between the left and right eyes. Occipital lobe lesions produce highly congruous deficits in the two eyes. As a general rule, the more anterior the lesion is in the optic radiations, the greater the amount of incongruity between the two eyes. Lesions of the optic tract just beyond the optic chiasm can sometimes produce bizarre, highly incongruous visual field deficits. For example, the deficit may be homonymous (on the same side of vision) and may respect the vertical meridian in both eyes, but there may be a superior wedge defect in one eye and an inferior wedge defect in the other eye.

Figure 10-14 presents examples of varying degrees of congruity. The top set of graphs *(A)* shows the left and right eyes of a patient with an incongruous superior quadrantanopsia produced by a lesion of the temporal lobe. The second set of graphs *(B)* shows the left and right eye visual fields for a patient with an incongruous left hemianopsia from a temporal lobe lesion. Note that the deficit in the left eye appears to be more extensive than the loss for the right eye. The third set of graphs *(C)* shows the visual fields of a patient with a parietal lobe lesion affecting the optic radiations. Here the deficit shows a greater amount of congruity, although the left eye has slightly greater damage than the right eye. The bottom graphs *(D)* show the left and right eyes of a patient with a quadrant deficit from an occipital lobe lesion. The extent of damage is virtually equivalent for the left and right eyes, revealing a high degree of congruity.

There are three potential caveats to the congruity evaluation of post-chiasmal lesions. First, the assessment of congruity is useful only if the visual field damage is less than a complete homonymous hemianopsia. The presence of a complete homonymous hemianopsia indicates that all of the fibers in the optic tract or optic radiations have been damaged at some point beyond the chiasm, but further localization cannot be deduced from visual field information. Second, the blind spot is located along the horizontal midline at 15° eccentricity in the temporal visual field. With small localized occipital lobe lesions, the blind spot can sometimes be contiguous with the deficit in the temporal visual field of one eye. This may cause a highly congruous deficit to appear to be somewhat incongruous. The visual

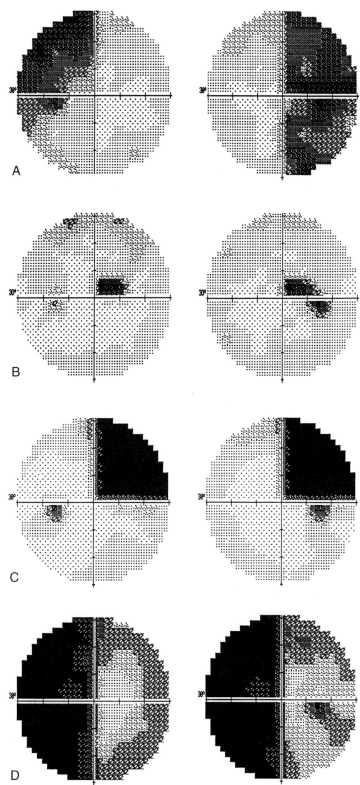

**FIGURE 10–13** Visual field deficits in disorders affecting the optic chiasm. *A,* Left and right eyes' visual fields of a patient with superior temporal visual field loss in pituitary adenoma. *B,* Small, localized homonymous visual field defect in the left and right eyes from an occipital lobe lesion. *C,* Homonymous superior quadrant deficit in both eyes. *D,* Total homonymous hemianopsia.

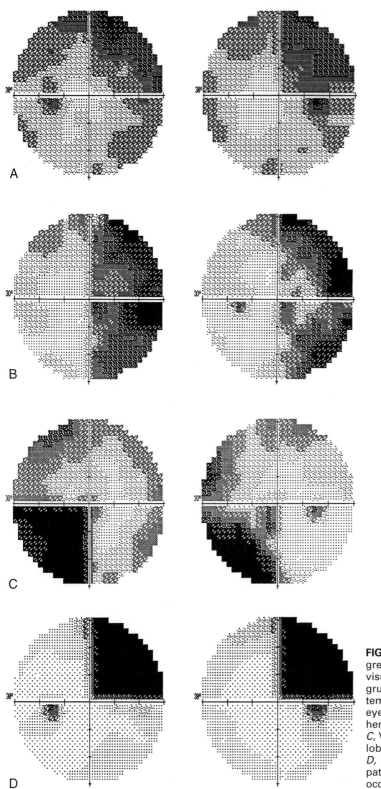

A

B

C

D

**FIGURE 10–14** Examples of varying degrees of congruity. *A,* Left and right eyes' visual fields of a patient with an incongruous superior quadrantanopsia in a temporal lobe lesion. *B,* Left and right eyes' visual fields of an incongruous left hemianopsia in a temporal lobe lesion. *C,* Visual fields of a patient with a parietal lobe lesion affecting the optic radiations. *D,* Left and right eyes' visual fields of a patient with a quadrant deficit from an occipital lobe lesion.

fields shown in Figure 10–13*B* are an excellent example of this caveat with the blind spot of one eye. Third, the temporal visual field extends farther than the nasal visual field. This difference in visual field extent may produce an appearance of differences between the two eyes. In addition, a "temporal crescent" may be present in one eye, which may produce the appearance of a difference between the two eyes. The temporal crescent is the outermost region of the temporal visual field that has only monocular representation. This third caveat is most pertinent to manual kinetic testing on the Goldmann perimeter because the differences are usually in the far periphery. Automated perimetry typically examines only the central 30°, where nasal and temporal visual field differences are minimal.

## PROGRESSION OF VISUAL FIELD LOSS

The determination of whether a patient's visual field improves, becomes worse, or remains stable over time is probably the most difficult aspect of interpretation of visual fields. Although several quantitative analysis procedures are available for evaluating visual field progression, none of them has been completely accepted by the clinical ophthalmic community. Thus, quantitative statistical analysis procedures may be helpful in monitoring a patient's visual field status, but they should be regarded with some caution at the present time.

Several important factors must be considered when evaluating a patient's visual field status over time. First, it is necessary to examine the test conditions present for each visual field examination. If test strategies, target sizes, or other test conditions are different from one examination to another, it is extremely difficult to compare the results. Second, it is important to determine whether there are any differences in patient characteristics from one visual field examination to another. Meaningful differences in pupil size, refractive corrections, visual acuity, or other factors (e.g., the upper lid was taped on one occasion and not on another occasion) can have a dramatic effect on the visual field results obtained on different visits, and an incorrect determination of visual field change may be assessed. Third, unless the visual field changes are dramatic, it is important to base judgments of visual field progression or stability on the entire series of visual field measurements that are available. It is not possible to distinguish subtle visual field changes from long-term variation on two visual field tests (e.g., comparing the current visual

field to the previous visual field). In particular, patients with moderate to advanced visual field loss can sometimes exhibit considerable variations from one visual field examination to another. Also, factors such as patient fatigue and experience can produce significant differences in visual field characteristics.[49–52] If it is suspected that a change in visual field loss has occurred, it is best to repeat the visual field examination on a separate visit to confirm the suspected change.

## SUMMARY

The examples of visual field loss presented in this chapter are only a small representative sample of the types of visual field loss which occur with common ocular and neurological disorders and are not intended to be comprehensive. A more detailed and extensive treatment of the myriad visual field deficits that are associated with the many disorders affecting the afferent visual pathways may be found in several texts.[7, 9]

## A SIMPLE "RECIPE" FOR VISUAL FIELD INTERPRETATION

In my experience, the most common error in visual field interpretation among novices occurs as a result of attending to specific details and nuances of the visual field prior to developing an overall global view, that is, not seeing the forest for the trees. To combat this tendency, I have developed a very simple four-step procedure for visual field interpretation. It is not intended to be comprehensive or to account for all cases but rather is meant to be a useful guide for those with limited background or experience in visual field interpretation to help avoid some of the common problems of misdiagnosis of visual field information.

**Step 1:** For each eye separately, determine whether the visual field is normal or abnormal. Automated perimetry statistical procedures provide excellent assistance with this task because they show both point-by-point and overall comparisons of the patient's test results with age-matched normal population values. If both eyes are normal, you are finished; if one or both eyes are abnormal, proceed to Step 2.

**Step 2:** Determine whether the visual field is abnormal in both eyes or in only one eye (I warned you that this was a simplistic approach!). If the visual field is abnormal in only one eye, your diagnostic dilemma has been reduced by half because it must be the consequence of a disorder occurring prior to the optic chiasm. If the visual fields of both eyes are abnormal, it means either that the deficit is at the chiasm or beyond *or* that the patient has bilateral retinal or optic nerve disease.

**Step 3:** This step is the most important component of defining the most likely locus of involvement along the visual pathways. Determine the general location of the visual field loss for each eye independently. Specifically, determine whether the visual field loss is in the superior or inferior hemifield, the nasal or temporal hemifield, or the central region. This is especially important for the nasal and temporal hemifield assessment. If the loss is extensive, determine where the *greatest* amount of visual field loss is present. What does this assessment tell you? If the visual field loss is bitemporal, then a chiasmal locus should be strongly suspected, especially if the deficit is in the superior temporal quadrant in each eye. If the visual field loss is nasal in one eye and temporal in the other eye, then a post-chiasmal locus should be suspected. Binasal defects or a nasal deficit in only one eye should lead you to suspect glaucoma, other optic neuropathies, or certain types of retinal disorders (e.g., retinal detachment or retinoschisis). A central deficit in one or both eyes should generate a suspicion of certain retinal disorders (e.g., macular degeneration or central serous choroidopathy) or an optic neuropathy. With this simple analysis, the general view of visual field properties has been generated, and a primary hypothesis (concerning locus of involvement along the visual pathways and the potential specific disease entity) and possibly one or more secondary hypotheses have been proposed, in order of likelihood.

**Step 4:** Now that you have a global picture of the visual field characteristics, look at the shape and features of the visual field loss. Does the defect respect either the horizontal or vertical meridians? What is the shape of the deficit (e.g., arcuate, candle-flame shaped, circular, pie-shaped, irregular)? Does the deficit "point" to the blind spot or to fixation? If there is visual field loss in both eyes, is it congruous or incongruous, symmetrical between the two eyes or asymmetrical? Do the edges of the defect have a steep or a gradually sloping profile? These and other specific features of the visual field

should provide confirming information for the primary or secondary hypotheses generated in step 3, or allow differentiation between the possible alternatives. However, attention to specific features of the visual field prior to getting the global view of the visual field from step 3 can sometimes lead to misinterpretation of visual field information. For example, a common error by novices is the misdiagnosis of subtle chiasmal visual field deficits due to the lack of awareness that the visual field loss is bitemporal.

This simple four-step approach to visual field analysis is not intended to cover all possible conditions but is rather meant to be a guide for the most typical kinds of visual field deficits and to avoid the most common pitfalls in the misinterpretation of visual field information. For greater detail concerning interpretation of patterns of visual field loss, the perimetry book by Harrington and Drake[9] contains a wealth of visual field examples and clinicopathological correlations.

# New Developments in Perimetry and Visual Field Testing

Perimetry testing and visual field testing have been useful and highly successful clinical diagnostic procedures for many years. The advent of automated perimetry has produced significant advances in the clinical efficacy of visual field testing, especially for general ophthalmic practitioners. However, there are limitations associated with these techniques that have prompted investigators to address these issues to improve the diagnostic utility of clinical perimetry and visual field testing. One of the areas that has received considerable attention in recent years is the application of additional tests of visual function to perimetry. In glaucoma and other ocular and neurological disorders, it has been reported that evidence of significant damage to the visual pathways can be present before any detectable abnormality is observed in visual field sensitivity (luminance increment thresholds). This is thought to be due to the fact that the increment threshold procedure used in automated static perimetry stimulates essentially all types of visual mechanisms. Thus, tremendous redundancy is seen in the response to a standard perimetry stimulus. A selective loss of a particular subpopulation of visual mechanisms or, alternatively, a moderate general loss for all visual mechanisms may not result in a detectable functional loss because of the redundancy that is present.

A number of new test procedures have recently been adapted for use in perimetric testing. Although the tests vary widely in terms of the particular visual function that is measured, each of them has a common theme: The tests are designed to provide a stimulus configuration that isolates the response of a particular subset of visual mechanisms. For example, the test procedure may attempt to isolate the responses of mechanisms sensitive to rapid stimulus changes by using a high-frequency flickering stimulus or a moving target.

There are two potential advantages to these approaches.[67] First, if certain ocular disorders produce *selective loss* to a particular subgroup of visual mechanisms early in the disease process, then a test designed to optimally stimulate these mechanisms is able to detect functional visual losses at an earlier stage of damage. Secondly, the procedures are *selective tests* that are designed to isolate the responses of a subpopulation of visual mechanisms. Thus, even if early losses are nonselective, the selective test procedures reduce the normal redundancy of the visual system and therefore are able to detect early losses more readily. Regardless of whether either or both of the two alternatives are correct, perimetric tests designed to stimulate and measure a subpopulation of visual mechanisms should perform better than standard visual field test procedures. Recently, several investigators have conducted perimetric evaluations of this type to assess specific visual functions. In the majority of instances, the test procedures have been directed toward the early detection of glaucomatous damage. Presented below are brief reviews of the most promising of these approaches to date.

## SHORT WAVELENGTH AUTOMATED PERIMETRY

Short wavelength automated perimetry (SWAP) is a visual field test procedure that utilizes a bright yellow background and a large, short-wavelength ("blue") stimulus to isolate and measure the sensitivity of short-wavelength chromatic mechanisms. The bright yellow background depresses the sensitivity of middle ("green") and long ("red") wavelength mechanisms, thereby allowing the sensitivity of the short-wavelength system to be measured using a large blue target. The test requires only modest modification of the Humphrey Field Analyzer, the most popular automated perimeter currently in

use, and the same test strategies, target presentation patterns, and other parameters that are used in standard automated perimetry can be employed for SWAP testing.[68-84]

Of all the new perimetric test procedures, SWAP has the most information available about its clinical efficacy and appears to be the most promising new test procedure to date. Although a number of other laboratories have investigated SWAP,[80-84] the largest amount of information has come from two independent laboratories at the University of California, Davis and the University of California, San Diego.[68-79] At both institutions, longitudinal studies of glaucoma patients, glaucoma suspects, and ocular hypertensives have now been conducted for approximately 8 years. Based on these investigations, the following results have been obtained: (1) About 15 to 20% of ocular hypertensives with normal visual fields on standard automated perimetry have abnormalities in their SWAP visual fields; (2) SWAP deficits in ocular hypertensives are predictive of the onset and location of future glaucomatous visual field loss on standard automated perimetry. SWAP deficits precede losses on standard automated perimetry by about 3 to 5 years; (3) localized SWAP deficits resemble the nerve fiber bundle type defects typically found in glaucoma for standard automated perimetry; (4) SWAP deficits are more prevalent in high-risk ocular hypertensives than in low- or medium-risk ocular hypertensives; (5) glaucoma patients with early visual field loss have larger SWAP deficits than those found for standard automated perimetry; and (6) in glaucoma patients, the rate of progression for SWAP deficits is twice as fast as the rate of progression for standard automated perimetry losses.

All of these findings provide strong evidence that SWAP is able to detect glaucomatous damage earlier than standard automated perimetry procedures. On the basis of these findings, commercially available automated perimeters are now being modified to allow SWAP testing to be performed as a standard clinical visual field test procedure.

## FLICKER AND TEMPORAL MODULATION PERIMETRY

Another procedure that has shown promise, especially for detection of early glaucomatous damage, is flicker perimetry, especially for high temporal frequencies. The rationale underlying flicker perimetry testing is that high temporal frequencies of flicker preferentially stimulate ganglion cells that project to the magnocellular layers of the lateral geniculate body (M-cell fibers). M-cell fibers consist primarily of large-diameter ganglion cell axons, which have been reported to be preferentially damaged in glaucoma. Thus, by presenting a stimulus that preferentially stimulates this group of nerve fibers, it is hoped that early glaucomatous losses can be more readily detected.

Two procedures have been introduced to perform flicker perimetry. The first method determines the highest frequency of flicker (the critical flicker frequency) that can be detected for a 100% contrast flicker target. Lachenmayr and his colleagues[85-88] have conducted the majority of work using this procedure. The second procedure consists of determining the minimum contrast needed to detect flicker for a fixed temporal frequency or group of frequencies. This procedure has been used primarily by Casson and co-workers[89-91] with temporal frequencies of 2, 8, and 16 Hz.

Both procedures have been shown to be effective in detecting glaucomatous visual field loss. In some ocular hypertensives, flicker deficits have been found in localized visual field locations in the presence of a normal visual field for conventional automated perimetry. In addition, recent evidence suggests that this form of perimetry has predictive value in distinguishing which ocular hypertensives with normal visual fields will develop glaucomatous visual field loss within several years.[89] Thus, results to date indicate that flicker perimetry is a useful adjunct to conventional automated perimetry, especially for detecting early glaucomatous losses.

In addition to its ability to detect early glaucomatous damage, flicker perimetry has another desirable feature as a clinical diagnostic test procedure. Recent investigations indicate that flicker detection thresholds are more resistant to the effects of blur, scattering, and image degradation than conventional automated perimetry.[88] Thus, the results of flicker perimetry in an elderly glaucoma or ocular hypertension patient with early cataract development can be more readily interpreted than those of conventional automated perimetry. One of the difficulties associated with the widespread clinical use of flicker perimetry is that the procedures cannot easily be implemented on existing automated perimeters. Specialized equipment must be constructed to perform flicker or temporal modulation perimetry.

## DISPLACEMENT AND MOTION DETECTION PERIMETRY

The ability to detect motion or small displacements of a stimulus at various locations in the

visual field has also been adapted for use as a perimetric test procedure. As with high temporal frequency flicker, the rationale underlying this test procedure is that motion is preferentially detected by M-cell mechanisms, which are putatively more susceptible to glaucomatous damage. Thresholds for detection of motion may therefore reveal early glaucomatous losses in localized visual field locations.

Two different approaches have been used to evaluate motion sensitivity of the visual field. The first method measures the minimum displacement of a small target superimposed on a uniform background that can be detected as movement.[92-95] Motion displacement thresholds are then determined for a number of visual field locations in a manner similar to traditional static perimetry. In this manner, motion sensitivity can be determined for small localized regions of the visual field. The second method presents a large display of random small dots moving in random directions (Brownian-like motion).[96-98] A "stimulus" is presented by briefly moving a small group of dots in the same direction. The patient's task is to detect this coherent direction of dot motion. A "motion coherence" threshold is determined by varying the percentage of dots within the small group that are moving in the same direction. This type of test procedure evaluates larger visual field regions but requires the combined input from a population of cells to be able to detect motion.

Recent studies of motion and displacement threshold perimetry indicate that it is able to detect subtle glaucomatous losses that are not evident with conventional automated perimetry.[92-98] Longitudinal studies need to be conducted to verify the clinical significance of these findings. However, motion and displacement perimetry have several desirable characteristics as clinical diagnostic test procedures. Motion detection is a very robust visual function, being only modestly affected by such factors as contrast, luminance, adaptation level, and target size. In addition, recent studies have indicated that, similar to flicker sensitivity, motion detection is very resistant to the effects of cataract, refractive error, and other forms of image degradation.[95, 99] The dynamic stimulus range for motion is also very large, especially for displacement of a single small target.

## HIGH-PASS RESOLUTION AND PATTERN DISCRIMINATION PERIMETRY

High-pass resolution perimetry is a perimetric procedure that utilizes a high-resolution video monitor to present ring optotypes that consist of a light central region surrounded by a dark annulus. The targets are high-pass filtered such that only high spatial frequencies are represented in the stimulus. Contrary to the situation for standard optotypes, high-pass resolution perimetry targets can be resolved at the same size that they can be detected. In high-pass resolution perimetry, target size is varied to determine the minimum size needed for detection of the stimulus at various visual field locations. The design of this type of stimulus is based on the premise that the stimulus configuration corresponds more closely to the center-surround arrangement of retinal ganglion cell receptive fields and that it therefore may be able to reveal glaucomatous ganglion cell losses more readily than conventional automated perimetry.[100-110]

Most of the studies to date have shown that high-pass resolution perimetry produces results comparable to but not better than conventional automated perimetry for detecting a variety of ocular disorders.[101-110] However, high-pass resolution perimetry has several practical advantages over conventional automated perimetry. First, the time required to perform high-pass resolution perimetry is considerably less than for conventional automated perimetry. In addition, the test procedure provides feedback to the patient and is more interactive than traditional automated perimetric test procedures. Because of this, patients prefer to be tested with high-pass resolution perimetry rather than standard automated perimetry.

Pattern discrimination perimetry (PDP) is a test procedure that was introduced by Drum and his colleagues.[111, 112] The stimulus consists of an alternating checkerboard pattern of light and dark dots presented on a background of a dynamic random pattern of light and dark dots. The patient's task is to detect the presence of the checkerboard target. The "coherence" of the stimulus is varied by changing the percentage of the target that is occupied by the alternating checkerboard pattern from 0% coherence (completely random dot pattern) to 100% (complete checkerboard). A coherence threshold is thereby determined for different visual field locations. The test is based on the premise that a combined population response of overlapping ganglion cell receptive fields is necessary to detect the stimulus at low coherence levels, and that if there is loss or drop-out of ganglion cells produced by glaucoma, a greater amount of coherence is needed for detecting the stimulus.

To date, existing studies suggest that PDP may be able to detect glaucomatous damage earlier than conventional automated perimetry test procedures can.[111-116] However, it appears that this test procedure may reveal different types of damage than that revealed by conventional automated perimetry because glaucomatous visual field abnormalities often are noted in different areas of the visual field for PDP and conventional automated perimetry. These investigations suggest that PDP may be useful for early detection of glaucomatous damage. However, this procedure has several potential disadvantages. First, the task is more difficult to perform than conventional automated perimetry, and some patients find it to be too demanding. Second, the response range is somewhat limited because even normal observers require a high degree of coherence in order to detect the stimulus; once a patient's detection thresholds are abnormal, there is a rather small interval before the maximum stimulus level (100% coherence) is reached, making it difficult to monitor progression of damage.

## Summary

At the present time, automated static perimetry with a white target superimposed on a white background remains the standard procedure for performing visual field evaluations. Although the new procedures previously described have several potential advantages to offer, further research and refinement of techniques are needed before they become accepted as standard clinical diagnostic test procedures. A similar situation was once present for automated static perimetry. Preliminary research on the clinical efficacy of automated perimetry began in the mid 1970s. Acceptance of automated perimetric testing as a routine clinical test procedure did not occur until the early to mid 1980s, and its use was not widespread until the mid to late 1980s. It was not until the 1990s that automated static perimetry was regarded as the "gold standard" for clinical visual field testing. In the future, some of these new visual field test procedures may enhance the sensitivity, specificity, efficiency, and patient acceptance of perimetric evaluation of the visual field.

In its current forms, perimetry is a very useful, noninvasive, clinical diagnostic test procedure for evaluation of the visual field. Early detection of ocular and neurological disorders, differential diagnosis and evaluation of existing visual dysfunction, monitoring of the status of ocular and neurological conditions, and assessment of the functional capabilities of patients are some of the important functions subserved by perimetric testing. This chapter emphasizes the value of visual field testing for clinical ophthalmic purposes and provides some helpful guidelines for conducting perimetric testing and interpreting visual field test results.

# References

1. Johnson CA, Keltner JL: Incidence of visual field loss in 20,000 eyes and its relationship to driving performance. Arch Ophthalmol 1983; 101:371-376.
2. Hedin A, Lovsund P: Effects of visual field defects on driving performance. Doc Ophthalmol Proc Series 1987; 49:541-548.
3. Szlyk JP, Alexander KR, Severing K, Fishman GA: Assessment of driving performance in patients with retinitis pigmentosa. Arch Ophthalmol 1992; 110:1709-1713.
4. Szlyk JP, Brigell M, Seiple W: Effects of age and hemianopic visual field loss on driving. Optom Vis Sci 1993; 70:1031-1037.
5. Marron JA, Bailey IL: Visual factors and orientation-mobility performance. Am J Optom Physiol Opt 1982; 59:413-426.
6. Anderson DR: Perimetry With and Without Automation. St. Louis: CV Mosby, 1987.
7. Choplin NT, Edwards RP: Visual Field Testing with the Humphrey Field Analyzer. Thoroughfare, NJ: Slack Inc., 1995.
8. Henson DB: Visual Fields. New York: Oxford University Press, 1993.
9. Harrington DO, Drake MV: The Visual Fields: Text and Atlas of Clinical Perimetry. St Louis: CV Mosby, 1990.
10. Frisen L: Clinical Tests of Vision. New York: Raven Press, 1990.
11. Greve EL: Single and Multiple Stimulus Static Perimetry: The Two Phases of Perimetry. The Hague: Dr. W. Junk Publishers, 1973.
12. Langerhorst CT: Automated Perimetry in Glaucoma. Amsterdam: Kugler Publications, 1988.
13. Drance SM, Anderson D: Automated Perimetry in Glaucoma. A Practical Guide. New York: Grune and Stratton, 1985
14. Lieberman MF, Drake MV: Computerized Perimetry: A Simplified Guide. Thorofare, NJ: Slack Inc., 1992.
15. Johnson CA: Evaluation of visual function. *In* Tasman W, Jaeger EA (eds): Duane's Foundations of Clinical Ophthalmology. Philadelphia: JB Lippincott, 1994.
16. Keltner JL, Johnson CA, Beck RW, et al.: The Optic Neuritis Study Group: Quality control functions of the Visual Field Reading Center (VFRC) for the Optic Neuritis Treatment Trial (ONTT). Controlled Clinical Trials 1993; 14:143-159.
17. Tate GW, Lynn JR: Principles of Quantitative Perimetry: Testing and Interpreting the Visual Field. New York: Grune and Stratton, 1977.
18. Aulhorn E, Harms H: Visual perimetry. *In* Jameson D, Hurvich LM (eds): Visual Psychophysics. Handbook of Sensory Physiology, Vol VII/4. New York: Springer-Verlag, 1972.
19. Boring EG: A History of Experimental Psychology. New York: Appleton-Century-Crofts, 1950.
20. Johnson CA, Keltner JL, Balestrery F: Effects of target size and eccentricity on visual detection and resolution. Vision Res 1978; 18:1217-1222.
21. Johnson CA, Keltner JL, Balestrery FG: Static and acuity

profile perimetry at various adaptation levels. Doc Ophthalmol 1981; 50:371-388.
22. Wall M, Kardon R, Moore P: Effects of stimulus size on test-retest variability. Perimetry Update 1992/93 (RP Mills, ed). Amsterdam: Kugler Publications, 1993, pp 371-376.
23. Uyama K, Matsumoto C, Okuyama S, Otori T: Influence of the target size on the sensitivity of the central visual field in patients with early glaucoma. Perimetry Update 1992/93 (RP Mills, ed). Amsterdam: Kugler Publications, 1993, pp 381-386.
24. Pennebacker GE, Stewart WC, Stewart JA, Hunt HH: The effect of stimulus duration upon the components of fluctuation in static automated perimetry. Eye 1992; 6:353-355.
25. Hart WM, Kosmorsky G, Burde RM: Color perimetry of central scotomas in diseases of the macula and optic nerve. Doc Ophthalmol Proc Series 1985; 42:239-246.
26. Hansen E, Olsen BT, Seim T, Wormald D: A modification of the Goldmann perimeter designed for colour perimetry. Doc Ophthalmol Proc Series 1985; 42:279-281.
27. Kitahara K, Kandatsu A, Tamaki R, Matsuzaki H: Spectral sensitivities on a white background as a function of retinal eccentricity. Doc Ophthalmol Proc Series 1987; 49:651-656.
28. Kitahara K, Kandatsu A, Noji J, Tamaka R: The usefulness of sensitivity measurements on a white background for detecting minor changes in visual disturbances in optic nerve diseases. Perimetry Update 1988/89 (A Heijl, ed). Amsterdam: Kugler and Ghedini Publishers, 1989, pp 39-44.
29. Flanagan JG, Hovis JK: Colored targets in the assessment of differential light sensitivity. Perimetry Update 1988/89 (A Heijl, ed). Amsterdam: Kugler and Ghedini Publishers, 1989, pp 67-76.
30. Mikelberg FS, Drance SM, Schulzer M, Wijsman K: The effect of miosis on visual field indices. Doc Ophthalmol Proc Series 1987; 49:645-650.
31. Rebolleda G, Munoz FJ, Fernandez Victorio JM, et al.: Effects of pupillary dilation on automated perimetry in glaucoma patients receiving pilocarpine. Ophthalmology 1992; 99:418-423.
32. Lindenmuth KA, Skuta GL, Rabbani R, Musch DC: Effects of pupillary constriction on automated perimetry in normal eyes. Ophthalmology 1989; 96:1298-1301.
33. Fankhauser F, Enoch JM: The effects of blur on perimetric thresholds. Arch Ophthalmol 1962; 68:120-131.
34. Benedetto M, Cyrlin MN: The effect of blur upon static perimetric thresholds. Doc Ophthalmol Proc Series 1985; 42:563-568.
35. Budenz DL, Feuer WJ, Anderson DR: The effect of simulated cataract on the glaucomatous visual field. Ophthalmology 1993; 100:511-517.
36. Wood JM, Wild JM, Smerdon DL, Crews SJ: Alterations in the shape of the automated perimetric profile arising from cataract. Graefe's Arch Clin Exp Ophthalmol 1989; 227:157-161.
37. van den Berg TJTP: Relation between media disturbances and the visual field. Doc Ophthalmol Proc Series 1987; 49:33-38.
38. Guthauser U, Flammer J, Niesel P: Relation between media disturbances and the visual field. Doc Ophthalmol Proc Series 1987; 49:39-42.
39. Baraldi P, Enoch JM, Raphael S: A comparison of visual impairment caused by nuclear (NC) and posterior subcapsular (PSC) cataracts. Doc Ophthalmol Proc Series 1987; 49:43-50.
40. Faschinger C: Computer perimetry in patients with corneal dystrophies. Doc Ophthalmol Proc Series 1987; 49:61-64.

41. Meyer DR, Stern JH, Jarvis JM, Lininger LL: Evaluating the visual field effects of blepharoptosis using automated static perimetry. Ophthalmology 1993; 100:651-658.

42. Patipa M: Visual field loss in primary gaze and reading gaze due to acquired blepharoptosis and visual field improvement following ptosis surgery. Arch Ophthalmol 1992; 110:63-67.

43. Zalta AH: Lens rim artifact in automated threshold perimetry. Ophthalmology 1989; 96:1302-1311.

44. Ruben JB, Lewis RA, Johnson CA, Adams C: The effect of Goldmann applanation tonometry on automated static threshold perimetry. Ophthalmology 1988; 95:267-270.

45. Saarinen J, Julesz B: The speed of attentional shifts in the visual field. Proceed Natl Acad Sci USA 1991; 88:1812-1814.

46. Werner EB, Krupin T, Adelson A, Feitl ME: Effect of patient experience on the results of automated perimetry in glaucoma suspect patients. Ophthalmology 1990; 97:44-48.

47. Wild JM, Dengler-Harles M, Searle AE, et al.: The influence of the learning effect on automated perimetry in patients with suspected glaucoma. Acta Ophthalmol 1989; 67:537-545.

48. Guttridge NM, Allen PM, Rudnicka AR, et al.: Influence of learning on the peripheral field as assessed by automated perimetry. Perimetry Update 1990/91 (RP Mills and A Heijl, eds). Amsterdam: Kugler and Ghedini Publishers, 1991, pp 567-576.

49. Johnson CA, Adams CW, Lewis RA: Fatigue effects in automated perimetry. Applied Optics 1988; 27:1030-1037.

50. Langerhorst CT, ven den Berg TJTP, Veldman E, Greve EL: Population study of global and local fatigue with prolonged threshold testing in automated perimetry. Doc Ophthalmol Proc Series 1987; 49:657-662.

51. Searle AET, Shaw DE, Wild JM, O'Neill EC: Within and between test learning and fatigue effects in normal perimetric sensitivity. Perimetry Update 1990/91 (RP Mills and A Heijl, eds). Amsterdam: Kugler and Ghedini Publishers, 1991, pp 533-538.

52. Hudson C, Wild JM, Searle AET, O'Neill EC: The magnitude and locus of perimetric fatigue in normals and ocular hypertensives. Perimetry Update 1992/93 (RP Mills, ed). Amsterdam: Kugler Publications, 1993, pp 503-508.

53. Demirel S, Vingrys AJ: Fixational instability during perimetry and the blindspot monitor. Perimetry Update 1992/93 (RP Mills, ed). Amsterdam: Kugler Publications, 1993, pp 515-520.

54. Vingrys AJ, Demirel S: Performance of unreliable patients on repeat perimetry. Perimetry Update 1992/93 (RP Mills, ed). Amsterdam: Kugler Publications, 1993, pp 521-526.

55. Eizenman M, Trope GE, Fortinsky M, Murphy PH: Stability of fixation in healthy subjects during automated perimetry. Can J Ophthalmol 1992; 27:336-340.

56. Johnson CA: The test logic of automated perimetry. ACTA:XXIV International Congress of Ophthalmology. Philadelphia: JB Lippincott, 1983, pp 151-155.

57. Johnson CA, Keltner JL: Optimal rates of movement for kinetic perimetry. Arch Ophthalmol 1987; 105:73-75.

58. Johnson CA, Keltner JL, Lewis RA: Automated kinetic perimetry: An efficient method of evaluating peripheral visual field loss. Applied Optics 1987; 26:1409-1414.

59. Ballon BJ, Echelman DA, Shields MB, Ollie AR: Peripheral visual field testing in glaucoma by automated kinetic perimetry with the Humphrey Field Analyzer. Arch Ophthalmol 1992; 110:1730-1732.

60. Barneby H, Yi L, Mills R: Automated peripheral perimetry: Kinetic versus suprathreshold static strategies. Perimetry Update 1990/91 (RP Mills and A Heijl, eds). Amsterdam: Kugler Publications, 1991, pp 423-432.

61. Lynn JR, Swanson WH, Fellman RL: Evaluation of automated kinetic perimetry (AKP) with the Humphrey Field Analyzer. Perimetry Update 1990/91 (RP Mills and A Heijl, eds). Amsterdam: Kugler Publications, 1991, pp 433-454.

62. Johnson CA: Role of automation in new instrumentation. Optom Vis Sci 1993; 70:288-298.

63. Heijl A, Lindgren G, Olssen J: Reliability parameters in computerized perimetry. Doc Ophthalmol Proc Series 1987; 49:593-600.

64. Katz J, Sommer A: Reliability indexes of automated perimetric tests. Arch Ophthalmol 1988; 106:1252-1254.

65. Keltner JL, Samuels S, Johnson CA, et al.: Factors affecting visual field and reliability indices in the Optic Neuritis Treatment Trial (ONTT). Invest Ophthalmol Vis Sci (Suppl) 1995; 36:S455 (ARVO abstract).

66. Asman P, Heijl A: Glaucoma Hemifield Test. Automated visual field evaluation. Arch Ophthalmol 1992; 110:812-819.

67. Johnson CA: Selective vs nonselective losses in glaucoma. J Glaucoma 1994; 3:S32-S44 (Feature Issue—Journal Supplement).

68. Sample PA, Martinez GA, Weinreb RN: Color visual fields: A five-year prospective study in suspect eyes and eyes with primary open angle glaucoma. Perimetry Update 1992/1993 (RP Mills, ed). Amsterdam: Kugler, 1993, pp 473-476.

69. Sample PA, Weinreb RN: Progressive color visual field loss in glaucoma. Invest Ophthalmol Vis Sci 1992; 33:2068-2071.

70. Johnson CA, Adams AJ, Casson EJ, Brandt JD: Progression of early glaucomatous visual field loss for blue-on-yellow and standard white-on-white automated perimetry. Arch Ophthalmol 1993; 111:651-656.

71. Johnson CA, Adams AJ, Casson EJ, Brandt JD: Blue-on-yellow perimetry can predict the development of glaucomatous visual field loss. Arch Ophthalmol 1993; 111:645-650.

72. Johnson CA, Adams AJ, Casson EJ: Blue-on-yellow perimetry: A five-year overview. Perimetry Update 1992/1993 (RP Mills, ed). Amsterdam: Kugler Publications, 1993, pp 459-466.

73. Sample PA, Boynton R, Weinreb R: Isolating the color vision loss in primary open angle glaucoma. Am J Ophthalmol 1988; 106:686-691.

74. Sample PA, Weinreb RN: Color perimetry for assessment of primary open-angle glaucoma. Invest Ophthalmol Vis Sci 1990; 31:1869-1875.

75. Johnson CA, Adams AJ, Twelker JD, Quigg JM: Age related changes of the central visual field for short wavelength sensitive (SWS) pathways. J Optical Soc Am 1988; 5:2131-2139.

76. Johnson CA, Adams AJ, Lewis RA: Automated perimetry of short-wavelength sensitive mechanisms in glaucoma and ocular hypertension. Preliminary findings. Perimetry Update 1988/89. Proceedings of the VIIIth International Perimetric Society Meeting. (A Heijl, ed). Amsterdam, Kugler & Ghedini, 1989, pp 31-37.

77. Adams AJ, Johnson CA, Lewis RA: S cone pathway sensitivity loss in ocular hypertension and early glaucoma has nerve fiber bundle pattern. Proceedings of the 10th Symposium of the International Research Group on Colour Vision Deficiencies (B Drum, J Moreland, and A Serra, eds). The Netherlands: Kluwer Academic Publishers, 1991, pp 535-542.

78. Johnson CA, Brandt JD, Khong AM, Adams AJ: Short wavelength automated perimetry (SWAP) in low, medium, and high risk ocular hypertensives: Initial baseline findings. Arch Ophthalmol 1995; 113:70–76.

79. Sample PA, Martinez GA, Weinreb RN: Short-wavelength automated perimetry without lens density testing. Am J Ophthalmol 1994; 118:632–641.

80. Hart WM, Silverman SE, Trick GL, et al.: Glaucomatous visual field damage. Luminance and color-contrast sensitivities. Invest Ophthalmol Vis Sci 1990; 31:359–367.

81. Flanagan JG, Trope GE, Popick W, Grover A: Perimetric isolation of the SWS cones in OHT and early POAG. Perimetry Update 1990/91 (RP Mills, A Heijl, eds). Amsterdam: Kugler, 1991, pp 343–345.

82. de Jong LAMS, Felius J, van den Berg TJTP, Greve EL: Blue-on-yellow perimetry in the detection of early glaucomatous damage. Invest Ophthalmol Vis Sci (Suppl) 1991; 32:1108 (ARVO abstract).

83. de Jong LAMS, Felius J, van den Berg TJTP, Greve EL: Comparison of color vision scores with visual field indices in white-on-white and blue-on-yellow automated perimetry in glaucomatous disease. Invest Ophthalmol Vis Sci (Suppl) 1993; 34:1267 (ARVO abstract).

84. Tamaki R, Kitahara K, Kandatsu A, Nishio Y: The vulnerability of the blue cone system in glaucoma. Perimetry Update 1990/91 (RP Mills, A Heijl, eds). Amsterdam: Kugler, 1991, pp 343–345.

85. Lachenmayr BJ, Drance SM, Douglas GR, Mikelberg FS: Light-sense, flicker and resolution perimetry in glaucoma: A comparative study. Perimetry Update 1990/91 (RP Mills and A Heijl, eds.). Amsterdam: Kugler and Ghedini, 1991, pp 351–356.

86. Lachenmayr BJ, Dramce SM, Chauhan BC, et al.: Diffuse and localized glaucomatous field loss in light-sense, flicker and resolution perimetry. Graefe's Arch Clin Exp Ophthalmol 1991; 229:267–273.

87. Lachenmayr B, Rothbacher H, Gleissner M: Automated flicker perimetry versus quantitative static perimetry in early glaucoma. Perimetry Update 1988/89 (A Heijl, ed). Amsterdam: Kugler and Ghedini, 1989, pp 359–368.

88. Lachenmayr BJ, Gleissner M: Flicker perimetry resists retinal image degradation. Invest Ophthalmol Vis Sci 1992; 33:3539–3542.

89. Casson EJ, Johnson CA, Shapiro LR: Longitudinal comparison of temporal-modulation perimetry with white-on-white and blue-on-yellow perimetry in ocular hypertension and early glaucoma. J Opt Soc Am A, 1993; 10:1792–1806.

90. Casson EJ, Johnson CA: Temporal modulation perimetry in glaucoma and ocular hypertension. Perimetry Update 1992/1993 (RP Mills, ed). Amsterdam: Kugler, 1993, pp 443–450.

91. Casson EJ, Johnson CA, Nelson-Quigg JM: Temporal modulation perimetry: The effects of aging and eccentricity on sensitivity in normals. Invest Ophthalmol Vis Sci 34:3096–3102.

92. Fitzke FW, Poinoosawmy D, Nagasubramanian S, Hitchings RA: Peripheral displacement thresholds in glaucoma and ocular hypertension. Perimetry Update 1988/89 (A Heijl, ed). Amsterdam: Kugler and Ghedini, 1989, pp 399–408.

93. Fitzke FW, Poinoosawmy D, Ernst W, Hitchings RA: Peripheral displacement thresholds in normals, ocular hypertensives and glaucoma. Doc Ophthalmol Proc Series 1986; 49:447–452.

94. Poinoosawmy D, Wu JX, Fitzke FW, Hitchings RA: Discrimination between progression and non-progression visual field loss in low tension glaucoma using MDT. Perimetry Update 1992/1993 (RP Mills, ed). Amsterdam: Kugler, 1993, pp 109–114.

95. Johnson CA, Marshall D, Eng K: Displacement threshold perimetry in glaucoma using a Macintosh computer system and a 21 inch monitor. Perimetry Update 1994/95 (RP Mills and M Wall, eds). Amsterdam: Kugler Publications, 1995, pp 91–96.

96. Silverman SE, Trick GL, Hart WM: Motion perception is abnormal in primary open-angle glaucoma and ocular hypertension. Invest Ophthalmol Vis Sci 1990; 31:722–729.

97. Bullimore MA, Wood JM, Swenson K: Motion perception in glaucoma. Invest Ophthalmol Vis Sci 1993; 34:3526–3533.

98. Wojciechowski R, Trick GL, Steinman SB: Topography of the age-related decline in motion sensitivity. Optom Vis Sci 1995; 72:67–74.

99. Whitaker D, Buckingham T: Oscillatory movement displacement thresholds: Resistance to optical image degradation. Ophthal Physiol Optics 1987; 7:121–125.

100. Frisen L: A computer graphics visual field screener using high-pass spatial frequency resolution targets and multiple feedback devices. Doc Ophthalmol Proc Series 1987; 49:441–446.

101. Sample PA, Ahn DS, Lee PC, Weinreb RN: High-pass resolution perimetry in eyes with ocular hypertension and primary open-angle glaucoma. Am J Ophthalmol 1992; 113:309–316.

102. Frisen L: High-pass resolution perimetry. Recent developments. Perimetry Update 1988/89 (A Heijl, ed). Amsterdam: Kugler and Ghedini, 1989, pp 369–376.

103. Dannheim F, Abramo F, Verlohr D: Comparison of automated conventional and spatial resolution perimetry in glaucoma. Perimetry Update 1988/89 (A Heijl, ed). Amsterdam: Kugler and Ghedini, 1989, pp 383–392.

104. House PH, Cooper RL, Bulsara M: Comparing long-term variability using the Humphrey Field Analyzer and the Ring Perimeter in glaucoma subjects and normal subjects. Perimetry Update 1992/1993 (RP Mills, ed). Amsterdam: Kugler, 1993, pp 63–72.

105. Kono Y, Maeda M, Yamamoto T, Kitazawa Y: A comparative study between high-pass resolution perimetry and differential light sensitivity perimetry in glaucoma patients. Perimetry Update 1992/1993 (RP Mills, ed). Amsterdam: Kugler, 1993, pp 409–414.

106. Wanger P, Martin-Boglind LM: High-pass resolution perimetry: Comparison between mean dB score and neural capacity in glaucoma diagnosis and follow-up. Perimetry Update 1992/1993 (RP Mills, ed). Amsterdam: Kugler, 1993, pp 415–418.

107. Wall M, Conway MD, House PH, Allely R: Evaluation of sensitivity and specificity of spatial resolution and Humphrey automated perimetry in pseudotumor cerebri patients and normal subjects. Invest Ophthalmol Vis Sci 1991; 32:3306.

108. Wall M: High-pass resolution perimetry in optic neuritis. Invest Ophthalmol Vis Sci 1991; 32:2525.

109. Bynke H: Evaluation of high-pass resolution perimetry in neuro-ophthalmology. Perimetry Update 1990/91. (RP Mills, A Heijl, eds). Amsterdam: Kugler, 1991, pp 143–149.

110. Lindblom B, Hoyt WF: High-pass resolution perimetry in neuro-ophthalmology. Ophthalmology 1992; 99:700.

111. Drum B, Breton M, Massof R, et al.: Pattern discrimination perimetry: A new concept in visual field testing. Doc Ophthalmol Proc Series 1987; 49:433–440.

112. Drum B, Severns M, O'Leary D, et al.: Selective loss of pattern discrimination in early glaucoma. Applied Optics 1989; 28:1135–1144.

113. Drum B, Severns M, O'Leary D, et al.: Pattern discrimi-

nation and light detection test different types of glaucomatous damage. Perimetry Update 1988/89 (A Heijl, ed). Amsterdam: Kugler, 1989, pp 341–347.

114. Nutaitis MJ, Stewart WC, Kelly DM, et al.: Pattern discrimination perimetry in patients with glaucoma and ocular hypertension. Am J Ophthalmol 1992; 114:297–301.

115. Stewart WC, Kelly DM, Hunt HH: Long-term and short-term fluctuation in pattern discrimination perimetry. Am J Ophthalmol 1992; 114:302–306.

116. Drum B, Bissett R: Optimizing dot size and contrast in pattern discrimination perimetry. Perimetry Update 1990/91. (RP Mills, A Heijl, eds). Amsterdam: Kugler, 1991, pp 373–380.

*David B. Elliott, BScOptom,*
*MCOptom, PhD, FAAO*

11

# Supplementary Clinical Tests of Visual Function

This chapter concentrates only on those supplementary tests of visual function (except visual field assessment, see Chapter 10) which are commercially available and have found widespread clinical use. Clinical testing of visual function has two major roles. First, with the aid of various objective techniques such as ophthalmoscopy and biomicroscopy, it can discriminate between diseased and normal eyes, assess disease progression, and evaluate the effects of intervention. Secondly, it is used as a surrogate measure of "real world" or functional vision performance. The epitome of this is when clinical tests are used (despite the paucity of supportive evidence) to decide whether people can see well enough to drive or join certain occupations and professional sports teams and whether their vision is bad enough to allow registration for legal blindness.

# What Makes a Good Test?

· · · · · · · · · · · · · · · · · · · · · · · ·

Commercialization of a clinical test probably occurs with inventor motivation and a company's belief that it can make a profit. Various aspects of the test considered at this stage are that the test should be perceived as being not too expensive given the information provided, should provide relatively quick and simple data collection (for both patient and clinician), and must not pose a hazard to patients. Important aspects of a test's performance (provided either before commercialization and/or after by independent researchers) are its validity, discriminative ability, and repeatability. These qualities are often described in the research literature and are also used by manufacturers to advertise a test's usefulness.

## VALIDITY

A test is valid if it measures what it says it measures. This is often indicated by how closely the results match those from a gold standard measurement. For example, the validity of new tonometers is often determined by how similar the results are to that of the Goldmann tonometer, and the validity of autorefractors is determined by how similar their results are to subjective refraction. Although this relationship is often described by the correlation coefficient between the two tests, a better description is provided by plotting frequency distributions of the differences between test and standard. For example, although a correlation coefficient of

0.97 between the equivalent sphere predicted by an autorefractor and subjective refraction does indicate that the two provide very similar results, knowing that 83% of autorefractor results are within $\pm 0.50$ D of subjective refraction and 96% are within $\pm 1.00$ D is much more meaningful.[1] Of course, this analysis can be used only if the gold standard and test are measured in the same units. For example, the validity of contrast sensitivity testing has been assessed by its relationship to various real world vision tasks. In this case, regression/correlation analysis would be appropriate.

## DISCRIMINATIVE ABILITY

Discriminative ability indicates how well a test discriminates between normal and abnormal eyes. In published results of clinical studies, it is often reported that a significant difference was found between a group of patients with an ocular abnormality and a control group. It should be noted that this only indicates that *on average* there is a difference between the groups. It does not indicate how well the test predicts whether an *individual patient* has the abnormality or not. If a test is used to discriminate between normal and abnormal, there are four possible outcomes. The test could indicate that an eye is abnormal and be correct (true positive) or incorrect (false positive or false alarm). A false alarm results in a patient being treated or referred for further testing for no reason. The test could also indicate that an eye is normal and be correct (true negative) or incorrect (false negative or miss). A "miss" results in patients not being treated or not being referred when they should have been. These results are usually described in terms of a test's sensitivity and specificity. Sensitivity is the proportion of abnormal eyes correctly identified, and specificity is the proportion of normal eyes correctly identified. In mathematical terms,

$$\text{Sensitivity} = \frac{\text{true positives}}{\text{true + false positives}}$$

$$\text{Specificity} = \frac{\text{true negatives}}{\text{true + false negatives}}$$

A test's sensitivity and specificity depend on the cut-off score chosen to differentiate normal and abnormal. For example, the sensitivity and specificity of visual acuity would change depending on whether the cut-off point for abnormality was chosen as 20/15 (6/4.5), 20/20 (6/6), or 20/25 (6/7.5). Using 20/15 would give the best sensitivity, as those abnormals with 20/20 or

20/25 would be correctly identified as abnormal. However, specificity would be poor, as normals with acuity of 20/20 or 20/25 would be classified as abnormal. Alternatively, sensitivity would be poorer and specificity better using 20/25 as the cut-off point. Plotting a graph of sensitivity against specificity helps to visualize the trade-off between specificity and sensitivity for different cut-off points and where the optimal cut-off point lies. This plot is called the receiver-operating characteristic (ROC) curve (Fig. 11–1).[2] Although the ROC curve can indicate the most efficient cut-off point, this is not always the most appropriate.[3] For example, if a test were being heavily relied on to determine whether a patient had a sight- (or life-) threatening disease that could be successfully treated, the test's sensitivity should be maximized. Although this would mean an increase in the number of false alarms, as few patients as possible with the disease would be missed. If early detection of the abnormality under consideration has little effect on the prognosis, a cut-off point providing relatively poor sensitivity may be chosen because a relatively high miss rate would not put patients at significant risk. This would then improve specificity, and relatively few normals would be wrongly treated or referred.

The end result of how well a test discriminates between normal and a particular disease also depends on the prevalence of the disease. For example, consider an optometrist who examines 10,000 patients and is using a test that detects an ocular disease whose prevalence is 0.1% (1 in 1000). Ten patients are likely to have the disease. If a test has 95% sensitivity and specificity (a very good test), then it is likely that 9 or all 10 abnormals would be detected. As 9990 do not have the disease, with a sensitivity of 95%, about 500 patients would be wrongly referred (or treated)! Despite an excellent test, about 1 in 50 of those referred would have the disease. If the cut-off criterion for this test were altered so that specificity was 99%, only 100 patients would be wrongly referred. The importance of using strict cut-off points (and tests with good specificity) is clear. Of course, changing the specificity to 99% would mean that sensitivity would be reduced and fewer of the 10 patients with the disease would be detected. The situation is much different if the same test were being used to detect a much more common disease with a prevalence of 10%. Of the 10,000 patients examined, 1000 would have the disease and 950 would be detected. As 9000 do not have the disease, 450 would be wrongly referred. In this case, many more patients would be referred and about two in three would have the disease. It is unfortunate for clinical tests that ocular diseases are rare (see Chapter 1).[3] To improve the situation, tests are particularly used when there are other suspicious symptoms or signs of a particular disease, because the prevalence of the disease in this subpopulation is much greater than in the population as a whole. For example, a practitioner is unlikely to check rigorously for possible glaucomatous fields in a 20 year old with no risk factors for glaucoma, but if the patient were 75 years old with a family history of the disease, visual fields would be mandated. In addition, treatment or referral is based not on the findings of one test but on a battery of tests.

## REPEATABILITY

Repeatability assesses the variability of results between testing occasions. Reliability has most

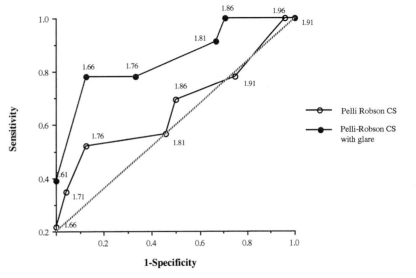

**FIGURE 11–1** A receiver-operating characteristic (ROC) curve for the Pelli-Robson chart with and without the brightness acuity tester (BAT). The plotted curve indicates their respective ability to discriminate between a group of 24 young normal and 23 older normal subjects. The dashed diagonal line indicates the zero discrimination level. The closer the ROC curve to the top left hand corner, the better the discrimination.

often been described in terms of correlation co-efficients. However, the correlation coefficient is determined in part by the range of values used, as well as by the relationship between the test and retest results.[4] A much better evaluation is the coefficient of repeatability (COR), which represents the 95% confidence limits of the difference between the test and retest scores. For example, correlation coefficients between test and retest visual acuity scores have been found to be 0.95 (unaided) and 0.90 (aided), respectively.[5] This suggests that the repeatability of the two tests is similar and may be slightly better for unaided acuity. However, COR results were $\pm 0.07$ logMAR (test and retest scores generally differ less than 3/4 of a line) for aided acuity and $\pm 0.21$ logMAR (within two lines) for unaided acuity, showing a much better repeatability for aided acuity. Given the greater variability of un-aided hyperopic acuity versus aided acuity, for example, this second analysis is intuitively correct. The high correlation coefficient found for unaided acuity is in part due to the much larger range of values used in its calculation (~20/200 (6/60) to 20/13 (6/4)), compared with the calculation involving aided acuity (~20/20 (6/6) to 20/13 (6/4)). Correlation coefficients are useful when comparing tests that do not use the same units. Concordance values (the percentage of patients getting exactly the same score on test and retest) have also been used to indicate that a test is reliable. However, normal patients all obtaining the same score on a test, or patients often obtaining exactly the same score on follow-up visits, indicates that the step sizes on the test are too big rather than that the test is some-how discriminative or repeatable.[6] A visual acuity chart containing only 20/20 (6/6) and 20/200 (6/60) lines would provide very high concordance but would be of very little value.

Repeatability results are also of value, as they indicate the size of a clinically significant change.[7] If a patient's contrast sensitivity has changed between examinations by 0.20 log unit, is this clinically important? Repeatability studies providing COR data indicate the size of the change in score due to chance. A significant change in score would then be anything larger than the COR (at least for tests with a continuous scale).[8] Unfortunately, relatively few studies have determined the size of a clinically significant change for optometric tests.

Repeatability appears to be the most important quality of a test, as it influences the others.[9] For example, if a test has poor repeatability and test results correlate poorly with retest results, it is unlikely that results from the test correlate highly with a gold standard measure. Therefore, its va-lidity is poor. If a test correlates poorly with itself, how can it correlate well with something else? Similarly, a test with poor repeatability likely has a large range of scores in normals. For an abnormal eye to be outside this large normal range would be more difficult, so good discriminative ability is less likely. Optical companies should be encouraged to provide repeatability data with any newly available test, so that it can be compared with the currently available tests.

## OBTAINING NORMAL DATA

Clinicians differ in the values they obtain using any device that requires the patient's subjective responses (perhaps because of differences in the amount of encouragement given to patients, among other factors).[10] Normative data provided with a chart may or may not be comparable to data a clinician would obtain from patients with normal vision. In objective electrophysiological testing, different equipment and procedures can also provide different results. It is therefore advisable for clinicians to obtain their own normative data. This provides good experience with the equipment and with interpretation of the results that are obtained. Because of probable age-related changes in test results, measurements should be collected from patients of each decade. Taking a mean for each decade gives an average score, and the mean $\pm 2$ standard deviations or the mean $\pm 3$ standard deviations provides the outer limits of normal scores and sets specificity at 95% or 99%, respectively.

## THE TESTS DISCUSSED

The following tests are discussed in this chapter: color vision, contrast sensitivity, disability glare, photostress recovery, potential vision assessment, the electroretinogram, and the visually evoked response. They represent the most commonly used supplementary clinical tests of vision (apart from visual fields, see Chapter 10). Although the electrophysiological tests do not provide direct information about vision per se, they are often used in combination with the psycho-physical tests. All tests are discussed in a similar format, including a brief history, clinical uses, and the theory or physiology underlying the test. Measurement procedure for individual tests is not provided, as this information is usually provided by the individual manufacturers.

# Color Vision Testing

. . . . . . . . . . . . . . . . . . . . . . .

## HISTORY

Wilson (1855) first suggested that the significant number of men with color vision deficits were unreliable in recognizing colored lights.[11] He also introduced the first color vision testing (for railway men in England) in 1853.[12] Holmgren was convinced that a train accident that occurred in Lagerlunda, Sweden, in 1875 was due to the driver's defective color vision. He subsequently convinced the Swedish State Railway and Royal Navy of the need to implement a color vision standard. Subsequent to a presentation at the Smithsonian Institute by Holmgren, a color vision standard was similarly adopted by the American Railway in 1877.[12] Holmgren is also credited with the invention of the first commercial color vision test, the Holmgren wool test. Interestingly, a review of the original documentation of the crash determined that Holmgren's belief that the crash was due to a color deficiency was probably unfounded.[11] This has also been shown for many accidents that were originally thought to be due to defective color vision.[11]

## RELEVANT PHYSIOLOGY

A simple linear zone model, combining the Young-Helmholtz trichromatic theory and Hering's opponent color theory, provides a reasonable first-order account of color vision deficiencies and normal color vision.[13] The first zone involves Helmholtz's proposition of three cone receptor types, each of which has its own photopigment: long wavelength–sensitive cones (red-catching, erythrolabe), medium wavelength–sensitive cones (green-catching, chlorolabe), and short wavelength–sensitive cones (blue-catching, cyanolabe). The information from this zone is sent to a second zone where three new opponent signals are generated: an achromatic signal or one of two antagonistic chromatic signals. The presence of a congenital or acquired color vision anomaly affecting either the photoreceptors or the channels results in variations in the ability to discriminate color.

## DEFINITIONS

Congenital color deficiency is found in both eyes equally and does not change over time. It is almost always a red-green deficiency and is far more common in males than females, as it is an X-linked disorder. Congenital blue-yellow deficiencies (tritanopia) are very rare, as they are not X-linked, and affect about 0.005% of the population. Eight percent (1 in 12) of the North American males and 0.5% of the female population are red-green color deficient. The possible outcomes for inheritance with the various combinations of color defective or normal parents and "carrier" mother are shown in Figure 11-2.[14]

Dichromats have the most severe form of color deficiency. They have a normal number of cones but just two pigment types, with either the red- or green-catching photopigment missing. Dichromats who lack the red-catching erythrolabe are called protanopes, and those that lack the green-catching chlorolabe are called deuteranopes. They are each found in about 1 in 100 males (1%). Dichromats have only an achromatic and a blue-yellow channel and have problems distinguishing reds from greens, oranges, or yellows, purples from blue, greens from browns, browns from reds, pinks from grays, blue-greens from grays, and oranges from greens.[14]

Anomalous trichromats tend to have a less severe form of color deficiency. They have all three photopigments, but the red- or green-catching photopigment's peak sensitivity is closer to the other than is normal. Protanomalous trichromats have a reduced sensitivity to red (i.e., the red-catching erythrolabe's sensitivity curve is closer to that of chlorolabe than normal), and deuteranomalous trichromats have a reduced sensitivity to green. The severity of this anomaly may range from near normal to almost dichromatic, depending on the extent of overlap. Deuteranomalous trichromats are more prevalent (5% of all males) than protanomalous trichromats (1% of males).

Acquired color defects are normally monocular or unequal in the two eyes, found about equally in males and females, can progress (or regress), and most often involve a blue-yellow discrimination loss accompanied by decreased vision.[14-16] Acquired defects may be due to the presence of an anomaly involving the internal components of the eye (lens, ocular media, retina), optic nerve, or the visual pathways. These anomalies are secondary to ocular or systemic pathologies, drugs, or toxic substances (Fig. 11-3). Köllner's rule suggests that blue-yellow discrimination loss can usually be attributed to diseases of the photoreceptors or the ocular media, whereas a red-green defect generally occurs with diseases of the visual pathway. The two main exceptions to Köllner's rule are central retinal dystrophies, which generally result in a red-green defect, and visual pathway lesions above the chiasm, which usually result in a blue-yellow defect.[16]

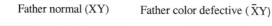

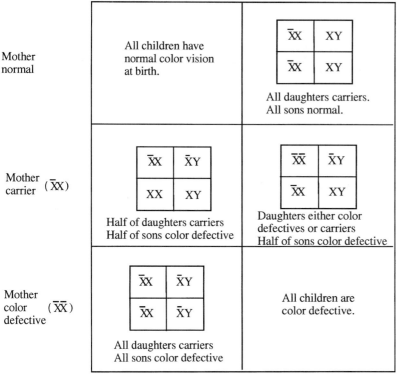

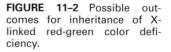

Father normal (XY)     Father color defective (X̄Y)

Mother normal

All children have normal color vision at birth.

| X̄X | XY |
|-----|-----|
| X̄X | XY |

All daughters carriers.
All sons normal.

Mother carrier (X̄X)

| X̄X | X̄Y |
|-----|-----|
| XX | XY |

Half of daughters carriers
Half of sons color defective

| X̄X̄ | X̄Y |
|-----|-----|
| X̄X | XY |

Daughters either color defectives or carriers
Half of sons color defective

Mother color defective (X̄X̄)

| X̄X | X̄Y |
|-----|-----|
| X̄X | X̄Y |

All daughters carriers
All sons color defective

All children are color defective.

**FIGURE 11–2** Possible outcomes for inheritance of X-linked red-green color deficiency.

Chromatopsia is a type of acquired defect in which white objects possess a color. The individual frequently perceives the white object as yellow (xanthopsia), red (erythropsia), blue (cyanopsia), or green (chloropsia). It can be associated with the presence of a lesion affecting either the optic pathway or the visual cortex, and in patients suffering from jaundice and central serous choroidopathy (xanthopsia), vitreal hemorrhages (erythropsia), and aphakia (cyanopsia). It is also a possible side effect of certain drugs, particularly digitalis.[14, 17] Digitalis poisoning (from the purple foxglove plant) has been suggested as linked to the predominance of yellow and the presence of scintillating whorls in the paintings of Vincent van Gogh.[18] It has been suggested that van Gogh was prescribed the drug for his epilepsy and/or his bouts of depression. Figure 11-4 shows van Gogh's last doctor, Dr. Paul Gachet, holding a purple foxglove plant.

## ASSESSING COLOR VISION

The objective of a color vision examination is to screen for a color deficiency, then to grade the severity and classify the type of defect if one is present. It is particularly important for certain occupations that mandate good color vision. This may be achieved through a series of clinical screening and grading tests. Screening tests utilize small color differences and attempt to categorize patients as normal or abnormal. In contrast, grading tests rely on several color difference steps. Vocational tests rely on color-matching abilities as well as color recognition.[16]

During color vision evaluation, the use of the proper quantity and quality of illumination is imperative. As the color temperature of the illuminant affects the colors of a test, color vision testing is normally performed under a Standard Illuminant Source C, in the form of the Macbeth easel lamp (Fig. 11-5). This simulates natural daylight conditions provided by direct sunlight and a clear sky. The use of a blue filter minimizes the amount of long wavelengths of light emitted from the tungsten bulb. Without this, the subsequent enhancement of the longer wavelength colors would cause a decrease in the detection of deuteranomalous individuals[15, 19] and an alteration in the rotation of the error axes when using arrangement tests.[20] Natural daylight is not recommended owing to its variability in both quality and quantity.

Because of the great expense associated with the MacBeth Easel Lamp, alternative sources are available. For example, a Kodak wratten #78AA filter (available from camera shops) placed in

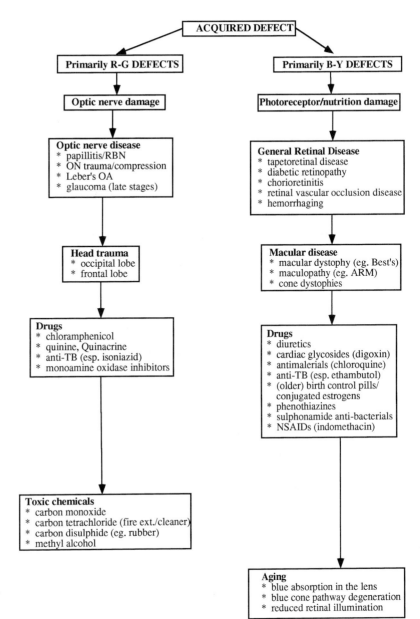

ACQUIRED DEFECT

**Primarily R-G DEFECTS**

Optic nerve damage

**Optic nerve disease**
* papillitis/RBN
* ON trauma/compression
* Leber's OA
* glaucoma (late stages)

**Head trauma**
* occipital lobe
* frontal lobe

**Drugs**
* chloramphenicol
* quinine, Quinacrine
* anti-TB (esp. isoniazid)
* monoamine oxidase inhibitors

**Toxic chemicals**
* carbon monoxide
* carbon tetrachloride (fire ext./cleaner)
* carbon disulphide (eg. rubber)
* methyl alcohol

**Primarily B-Y DEFECTS**

Photoreceptor/nutrition damage

**General Retinal Disease**
* tapetoretinal disease
* diabetic retinopathy
* chorioretinitis
* retinal vascular occlusion disease
* hemorrhaging

**Macular disease**
* macular dystrophy (eg. Best's)
* maculopathy (eg. ARM)
* cone dystrophies

**Drugs**
* diuretics
* cardiac glycosides (digoxin)
* antimalerials (chloroquine)
* anti-TB (esp. ethambutol)
* (older) birth control pills/
  conjugated estrogens
* phenothiazines
* sulphonamide anti-bacterials
* NSAIDs (indomethacin)

**Aging**
* blue absorption in the lens
* blue cone pathway degeneration
* reduced retinal illumination

**FIGURE 11–3** An approximate differentiation of acquired color deficiencies into red-green and blue-yellow types.

## CLINICAL TESTS

### Anomaloscope

The anomaloscope is the gold standard measure of color vision, and it is often used to assess the validity of new tests. It provides the only clinical front of the patient's eye in conjunction with a 100-watt incandescent light source has proven to be a close approximation to the Illuminant C.[20] Standard fluorescent lights should be avoided, although some high-quality types have reasonable color-rendering properties.[21]

method of identifying anomalous trichromatic and dichromatic red-green deficiencies and can reliably identify protans and deutans.[22] It is not often used clinically, however, as it is expensive and requires an experienced clinician and regular calibration. The patient generally observes a circular target in which one half contains a spectral yellow light. The patient's task is to mix spectral red and green lights on the other half to match the yellow (Rayleigh match). Some anomaloscopes also allow the evaluation of tritan deficiencies using a desaturated blue-green test field to match with a blue and green mix (Moreland match). This match was developed to minimize the discrepancies associated with macular pig-

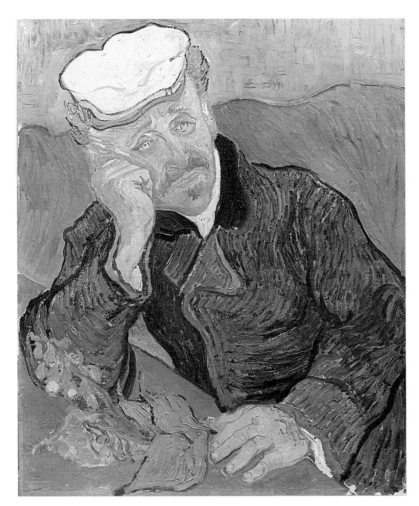

**FIGURE 11–4** *Le Docteur Paul Gachet (1828–1909)* (1890) by Vincent van Gogh (1853–1890). (Courtesy of the Réunion des Musées Nationaux, Paris.)

ment and aging changes.[22] Recently, advancements with the anomaloscope have focused on establishing a smaller, less expensive instrument that still matches the standard results obtained with the Nagel anomaloscope.[23, 24]

## Pseudoisochromatic Plates

These are the most widely used screening tests for abnormal color vision because of their quick and easy administration, efficiency, and low cost. They screen mainly for red-green deficiencies. Each pseudoisochromatic plate is crowded with colored spots. The color and position of the spots are arranged so that patients with normal color vision can see a figure, whereas color defectives cannot. The colors chosen are therefore those that look the same to red-green color defectives (pseudoisochromatic colors). Many types of isochromatic plates are available, although the most commonly used and most efficient remain the Ishihara plates (Fig. 11–6).[16] The full version of the test contains 38 plates, although there are

abridged versions containing 24 and 14 plates. Unfortunately, the selection of plates in these abbreviated versions appears to have been made on a purely economic basis, as they do not include what are regarded as the most efficient plates. Birch[16] suggests that if a rapid screening is required, it is better to select plates from the full version, such as plates 2, 3, 5, 9, 12, and 16. The full version consists of two sections: the first 25 plates contain numerals, and the rest contain pathways and are used for patients who cannot read letters, such as young children. The patient's task with the latter is to trace the pathway. Plate 1 is a demonstration plate that should be read by all literate patients and can be used to identify malingerers. Different designs of pseudoisochromatic plates follow and include transformation (plates 2 to 9), vanishing (10 to 17), and hidden digit (18 to 21) plates. Normal trichromats can see numbers on all but the hidden digit plates. Patients with red-green color deficiency do not see a number on the vanishing plates, see a different number than do normals on the trans-

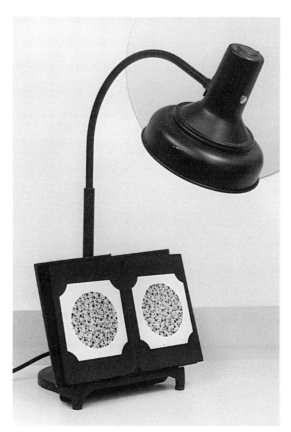

**FIGURE 11–5** The MacBeth Easel Lamp provides an approximation to the CIE standard illuminant C and is often used to provide illumination for plate color vision tests.

formation plates, and *can* see a number on the hidden digit plates. The pass/fail criteria are different for the various versions of the test,[16] but this information is included in the test manual. Classification plates, which attempt to differentiate protans and deutans, are plates 22 to 25. Two numbers are shown on each plate. The right hand number (blue-purple) is not seen or is seen less well by deutans, and the left hand number (red-purple) is not seen or is less well seen by protans. Even though the Ishihara test is efficient at screening for red-green defects, it cannot be used to classify the severity of a color vision deficiency. Other limitations of this test include its inability to screen for blue-yellow deficiencies and the fading of colors with time. The administration of the test requires an Illuminant C source, incident at 45° to the plate. The observer is allotted only 3 seconds to view each plate located 75 cm (arm's length) away.

## Arrangement Tests

These are an important tool in the analysis of both congenital and acquired color deficiencies.

Unlike the pseudoisochromatic plates, arrangement tests are not designed to screen for color deficiencies.[14-16] Indeed, color defectives can "pass" the test. Instead, the various arrangement tests evaluate the severity of hue discrimination. The patient's task is to arrange a series of colored caps in order with respect to one or two reference caps.

The origination of the first arrangement test, in 1943, was based on the classification of color proposed by the artist Munsell in 1901. Munsell had formulated a classification system for color in order to make both the teaching and recording of color much easier.[15] The most popular arrangement test is the Farnsworth D-15, which is capable of detecting moderate and severe color discrimination loss due to red-green, blue-yellow, or monochromatic color deficiencies.[15] Fifteen colored papers are placed in 12-mm caps, each of which subtends an angle of 1.5° at 50 cm. The patient's task is to arrange the 15 colored caps in order compared to the reference cap, and although there is no time limit, normally the task is completed within 2 minutes (Fig. 11–7). Patients with severe arthritis can have problems performing the test. The scoring diagram and the commonly found mistakes made by patients with color deficiency are shown in Figure 11–8. An individual with normal color vision is permitted two minor mistakes. A patient "fails" the test if the color circle is crossed at least twice.[14] The desaturated derivatives of the D-15 test (using paler colors) can be used to provide a more sensitive assessment of the severity of hue discrimination.[14]

The Farnsworth-Munsell 100 hue test is rarely

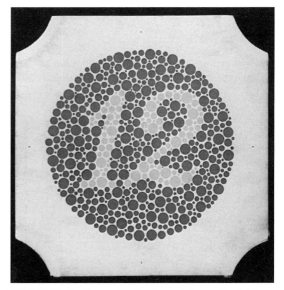

**FIGURE 11–6** Example of a test plate on the Ishihara pseudoisochromatic plate test.

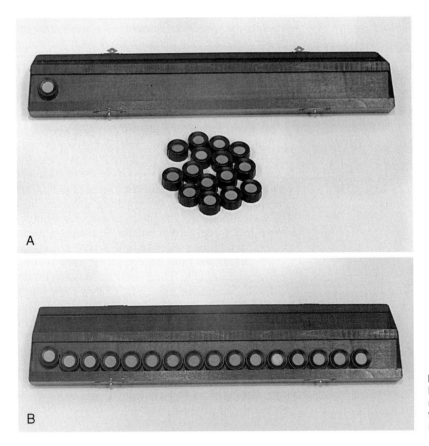

**FIGURE 11–7** *A,* Farnsworth D-15 panel test with color caps mixed together in front of the tray. *B,* With the color caps arranged in order in the tray.

used in clinical practice and is essentially limited to educational institutions and specialized clinics. Although it provides the most sensitive assessment of hue discrimination of available tests, it is an expensive and time-consuming procedure, can produce somewhat variable results, and has a marked learning effect.[14]

## Lantern Tests

These were first introduced in the 1890s in order to disqualify individuals with color deficiencies from working on the railroads. Soon after their origination, they were also adopted as a color vision testing method in the Navy, Armed Forces, and navigational transportation. The lantern tests that were developed at that time are still used today. Unfortunately, most of the data relating to the tests' validity have been submitted for government, rather than scientific, publication. Thus, there is a lack of scientific literature comparing the efficiency of lantern tests to the standard battery of color vision tests. Nonetheless, the protective legislation governing the use of

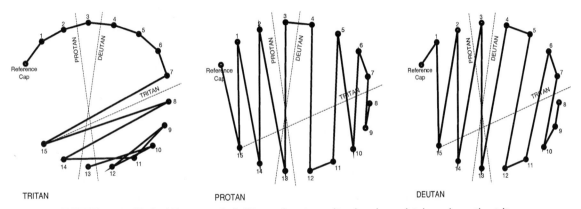

**FIGURE 11–8** Typical Farnsworth D-15 panel test results showing mistakes along the tritan, protan, and deutan axes.

lantern tests has enabled their continued widespread use in occupational color vision testing.[11, 12] Lantern tests are color-naming tests, and the two most commonly used in North America are the Farnsworth and Holmes-Wright.

## Summary

It is important to realize that no single color vision test is capable of screening, diagnosing, and grading the severity of acquired or congenital color vision defects, and it is recommended that a test battery be used. When screening for congenital color deficiency, a plate test such as the Ishihara should be used to help separate individuals with normal color vision from those with a deficiency. If a patient is determined to be color deficient, an arrangement test such as the D-15 should be used to better grade the severity of the deficiency and specifically classify it. Patients who fail the Ishihara and then pass the D-15 have a mild red-green defect and are unlikely to have trouble with most occupations.[14] When evaluating the extent of and monitoring an acquired color deficiency, a D-15 and one of the pseudoisochromatic tests (e.g., Ishihara if a red-green deficiency is present) are recommended.

## CLINICAL USES

### Detecting Color Deficiencies in Children

Owing to the increased use of color as a teaching aid in schools, it is important to perform color vision screenings on children soon after they begin school. A child with a color deficiency could otherwise be labeled as being "academically delayed." Teachers should be trained to realize that a child experiencing difficulty with colored tasks may possess poor color discrimination. In addition, following the identification of a child with a color vision deficiency, it is important that other teaching techniques that do not stress color be employed.[16]

### Counseling Young Congenital Color Defectives

All hereditary color defectives should be reassured about their condition: that they are not color blind, that it is not a disease, and that the condition will always be present but will not get worse. Young color defectives and their parents should be counseled that their condition lessens

their chances of joining certain occupations, such as aviation, law enforcement, and fire fighting. The more severe the color deficiency, the more unlikely their chances of joining these occupations successfully. In addition to these occupations, the presence of a color deficiency results in greater difficulty in pursuing a career that stresses the ability to discriminate color. Such careers include histology, chemistry, photography, the paint and textiles industries, interior decorating, electronics, dentistry, and optometry. A protanopic optometrist, for example, may have trouble detecting subtle retinal or choroidal hemorrhages and discriminating them from retinal or choroidal pigmentation.[14] Again, the extent of this handicap depends on the severity of the color deficiency. Patients can also be warned that certain everyday tasks, such as choosing an appropriate tie for a shirt, wearing matched socks, choosing ripe fruit, and differentiating green, brown, and red billiard balls, may be difficult. More importantly, protanopes should be especially warned that they will experience greater problems when driving. Protan drivers are involved in twice as many rear-end accidents as color normals or deutans and have greater difficulty with red signal lights.[16]

### Counseling Patients with Acquired Color Deficiency

In patients with acquired color deficiencies, color problems can be ignored because other aspects of vision, such as acuity or visual fields, are reduced and take precedence. Although these latter tests may be more routinely measured in patients with ocular abnormality and may be more important from a diagnostic perspective, color vision is an important part of the assessment of a patient's real world vision. Color vision assessment can provide useful information in any patient with reduced vision due to ocular disease and, obviously, in any patient who complains of color vision problems. An extreme example is the effect of acquired color vision changes on the lives of artists. The effects of cataract (presumably blue light absorbing nuclear cataract) on the color in the later paintings of the impressionist Claude Monet were appreciable and immensely annoying to Monet.[25, 26] Patients with acquired color deficiency should be informed of whether the problem is likely to reverse (e.g., optic neuritis, many drug-induced conditions, or cataract if surgically removed) or persist (e.g., age-related maculopathy or diabetic retinopathy). Many of these patients are older and may not need counseling about careers. Most of those who have acquired color deficiency when young, such as patients with retinitis pigmentosa, have been counseled about careers because of the poor prognosis of their acuity and visual fields. Young insulin-dependent diabetics, however, may retain good acuity yet have significant color problems. They should be warned of the likelihood of color vision changes and counseled about career paths. Older acquired color defectives need counseling about the effect of their changed vision on everyday activities. Unlike congenital color defectives, these patients had normal color vision and now have to adapt. Particular examples of advice for patients with acquired color vision deficiency include suggesting that diabetics with a color deficiency monitor their blood sugar levels using blood glucose tests such as the Chemstrip bG, rather than trying to differentiate the colors on urine glucose tests.[14] Similarly, elderly individuals should be warned of possible difficulty in differentiating certain colored tablets.

### Prescribing Colored Filters

Colored filters can help a relatively small number of patients with a hereditary color deficiency who wish to perform a specific color discrimination task better. For example, they can help color defectives distinguish red from green more easily, which may be useful for the particular occupation or hobby they are involved in. Although improvements in color vision may be suggested by improved scores on the Ishihara test, color discrimination on the Farnsworth-Munsell 100 hue test tends to get worse, and the D-15 shows a change in the axis of confusion.[16] They do not "cure" color defects because some color discriminations become easier whereas others worsen.[14, 16] The most commonly used filter is the X-Chrom lens, which is a dyed, deep red contact lens that is fitted monocularly.

### Aid in Differentiating Optic Nerve and Macular Disease

Color vision tests can be used in certain cases to differentiate an optic nerve problem from a subtle maculopathy. An optic nerve problem is likely to produce a monocular red-green acquired deficiency, which is best detected using the Ishihara or other pseudoisochromatic plate and graded with the D-15. A unilateral maculopathy is likely to produce a monocular blue-yellow deficiency. Subtle blue-yellow defects are likely to be missed using the D-15 tests, and the Farnsworth D-15 is

likely to be less sensitive than the desaturated D-15 tests.

# Contrast Sensitivity

### HISTORY

Low contrast letter charts are literally antique. Bjerrum made low contrast letter charts of 9, 20, 30, and 40% contrast in Copenhagen in 1884.[27] British ophthalmologist George Berry also published papers of such measurements in patients with tobacco amblyopia and retrobulbar neuritis in the 1880s. The first commercially available test seems to have been George Young's contrast sensitivity test apparatus, available from J. Weiss of London in the 1920s. The great impetus to present-day contrast sensitivity measurement came in the late 1950s and 1960s with the work of Campbell and Robson. An extensive and fascinating review of the history of contrast sensitivity is given by Robson.[27] A piece of work not included in Robson's review, but deserving of mention, is that of Fortuin.[28] His measurement of "visual power" included visual acuity and letter contrast sensitivity at various illumination levels.

### DEFINITIONS

Contrast sensitivity is the reciprocal value of the smallest distinguishable contrast. Prior to the use of sine-wave gratings to measure contrast sensitivity, contrast was calculated in terms of Weber contrast. Weber contrast is defined as $(L_t-L_b)/L_b$, where $L_b$ and $L_t$ are the luminance of the background and target, respectively. Currently, the Weber fraction is generally used when calculating the contrast of letters or similar targets. Michelson contrast is defined as

$$(L_{max} - L_{min})/(L_{max} + L_{min})$$

and is generally used when calculating contrast for repetitive stimuli such as sine-wave gratings. $L_{max}$ and $L_{min}$ are the luminance of the "light" and "dark" regions of the grating, respectively. Although the term *contrast sensitivity* applied to letters predates contrast sensitivity of sine-wave gratings by many years,[28] because of the large body of recent literature on contrast sensitivity using gratings, contrast sensitivity of letters is now often termed *letter contrast sensitivity* to avoid confusion.

A plot of contrast sensitivity over a range of spatial frequencies gives the contrast sensitivity function. A normal photopic contrast sensitivity

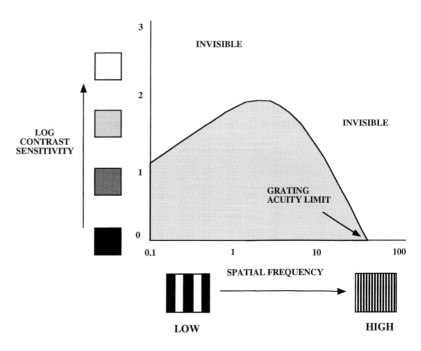

**FIGURE 11–9** A typical photopic contrast sensitivity function. The grating acuity limit is shown as the highest spatial frequency grating that can be detected at maximum contrast.

function is shown in Figure 11-9. It shows a clear peak at intermediate spatial frequencies, between about 2 to 6 cycles/deg, a rapid fall-off in sensitivity at higher spatial frequencies, and a more gradual fall at lower frequencies. Anything in the area outside the curve is invisible to the human eye.

## RELEVANT PHYSIOLOGY

The neural and optical attenuation of high spatial frequency contrast sensitivity is about the same, so that either or both are the cause of the high spatial frequency drop-off.[29] For example, the optical quality of the eye limits resolution to about the same level as the foveal spacing of cones.[30] Low spatial frequency decline is due to neural attenuation. Campbell and Robson (1968)[31] first suggested that the contrast sensitivity function was an envelope of contrast sensitivity functions of several independent parallel detecting mechanisms. Each channel is highly sensitive to some particular spatial frequency and virtually insensitive to all spatial frequencies differing by a factor of two (Fig. 11-10). These channels could be due to a series of ganglion cells that have receptive fields of different sizes, so that they are maximally sensitive to different spatial frequencies. The spatial frequency "tuning" of each channel is thought to be due to the characteristic center-surround organization of ganglion cell receptive fields (Fig. 11-11). Stimulation of the receptors in the center of the field produces an

increase in the cell's response, whereas stimulation of the surround area causes a decrease. Stimuli smaller than the center receptive field (higher frequency) produce only a partial response from the ganglion cell. Stimuli larger than the center receptive field also stimulate the inhibitory surround area, so that the overall response from the ganglion cell is progressively reduced. The contribution of the magnocellular and parvocellular pathways is controversial, but it is most likely that both contribute, with the parvocellular contribution increasing with spatial frequency.[32]

## MEASURING CONTRAST SENSITIVITY

A new clinical test must first provide additional information to that already provided by a traditional test (in this case, visual acuity). The point where the contrast sensitivity function intercepts the x-axis indicates the finest pattern just detectable at maximum contrast, which corresponds to visual acuity. Visual acuity can therefore be predicted approximately from the contrast sensitivity function. However, the reverse is not possible. As clinicians, accustomed to always thinking of a patient's level of vision in terms of visual acuity, it can be difficult to comprehend how vision can be poor if acuity is normal. However, just as the quality of sound is not determined by the highest pitched note heard, so the quality of vision is not determined solely by the smallest

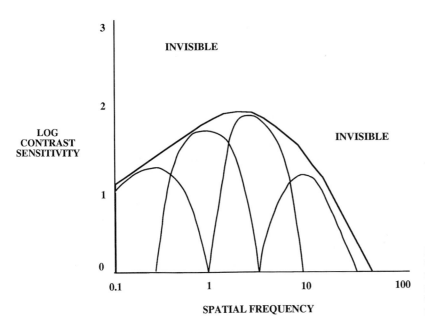

LOG CONTRAST SENSITIVITY

INVISIBLE

INVISIBLE

SPATIAL FREQUENCY

**FIGURE 11–10** Four channels with their own contrast sensitivity functions are shown summed together to illustrate the channel theory of the contrast sensitivity function.

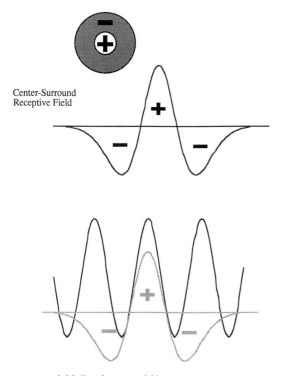

Center-Surround Receptive Field

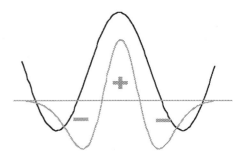

1. High frequency yields weak response

2. Medium frequency yields strong response

3. Low frequency yields weak response

**FIGURE 11–11** The spatial frequency "tuning" of each channel of the contrast sensitivity function is thought to be due to the characteristic center-surround organization of ganglion cell receptive fields. Stimulation of the photoreceptors in the center causes an increase in the cell's response, whereas stimulation of the surround area causes a decrease. This renders particular receptive fields more responsive to some spatial frequencies than to others.

detail that can be resolved at the highest contrast. The loss of low-frequency sound produces a "thin" sound, which has lost its "body" (try it on a hi-fi system with a graphic equalizer). The loss of low-frequency spatial frequencies similarly produces a thin, "washed-out" picture of the world, yet acuity remains the same.

Following this theme, numerous studies have shown that contrast sensitivity provides useful information about functional or real world vision which is not provided by visual acuity.[33-39] Contrast sensitivity has been shown to correlate better than visual acuity with various functional vision tasks, including mobility-orientation, balance control, driving, face perception, reading performance, and a patient's perceived visual disability.[33-36] Using contrast sensitivity in combination with visual acuity therefore gives the clinician a much better idea of how well a patient actually "sees" in the real world.

Contrast sensitivity can also show defects when acuity is normal, particularly for disorders of the visual pathways.[37-39] An advantage to measuring contrast sensitivity at high spatial frequencies is that it can provide a more sensitive measure of blur than acuity.[40] Because of the steepness of the contrast sensitivity function near the high spatial frequency cut-off, a blur-induced loss of acuity involves a relatively larger loss of contrast sensitivity. Unfortunately, previous clinical measures of high spatial frequency contrast sensitivity have been so unreliable as to be less sensitive to refractive blur than acuity.[41] A "small letter" contrast sensitivity measure such as proposed by Rabin (1994)[40] has had little evaluation, and little is known of its clinical usefulness. However, it may provide a more sensitive assessment than does visual acuity of disorders that affect high spatial frequency, such as early cataract, refractive surgery, and contact lens–induced corneal edema.

Whether one or many measures of contrast sensitivity should be taken is controversial.[42-45] Visual acuity measures have been shown to be highly correlated with high spatial frequency contrast sensitivity, so it may not be necessary to measure contrast sensitivity at these frequencies.[10, 46] It has been suggested that in addition to acuity, only a single measure of contrast sensitivity, at or near the peak of the contrast sensitivity function, may be sufficient.[10, 42, 46] This is the rationale behind the development of the Pelli-Robson chart. Linked to this controversy is whether contrast sensitivity should be measured by gratings or letters.[43-45] Despite all the theoretical arguments, in the end it is a matter of which types of chart "work,"[45] that is, which charts best discriminate normal from diseased eyes and

which best predict functional vision loss. More research is required in this area. At the present time, the most used letter charts are the Pelli-Robson and Regan charts, and the most used grating charts are the Vistech series. Letter charts clearly have the edge at the moment, as the Vistech has been shown to provide unreliable results, unlike both letter charts.[9, 47] As stated in the introduction, the repeatability of a test to a reasonable degree determines other properties of a test, such as its validity and discriminative ability.[9]

The American Academy of Ophthalmology has suggested the following important test design principles for contrast sensitivity and glare tests.[48] Tests that are consistent with these three principles of test design provide reliable data, unlike those that do not:[9]

1. The test should use a forced-choice psychophysical method. Tests generally attempt to determine a threshold value, that is, the point between always seen and not seen. Unfortunately, because of "internal noise" (such as random firing of neural cells within the visual system), this changeover is a gradual one and is known as the psychometric function (Fig. 11–12). This makes it difficult for a patient to state definitely whether or not he or she can see a target. Some patients are cautious and state that they can see a target only when they are absolutely sure, whereas others are more confident (Fig. 11–12). A threshold can therefore vary depending on the type of patient (cautious or otherwise) and can change between examinations of a particular patient by a change in his or her degree of caution. This problem can be removed by using forced-choice psychophysical methods, in which the patient is typically forced to state what or where a target is. However, the suggestion that any forced-choice task is good must also be avoided, as great care must be taken when there are only a small number of choices. For example, a patient with his or her eyes closed can get 50% of presentations correct in a two-alternative forced-choice method! Letter targets are particularly useful in this regard, as they provide a choice of 26 or 10 patient responses. Many clinical charts use just the 10 Sloan letters of D, H, N, V, R, Z, S, K, O, and C or the 10 British Standard letters of D, H, N, V, R, Z, F, P, E, and U, as they have been shown to have similar legibility (at high contrast). Letters also have the advantage of being very familiar to both patient and clinician.

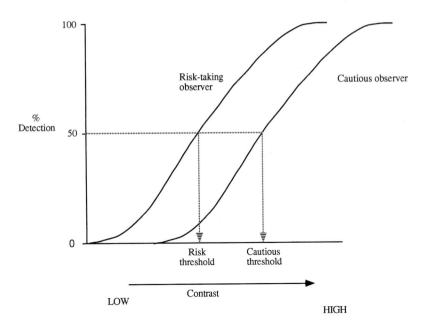

FIGURE 11–12 As the contrast of a target increases, a subject is more likely to see the target. There is no sharp division between visible and invisible, and the plot of detection versus contrast follows an S-shaped curve or psychometric function. The threshold value can be influenced by a subject's criterion of threshold. For example, a cautious observer might wait until he is absolutely certain he can see the target and therefore has a higher contrast threshold than a more risk-taking observer.

2. Test targets should follow a uniform logarithmic progression. This scale of progression provides equal perceptual steps.
3. Several trials should be used at each level, and step sizes should be smaller than the variability inherent in patients with normal vision.

## CONTRAST SENSITIVITY CHARTS

Contrast sensitivity is becoming more widely used in clinical practice. For example, in a recent survey of ophthalmologists of the American Society of Cataract and Refractive Surgery, 29% of respondents were using contrast sensitivity as part of their routine assessment of cataract.[49] Most of these were using the Vistech 6500 contrast sensitivity system. A new version of the Vistech chart incorporates some of the design features suggested by the American Academy of Ophthalmology which were missing in the original. In addition, a spin-off from the Vistech, the CSV-1000, has recently been shown to have superior repeatability to the original Vistech.[50]

The Pelli-Robson chart is an 86 × 63 cm chart that is hung 1 m from the patient's eye (Fig. 11-13). The chart measures the contrast threshold of letters of a fixed size. The letters are equivalent to 6/270 Snellen letters, and the chart gives an indication of contrast sensitivity just below the peak of the curve at 0.5 to 2 cycles/deg. Within each triplet, the letters have the same contrast, and the contrast in each successive triplet decreases by a factor of 0.15 log units. The patient is asked to read as far down the chart as he or she can. Incorrectly identifying the letter C as an O is a common error and can be counted as correct. The chart is becoming more popular because of its good repeatability and correlation with several real world tasks. It is also easy to use and relatively inexpensive. One disadvantage is that threshold can vary de-

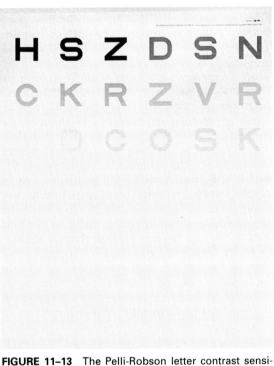

FIGURE 11–13 The Pelli-Robson letter contrast sensitivity chart. (From Clement Clarke Inc., Columbus, Ohio.)

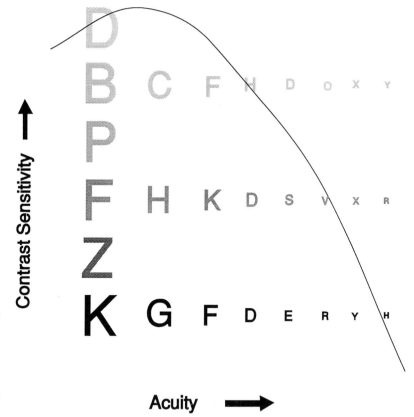

FIGURE 11-14 A schematic representation of the difference between letter-contrast sensitivity measurements (e.g., Pelli-Robson charts) and low-contrast acuity measurements (e.g., Bailey-Lovie, Regan). The line represents a typical contrast sensitivity function.

pending on how long patients are allowed to look at the chart as they near threshold.[10]

Low contrast acuity charts measure the smallest letter that can be resolved at a fixed contrast, and they do not measure contrast sensitivity (Fig. 11-14). It is very difficult to state what spatial frequencies the charts are measuring, because this depends on the visual acuity threshold. If only the large letters at the top of the chart can be seen, the score gives an indication of contrast sensitivity at intermediate spatial frequencies. If a patient can see the small letters at the bottom of the chart, the score gives an indication of higher spatial frequencies. The two most popular commercially available charts are the 10% (Michelson) contrast Bailey-Lovie charts (Fig. 11-15) and the 50%, 25%, 11%, and 4% (Weber) contrast Regan charts. They have also been shown to provide repeatable results.

## CLINICAL USES

### Screening for Visual Pathway Disorders

In some of these cases, both visual acuity and ophthalmoscopy can be normal, whereas contrast sensitivity at low frequencies is reduced.[37-39]

This is true of optic neuritis, multiple sclerosis, Parkinson's disease, papilledema, and any compressive lesion of the visual pathway. Because of the low incidence of such diseases and the fact that contrast sensitivity need not always be reduced in them, it is debatable whether routine contrast sensitivity screening by optometrists is worthwhile. However, because of the speed and ease of contrast sensitivity measurement and the relatively low cost of contrast sensitivity charts, coupled with the possible drastic outcome of certain visual pathway disorders, some clinicians believe that using contrast sensitivity as part of a battery of tests in routine screening is worthwhile.[37-39]

The value of currently available contrast sensitivity tests in glaucoma screening is still to be determined,[50] but most recent results are not promising.[39, 51] Arden[51] suggests that although contrast sensitivity testing in diabetics may be useful to explain symptoms of poor vision when visual acuity is normal, it provides no information regarding patient management. Unless a reduction in contrast sensitivity is shown to be indicative of pre-proliferative retinopathy or an important systemic diabetic abnormality, for which there is only very limited evidence,[52] its role as a screening device in diabetics appears limited.

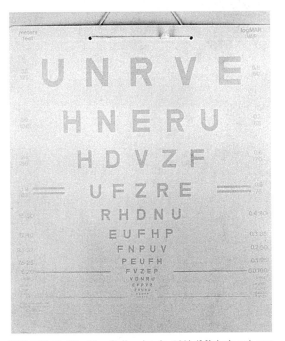

**FIGURE 11-15** The Bailey-Lovie 10% (Michelson) contrast logMAR charts. (From Dr. Ian Bailey, School of Optometry, UC Berkeley, California.)

## Explaining Symptoms of Reduced Vision in a Patient with Good Visual Acuity

Contrast sensitivity at low and intermediate spatial frequencies can be reduced when visual acuity is normal in patients with visual pathway disorders, diabetic retinopathy, or glaucoma. It can also provide important information about real world vision, so that it can be used to explain symptoms of poor vision in patients with good acuity. This can be important to the patient who has been told his or her vision is fine (because of good visual acuity) when he or she knows that it is not.[39] Such patients can also be counseled that their vision is likely to be worse in low contrast situations, such as at dawn and at dusk, in fog, or in heavy rain.

### Justify Cataract Referral in Patients with Good Visual Acuity

The decision to refer a cataract patient is generally influenced by the patient's claim that the reduced vision is interfering with his or her lifestyle. This may be because of the patient's personality, occupation, or hobbies. Contrast sensitivity measurement can help in two ways. A normal low frequency contrast sensitivity in a patient with poor visual acuity (perhaps 20/60 [6/18] or worse) can explain why a patient is not experiencing serious problems and need not necessarily be referred.[39] Perhaps more importantly, a reduced low frequency contrast sensitivity in a patient with reasonable visual acuity (20/40 [6/12] or better) who is experiencing significant problems can help to justify referral.[53]

## Providing Additional Information About a Patient's Visual Function

Contrast sensitivity at low spatial frequencies or at the peak of the contrast sensitivity function provides useful information about real world vision. Two patients could have the same visual acuity, such as 20/40 (6/12), yet one patient could have contrast sensitivity loss only at high spatial frequencies (hence the visual acuity loss) and the other could have contrast sensitivity loss at all spatial frequencies. Despite having the same visual acuity as the first patient, the second patient is much more likely to suffer from and complain about visual problems. In patients with reduced visual acuity due to ocular disease other than cataract, contrast sensitivity measurements can therefore be used to help explain symptoms of poor or deteriorating vision.

## In Low Vision Examinations

Because contrast sensitivity is correlated with reading speed,[33] reduced contrast sensitivity can explain a poor response to an optical aid by a low vision patient and suggest the need for a contrast-enhancing CCTV. Indeed, Whittaker and Lovie-Kitchin[54] suggest that poor contrast sensitivity measurements are a useful indicator that a low vision patient will not benefit from optical devices. In this respect, it can be more useful to provide a monocular optical aid to the eye with the better contrast sensitivity rather than to the eye with the better visual acuity.

# Disability Glare Testing

### HISTORY

Helmholtz in 1852 appears to have been the first to mention the effect of glare on vision, and Depène's work in 1890 is probably the first documented result of this effect. Depène showed that a glare source (a candle!) has lessening effects on acuity with increasing glare angle (the angle between the glare source and the acuity chart or other target). Holladay's work in 1926 represents the first classic study of glare. David Miller and Ernst Wolf produced the first commercially available glare tester in the early 1970s. When only three were sold, test production was discontinued.[55] Subsequently, the enthusiasm for glare testing of ophthalmologist Princeton Nadler led to the production of a simpler, less expensive version of the test, the Miller-Nadler Glare Tester, which was much more popular.[55]

## DEFINITIONS

Lucretius provided a description of glare nearly 2000 years ago: "Bright things the eyes eschew and shun to look upon; the sun even blinds them, if you persist in turning towards it, because its power is great and idols are borne through the clear air with great downward force, and strike the eyes and disorder their fastenings." A good definition of glare is "a strong, unpleasant light." Glare sources can be direct, such as the sun and lamps, or indirect, such as surfaces that are too bright. The latter includes reflections of primary sources in glossy materials or off water, that is, veiling reflections. Glare effects can be separated into two classes, *disability glare,* which reduces visual function, and *discomfort glare,* which makes vision uncomfortable. Discomfort glare is not discussed further as it is not well understood, is difficult to quantify, and has no commercially available measuring techniques.

## RELEVANT PHYSIOLOGY

Disability glare tests measure the reduction in a patient's vision due to a glare source. Light from the glare source is scattered within the patient's eye, and the forward scatter produces a veiling luminance on the retina that reduces the contrast of the retinal image. Miller and Nadler have used special inverse holograms to provide a clever illustration that ocular media opacification is due to light scatter rather than the "stopping" or absorption of light. The holograms collect the scattered light from a cataract and recreate a sharp image.[55] The physics behind ocular media transparency is well explained by Miller and Benedek.[56] Light scatter occurs when the spacing between elements of different refractive index becomes comparable to or greater than the wavelength of light. In this way, "lakes" of corneal edema and water clefts and vacuoles in the lens scatter light once they become comparable in size to the wavelength of light. Large particle

light scatter also occurs when the elements themselves become comparable in size to 500 nm. This occurs with aggregation of protein molecules in the lens nucleus (the effect possibly being enhanced by syneretic changes) and with the posterior migration of epithelial cells containing many large organelles in posterior subcapsular cataract.

In the young eye, forward light scatter can be attributed to comparable contributions from the cornea, lens, and retina.[57] In addition, scattered light filters through the iris in light-eyed patients.[58] The Stiles-Holladay approximation indicates that light scatter is inversely proportional to the square of the glare angle. With increasing age, there is a relative increase in the amount of light scatter from the lens, although the angular dependency remains similar.[59] In the following clinical conditions where disability glare can be a problem, the site of the increase in light scatter is indicated: corneal edema (corneal epithelium) and opacity, refractive surgery (corneal epithelium), cataract (particularly posterior subcapsular cataract), cataract surgery (capsular remnants), and retinitis pigmentosa and other retinal disorders leaving a large reflective area on the retina. Light scatter within the retina may also be increased in conditions such as macular edema.

## MEASURING DISABILITY GLARE

Disability glare tests measure the reduction in contrast sensitivity or visual acuity due to a glare source. As most disability glare tests use peripherally placed glare sources, the tests measure wide-angle light scatter. Paulsson and Sjöstrand first suggested that contrast sensitivity measurements with and without glare could be used to provide a clinical quantification of light scatter by using a suitable equation.[60] A recent paper questioning the validity of this equation has led some authors to doubt the validity of the method itself and suggest that some disability glare measures are influenced by neural changes. This is highlighted by the fact that improvement in contrast sensitivity can sometimes be obtained with a glare source in young subjects. However, this is a matter of some controversy.[61, 62] Several strategies have been suggested which attempt to ensure that disability glare results reflect changes in light scatter only.[62]

A number of so-called disability glare tests actually measure the level of contrast sensitivity or acuity under glare conditions. They do not measure disability glare in its true sense, as they are dependent on the neural system as well as on the ocular media. Such measures cannot be used to calculate the amount of light scatter.[60] In patients with normal neural function, however, this measure has been shown to be highly correlated with wide-angle light scatter[53] and is probably the most useful score to use in such patients.

When measuring visual function in patients with cataract and an abnormal retinal/neural system, disability glare must be measured as the difference in contrast sensitivity or visual acuity caused by the glare source. In this way, the scores depend less on the neural system and more closely indicate the level of intraocular light scatter. In these patients tests that measure visual function behind a cataract should also be used.

## GLARE TESTS

Simple glare tests include measuring visual acuity when the chart is placed in front of a window against the incoming light or while directing a penlight into the patient's eye. In these situations, using a logMAR chart would provide a more reliable result than using a traditional Snellen chart (see Chapter 2). In a recent survey of ophthalmologists, the most commonly used glare tests in clinical practice were the Miller-Nadler Glare Tester and the Brightness Acuity Tester.[49] The Miller-Nadler Glare Tester has reasonable test-retest reliability, but it is not sensitive to small light scatter changes owing to its large step sizes (in log contrast sensitivity terms) at low contrast levels.[9]

The Brightness Acuity Tester (Fig. 11-16) has the form of an illuminated hemispherical bowl which is placed close to the eye. It has a central aperture through which a chart can be viewed. The glare source subtends a visual angle of 8° to 70° at a vertex distance of 12 mm. The medium intensity setting is preferred for cataract patients, as the high intensity setting has been reported to give poor predictions of visual acuity measured outdoors and reduces contrast beyond a chart's limits for some patients with early cataract.[53] The low intensity setting has a minimal effect. The Brightness Acuity Tester can be used with contrast sensitivity charts,[12] low contrast acuity charts, and conventional high contrast visual acuity charts.[53, 63] Low contrast charts provide a more sensitive measure of disability glare than high contrast charts.[9, 53, 63] Measuring traditional high contrast visual acuity with the Brightness Acuity Tester, however, has the advantage that the score is universally understood. This is well illustrated by the scoring systems used by the Miller-Nadler and Vistech tests, as they provide charts that convert their contrast sensitivity scores into equivalent outdoor Snellen visual acuity values. Glare measurements using the Bright-

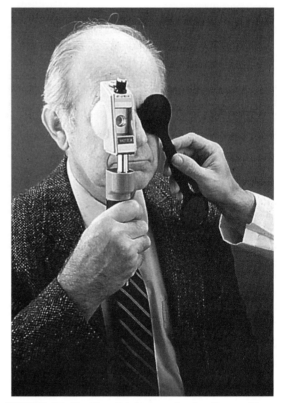

**FIGURE 11–16** The Brightness Acuity Tester. (From Mentor O & O Inc, Norwell, Massachusetts.)

ness Acuity Tester and logMAR acuity charts have been shown to have good reliability and discriminative ability.[9, 63] Of the Regan low contrast charts, the 25% contrast chart seems to be the most appropriate for assessing disability glare in early cataract.[9, 63]

## CLINICAL USES

### To Determine When to Refer for Cataract Surgery and Nd:YAG Capsulotomy

It is now well established that visual acuity can be an inadequate measure of visual function in cataract. Many studies have shown little or no correlation between visual acuity and glare scores in cataract.[53, 63, 64] Research is still required to determine whether glare tests provide any significant information about functional vision beyond acuity,[53, 64] but several case reports strongly suggest that they do, at least for some patients. An example is the case reported by Rubin in 1972.[65] A healthy, 45-year-old prison guard complained of a gradual decrease in vision over the previous year. The vision loss occurred particularly in bright sunlight, when guarding prisoners outside. The loss of vision had recently become so great as to allow two convicts to escape! His visual acuity was 20/20 (6/6) in each eye. However, careful examination found small posterior subcapsular cataracts and visual acuity of 20/200 (6/120) in bright light levels. Posterior subcapsular cataracts give much greater levels of disability glare than other types of cataract.[53, 60, 65] This is probably because of the dramatic effect on vision with these centrally positioned cataracts due to pupillary constriction in bright light levels.[65] There are no definitive levels of glare scores at which a patient should be referred. Referral should be based primarily on patient symptoms and the presence of cataract or posterior capsule remnants.[53, 64] High glare scores provide justification for referral, particularly in a patient with good or reasonable acuity.

## Before and After Surgery

Disability glare assessment can document any change in disability glare due to cataract surgery or vitrectomy and any significant increase in glare after refractive surgery.

## In Patients with Symptoms of Glare

Disability glare assessment can indicate whether such symptoms are due to significant disability glare (as opposed to discomfort glare or increased photostress, for example) and can quantify the degree of any problem for subsequent monitoring.

## Prescribing Tints

Disability glare is determined by the difference between contrast sensitivity without and with veiling glare.[60] Prescribing a tint does not automatically improve vision; although a tint cuts down the amount of scattered light, it also reduces the luminance of the object of regard.[66] The net effect on disability glare is zero. The optimal method by which disability glare may be alleviated is to reduce stray light reaching the eye from a glare source without affecting the object of interest. This can be achieved with visors, broad-brimmed hats, graduated tints, and polarized lenses, or, in some circumstances, the patient may select a type of tint that is specific for the offending glare source.

It is a commonly held belief that intraocular light scatter includes a relatively large amount of blue scatter (Rayleigh scatter). However, visible light scatter in normal and cataractous eyes appears to be essentially wavelength-independent.[57, 58, 67] There seems to be no rationale for prescribing blue-absorbing tints. Also note that nuclear cataract already provides a patient with his or her own built-in blue-absorbing filter. One special type of light/radiation scatter which is wavelength dependent is fluorescence, in which invisible ultraviolet radiation is converted to scattered visible light. Autofluorescence has been shown to increase with age and in crystalline lenses with nuclear and cortical cataract, so it has been suggested that ultraviolet absorbing tints improve vision in these patients.[68] However, disability glare tests are unlikely to indicate the extent of this loss, as glare tests generally contain relatively little ultraviolet radiation. Disability glare scores can perhaps help to determine whether to prescribe a tint to patients with centrally placed opacities. In these patients, a tint may help disability glare by reducing pupil constriction. However, given the relatively small changes in pupil size under photopic conditions,[69] the density of such a tint may have to be high.

# Photostress Recovery Testing

## HISTORY

Although it is a well known clinical technique, photostress recovery testing (PSRT) has a fairly recent and limited appearance in the research literature. Bailliart was probably the first to report the technique in 1954.[70] Since then, a small number of papers discussing its clinical usefulness have appeared.

## DEFINITIONS

Photostress testing determines the rate of photoreceptor visual pigment resynthesis by bleaching the foveal cone photopigments and thereby causing a temporary state of retinal insensitivity perceived as a central scotoma. The time required to regain high spatial resolution is taken as an index of the photochemical capability of the macula. Usually visual acuity is measured, and then the eye is exposed to a bright light source. A PSRT score is obtained by timing how long it takes for acuity to recover to its normal or near normal level.

## RELEVANT PHYSIOLOGY

Brindley has shown that long-lasting after-images (longer than 15 seconds) produced by brief light flashes (less than about 5 seconds) are due to photochemical changes in the receptors.[71] It is suggested that neural effects contribute to the first 15 seconds of an after-image.[71] Mammalian cone photopigments have not been isolated. However, it is assumed that cone photopigment regeneration is similar to rod photopigment regeneration.[72] The light sensitivity of the visual pigments is due to a chromophore, vitamin A aldehyde (retinal), which is bound to the visual pigment protein (opsin). Rod and cone photopigments differ only by the opsin they contain. The difference is still only slight, as genes encoding for rhodopsin and the cone opsins show approximately 40% identity.[73] The basic dynamics of cone pigment regeneration are similar to those for rhodopsin, except that bleached cone pigment molecules return to their regenerated state more quickly. Light absorption by rhodopsin leads to the separation of the retinal chromophore from opsin. This process is called bleaching, as it results in the loss of rhodopsin's purple color. The regeneration cycle of rhodopsin is shown in Figure 11–17 (adapted from Dowling[72]). The II-*cis* retinal and all-*trans* retinal are isomers, in that the backbone of the molecule changes shape but its composition remains unaltered. All-*trans* retinal may be reversibly converted to all-*trans* vitamin A or be isomerized to II-*cis* retinal, in which case it can combine spontaneously with opsin to form rhodopsin. II-*cis* retinal may be reduced to II-*cis* vitamin A.

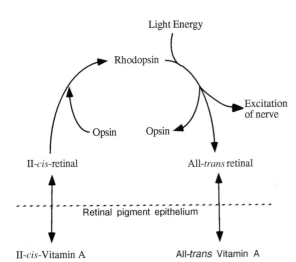

**FIGURE 11–17** The regeneration cycle of rhodopsin. (Reprinted by permission of the publisher from The Retina by John E. Dowling, Cambridge, MA: Harvard University Press. Copyright © 1987 by John E. Dowling.)

Most vitamin A is transported to the retinal pigment epithelium (RPE) and stored there.

There are several possible causes of prolonged recovery time.[74] The RPE ingests and destroys membranes shed by receptor cells as well as storing and transporting vitamin A. Therefore, any interference between the RPE/receptor complex (such as with age-related maculopathy, angioid streaks, choroideremia, serous retinal detachment, or pigment epithelium retinopathy) disturbs these processes and slows the regeneration of photopigments.[74-76] Also the receptors' high metabolic activity depends on the integrity of the underlying choriocapillaris. Disruption of this metabolic activity, such as with hypoxia[77] or in patients with impaired retinal vascular supply (e.g., diabetics and hypertensives), can lead to longer recovery times.[76]

## MEASURING PSRT

The most commonly accepted clinical technique is to time a patient's recovery to within one line of pre-adaptation visual acuity after a 10-second exposure to a bright light source. Textbooks suggest slight differences in technique. The light source could be a direct ophthalmoscope,[78, 79] penlight,[80] indirect ophthalmoscope,[80] or Brightness Acuity Tester,[79] and patients should read one line larger than pre-adaptation acuity[78, 79] or three letters of pre-adaptation acuity.[80] Despite the differences in technique suggested, all these texts suggest abnormal values as greater than 50 seconds. The source of these normal figures is sometimes not given,[79, 80] but they are probably based on results from normal subjects by Glaser et al.[70] They used a penlight 2 to 3 cm from the cornea and asked patients to read one line larger than their pre-adaptation acuity. Other studies have found the upper limit of normal to be 60 seconds (direct ophthalmoscope light for 15 seconds[81]; "dimmed" direct ophthalmoscope light for 30 seconds[82]) and 70 seconds (flashlight from Goldmann-Weekers adaptometer).[83] Recent unpublished studies with 34 subjects with healthy eyes (age range 19 to 67 years) have found upper limits of normal of 8 seconds with the Brightness Acuity Tester (high illuminance setting of 1300 cd/m²) and 40 seconds with a penlight using Glaser's procedure. A single figure for the upper limit of normal is also questionable, as several studies have found significant increases in PSRT with age.[70, 83, 84]

The non-standardization of the technique may be due to its relatively infrequent use. Because patients with early maculopathy often show extremely long recovery times, an exact value of the upper limit of normal may not be essential. Glaser found an average recovery time of 63 patients with maculopathy of 150 seconds, with the longest time being 8 minutes.[70] However, standardization would certainly provide a more sensitive test. This is best achieved by each clinician obtaining his or her own normative data, as suggested in the introduction of this chapter. This also provides the clinician with good experience with the test. Given the variability of light output from penlights[70] and the low PSRT scores using the Brightness Acuity Tester, a direct ophthalmoscope or transilluminator may be the best light source to use.[78] The present standard of a 10-second duration seems reasonable. From Brindley's work, the duration of exposure should not be much more than 5 seconds but sufficient to give a PSRT time greater than 15 seconds.[71] It seems advisable to have the post-photostress task as reading about two-thirds of the line larger than the pre-stress value, given that visual acuity measurements are not exactly reproducible and that retest measurements can be a line or more worse than test measurements.[85]

## CLINICAL USES

### Differentiating Macular from Optic Nerve Disease

The cause of central vision loss can occasionally be difficult to diagnose, as optic nerve disorders and subtle maculopathies can give inconclusive funduscopic findings. As optic nerve disorders, such as optic neuritis and ischemic optic neuropathy (and other abnormalities such as amblyopia), do not affect the photochemical processes in the photoreceptors, recovery times remain normal.[70, 78] A long recovery time suggests a macular problem.

### Monitoring Macular Disease

PSRT can aid in monitoring the recovery or progression of maculopathies such as early cystoid macular edema, idiopathic central serous chorioretinopathy, and chloroquine or solar burn effects on the macula.[80]

### Possible Future Uses

A series of research studies in Denmark has shown that nyctometry, which is basically a very standardized form of PSRT, can help in determining which patients with early diabetic retinopathy are likely to progress to severe proliferative diabetic retinopathy and subsequent vision loss.[86]

# Potential Vision Assessment

## HISTORY

The history of potential vision assessment is linked with that of cataract surgery. Early descriptions of cataract surgery ("couching" or dislocating the lens) are found in the writings of Celsus (AD 29) and Paullus of Aegina (7th century AD).[87] Even at this stage it is possible that a potential vision assessment was performed, as it was noted that if a patient had no light perception, the operations were frequently unsuccessful because of underlying ocular disease. Helmholz's (or Purkinje's[88] or Babbage's[87]) invention of the ophthalmoscope around 1850 did not immediately improve potential vision assessment, as surgeons continued to wait for cataracts to "ripen" (become completely opaque) until as late as the early 1900s.[89] The assessment of potential vision at this time was merely to check preoperatively for light perception and light projection.[89] With the invention of the intraocular lens implant by Harold Ridley in 1949 and ever-increasing improvements in its design and in cataract surgery, it became increasingly common to extract more immature cataracts. This made it possible for improved assessment of potential vision. In addition, this earlier stage of extraction, coupled with greater patient expectations, created a need for more accurate assessments of potential vision. An improvement in acuity from light perception to 20/40 (6/12) may delight a patient, unlike a change from 20/60 (6/18) to 20/40 (6/12). By the early 1980s, several potential acuity meters were made commercially available.[90] Le Grand used interference fringes in Maxwellian view to obtain a value of retinal visual acuity many years earlier in 1935.[29]

## DEFINITIONS

Potential vision assessment predicts the neural vision behind cataracts or other media opacities and thus the potential vision after cataract or other surgery.

## UNDERLYING THEORY

Many different techniques are used to assess potential vision behind media opacities. The most commonly used technique, and the only one to measure potential acuity, uses Maxwellian-view projection systems to image a small light source or sources in the eye's entrance pupil. The clinician can control the position of the highly localized Maxwellian beam so that it avoids any cataract or other localized opacity. In this way the estimate of potential visual acuity should be unaffected by intraocular light scattering. A single channel Maxwellian-view system is used in the Potential Acuity Meter (PAM) to project a letter acuity chart onto the retina (Fig. 11–18). This is therefore a highly developed technological improvement of the clinical pinhole test (see Chapter 2). In this test the patient looks at a Snellen chart and moves a single or multiple pinholes around in front of his or her eye and tries to obtain the optimal acuity. In this case, the "point source" is at the pinhole in front of the eye rather than in the entrance pupil, the patient rather than the practitioner attempts to find a clear area in the lens, and the retinal illuminance of the chart is lower. Another type of Maxwellian-view system uses two channels to produce an interference fringe on the retina (Fig. 11–19). By increasing the spatial frequency of the interference pattern, a measure of grating acuity can be obtained. The Rodenstock retinometer uses a coherent helium-neon laser to produce an interference pattern (Fig. 11–20), whereas the Haag-

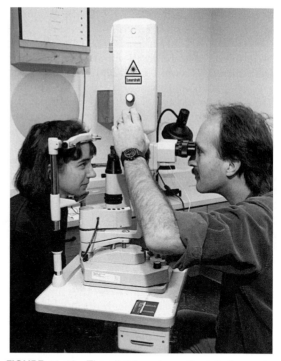

**FIGURE 11–19** The clinician steers the interferometer beam through a clear part of a patient's lens using the slit-lamp biomicroscope.

Streit visometer and the IRAS interferometer use two high-frequency square-wave gratings at slightly different orientations (moiré fringes). The spatial frequency of the interference patterns is varied by either changing the separation distance between the two coherent laser beams or changing the orientation of the two high-frequency gratings. It should be noted that as the non-laser beams pass through the pupil, they are not simple point light sources but imaged diffraction patterns of the objects used.[91] In the case of the PAM, the letter chart image is not a 0.15-mm diameter point source image as claimed but a much larger cross-like diffraction pattern.[91]

Several techniques are available which provide a qualitative assessment of vision. Somewhat crude techniques include the light projection, two-light discrimination, Maddox rod, and transilluminated Amsler tests.[92] Although they are likely to be rarely used, they may still be of value when a dense cataract is encountered. The rationale behind these techniques is that if a bright enough light is used, it can penetrate even a dense cataract and can provide an indication that the retina, and particularly the macula, is functioning. In the Maddox rod test, a bright light is shone through the Maddox rod and the patient is asked if all of the line is seen or if a part is

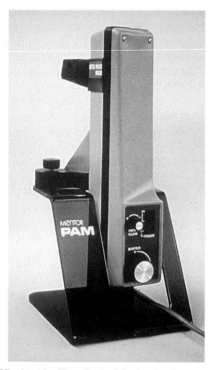

**FIGURE 11–18** The Potential Acuity Meter (PAM). (From Mentor O & O Inc, Norwell, MA.)

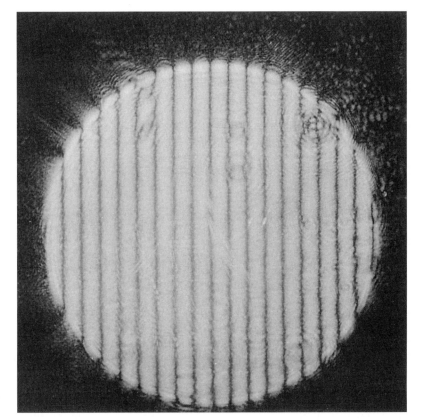

**FIGURE 11–20** An interference fringe pattern produced by the Rodenstock retinometer.

missing. A distortion or break in the middle of the line can indicate a macular abnormality.

Other qualitative techniques include electrophysiology, B-scan ultrasonography, and entoptic phenomena. The relevant physiology of visual evoked potentials and electroretinography is discussed below. Ultrasonography uses inaudible (to humans) high-frequency sound waves that echo back from the various interfaces within the eye. B-scan ultrasonography provides a two-dimensional cross-sectional view of the eye's internal structures. It can be used to indicate the presence behind dense cataract of intravitreal disorders, such as vitreous hemorrhage or proliferative retinopathy with traction, retinal or choroidal detachment, and intraocular tumors or foreign bodies.[92] Blue-field entoptoscopy (BFE) has the patient describe the presence or absence, number, position, and possibly the speed of leukocytes flowing in parafoveal capillaries. Unlike erythrocytes, leukocytes do not contain hemoglobin and therefore are seen in the strong blue light of the instrument.

## MEASURING POTENTIAL VISION

The literature evaluating the usefulness of the various potential acuity tests is somewhat confus-

ing.[64] It suggests that the ability of the tests to correctly indicate which patients will have a poor outcome postoperatively ranges between a very poor 20% to a superb 100%. Similarly, their ability to correctly predict those patients who will achieve a good surgical outcome has been suggested as ranging between 22% and 90%, although mainly between 70% and 90%. All the potential acuity meters, particularly the PAM, underpredict postoperative acuity when the cataracts or capsular thickening are dense and a large clear window in the lens cannot be found.[64, 92] The PAM suggests a poor visual acuity because it is unable to penetrate the cataract, yet postoperative acuity is often normal. (Remember that the PAM has a larger point source image in the entrance pupil than the 0.15-mm diameter claimed.[91]) Reduced potential acuity scores are also obtained when the light is directed through the edge of the pupil (e.g., around a posterior subcapsular cataract or capsular thickening) owing to lateral chromatic aberration (white light interferometers, PAM) and other off-axis aberrations (PAM).[91] The interferometers' accuracy at attempting to predict acuity is reduced because they use a grating target, and patients with various maculopathies and amblyopia demonstrate higher grating acuity than letter acuity. Not surprisingly, it has been shown that the interferometers overestimate post-operative acuity in patients with maculopathies and amblyopia.[93, 94] The PAM, although better than the interferometers, has also been shown to overestimate potential acuity in patients with cystoid macular edema and macular holes.[93, 94] Given that the most unwanted result when using these tests is an overprediction of postoperative acuity, the PAM may be the preferred test. It appears to provide a reasonable assessment of dry age-related maculopathy[94, 95] and may indicate the worst acuity that is likely postoperatively. This is despite its lack of penetration of moderately dense cataract and the reduced scores obtained when directing the light through the pupil edge. The Randwal IRAS interferometer, being hand-held and portable, is of particular value in assessing bedridden patients or patients confined to a wheelchair or when examining patients in nursing homes or hospitals.

The electroretinogram (ERG) reflects only gross retinal function, and a patient may have a macula or optic pathway abnormality and have a normal ERG response. Its usefulness in preoperative evaluation is therefore limited. The visual evoked potential (VEP) is much more useful, as it reflects primarily macular function. Pattern VEPs are significantly affected by the cataract, so a flash VEP is used in preoperative evaluation. A high-intensity 10-Hz flickering flash appears to be the optimal stimulus and the smaller, second peak in the wave complex is thought to best reflect macular function.[96] The flash VEP may be able to obtain a more useful result in dense cataracts than the PAM.[96] The Agency for Health Care Policy and Research report indicated that results from studies using BFE and electrophysiological techniques are also varied, with results similar to those with the potential acuity instruments.[64] It should be noted that the BFE uses a parafoveal stimulus. There is much less literature describing the usefulness of the various crude qualitative techniques. The Maddox rod has been compared favorably with the retinometer, but two-light discrimination compared less well with the BFE.[64]

## CLINICAL USES

### Predicting Potential Acuity Before Cataract Surgery

Cataract extraction with intraocular lens implantation is an extremely successful operation, and post-operative visual acuities of 20/40 (6/12) are obtained in about 90% of cases.[64] The most common cause of "unsuccessful" surgery is underlying retinal or neural disease.[64, 97] The huge success of the operation has led to patients feeling assured that vision will return to normal after the operation, and those who obtain little improvement due to underlying age-related maculopathy postoperatively can be bitterly disappointed.[97] Subtle maculopathies can give inconclusive funduscopic findings in patients with clear media, so that determining the state of the macula behind a cataract is particularly difficult. Potential acuity measurements therefore provide important prognostic information regarding cataract surgery, although their limitations as reported earlier should be considered. A battery of tests or procedures should be used to predict postoperative vision. For early and moderate cataract (up to 20/120 [6/36] or so), a PAM should be used to augment the information obtained from history, ophthalmoscopy, biomicroscopy, and pupillary reflexes. For more dense cataracts with which a view of the posterior pole is not available, the more rudimentary techniques such as light projection or Maddox rod testing should be used, in addition to history and pupillary reflexes and VEP, ERG, and especially B-scan imaging, if available. In all cases, the older the patient, the greater the likelihood of neural disease behind a dense cataract. It might be anticipated that cataract surgery would still be performed on patients with both cataract and age-related maculopathy, as improvements in vision could still improve quality of life. There would likely be significant improvements in disability glare, contrast sensitivity, and the patient's response to magnification, even if visual acuity improvements were minimal. However, this does not seem to be the case, as cataract is still found as a primary diagnosis in low vision patients and is the secondary diagnosis in over 50% of cases.[98]

### Other Prognostic Uses

Potential Acuity Meters can also provide useful prognostic information in a traumatized eye and prior to Nd:YAG capsulotomy, penetrating keratoplasty, and vitrectomy. As with cataract, the density of the opacity determines the type of tests used.

Levi and Feldman[99] suggest the use of the PAM as an aid in suspected malingering. It is explained to the patient that the test is designed to circumvent the eye problem and provide an indication of vision had the injury or other problem not occurred.

# Visual Evoked Potentials

## HISTORY

The measurement of evoked brain potentials was first mentioned by Richard Caton in 1875, when he described potentials evoked by head turning and mastication, as well as VEPs.[100] The next major advances in the measurement of VEPs were technological ones: the photographic superimposition and later averaging techniques developed by Dawson in 1947 and 1951.[100] These made many small potentials, which had previously been undetectable, accessible. Unfortunately, the flash VEP gave somewhat disappointing results, and it was not until the pattern VEP was introduced by Halliday and co-workers in the early 1970s that VEPs gained clinical recognition.[100]

## DEFINITIONS

The electrical activity of the brain elicited by visual stimulation is referred to as the VEP. VEPs are recorded by surface electrodes placed onto the scalp surface over the occipital cortex. The electrical activity evoked by a changing visual stimulus (a flash of light or a changing pattern) is monitored by the waveform it generates. The components of the waveform are measured in terms of amplitude in microvolts ($\mu$V) and peak latency in milliseconds (msec).

## RELEVANT PHYSIOLOGY

Although the VEP is often interpreted to reflect the visual system as a whole, it reflects primarily macular function. Macular representation in the visual cortex is extensive owing to the minimal or absent convergence between central retinal cones and their corresponding bipolar and ganglion cells. Peripheral representation in the cortex is much less because numerous peripheral photoreceptors converge onto a few bipolar cells, which converge onto still fewer ganglion cells. A surface electrode placed 2 to 5 cm above the inion (the bony ridge just above the base of the skull) transmits a predominantly macular response. There is considerable controversy about detailed localization for sources of VEPs, and, as Regan suggests, this may be like seeking the pot of gold at the end of the rainbow.[101]

## MEASURING VEPs

The VEP is usually recorded between an active electrode placed on the scalp over the visual cortex and a reference scalp electrode over a less visually active area (e.g., 2.5 cm higher along the midline or on some neutral position like the ear, mastoid, or forehead). The potential between these two electrodes is then amplified and displayed on a monitor or oscilloscope. Because the VEP response is time-locked to the stimulus, the amplified signal can be improved by using averaging and filtering procedures. A ground electrode is placed on an electrically neutral place, such as the earlobe. The placement of the active electrodes is important for accurate VEP recordings. Although some systems place the electrodes at fixed distances from bony landmarks (typically the inion), the most commonly used system of electrode placement is the International 10-20 System.[102] This has also recently been endorsed in the International Society of Clinical Electrophysiology of Vision (ISCEV) draft standards.[103] Measurements are made as a percentage of the distance along the midline between the inion and nasion (bridge of the nose) and are equally applicable to babies and adults. Interelectrode distances are 10% or 20% of the measurement between the two bony landmarks.

Differences in amplitude and/or latency between the patient and age-matched normal data may signify a disturbance of the visual pathway. Additionally, it can be important to look for differences in waveform between the two eyes and the two hemispheres. Each testing center should develop its normative VEP data using its own equipment because technical factors may affect latencies. In recent years, researchers have attempted to standardize VEP recording techniques so that test results may be compared between different clinics,[104] and ISCEV is currently completing the final stages of a draft paper on standards for VEPs.[103]

## VEP TECHNIQUES

### Flash VEP

This is elicited by a standard Ganzfeld flash, similar to that used for ERG recording. The ISCEV draft paper suggests the use of the standard flash defined in the ERG standards. The flash VEP is particularly used to assess neural function of patients with opaque media.

## Pattern VEP

The pattern VEP maintains constant overall luminance, whereas a number of other stimulus variables are adjustable, including contour, contrast, color, spatial frequency, stimulus field size, and stimulus orientation. The pattern VEP gives more information about visual function than the flash VEP. Two principal modes of pattern presentation are currently in use: pattern reversal and pattern onset-offset.

### Pattern Reversal

The stimulus is an alternating black and white check or black and white grating pattern in which there is no overall change in luminance. The stimulus is defined as either the spatial frequency of the bars or gratings or the visual angle of a check. A typical waveform produced is shown in Figure 11–21. ISCEV recommends measuring the amplitude of the P100 component from the preceding N75 peak.[103] The latency of the P100 component is particularly useful clinically, as it shows small intersubject variability and interocular range.[103]

### Pattern Onset-Offset

The stimulus is a black and white check or black and white grating pattern which alternates with a blank gray field of the same mean luminance as the pattern. There should be no overall change in luminance as the pattern appears or disappears. ISCEV recommends a time sequence of a 200-ms pattern separated by at least a 400-ms gray background.[103] Amplitudes are again measured from the preceding peak. Although the

pattern onset-offset has a larger intersubject variability than pattern reversal VEPs, it often shows a small intrasubject variability.[103]

### Transient or Steady State

Both types of pattern VEP can be further subdivided by the stimulus repetition rate into either transient or steady state. At reversal speeds below 2 Hz, the transient pattern VEP is measured. When stimulus presentation is increased to a higher rate, responses begin to overlap and become sinusoidal at about 8 Hz and are said to have reached a "steady state."[101] Steady-state potentials are used less often clinically; in many kinds of visual loss, the response is nonrecordable.

## CLINICAL USES

### Early Diagnosis of Optic Neuritits

The onset of optic neuritis is typically between 18 and 45 years of age, and the patient experiences a sudden, unilateral vision loss and possibly painful eye movement. Very often, there are no appreciable optic nerve head changes in the early stages. Signs that can help in diagnosis include a Marcus-Gunn pupil and tenderness of the upper lid near the insertion of the superior rectus. Myelin sheath breakdown in optic neuritis slows the conduction of the nerve impulse to the visual cortex, and the pattern VEP waveform shows a long latency.[105] Delayed pattern VEPs can be found even in the absence of other clinical evidence of visual pathway damage, making them an important diagnostic tool.[106-108] Other

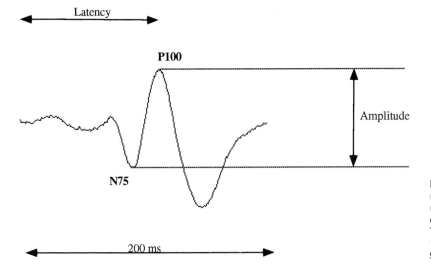

**FIGURE 11–21** A 1-Hz pattern-reversal visual evoked potential using 16-minute high contrast checks from a normal subject. The latency of the P100 wave is 112 ms, and the amplitude is 9 μV.

tests to aid in diagnosis include central red field testing or red cap tests and contrast sensitivity.[37, 38] The increase in latency of the pattern VEP may improve in some patients and may even return to normal.[109] In other patients, the increase in latency of the pattern VEP may persist even after acuity has returned. Optic neuritis occurs in approximately 70% of all cases of multiple sclerosis and is the presenting feature in about 25%.

## Diagnosis of Other Optic Nerve Disorders

Gross distortion of the VEP waveform is the dramatic effect of compressive lesions and trauma of the optic nerve. Although the VEP can be delayed by such lesions, the size of the delay is much smaller than in optic neuritis.[110] Hereditary optic atrophies also show markedly abnormal VEPs.

## Diagnosis of Ocular Albinism

Oculocutaneous albinism is diagnosed readily on the basis of clinical and ophthalmic examination. Although patients with ocular albinism may have characteristically reduced visual acuity, nystagmus, pale fundi, iris transillumination defects, and strabismus, the condition it is not easily diagnosed owing to the variable expressivity of the disease.[111, 112] Regardless of albino genotype or phenotype, all forms of albinism are characterized by VEP asymmetry between the right and left occipital hemispheres.[111] The asymmetry occurs as a result of an erroneous decussation of temporal retinal fibers at the optic chiasm. To detect asymmetry, electrodes are placed on either side of the midline, and a multichannel VEP is recorded. Apkarian has been able to achieve nearly 100% detection rate for VEP asymmetry in albinos with no false positives in normal controls, heterozygote family members, and non-albino patients with comparable albino symptoms (e.g., nystagmus, retinal hypopigmentation).[111] Because of different maturation rates of the various VEP responses, Apkarian suggests using flash VEPs for albino suspects under 3 years old, both flash and pattern onset between 3 and 6 years, and just pattern onset after the age of 6.[111]

## Diagnosis of Psychogenic Vision Loss

Some patients complain of poor vision and present with reduced visual acuity yet show no signs of refractive error (or refractive error change) or ocular disease. In this case, the patient may be suspected of a psychogenic disorder such as ocular hysteria or malingering.[113] Before a diagnosis of a psychogenic disorder can be made, organic dysfunction must first be ruled out. Several conditions can produce visual symptoms in the absence of overt disease, and the VEP may be used to detect such conditions. When little or no ocular anomaly is observable to the clinician, abnormal VEPs may be generated by Stargardt's macular degeneration, Leber's congenital amaurosis, rod monochromatism, retrobulbar optic neuritis, and amblyopia.[113] In addition to the VEP, other supplementary tests such as the ERG, color vision, visual fields, and dark adaptation can be used in the differential diagnosis. It should be remembered, however, that a normal VEP can be recorded in a patient who is cortically blind.

## Assessment of Newborns, Infants, and Young Children, Including Early Diagnosis, Assessing Prognosis, and Monitoring Treatment of Amblyopia

The ability to assess the state of the visual system in preverbal children and those with developmental disabilities makes the VEP a potentially useful tool for the early diagnosis of some visual dysfunctions. Early detection is important so that they may be treated while there is maximum plasticity within the visual system, that is, within the first year of life.[114] The sweep VEP is most commonly used when testing the acuities of infants and individuals who cannot cooperate for standard vision assessment.[101] This technique is particularly advantageous because factors such as poor motor coordination, abnormal eye movements, and poor or absent verbal skills do not affect the estimated acuity.[115] The technique uses a pattern reversal stimulus of black and white bars that are changed in size from wide to narrow widths.[116] Fourier analysis bypasses the time-consuming process of averaging, making this technique much quicker than transient VEP extrapolation. The sweep technique generates a plot of amplitude versus spatial frequency. At higher frequencies, the sweep VEP amplitude/spatial frequency function is linear, and extrapolation to zero amplitude voltage provides an estimate of acuity. Amblyopia may be detected, the prognosis assessed, and patching therapy monitored using the VEP.[96] Infants treated for unilateral congenital cataract also may benefit from the VEP, as it monitors visual function after surgery and contact lens correction.[117]

## Other Possible Uses

Using multichannel recordings, vertical and horizontal half and quandrantic field patterns may be used to test for visual field defects. However, because the VEP primarily reflects macular function, testing for defects is limited to the central 5°. In addition, the accuracy of results depends upon good fixation.

## Possible Future Uses

Recent research has suggested that various specialized forms of pattern VEPs may be useful in the early detection of primary open-angle glaucoma.[101, 118]

# The Electroretinogram

. . . . . . . . . . . . . . . . . . . . . . . . . . .

## HISTORY

Dewar and McKendrick[119] acknowledge Holmgren (1865) as the first to observe an electrical fluctuation from the eye by the action of light. Their own paper draws a fascinating picture of scientific breakthrough as they, among many other things, determined the electrical signal's intraretinal origin. In one experiment they determined the electrical signal to moonlight from a frog eye. This was to rule out the possibility that heat, rather than light, was the stimulus causing the electrical fluctuations to their gas flame stimulus. In 1877, Dewar made initial recordings of this electrical response in humans. Granit's work in 1933 was also a milestone, as he broke down the electroretinogram (ERG) waveform into three components: PI, PII, and PIII.[120] The ERG was not used effectively as a clinical procedure until the development of a corneal contact lens electrode by Riggs in 1941, and subsequently, Karpe in 1945 began to analyze normal versus pathological responses of the retina.[120]

## DEFINITIONS

The ERG represents a composite of electrical potentials developed in several retinal cells in response to light stimulation. It consists of three main waves known as a, b, and c (see Fig. 11–22), which correspond to Granit's PI, PII, and PIII components. In addition to the components already mentioned, there exists a series of wavelets on the ascending portion of the b-wave, the oscillatory potentials, which become noticeably dominant under mesopic conditions.

## RELEVANT PHYSIOLOGY

In the human retina, light induces a hyperpolarization of photoreceptors, resulting in the negative portion of the ERG, or the a-wave. The positive b-wave is created by an elevation of extracellular potassium from the bipolar cells depolarizing the Müller cells.[121, 122] The c-wave develops about 2 seconds after the presentation of a visual stimulus and is thought to be due to RPE input and hyperpolarization of the distal portion of the Müller cells. The origin of the oscillatory potentials still remains uncertain, but it is known that they have a different origin than the b-wave.[123, 124] Current research indicates that the inner plexiform layer is the source of the oscilla-

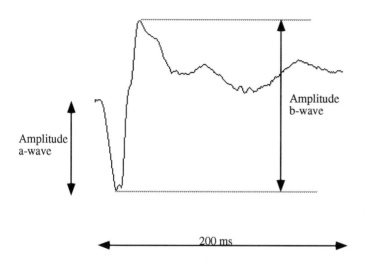

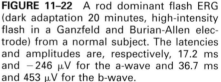

FIGURE 11–22 A rod dominant flash ERG (dark adaptation 20 minutes, high-intensity flash in a Ganzfeld and Burian-Allen electrode) from a normal subject. The latencies and amplitudes are, respectively, 17.2 ms and −246 μV for the a-wave and 36.7 ms and 453 μV for the b-wave.

tions, with possible bipolar or amacrine cell involvement.[123, 124]

## MEASURING THE ERG

Prior to recording the ERG, the pupil should be fully dilated to allow maximal retinal stimulation. The state of retinal adaptation and the characteristics of the Ganzfeld light stimulus determine what type of retinal cells are assessed by the ERG. For example, a rod-isolated (scotopic) ERG is best elicited after 30 minutes of dark adaptation using dim, slow frequency white flashes and no background light. A cone-isolated (photopic) ERG is best elicited after 10 minutes of light adaptation using a white stimulus flickering at 30 Hz against a background light. Colored stimuli can be used to record ERGs, but they create problems of standardization.[125] There are a number of recording electrode types.[120] The ERG is usually recorded between an active electrode embedded in a contact lens on the cornea (Fig. 11-23) or on the eyelid, and a reference electrode on the patient's forehead. Alternatively, the reference electrode can be situated in a speculum surrounding the contact lens. The potential between these two electrodes is then amplified

and displayed on a monitor screen or oscilloscope. A ground electrode is placed on an electrically neutral place (e.g., the earlobe). The c-wave is difficult to measure clinically and even with adequate new techniques, the variable c-wave does not isolate the response of the RPE from damage that may be occurring at the level of the photoreceptor. Therefore, it is just the biphasic responses of the a- and b-waves which are measured in the clinic. In 1989, ISCEV published standards for the clinical ERG.[125] ISCEV suggests that anyone measuring clinical ERGs should use the ISCEV standard or demonstrate that their alternative techniques produce signals equivalent in basic waveform, amplitude, and physiological significance to the standard. A detailed description of ERG equipment and clinical procedure is provided by Sutija and Sherman.[120]

Measures of both wave amplitude and time characteristics may be considered in the evaluation of the ERG, as these parameters are often selectively reduced in various disease processes. The principally used measures are the amplitudes of the a- and b-waves, measured in microvolts. Measures of the time from the onset of the stimulus to the initial response (latency) or peak amplitude (implicit time) are also used. An ERG can be considered abnormal by comparison with age-matched normative data, or if a suspect eye shows a 25% reduction from the other, presumably healthy eye. The variability of the ERG amplitude makes this latter comparison a risky one.

## MORE SPECIALIZED TYPES OF ERG

The full-field flash ERG is representative of the overall function of the outer and mid-retina, so it is poor at assessing localized retinal disturbances such as at the fovea. Focal ERGs can be used to assess localized areas of the retina. Problems have existed in recording the focal ERG because the optical media scatters the stimulus light and stimulates areas of the retina outside the area of regard. It is also difficult to extract a useful ERG signal from a small area of stimulation. A vast, brightly illuminated surround can be used to avoid the effects of light scatter or an adapted ophthalmoscope can be used to provide the stimulus.[120] The pattern ERG can similarly be used for recording more localized retinal function. The target used for a pattern ERG is a reversing checkerboard pattern, so that unlike the flash ERG, the overall luminance level remains constant. The pattern ERG is produced in response to the local changes in luminance. The pattern ERG can be divided into two portions, a negative wave, referred to as N95, preceded by an early

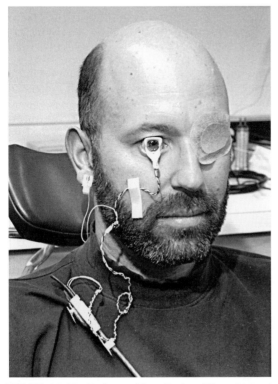

**FIGURE 11-23** Patient with a Burian-Allen electrode on the cornea, with an ear electrode serving as ground.

positive wave P50 (Fig. 11–23). Comparison of the pattern ERG and the focal ERG suggests that they are generated by separate retinal structures. Although currently still under debate, the origin of the pattern ERG is believed to be the inner retina, specifically the retinal ganglion cells.[126] The practical problems encountered when trying to record reliable pattern ERG results are discussed by Berninger and Arden.[127] The ISCEV standards mentioned previously cover only full-field flash ERG.[125]

## CLINICAL USES

The ERG is a costly test in terms of time and money, compared with more conventional methods of examination. However, it serves as a powerful diagnostic and prognostic tool in certain retinal conditions for which more conventional procedures are ineffective. The objective nature of the ERG is an advantage, as some of these conditions can be found in the very young and people with developmental disabilities. New advances are drawing attention to the diagnostic abilities of the ERG, which may serve to increase its utility for the future.

### Differential Diagnosis of Retinal Disease

Retinal degenerations can be difficult to classify because of the number and variety of fundus presentations. The ERG amplitude can be absent or reduced by certain disorders of the choroid (e.g., choroidemia, gyrate atrophy), Bruchs' membrane (e.g., degenerative myopia), the RPE-photoreceptor complex (e.g., retinitis pigmentosa [RP] and RP-associated syndromes), the photoreceptors (e.g., fundus albipunctatus, rod monochromatism, congenital stationary night blindness type I), and bipolar cells (congenital stationary night blindness type II).[128] When overall outer and mid-retinal function is compromised, both the a- and b-waves are affected. If both rods and cones are affected, then both the scotopic and photopic ERGs may be abnormal. Retinitis pigmentosa preferentially affects the rods, so that the scotopic ERG is characteristically absent or reduced and delayed in latency even in the early stages of the disease.[129] The lack of such results aid in the diagnosis of pseudoretinitis pigmentosa (e.g., trauma or chorioretinitis).[130] As complete rod monochromats have no cones, they do not show a photopic ERG response, whereas the scotopic response is normal or near normal. When the defect is at the mid-

retinal layers, only the b-wave may be affected, thus producing a negative ERG (e.g., congenital stationary night blindness type II and juvenile retinoschisis).[128]

### Differential Diagnosis of Patients with Night Blindness

The most common cause of symptoms of "night blindness" is probably night (empty field) myopia or slightly undercorrected myopia. However, various retinal degenerations can cause symptoms of night blindness, most commonly appearing in the teenage or early adult years. These include retinitis pigmentosa, choroideremia, gyrate dystrophy, and congenital stationary night blindness.

### Differential Diagnosis of Infants with Nystagmus, Poor Vision, and Normal Appearing Fundi

Congenital nystagmus and poor vision can be due to fairly easily diagnosed conditions such as corneal opacities, cataracts, and retinopathy of prematurity. The ERG can help in the differential diagnosis of various congenital and childhood forms of pigmentary retinal dystrophy and also rule out other causes such as cortical blindness and optic atrophy or hypoplasia.[131] In Leber's congenital amaurosis (in which the fundi can appear normal) and juvenile and early-onset retinitis pigmentosa, the ERG is characteristically extinguished.[130] The ERG can also be used in the differential diagnosis of patients with congenital stationary night blindness, rod and cone monochromatism, and hereditary cone dystrophy. More detailed information is provided by Lambert and colleagues.[131]

### Other Uses

The ERG may be used to evaluate possible adverse effects on the retina of drug therapy,[132] and in combination with the VEP and ultrasonography, the ERG can provide useful prognostic information after traumatic damage to the eye.[133]

### Possible Future Uses

Recent research has shown the pattern ERG to have prognostic value in determining which ocular hypertensive patients are likely to progress to glaucoma.[132, 134, 135] Oscillatory potentials have been shown to predict the risk of iris neovascularization (and subsequent neovascular glaucoma and vision loss) after central vein occlusion by providing an index of the extent of ischemic damage.[136] Oscillatory potentials and pattern ERGs have also been shown to determine which patients with early diabetic retinopathy are likely to progress to severe proliferative diabetic retinopathy and subsequent vision loss.[137, 138] It is possible that these prognostic ERG indicators may aid in the decision of whether to treat such patients prophylactically with panretinal photocoagulation.

# References

1. Elliott DB, Wilkes R: A clinical evaluation of the Topcon RM-6000 autorefractor. Clin Exp Opt 1989; 72:150–153.
2. Swets JA, Pickett RM: Evaluation of diagnostic systems. Methods from signal detection theory. London: Academic Press, 1982.
3. Reeves BC: Unfortunately diseases are rare. Optician 1989; 197(5208):18–24.
4. Bland JM, Altman DG: Statistical methods for assessing agreement between two methods of clinical measurement. Lancet 1986; 1:307–310.
5. Elliott DB, Sheridan M: The use of accurate visual acuity measurements in clinical anti-cataract formulation trials. Ophthal Physiol Opt 1988; 8:397–401.
6. Bailey IL, Bullimore MA, Raasch TW, Taylor HR: Clinical grading and the effects of scaling. Invest Ophthalmol Vis Sci 1991; 32:422–432.
7. Reeves BC, Hill AR, Aspinall PA: The clinical significance of change. Ophthal Physiol Opt 1987; 7:441–446.
8. Elliott DB, Bullimore MA, Bailey IL: Improving the reliability of the Pelli-Robson contrast sensitivity test. Clin Vis Sci 1991; 6:471–475.
9. Elliott DB, Bullimore MA: Assessing the reliability, discriminative ability, and validity of disability glare tests. Invest Ophthalmol Vis Sci 1993; 34:108–119.
10. Elliott DB, Whitaker D: Clinical contrast sensitivity chart evaluation. Ophthal Physiol Opt 1992; 12:275–280.
11. Vingrys AJ, Cole BL: Are colour vision standards justified in the transport industry? Ophthal Physiol Opt 1988; 8:257–274.
12. Vingrys AJ, Cole BL: Origins of colour vision standards within the transport industry. Ophthal Physiol Opt 1990; 10:8–15.
13. Hurvich LM: Color Vision. Sunderland, MA: Sinauer Associates Inc., 1981.
14. Adams AJ, Portnoy GH: Colour deficiency. In Amos JF (ed): Diagnosis and Management of Vision Care. Boston: Butterworths, 1987.
15. National Research Council: Procedures for testing colour vision: Report of working party 41 of the National Research Council. Washington, DC: National Academy Press, 1981.
16. Birch J: Diagnosis of Defective Colour Vision. Oxford: Oxford University Press, 1993.
17. Dubois-Poulsen A: Acquired dyschromatopsias. Mod Probl Ophthalmol 1972; 11:84–93.
18. Lee TC: Van Gogh's vision—Digitalis intoxication? JAMA 1981; 245:727–729.
19. Hardy LH, Rand G, Rittler MC: Effect of quality of illumination on results of the Ishihara test. J Opt Soc Am 1946; 36:86–94.
20. Higgins KE, Moskowitz-Cook A, Knoblauch K: Colour vision testing: An alternative 'source' of illuminant C. Mod Probl Ophthalmol 1978; 19:113–121.
21. Richards OW, Tack TO, Thomé C: Fluorescent lights for colour vision testing. Am J Optom Arch Am Acad Optom 1971; 43:747–753.
22. Moreland JD, Kerr J: Optimisation of a Rayleigh type equation for the detection of tritanomaly. Vis Res 1979: 19:1369–1375.
23. Pokorny J, Smith VC, Lutze M: A computer controlled briefcase anomaloscope. In Drum B, Verriest G (eds): Colour Vision Deficiencies IX. Dordrecht: Kluwer Academic Publishers, 1989, pp 515–522.
24. Drum B, Sternheim C, Severns M: Anomaloscope plate test field trial: Comparison with four other tests of congenital red-green colour vision deficiencies. In Drum B, Moreland JD, Serra A (eds): Colour Vision Deficiencies X. Dordrecht: Kluwer Academic Publishers, 1991, pp 77–84.
25. Ravin JG: Monet's cataracts. JAMA 1985; 254:394–399.
26. Elliott DB, Skaff A: Vision of the famous: The artist's eye. Ophthal Physiol Opt 1993; 13:82–90.
27. Robson JG: Contrast sensitivity: One hundred years of clinical measurement. In Shapley R, Lam DM-K (eds): Contrast Sensitivity. Cambridge: MIT Press, 1993, p 253.
28. Fortuin GJ: Visual power and visibility. Philips Res Rep 1951; 6:251, 347.
29. Campbell FW, Green DG: Optical and retinal factors affecting visual resolution. J Physiol 1965; 181:576–593.
30. Snyder AW, Miller WH: Photoreceptor diameter and spacing for highest resolving power. J Opt Soc Am 1977; 67:696–698.
31. Campbell FW, Robson JG: Application of Fourier analysis to the visibility of gratings. J Physiol 1968; 197:551.
32. Kulikowski JJ: The role of P and M Systems: (c) Psychophysical aspects. In Kulikowski JJ, Dickinson CM, Murray IJ (eds): Seeing Contour and Colour. Oxford: Pergamon Press, 1989, p 232.
33. Leat SJ, Woodhouse JM: Reading performance with low vision aids: Relationship with contrast sensitivity. Ophthal Physiol Opt 1993; 13:9–16.
34. Rubin GS, Roche KB, Prasada-Rao P, Fried LP: Visual impairment and disability in older adults. Optom Vis Sci 1994; 71:750–760.
35. Turano K, Rubin GS, Herdman SJ, et al: Visual stabilization of posture in the elderly: Fallers versus non-fallers. Optom Vis Sci 1994; 71:761–769.
36. Wood JM, Dique T, Troutbeck R: The effect of artificial visual impairment on functional visual-fields and driving performance. Clin Vis Sci 1993; 8:563–575.
37. Regan D: Low-contrast letter charts and sinewave grating tests in ophthalmological and neurological disorders. Clin Vis Sci 1988; 2:235–250.
38. Storch RL, Bodis-Wollner I: Overview of contrast sensitivity and neuro-ophthalmic disease. In Nadler MP, Miller D, Nadler DJ (eds): Glare and Contrast Sensitivity for Clinicians. New York: Springer-Verlag, 1990, p 85.
39. Elliott DB, Whitaker D: How useful are contrast sensitivity charts in optometric practice? Optom Vis Sci 1992; 69:378–385.
40. Rabin J: Optical defocus: Differential effects on size and contrast letter recognition thresholds. Invest Ophthalmol Vis Sci 1994; 35:646–648.
41. Bradley A, Hook J, Haeseker J: A comparison of clinical acuity and contrast sensitivity charts: Effect of uncorrected myopia. Ophthal Physiol Opt 1991; 11:218–226.
42. Legge GE, Rubin GS: Contrast sensitivity function as a screening test: A critique. Am J Optom Physiol Opt 1986; 63:265–270.

43. Leguire LE: Do letter charts measure contrast sensitivity? Clin Vis Sci 1991; 6:391–400.

44. Pelli DG, Robson JG: Are letters better than gratings? Clin Vis Sci 1991; 6:409–411.

45. Regan D: Do letter charts measure contrast sensitivity? Clin Vis Sci 1991; 6:401–408.

46. Pelli DG, Robson JG, Wilkins AJ: The design of a new letter chart for measuring contrast sensitivity. Clin Vis Sci 1988; 2:187–199.

47. Rubin GS: Reliability and sensitivity of clinical contrast sensitivity tests. Clin Vis Sci 1988; 2:169–177.

48. American Academy of Ophthalmology: Contrast sensitivity and glare testing in the evaluation of anterior segment disease. Ophthalmology 1990; 97:1233–1237.

49. Koch DD, Liu JF: Survey of the clinical use of glare and contrast sensitivity testing. J Cataract Refract Surg 1990; 16:707–711.

50. Pomerance GN, Evans DW: Test-restest reliability of the CSV-1000 contrast test and its relationship to glaucoma therapy. Invest Ophthalmol Vis Sci 1994; 35:3357–3361.

51. Arden GB: Testing contrast sensitivity in clinical practice. Clin Vis Sci 1988; 2:213–224.

52. Dhanesha U, Gilchrist J, Miles D, et al: Loss of visual function associated with microalbuminuria in diabetes-mellitus—a pilot study. Acta Ophthalmol 1991; 69:521–526.

53. Elliott DB: Evaluating visual function in cataract. Optom Vision Sci 1993; 70:896–902.

54. Whittaker SG, Lovie-Kitchin J: Visual requirements for reading. Optom Vis Sci 1993; 70:54–65.

55. Miller D, Nadler MP: Light scattering: Its relationship to glare and contrast in patients and normal subjects. *In* Nadler MP, Miller D, Nadler DJ (eds): Glare and Contrast Sensitivity for Clinicians. New York: Springer-Verlag, 1990, p 24.

56. Miller D, Benedek GB: Intraocular Light Scattering. Springfield, IL: Charles C Thomas, 1973.

57. Vos JJ: Disability glare—a state of the art report. CIE 1984; 3:39.

58. van den Berg TJTP, IJspeert JK, de Waard PWT: Dependence of intraocular straylight on pigmentation and light transmission through the ocular wall. Vis Res 1991; 31:1361–1367.

59. de Waard PW, Ijspeert JK, van den Berg TJTP, de Jong PT: Intraocular scattering in age-related cataracts. Invest Ophthalmol Vis Sci 1992; 33:618–625.

60. Paulsson LE, Sjöstrand J: Contrast sensitivity in the presence of a glare light. Invest Ophthalmol Vis Sci 1980; 19:401–406.

61. van den Berg TJTP: On the relation between intraocular straylight and visual function parameters. Invest Ophthalmol Vis Sci 1994; 35:2659–2661.

62. Whitaker D, Steen R, Elliott DB: On the relation between intraocular straylight and visual function parameters—reply. Invest Ophthalmol Vis Sci 1994; 35:2660–2661.

63. Regan D, Giaschi DE, Fresco BB: Measurement of glare sensitivity in cataract patients using low-contrast letter charts. Ophthal Physiol Opt 1993; 13:115–123.

64. Cataract Management Guideline Panel: Cataract in adults: Management of functional impairment. Clinical Practice Guideline, Number 4. Rockville, MD: U.S. Department of Health Care Policy and Research. AHCPR Pub. No. 93-0542. Feb. 1993.

65. Rubin ML: The little point that isn't there. Surv Ophthalmol 1972; 17:52–55.

66. Steen R, Whitaker D, Elliott DB, et al.: Effect of filters on disability glare. Ophthal Physiol Opt 1993; 13:371–376.

67. Whitaker D, Steen R, Elliott DB: Light scatter in the normal young, elderly and cataractous eye demonstrates

68. little wavelength dependency. Optom Vision Sci 1993; 70:963–968.

68. Zigman S: Vision enhancement using a short wavelength light-absorbing filter. Optom Vis Sci 1990; 67:100–124.

69. Winn B, Whitaker D, Elliott DB, Phillips NJ: Factors affecting light adapted pupil size in normal human subjects. Invest Ophthalmol Vis Sci 1994; 35:1132–1137.

70. Glaser JS, Savino PJ, Sumers KD, et al.: The photostress recovery test in the clinical assessment of visual function. Am J Ophthalmol 1977; 83:255–260.

71. Brindley GS: The discrimination of after-images. J Physiol 1959; 147:194–203.

72. Dowling JE: The Retina. Cambridge: Belknap Press, 1987.

73. Nathans J, Piantanida TP, Eddy RL, et al.: Molecular genetics of inherited variation in human color vision. Science 1986; 232:203–210.

74. Collins M, Brown B: Glare recovery and age related maculopathy. Clin Vis Sci 1989; 4:145–153.

75. Alpern M, Krantz DH: Visual pigment kinetics in abnormalities of the uvea-retinal epithelium interface in man. Invest Ophthalmol Vis Sci 1983; 20:183–203.

76. Wu G, Welter JJ, Santos S, et al.: The macular photostress test in diabetic retinopathy and age-related macular degeneration. Arch Ophthalmol 1990; 108:1556–1558.

77. Tengroth B, Hogman B, Linde C-J, et al.: Readaptation time after photostress—readaptation time as a function of oxygen concentration. Arch Ophthal 1976; 54:507–516.

78. Patorgis CJ: Photostress recovery testing. *In* Eskridge JB, Amos JF, Bartlett JD (eds): Clinical Procedures in Optometry. Philadelphia: JB Lippincott, 1991, p 482.

79. Alexander LJ: Primary Care of the Posterior Segment, 2nd ed. p 17. Norwalk, CT: Appleton and Lange, 1990, p 17.

80. Kanski JJ: Clinical Ophthalmology: A Systematic Approach, 2nd ed. London: Butterworth and Company Ltd. 1989, p 442.

81. Magder H: Test for central serous retinopathy based on clinical observations and trial. Am J Ophthalmol 1960; 49:147–150.

82. Chilaris GA: Recovery time after macular illumination as a diagnostic and prognostic test. Am J Ophthalmol 1962; 53:311–314.

83. Severin SL, Tour RL, Kershaw RH: Macular function of the photostress test 1. Arch Ophthalmol 1967; 77:2–7.

84. Elliott DB, Whitaker D: Changes in macular function throughout adulthood. Doc Ophthalmol 1991; 76:251–259.

85. Lovie-Kitchin JE: Validity and reliability of visual acuity measurements. Ophthal Physiol Opt 1988; 8:363–370.

86. Frost-Larsen K, Larsen H-W: Macular recovery time recorded by nyctometry—A screening method for selection of patients who are at risk of developing proliferative diabetic retinopathy—Results of a 5 year follow-up. Acta Opthalmol (Suppl)1985; 63:39–47.

87. Grom E: An enquiry into the history of the crystalline lens. *In* Bellows JG (ed): Cataract and Abnormalities of the Lens. New York: Grune and Stratton, 1975, p 1.

88. Weale R: On the invention of the ophthalmoscope. Doc Ophthalmol 1994; 86:163–166.

89. May CH: Diseases of the Eye, 9th ed. New York: W Wood and Co, 1920.

90. Lotmar W: Apparatus for measurement of retinal visual acuity by moire fringes. Invest Ophthalmol Vis Sci 1980; 19:393–400.

91. Bradley A, Thibos L, Still D: Visual acuity measured with

clinical Maxwellian-view systems: Effects of beam entry location. Optom Vis Sci 1990; 67:811–817.

92. Hurst MA, Douthwaite WA, Elliott DB: Assessment of retinal and neural function behind a cataract. *In* Douthwaite WA, Hurst MA (eds): Cataract Detection, Measurement and Management in Optometric Practice. Oxford: Butterworth-Heinemann Ltd, 1993, p 46.

93. Faulkner W: Laser interferometric prediction of postoperative visual acuity in patients with cataract. Am J Ophthalmol 1983; 95:626–636.

94. Barrett BT, Davison PA, Eustace PE: The effects of posterior segment disorders on oscillatory displacement thresholds, and on acuities as measured using the potential acuity meter and laser interferometer. Ophthal Physiol Opt 1994; 14:132–138.

95. Alio JL, Artola A, Ruiz-Mareno JM, et al.: Accuracy of the potential acuity meter in predicting the visual outcome in cases of cataract associated with macular degeneration. Eur J Ophthalmol 1993; 3:189–192.

96. Sherman J, Sutija VG: Visual-evoked potentials. *In* Eskridge JB, Amos JF, Bartlett JD (eds): Clinical Procedures in Optometry. Philadelphia: JB Lippincott, 1991, p 514.

97. Bernth-Petersen P: Outcome of cataract surgery III. Influence of age, macular disease and type of correction. Acta Ophthalmol 1982; 60:455–460.

98. Leat SJ, Rumney NJ: The experience of a university-based low vision clinic. Ophthal Physiol Opt 1990; 10:8–15.

99. Levi L, Feldman RM: Use of the Potential Acuity Meter in suspected functional visual loss. Am J Ophthalmol 1992; 114:502–503.

100. Halliday AM: Evoked brain potentials: How far have we come since 1875? *In* Barber C (ed): Evoked Potentials. Baltimore: University Park Press, 1980, p 3.

101. Regan D: Human Brain Electrophysiology. New York: Elsevier, 1989.

102. Jasper HH: The ten-twenty electrode system of the international federation. Electroenceph Clin Neurophysiol 1958; 10:371–375.

103. ISCEV VEP standards (in press).

104. Brigell M, Kaufman DI, Bobak P, et al.: The pattern visual evoked potential: A multi-center study using standardized techniques. Doc Ophthalmol 1994; 86:65–79.

105. Halliday AM, McDonald WI, Mushin J: Visual evoked response in diagnosis of multiple sclerosis. Br Med J 1973; 4:661–664.

106. Asselman P, Chadwick DW, Marsden CD: Visual evoked responses in the diagnosis and management of patients suspected of multiple sclerosis. Brain 1975; 98:261–282.

107. Duwaer AL, Spekreijse H: Latency of luminance and contrast evoked potentials in multiple sclerosis patients. Electroenceph Clin Neurol 1978; 45:244–258.

108. van Diemen HAM, Lanting P, Koetsier JC, et al.: Evaluation of the visual system in multiple sclerosis: A comparative study of diagnostic tests. Clin Neurol Neurosurg 1992; 94:191–195.

109. Jones SJ: Visual evoked potentials after optic neuritis. J Neurol 1993; 240:489–494.

110. Halliday AM: Visually evoked responses in optic nerve disease. Trans Ophthalmol Soc UK 1976; 96:372–376.

111. Apkarian P: A practical approach to albino diagnosis. Ophthal Ped Genet 1992; 13:77–88.

112. Bouzas EA, Caruso RC, Drews-Bankiewicz MA, et al.: Evoked potential analysis of visual pathways in human albinism. Ophthalmology 1994; 101:309–314.

113. Maino JH: Ocular hysteria and malingering. *In* Amos JF (ed): Diagnosis and Management of Vision Care. Boston: Butterworths, 1987, p 409.

114. Haegerstrom-Portnoy G: New procedures for evaluating

vision functions of special populations. Optom Vis Sci 1993; 70:306–314.

115. Odom JV, Green M: Visually evoked potential (VEP) acuity: Testability in a clinical pediatric population. Acta Ophthalmol 1984; 62:993–998.

116. Tyler CW, Apkarian P, Levi DM, et al.: Rapid assessment of visual function: An electronic sweep technique for the pattern visual evoked potential. Invest Ophthalmol Vis Sci 1979; 18:703–713.

117. McCulloch DL, Skarf B: Pattern reversal visual evoked potentials following early treatment of unilateral, congenital cataract. Arch Ophthalmol 1994; 112:510–518.

118. Parisi V, Bucci MG: Visual evoked potentials after photostress in patients with primary open-angle glaucoma and ocular hypertension. Invest Ophthalmol Vis Sci 1992; 33:436–442.

119. Dewar J, McKendrick JG: On the physiological action of light. Trans Ophth Soc Edinburgh 1873; 27:141–168.

120. Sutija VG, Sherman J: Electroretinography. *In* Eskridge JB, Amos JF, Bartlett JD (eds): Clinical Procedures in Optometry. Philadelphia: JB Lippincott, 1991, p 505.

121. Noell WK: The origin of the electroretinogram. Am J Ophthalmol 1954; 38:78–90.

122. Newman EA: Current source-density analysis of the b-wave of the frog retina. J Neurophys 1980; 43:1355.

123. Ogden JE: The oscillatory waves of the primate electroretinogram. Vision Res 1973; 13:1059–1066.

124. Heynen H, Wachtmeister L, van Norren D: Origin of oscillatory potentials in the primate retina. Vision Res 1985; 25:1365–1373.

125. Marmor MF, Arden GB, Nilsson SE, et al.: Standard for electroretinography. Arch Ophthalmol 1989; 107:816–819.

126. Hollander H, Bisti S, Maffei L, et al.: Electroretinographic responses and retrograde changes of retinal morphology after intercranial optic nerve section. A quantitative analysis in the cat. Exp Brain Res 1984; 55:483–493.

127. Berninger TA, Arden GB: The pattern electroretinogram. Eye (Suppl) 1988; 2:257–283.

128. Jiménez-Sierra JM, Ogden TE, van Boemel: Inherited Retinal Diseases. A Diagnostic Guide. St. Louis: CV Mosby, 1989.

129. Bersen EL: Retinitis pigmentosa and allied retinal disease: electrophysiologic findings. Trans Am Acad Ophth Otol 1976; 81:659.

130. Heckenlively JR: Retinitis Pigmentosa. Philadelphia: JB Lippincott, 1988.

131. Lambert SR, Taylor D, Kriss A: The infant with nystagmus, normal appearing fundi, but an abnormal ERG. Surv Ophthalmol 1989; 34:173–186.

132. Arden GB: An overview of the uses and abuses of electrodiagnosis in ophthalmology. Int J Psychophys 1994; 16:113–119.

133. Crews SJ, Hillman JS, Thompson CRS: Electrodiagnosis and ultrasonography in assessment of recent major trauma. Trans Ophthalmol UK 1975; 95:315–321.

134. Trick GL, Bickler-Bluth M, Cooper DG, et al: Pattern reversal electroretinogram (PRERG) abnormalities in ocular hypertension: Correlation with glaucoma risk factors. Curr Eye Res 1988; 7:201–206.

135. Pfeiffer N, Tillmon B, Bach M: Predictive value of the pattern electroretinogram in high-risk ocular hypertension. Invest Ophthalmol Vis Sci 1993; 34:1710–1715.

136. Kaye SB, Harding SP: Early electroretinography in unilateral central retinal vein occlusion as a predictor of rubeosis iridis. Arch Ophthalmol 1988; 106:353–356.

137. Bresnick GH, Korth K, Groo A, et al.: Electroretinographic oscillatory potentials predict progression of diabetic retinopathy. Arch Ophthalmol 1984; 102:1307–1311.

138. Arden GB, Hamilton AMP, Wilson-Holt J, et al.: Pattern

electroretinograms become abnormal when background diabetic retinopathy deteriorates to a pre-proliferative stage: Possible use as a screening test. Br J Ophthalmol 1986; 70:330–335.

## ACKNOWLEDGMENTS

I thank the following faculty (from the School of Optometry, Waterloo, unless indicated) for valuable comments and discussion on certain sections of this chapter: David Whitaker (Aston University, UK), Jeff Hovis, Michael Doughty (Glasgow, UK), Lisa Prokopich, Marlee Spafford, and Trefford Simpson. I also thank the following students for providing extensive literature surveys and valuable comments: Kim Burgera, Selena Friesen, Ana Juracic, and Stephanie Millar.

# Index

Note: Page numbers in *italics* refer to illustrations; page numbers followed by t refer to tables.